THE ENCYCLOPEDIA OF

CHILD ABUSE
THIRD EDITION

Robin E. Clark, Ph.D.
and
Judith Freeman Clark
with
Christine Adamec

Introduction by
Richard J. Gelles, Ph.D.

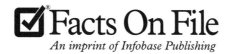

Facts On File
An imprint of Infobase Publishing

The Encyclopedia of Child Abuse, Third Edition

Facts On File, Inc.
An imprint of Infobase Publishing
132 West 31st Street
New York NY 10001

ISBN 13: 978-0-8160-6677-3
ISBN 10: 0-8160-6677-9

Library of Congress Cataloging-in-Publication Data

Clark, Robin E.
The encyclopedia of child abuse / Robin E. Clark and Judith Freeman Clark with Christine Adamec; introduction by Richard J. Gelles.—3rd ed.
p. cm.
Includes bibliographical references and index.
ISBN 0-8160-6677-9 (hardcover: alk. paper)
1. Child abuse—United States—Dictionaries. 2. Child abuse—Dictionaries. I. Clark, Judith Freeman. II. Adamec, Christine A. 1949— III. Title.
HV6626.5.C57   2000
362.76′0973′03—dc21   00-035384

Facts On File books are available at special discounts when purchased in bulk quantities for businesses, associations, institutions, or sales promotions. Please call our Special Sales Department in New York at (212) 967-8800 or (800) 322-8755.

You can find Facts On File on the World Wide Web at http://www.factsonfile.com

Text and cover design by Cathy Rincon

Printed in the United States of America

VB Hermitage 10 9 8 7 6 5 4 3 2 1

This book is printed on acid-free paper.

CONTENTS

PREFACE

Child abuse and neglect have many different dimensions. Though we often think of child abuse only in terms of physical violence, various forms of psychological threats, coercion, sexual exploitation and even folk medicine practices can also produce serious and long-lasting damage. The range of actions classified as child abuse or neglect is constantly changing as a result of social and economic conditions, political ideology, advances in medicine, improvements in communication and melding of cultures. Absence of a single, explicit and universally accepted definition of abuse makes studies of it difficult. Yet, child abuse and neglect are not simply cultural inventions. As international concern for the plight of children grows, those concerned with preventing abuse and neglect are beginning to find more and more common ground for collaboration.

The Encyclopedia of Child Abuse reflects the struggle to define, prevent and treat this problem. Entries reflect the range of disciplines (including law, medicine, psychology, sociology, economics, history, education and others) that contribute to our understanding of child maltreatment as well as the scope of debate within and among disciplines. Where there is disagreement on a particular point, we have tried to identify the different arguments. Obviously, it is not possible to present an exhaustive discussion of each of the hundreds of topics included in this book. For those who wish to explore a topic in depth, we make suggestions for further reading at the end of selected entries. An extensive bibliography is also included at the back of the book.

Space and time considerations forced us to be selective in choosing the topics we discussed. In attempting to present an overall view of child abuse and neglect, we chose topics that we felt would give the reader a grasp of the central issues.

Information presented in this book comes from the most up-to-date sources available at the time of writing. We have attempted to present material in clear language that does not require specialized knowledge of medicine, law or other disciplines. Our use of "simple" language should not be construed as simplistic. We believe professionals and general readers alike will find the book contains a wealth of useful information.

Though we have attempted to present child abuse and neglect from an international perspective, readers will notice that most statistical information comes from the United States. This is a reflection of the availability of such information rather than a statement of relative importance.

In selecting entries, we chose not to include biographies of individuals who have contributed to the understanding and/or prevention of child abuse and neglect. The list of these individuals is long, and new names are constantly being added. Such a listing, though important, is beyond the scope of this book. Biographical information is included only when it is relevant for the understanding of a particular case, concept or contribution.

In this third edition of *The Encyclopedia of Child Abuse*, we have both updated older entries and included new entries. For example, we offer a new entry on abusers, with an analysis of those individuals who neglect or physically or sexually maltreat children. We also offer a new entry on adults abused as children, because numerous studies have documented that child abuse often has a lifelong effect; for example, adults abused as children have a greater risk of substance abuse in adulthood, as well as risks for psychiatric problems such as depression and anxiety disorders.

Adults abused as children also have a greater risk for suicide than individuals who were not abused in childhood. Childhood abuse has a long reach in its effects, and adults abused as children are more likely to be victimized in adulthood with sexual and physical abuse. Not all adults abused as children grow up to abuse their own children, but the risk is elevated, and as many as 40% will be abusive to their children. Without intervention the cycle may continue when their children grow up.

We also offer a new entry on sexual abuse of children and adolescents that was perpetrated by members of the clergy, peaking in the 1970s to 1980s. This discovery shocked millions of people worldwide and rocked the Catholic Church, as well as other churches which discovered incidents of sexual abuse.

Other new entries include bullying, central registries of abuse, guilt and shame, pediatricians and statutory rape. We have also heavily rewritten many entries, such as burns, civil commitment laws, family preservation, fetal alcohol syndrome, foster care, Munchausen syndrome by proxy, parental substance abuse, sexual trafficking and shaken infant syndrome, to name just a few.

This third edition includes two new appendixes, including an appendix on state-by-state laws on the involuntary termination of parental rights and an appendix with state-by-state definitions of abuse, physical abuse, neglect, sexual abuse and emotional abuse.

We hope users of this book will be stimulated to learn more about child abuse and neglect. Only through a better understanding of the complex and often misunderstood phenomenon of child abuse can we hope to prevent it.

ACKNOWLEDGMENTS

Over the months that the third edition of this book was researched and written, we contacted dozens of organizations to ask for information about child abuse and neglect. In particular, staff at the Clearinghouse on Child Abuse and Neglect Information; the House of Representatives Subcommittee on Children, Youth and Families; staff of the American Association for Protecting Children; and staff of the Incest Survivors Resource Network deserve special acknowledgment. Countless individuals at other public- and private-sector agencies answered our mail and telephone inquiries and sent us statistics and facts on hundreds of topics. Although it is impossible to mention each person by name, a sincere thank-you goes to these people for their cooperation and assistance.

Kate Kelly, our former editor, was unfailingly cheerful throughout all stages of the original project; her suggestions were thoughtful and her editorial comments helpful. Elizabeth Frost Knappmann of New England Publishing Associates deserves mention for her efforts on our behalf.

Friends and colleagues have been generous with support and encouragement during the time that we researched and wrote this book. Janet Logan and Susan Carter Sawyer are among those who were especially helpful to us.

Members of our family have been patient as we completed our work. We are grateful for their understanding and, in particular, would like to acknowledge the support of our mothers, Martha Clark and Elizabeth Bartlett. Finally, a very special thanks to Tim and Stephanie.

INTRODUCTION
CHILD ABUSE—AN OVERVIEW

Today, child abuse and neglect is widely recognized as a major social problem and policy issue in the United States and throughout much of the world. During the last 50 years, the United States and many of the world's nations have responded to child abuse and neglect with legislative efforts, a variety of programs and interventions, and organizational efforts to identify, respond to and prevent the abuse and neglect of dependent children. Today, there are innumerable local, national and international organizations, professional societies and advocacy groups devoted to preventing and treating child abuse and neglect.

The Social Transformation of Child Abuse and Neglect

While international concern about child maltreatment is relatively new, child abuse and neglect is not a recent phenomenon. The maltreatment of children has manifested itself in nearly every conceivable manner—physically, emotionally, sexually and by forced child labor (Ten Bensel, Rheinberger and Radbill, 1997). Historians have been able to document the occurrence of various forms of the mistreatment of children back to the beginnings of recorded history. In some ancient cultures, children had no rights until the right to live was bestowed upon them by their fathers. The right to live was sometimes withheld by fathers, and newborns were abandoned or left to die. Although we do not have the means to know how commonplace abandonment or killing was, we do know that infanticide was widely accepted among ancient and prehistoric cultures. Newborns and infants could be put to death because they cried too much, because they were sickly or deformed, or because of some perceived imperfection. Girls, twins and children of unmarried women were the special targets of infanticide (Robin, 1980).

Many societies subjected their offspring to survival tests. Some Native Americans threw their newborns into pools of water and rescued them only if they rose to the surface and cried. German parents also plunged children into icy waters as a test of fitness to live (Ten Bensel, Rheinberger and Radbill, 1997). Greek parents exposed their children to natural elements as a survival test.

Survival tests and infanticide were not the only abuses inflicted by generations of parents. From prehistoric times to the present, children have been mutilated, beaten and maltreated. Such treatment was not only condoned but was often mandated as the most appropriate child-rearing method. Children were, and continue to be, hit with rods, canes and switches. Boys have been castrated to produce eunuchs. Girls have been, and continue to be, subjected to genital surgery or mutilation as part of culturally approved ritual. Colonial parents were implored to "beat the devil" out of their children (Greven, 1991; Straus, 1994).

Summing up the plight of children from prehistoric times until the present, David Bakan comments that "Child abuse thrives in the shadows of privacy and secrecy. It lives by inattention" (Bakan, 1971).

The Discovery of Childhood, Children and Abuse and Neglect

Although abuse and neglect of children was sometimes condoned, and most of the time occurred within the intimacy and privacy of the home, social concern for children, their plight and their rights coexisted with the occurrence of maltreatment. Concern for the rights and welfare of children has waxed and waned over the centuries, but there has always been some attempt to protect children from mistreatment.

Six thousand years ago, children in Mesopotamia had a patron goddess to look after them. The Greeks and Romans had orphan homes. A variety of historical accounts mention some form of "fostering" for dependent children. The absolute rights of parents were limited by legislation. Samuel Radbill (1980) reports that child protection laws were enacted as long ago as 450 B.C.E. Attempts were made to modify and restrict fathers' complete control over their children. Anthropologists note that virtually all societies have had mores, laws or customs that regulate sexual access to children.

The Renaissance marked a new morality regarding children. Children were seen as a dependent class in need of the protection of society. At the same time, however, the family was expected to teach children the proper rules of behavior. Moreover, this was a historical period in which the power of the father increased dramatically. This dialectic—concern for children and increased demands and power of parents to control children—has been a consistent theme throughout history.

Defining childhood as a separate stage and children as in need of protection did not reduce the likelihood of maltreatment. In Colonial America, Puritan parents were instructed by leaders, such as Cotton Mather, that strict discipline of children could not begin too early (Greven, 1991).

The enlightenment of the 18th century brought children increased attention, services and protection. The London Foundling Hospital, established during the 18th century, not only provided medical care but also was a center of the moral reform movement on behalf of children (Robin, 1982).

In the United States, the case of Mary Ellen Wilson is usually considered the turning point in concern for children's welfare. In 1874, the then eight-year-old Mary Ellen lived in the home of Francis and Mary Connolly but was not the blood relative of either. Mary Ellen was the illegitimate daughter of Mary Connolly's first husband. A neighbor noticed the plight of Mary Ellen, who was beaten with a leather thong and allowed to go ill-clothed in bad weather. The neighbor reported the case to Etta Wheeler—a "friendly visitor" who worked for St. Luke's Methodist Mission. (In the mid-1800s, child welfare was church-based rather than government-based.) Wheeler turned to the police and the New York City Department of Charities for help for Mary Ellen Wilson and was turned down—first by the police, who said there was no proof of a crime, and second by the charity agency, which said they did not have custody of Mary Ellen. The legend goes on to note that Henry Bergh, founder of the Society for the Prevention of Cruelty to Animals, intervened on behalf of Mary Ellen and the courts accepted the case because Mary Ellen was a member of the animal kingdom. In reality, the court reviewed the case because the child needed protection. The case was argued, not by Henry Bergh, but by his colleague, Elbridge Gerry. Mary Ellen Wilson was removed from her foster home and initially placed in an orphanage. Her foster mother was imprisoned for a year, and the case received detailed press coverage for months. In December 1874, the New York Society for the Prevention of Cruelty to Children was founded (Nelson, 1984; Robin, 1982). This was the first organization that focused on child maltreatment in the United States.

Protective societies appeared and disappeared during the next 80 years. The political scientist Barbara Nelson (1984) notes that by the 1950s public interest in child maltreatment was practically nonexistent in the United States (and much of the world, for that matter). Technology paved the way for the rediscovery of physical child abuse. In 1946, the radiologist John Caffey reported on six cases of children who had multiple long bone fractures and subdural hematomas (Caffey, 1946).

It would take nine more years before the medical profession would begin to accept that such injuries were the result of actions by children's caretakers. In 1955, P. V. Wooley and W. A. Evans not only concluded that the X-rays revealed a pattern of injuries but that the injuries were committed willfully (Wooley and Evans, 1955). Wooley and Evans went on to criticize the medical profession for its reluctance to accept the accumulating evidence that long-bone fractures seen on X-rays were indeed inflicted willfully.

In 1958, C. Henry Kempe and his colleagues formed the first hospital-based child protective team at Colorado General Hospital in Denver. Kempe and his colleagues would publish their landmark article, "The Battered Child Syndrome," in the *Journal of the American Medical Association* in July 1962. Kempe's and his multidisciplinary colleagues' article was accompanied by a strong editorial on the battered child. The article and the editorial were the beginning of the modern concern for child abuse and neglect, a concern that has grown and expanded both nationally and internationally in the past four decades.

Prevention and Treatment Efforts

The United States Children's Bureau was founded in 1912 as an agency in the Department of Labor. (The bureau was later moved to the newly created Department of Health, Education, and Welfare, which was subsequently renamed the Department of Health and Human Services.) The Children's Bureau was founded by an act of Congress with a mandate to disseminate information on child development; it also acquired the budget and mandate to conduct research on issues concerning child development. The Children's Bureau has engaged in a variety of activities regarding child maltreatment and participated in the earliest national meetings on child abuse, sponsored by the Children's Division of the American Humane Association. After the publication of Kempe and his colleagues' 1962 article, the Bureau convened a meeting in 1963 that drafted a model child abuse reporting law. By 1967, all 50 states and the District of Columbia had enacted mandatory reporting laws based on the Bureau's model. In 1974, Congress enacted the Child Abuse Prevention and Treatment Act and created the National Center on Child Abuse and Neglect (Nelson, 1984). Today, the Office of Child Abuse and Neglect remains within the Children's Bureau and continues to coordinate the federal effort to prevent and treat the abuse and neglect of children in the United States.

The Definitional Dilemma

One of the most enduring problems in the field of child abuse and neglect has been the development of a useful, clear, acceptable and accepted definition of "abuse" and "neglect." Defining what is and is not abuse and neglect is at the core of research, intervention, prevention and social policy. Researchers must have a definition of abuse and neglect in order to engage in the most basic studies of extent, risk factors and causes. Those who are required to report child maltreatment need a benchmark or standard to determine what should be reported and what should not. And yet, there still is not a widely accepted definition of abuse and neglect. There is considerable variation across the 50 state definitions that are included in laws mandating reporting.

At the core of the definition problem is deciding what constitutes appropriate and inappropriate parent and caretaker behavior. Is a spanking an appropriate and even necessary method of disciplining children, or is it physical abuse? Most people agree that an adult having sexual intercourse with a minor child is sexual abuse. But what if the child is 13, 14 or even 17 years of age? Legally a 17-year-old is a child, but if the sex is consensual, is it abuse? Most people agree that appropriate parent behavior includes providing food and shelter for children. But what if poverty limits a parent's ability to provide—is this neglect? There is an infinite set of questions and dilemmas about where to draw the line between appropriate and acceptable behavior versus inappropriate and unacceptable behavior. There is general agreement at the extremes as to what is appropriate and inappropriate, but the middle area is subject to intense debate. The debate deepens when we consider cultural variations, both within our own society and across societies. In some cultures, female genital cutting (or what is called female circumcision or genital mutilation) is acceptable and even mandated. In the United States, cutting the genitals of females is considered abusive. Male circumcision is accepted in the United States and many other nations.

What is defined as abuse and neglect varies across societies, cultural groups and even across historical time. Kempe and his colleagues' first focus was restricted to physical abuse, or what they called "the battered child." In the subsequent 50 years, as concern for children's well-being expanded, so, too, did the definition of child abuse and neglect. The expansion of the definition can be seen in changes in how child abuse and neglect have been defined in the Federal Child Abuse Prevention and Treatment Act. In the 1974 version of the law, abuse and neglect were defined as:

The physical or mental injury, sexual abuse, negligent treatment, or maltreatment of a child under the age of eighteen by a person who is responsible for the child's welfare under circumstances which indicate that a child's health and welfare is harmed or threatened thereby (Public Law 93-237).

The Child Abuse Prevention and Treatment Act of 1984 defined child abuse and neglect as:

The physical or mental injury, sexual abuse or exploitation, negligent treatment, or maltreatment of a child under the age of eighteen or the age specified by the child protection law of the state in question, by a person (including an employee of a residential facility or any staff person providing out-of-home care) who is responsible for the child's welfare under circumstances which indicate that the child's health or welfare is harmed or threatened thereby, as determined in regulations prescribed by the Secretary.

The federal definition was expanded in 1988 to indicate that the behavior had to be avoidable and nonaccidental. This new clause attempted to address the issue of intent; however, it still provided no clear guidance as to how to classify or categorize cases based on intent.

The most recent authorization of the Child Abuse Prevention and Treatment Act, signed into law in 2003, defined child abuse and neglect as

the term "child abuse and neglect" means, at a minimum, any recent act or failure to act on the part of a parent or caretaker, which results in death, serious physical or emotional harm, sexual abuse or exploitation, or an act or failure to act which presents an imminent risk of serious harm;

the term "sexual abuse" includes

(A) the employment, use, persuasion, inducement, enticement, or coercion of any child to engage in, or assist any other person to engage in, any sexually explicit conduct or simulation of such conduct for the purpose of producing a visual depiction of such conduct; or
(B) the rape, and in cases of caretaker or interfamilial relationships, statutory rape, molestation, prostitution, or other form of sexual exploitation of children, or incest with children;

the term "withholding of medically indicated treatment" means the failure to respond to the infant's life-threatening conditions by providing treatment (including appropriate nutrition, hydration, and medication) which, in the treating physician's or physicians' reasonable medical judgment, will be most likely to be effective in ameliorating or correcting all such conditions, except that the term does not include the failure to provide treatment (other than appropriate nutrition, hydration, or medication) to an infant when, in the treating physician's or physicians' reasonable medical judgment —

the infant is chronically and irreversibly comatose; the provision of such treatment would —

merely prolong dying;
not be effective in ameliorating or correcting all of the infant's life-threatening conditions; or
otherwise be futile in terms of the survival of the infant; or

the provision of such treatment would be virtually futile in terms of the survival of the infant and the treatment itself under such circumstances would be inhumane

Source: (U.S.C. Title 42, Chapter 67, Subchapter I, § 5106g)

That the federal government has a legal definition of child abuse and neglect still does not settle the matter. First, each state has its own legal definition of child maltreatment and those definitions do vary. Second, child welfare caseworkers and family and juvenile court judges vary in how they apply the state definitions during the course of child abuse and neglect investigations and court actions. Thirdly, researchers must "operationalize" the definitions; that is, they must determine how they will actually measure child abuse and neglect. Here too, there is considerable variation in how the concept "child abuse and neglect" is operationally defined. Finally, legal definitions and research operationalizations do not result in definitions that can be applied across cultures and subcultures.

All of the above problems actually arise out of the fact that there is no universal standard for what constitutes optimal child rearing. Thus, there is no universal standard for what constitutes child abuse and neglect (Korbin, 1981). David Finkelhor and Jill Korbin (1988) propose that a definition of child abuse and neglect that could be applied across subcultures and cultures should have two objectives: (1) it should distinguish child abuse clearly from other social, economic and health problems; and (2) it should be sufficiently flexible to apply to a range of situations in a variety of social and cultural contexts. The later recommendation is a caution that some of what is considered child abuse in Western societies has very little meaning in other societies and vice versa.

Finkelhor and Korbin (1988) propose the following definition of child abuse and neglect for cross-cultural research and study: "Child abuse is the portion of harm to children that results from human action that is proscribed (negatively valued), proximate (the action is close to the actual harm—thus deforesting land that results in child

harm does not meet this definition), and preventable (the action could have been prevented)."

The Extent of Child Abuse and Neglect

As explained in the previous section, child abuse and neglect is a general term that covers a wide range of acts of commission and omission, either carried out by a child's caretaker or allowed to happen, that result in a range of injuries ranging from death, to serious disabling injury, to emotional distress, to malnutrition and illness.

Child abuse and neglect can take many and varied forms. The Office on Child Abuse and Neglect classifies the various forms of maltreatment into six major types (see National Center on Child Abuse and Neglect [NCCAN], 1988):

1. *Physical Abuse:* Acts of commission that result in physical harm, including death, to a child.
2. *Sexual Abuse:* Acts of commission including intrusion or penetration, molestation with genital contact or other forms of sexual acts in which children are used to provide sexual gratification for a perpetrator.
3. *Emotional Abuse:* Acts of commission that include confinement, verbal or emotional abuse or other types of abuse such as withholding sleep, food or shelter.
4. *Physical Neglect:* Acts of omission that involve refusal to provide health care, delay in providing health care, abandonment, expulsion of a child from a home, inadequate supervision, failure to meet food and clothing needs, and conspicuous failure to protect a child from hazards or danger.
5. *Educational Neglect:* Acts of omission and commission that include permitting chronic truancy, failure to enroll a child in school and inattention to specific education needs.
6. *Emotional Neglect:* Acts of omission that involve failing to meet the nurturing and affection needs of a child, exposing a child to chronic or severe spouse abuse, allowing or permitting a child to use alcohol or controlled substances, encouraging the child to engage in maladaptive behavior, refusal to provide psychological

care, delays in providing psychological care and other inattention to the child's developmental needs.

Prevalence

Various methods have been used in attempts to achieve an accurate estimate of child abuse and neglect in the United States, including tabulating official reports of child maltreatment received by state child welfare agencies, as well as self-report surveys.

The Office on Child Abuse and Neglect has conducted three surveys designed to measure the national incidence of reported and recognized child maltreatment (Burgdorf, 1980; NCCAN, 1988; NCCAN, 1996). (A fourth study is under way as of 2006, but results are not yet available.) The surveys assessed how many cases were known to investigatory agencies, professionals in schools, hospitals and other social service agencies. A total of 2.9 million children were known by the agencies surveyed in 1993 (see table).

A second source of data on the extent of child maltreatment comes from the National Child Abuse and Neglect Data System (NCANDS). NCANDS is a national data collection and analysis project carried out by the U.S. Department of Health and Human Services, Office of Child Abuse and Neglect. In 2004, states received nearly 3 million reports of child maltreatment. (Only 38 states provided data on the number of reports received in 2004, totaling 2,043,523 reports.) Of these reports, 872,088 children were indicated or substantiated for maltreatment. Data on type of maltreatment were available for 49 states and the District of Columbia (Alaska did not report data on types of abuse). Of 872,088 victims of maltreatment, 152,250 experienced physical abuse, 544,050 experienced neglect, 84,398 experienced sexual abuse, 61,272 experienced psychological maltreatment and the remainder were subjected to medical neglect or other forms of maltreatment (U.S. Department of Health and Human Services, 2006).

Social science surveys of the use of violence against children by parents and caregivers provide estimates of children's experiences with violence. The National Family Violence Surveys (NFVS),

ESTIMATES OF THE TOTAL NUMBER OF MALTREATED CHILDREN, 1993

Maltreatment Type	Total Number of Cases
Physical Abuse	614,000
Sexual Abuse	300,200
Emotional Abuse	532,200
Neglect	961,300
Physical Neglect	1,335,100
Emotional Neglect	584,100
Educational Neglect	397,300
Seriously Injured Children	565,000

Source: National Center on Child Abuse and Neglect, 1996.
Note: Children who experience more than one type of abuse or neglect are reflected in the estimates for each applicable type. As a result, the estimates for the different types of maltreatment sum to more than the total number of maltreated children.

FREQUENCY OF PARENTAL VIOLENCE TOWARD CHILDREN

Percentage of Occurrences in Past Year

Violent Behavior	Once	Twice	More Than Twice	Total	Percentage of Occurrences Ever Reported
Threw something at child	1.5	.7	.9	3.1	4.5
Pushed, grabbed or shoved child	5.8	7.5	14.9	28.2	33.6
Slapped or spanked child	8.1	8.5	39.1	55.7	74.6
Kicked, bit or hit with fist	.7	.5	.3	1.5	2.1
Hit or tried to hit child with something	2.4	2.0	5.3	9.7	14.4
Beat up child	.3	.1	.2	.6	1.0
Burned or scalded child	.2	.1	.1	.4	.6
Threatened child with knife or gun	.1	.1	0	.2	.3
Used a knife or gun	.1	.1	0	.2	.2

Source: Second National Family Violence Survey, Richard J. Gelles and Murray A. Straus, 1989.

conducted by Murray Straus and his colleagues, interviewed two nationally representative samples of families: 2,146 family members in 1976 (Straus, Gelles and Steinmetz, 1980) and 6,002 family members in 1985 (Gelles and Straus, 1988). The surveys measured violence and abuse by asking respondents to report their behaviors toward their children during the previous 12 months. "Mild" forms of violence, such as that thought of as "physical punishment" by most people, was the type reported most commonly. More than 80% of the parents/caregivers of children three years to nine years of age reported hitting their children at least once during the previous year. Among older children, the reported rates were lower: 67% of the parents/caregivers of preteens and young adolescents reported hitting their youngsters during the previous year and slightly more than 33% of caregivers/parents of teenagers 15 years to 17 years of age reported hitting their adolescents during the prior year.

Even with the most severe forms of violence, the reported rates were surprisingly high. Slightly more than 20 parents in 1,000 admitted to engaging in an act of "abusive violence" during the year prior to the 1985 survey. Abusive violence, which was defined as an act that had a high probability of injuring the child, included kicking, biting, punching, beating, hitting or trying to hit a child with an object, burning or scalding, and threatening to use or using a gun or a knife. Seven children in 1,000 were hurt as the result of an act of violence directed at them by a parent or caregiver during the previous year. Based on these findings, it is projected that 1.5 million children in the United States under the age of 18 years who live with one or both parents are victims of acts of abusive physical violence each year, and 450,000 children are injured annually as a result of parental violence.

In a more recent telephone survey of 900 parents regarding children's experiences with violence in the home, more than 28% of parents of two- to eight-year-old children reported using an object to spank their child's bottom (Straus and Stewart, 1999). Nearly three-quarters (74%) of children under the age of five years had been hit or slapped by their parent(s) (Straus and Stewart, 1999).

Finkelhor and his colleagues conducted a national survey of child victimization in 2002–03 (Finkelhor, Ormrod, Turner and Hamby, 2005). The survey collected data on children from two to 17 years of age. Interviews were conducted with parents and youth. Slightly more than one in seven children (138 per 1,000) experienced child maltreatment. Emotional abuse was the most frequent type of maltreatment. The rate of physical abuse (meaning that children experienced physical harm) was 15 per 1,000, while the rate of neglect was 11 per 1,000. The overall projected extent of maltreatment was 8,755,00 child victims (Finkelhor, Ormrod, Turner and Hamby, 2005).

An examination of NCANDS's data on reports of child maltreatment reveals that the number of sustantiated reports of sexual abuse cases has declined 40% from 1992 to 2000—from 150,000 cases to 89,500 cases (Finkelhor and Jones, 2004). There are a number of plausible explanations for this drop, and, in fact, there are probably many factors that led to the decline. However, Finkelhor and Jones conclude that at least part of the decline is due to a true overall decline in the occurrence of child sexual abuse.

Child Homicide. NCANDS estimated that 1,500 children were killed by parents or caregivers in 2004 (U.S. Department of Health and Human Services, 2006). Expressed in rates, 2.03 children per 100,000 children under 18 years of age are victims of fatal child abuse and neglect. This rate is slightly higher than the rate of 1.84 in 2000. Forty-five percent of child maltreatment fatalities were children under the age of one, while 38% of the victims were between one and three years of age. Nearly 78% of the perpetrators were either one or both parents.

The varied estimates of the prevalence of child abuse and neglect most likely underestimate the true extent of child maltreatment. Given that caretakers carry out most maltreatment in the privacy of the home, much abuse and neglect goes undetected. Moreover, the lack of a cultural consensus about which acts constitute abuse and neglect and which acts are designated appropriate discipline techniques makes it difficult to assess the true level of the mistreatment of children. The above estimates of maltreatment, including the estimate of child homicide, should be considered a lower boundary of the full extent of abuse and neglect in the United States.

Risk and Protective Factors

The first research articles on child abuse and neglect characterized offenders as suffering from various forms of psychopathology (see for example, Bennie and Sclare, 1969; Galdston, 1965; Steele and Pollock, 1974). Thus, the initial approach to explaining, understanding and treating maltreatment was to identify the personality or character disorders that were thought to be associated with abuse and neglect. There were many methodological problems that limited studies that attempted to develop psychological profiles of caretakers who maltreated their children. Most early studies had small samples and no, or inappropriate, comparison groups. Collectively, the studies failed to develop a consistent profile of abusers.

Current theoretical approaches tend to recognize the multidimensional nature of abuse and neglect and locate the roots of child maltreatment in psychological, social, family, community and societal factors.

Researchers have identified both risk and protective factors for abuse and neglect. The following are the major risk and protective factors:

Age. One of the most consistent risk factors is the age of the offender. According to NCANDS data on reported and investigated child maltreatment, the modal age of perpetrators is 30 to 39. However, the modal age for female perpetrators—mostly mothers—is 20 to 29 (U.S. Department of Health and Human Services, 2006).

Sex. Mothers are the most likely offenders in acts of child homicide, accounting for 31.3% of all child homicide perpetrators in 2004 (U.S. Department of Health and Human Services, 2006). Women were the perpetrators in 57.8% of child maltreatment homicides (U.S. Department of Health and Human Services, 2006). Of course, women's higher rate of fatal and nonfatal abuse and neglect is not surprising, given that women spend more time caring for children and are delegated far more responsibility for raising children than men.

Income. Although most poor parents do not abuse or neglect their children, self-report surveys and official report data find that the rates of child maltreatment, with the exception of sexual abuse, are higher for those whose family incomes are below the poverty line than for those whose income is above the poverty line. (Pelton, 1994; Waldfogel, 1998)

However, the impact of poverty varies by the age of the child victim and the type of abuse. Child abuse rates are higher for infants who live in high-poverty counties compared to infants growing up in low-poverty counties (Wulczyn, Barth, Yuan, Harden and Landsverk, 2005). The county poverty rate made less of a difference in terms of maltreatment for children older than one year of age. Living in a high-poverty county increased the risk of physical abuse for all children, irrespective of age; however, only one-year-olds had significantly higher rates of neglect in high-poverty versus low-poverty counties. For children older than one, the poverty rate of a county did not make a large difference in terms of the risk of child neglect.

Race. Both official report data and self-report survey data often report that child abuse is over-represented among minorities. However, both the second and the third study of the National Incidence and Prevalence of Child Abuse and Neglect (National Center on Child Abuse and Neglect, 1988; 1996) found no significant relationship between the incidence of maltreatment and the child's race/ethnicity. There was no significant relationship for any of the subcategories of maltreatment. NCANDS data and the two National Family Violence Surveys, however, found stronger relationships between race/ethnicity and violence toward children. According to the most recent NCANDS data, African-American children experienced the highest rates of maltreatment (19.9 per 1,000), followed by Pacific Island (17.6), and Native American children (15.5). The lowest rates were for whites (10.7), Hispanic (10.4), and Asian children (2.9) (U.S. Department of Health and Human Services, 2006).

Wulczyn and his colleague's (Wulczyn, Barth, Yuan, Harden and Landsverk, 2005) found a much more nuanced relationship between multiple variables in their examination of NCANDS data. Here again, age was a major factor in differentiating the risk of child maltreatment. The rate of maltreatment for African-American children, one year of ago and living in high-poverty counties, was significantly higher than the rate for white or Hispanic children. However, for older children, the race of a child was not a major risk predictor (although the rate of victimization was still highest for African-American children). The same age-specific pattern was found in the low-poverty counties; however, here the rate for older African-American children was higher than for older white or Hispanic children.

Situational and Environmental Factors

Stress. Unemployment, financial problems, being a single parent, being a teenage mother and sexual difficulties are all factors that are related to child maltreatment, as are a host of other stressor events (Burrell, Thompson and Sexton, 1994; Gelles and Straus, 1988; Gelles, 1989; Parke and Collmer, 1975; Straus et al., 1980).

Social isolation and social support. The data on social isolation are somewhat less consistent than are the data for the previously listed risk factors. First, because so much of the research on child abuse and neglect is cross-sectional, it is not clear whether social isolation precedes maltreatment or is a consequence of it. Second, social isolation has been crudely measured and the purported correlation may be more anecdotal than statistical. Nevertheless, researchers often agree that parents who are socially isolated from important sources of social support are more likely to maltreat their children. (Wolfe and St. Pierre, 1989) Part of the explanation for the correlation between social isolation and child maltreatment may be the poor social skills of the caregivers (Azar, Povilaitis, Lauretti and Pouquette, 1998).

Social support appears to be an important protective factor. One major source of social support is the availability of friends and family for help, aid and assistance. The more a family is integrated into the community and the more groups and associations they belong to, the less likely they are to be violent (Straus et al., 1980).

The intergenerational transmission of violence. The notion that abused children grow up to be abusing parents and violent adults has been widely expressed in the child abuse and family violence literature (Gelles, 1980). Kaufman and Zigler (1987) reviewed the literature that tested the hypothesis of intergenerational transmission of violence toward children and concluded that the best estimate of the rate of intergenerational transmission appears to be 30% (plus or minus 5%). Although a rate of 30% is substantially less than the majority of abused children, the rate is considerably more than the 2–4% rate of abuse found in the general population (Straus and Gelles, 1986; Widom 1989). Egeland and his colleagues (Egeland, Jacobvitz and Papatola, 1987) examined continuity and discontinuity of abuse in a longitudinal study of high-risk mothers and their children. They found that mothers who had been abused as children were less likely to abuse their own children if they had emotionally supportive parents, partners or friends. In addition, the abused mothers who did not abuse their children were described as "middle class" and "upwardly mobile," suggesting that they were able to draw on economic resources that may not have been available to the abused mothers who did abuse their children.

Evidence from studies of parental violence indicates that although experiencing violence in one's family of origin is often correlated with later violent behavior, such experience is not the sole determining factor. When the intergenerational transmission of violence occurs, it is likely the result of a complex set of social and psychological process.

Research on Victims

Compared to research on offenders, there has been somewhat less research on victims of child abuse and neglect that focuses on factors that increase or reduce the risk of victimization. Most research on victims examines the consequences of victimization (e.g., depression, psychological distress, suicide attempts, symptoms of post-traumatic stress syndrome, etc.) or the effectiveness of various intervention efforts.

The very youngest children are at the greatest risk of being abused, especially by lethal forms of violence (U.S. Department of Health and Human Services, 2006; Wulczyn, Barth, Yuan, Harden and Landsverk, 2005). However, older children are at the greatest risk of nonlethal physical abuse and the youngest children (one to three years of age) have the highest rate of being reported for child neglect (U.S. Department of Health and Human Services, 2006).

Early research suggested that there were a number of factors that raise the risk of a child being abused. Low birth weight babies (Parke and Collmer, 1975), premature children (Elmer, 1967; Newberger et al., 1977; Parke and Collmer, 1975; Steele and Pollock, 1974) and handicapped, retarded or developmentally disabled children (Friedrich and Boriskin, 1976; Gil, 1970; Steinmetz, 1978) were all described as being at greater risk of being abused by their parents or caretakers. However, a review of studies that examines the child's role in abuse calls into question many of these findings (Starr, 1988). One major problem is that few investigators used matched comparison groups. Secondly, newer studies fail to find premature or handicapped children at higher risk for abuse (Egeland and Vaughan, 1981; Starr et al., 1984).

Factors Associated with Sexual Abuse of Children

There has been a great deal of research on the characteristics of sexual abusers, but current research has failed to isolate characteristics, especially demographic, social or psychological characteristics, that discriminate between sexual abusers and nonabusers (Black, Heyman and Slep, 2001; Quinsey, 1984).

One of the key questions raised in discussions about sexual abuse is whether all children are at risk for sexual abuse or whether some children, because of some specific characteristic (e.g., age or poverty status), are at greater risk than others are. Current research is unclear as to definitive factors that can predict future sexual abuse. Finkelhor, Moore, Hamby and Straus (1997) found that a child's sex does not necessarily predict later victimization. However, Sedlak (1997) asserts that female children are at an increased risk for sexual abuse, and the relationship between a child's sexual victimization and age is also associated with family structure and race.

Explaining the Abuse and Neglect of Children

Risk and protective factors do not, in and of themselves, explain why parents and caretakers abuse and neglect their children. The earliest explanatory theories and models focused on intra-individual factors to explain maltreatment. These models included a psychopathological explanation that explained abuse and neglect as a function of individual psychopathology. Other models proposed that maltreatment arose out of mental illness or the use and abuse of alcohol and illicit drugs.

Later theories added social, cultural and environmental factors to the models. The major multi-dimensional models include:

Social learning theory. Social learning theory proposes that individuals who experienced abuse and neglect as children are more likely to maltreat their own children than individuals who experienced no abuse or neglect. Children who either experience abuse themselves or who witness violence between their parents are more likely to use violence when they grow up. This finding has been interpreted to support the idea that family violence and caretaking is learned. The family is the institution and social group where people learn the roles of husband and wife, parent and child. The home is the prime location where people learn how to deal with various stresses, crises and frustrations. In many instances, the home is also the site where a person first experiences violence and abuse. Not only do people learn violent behavior, but also they learn how to justify being violent. For example, hearing father say "this will hurt me more than it will hurt you," or mother say, "you have been bad, so you deserve to be spanked," contributes to how children learn to justify violent behavior.

Social situational/stress and coping theory. Social Situational/Stress and Coping Theory explains why maltreatment occurs in some situations and not others. The theory proposes that abuse and neglect occur because of two main factors. The first is structural stress and the lack of coping resources in a family. For instance, the association between low income and child abuse indicates that an important contributor to the risk of abuse is inadequate financial resources. The second factor is the cultural norm concerning the use of force and violence. In contemporary American society, as well as many societies, violence in general, and violence toward children in particular is normative (Straus, 1994). Thus, individuals learn to use violence both expressively and instrumentally as a means of coping with a pileup of stressor events.

Ecological theory. Garbarino (1977) and Belsky (1980; 1993) propose an ecological model to explain the complex nature of child maltreatment. The ecological model proposes that violence and abuse arise out of a mismatch of parent to child or family to neighborhood and community. For example, parents who are under a great deal of social stress and have poor coping skills may have a difficult time meeting the needs of a child who is hyperactive. The risk of abuse and violence increases when the functioning of the children and parents is limited and constrained by developmental problems such as children with learning disabilities and social or emotional handicaps, and when parents are under considerable stress or have personality problems, such as immaturity or impulsiveness. Finally, if there are few institutions and agencies in the community to support troubled families, then the risk of abuse is further increased.

Exchange theory. Exchange theory proposes that child rearing and child abuse is governed by the principle of costs and benefits. Abuse is used when the rewards are perceived as greater than the costs (Gelles, 1983). The private nature of the family, the reluctance of social institutions and agencies to intervene—in spite of mandatory child abuse reporting laws—and the low risk of other interventions reduce the costs of abuse and neglect. The cultural approval of violence as both expressive and instrumental behavior raises the potential rewards for violence. The most significant reward is social control, or power.

Sociobiology theory. A sociobiological, or evolutionary perspective of child maltreatment, suggests that the abuse and neglect of human or nonhuman primate offspring is the result of the reproductive success potential of children and parental investment. The theory's central assumption is that natural selection is the process of differential reproduction and reproductive success (Daly and Wilson, 1980). Males can be expected to invest in offspring when there is some degree of parental certainty (how confident the parent is that the child is their own genetic offspring), while females are also inclined to invest under conditions of parental certainty. Parents recognize their offspring and avoid squandering valuable reproductive effort on someone else's offspring. Thus, Daly and Wilson (1985) conclude that parental feelings are more readily and more profoundly established with one's own offspring than in cases where the parent-offspring relationship is artificial. Children not genetically related to the parent (e.g., stepchildren, adopted or foster children) or children with low reproductive potential (e.g., handicapped or retarded children) are at the highest risk for infanticide and abuse (Burgess and Garbarino, 1983; Daly and Wilson, 1980; Hrdy, 1979). Large families can dilute parental energy and lower attachment to children, thus increasing the risk of child abuse and neglect. (Burgess & Drais-Parrillo, 2004).

Attachment Theory. Attachment theory describes the propensity of individuals to form a strong emotional bond with a primary caregiver who functions as a source of security and safety (Bowlby, 1973). The theory proposes that there is a clear association between early attachment experiences and the pattern of affectionate bonds one makes throughout one's lifetime. If an individual has formed strong and secure attachments with early caregivers, later adult relationships will also have secure attachments. On the other hand, if an individual has formed insecure, anxious or ambivalent attachments early on, later adult attachments will be replicated similarly. Therefore, according to the theory, attachment difficulties underlie adulthood relational problems. Bowlby (1988) posits that anxiety and anger go hand-in-hand as responses to risk of loss and that anger is often functional. For certain individuals with weak and insecure attachments, the functional reaction to anger becomes distorted and is manifested by violent acts against one's partner.

A model of sexual abuse. Finkelhor (1984) reviewed research on the factors that have been proposed as contributing to sexual abuse of children and developed what he calls the "Four Precondition Model of Sexual Abuse." His review suggests that all the factors relating to sexual abuse can be grouped into one of four preconditions that must be met before sexual abuse can occur. The preconditions are:

1. A potential offender needs to have some motivation to abuse a child sexually.
2. The potential offender has to overcome internal inhibitions against acting on that motivation.
3. The potential offender has to overcome external impediments to committing sexual abuse.
4. The potential offender or some other factor has to undermine or overcome a child's possible resistance to sexual abuse.

Summary. The intra-individual models of child abuse and neglect dominated the first decade of research, practice and policy. Although some professions still subscribe to psychopathological explanations for child maltreatment, such narrow models eventually gave way to more multidimensional approaches that included psychopathology, but also considered social, environmental and cultural factors. Current theoretical approaches tend to be based on the ecological model of child maltreatment (National Research Council, 1993).

The Consequences of Maltreatment

The consequences of child abuse and neglect differ by the age of the child. During childhood some of the major consequences of maltreatment include problematic school performance and lowered attention to social cues. Researchers have found that children whose parents are "psychologically unavailable" function poorly across a wide range of psychological, cognitive and developmental areas (Egeland and Sroufe, 1981). Physical aggression, antisocial behavior and juvenile delinquency are among the most consistently documented consequences of abuse in adolescence and adulthood (Aber et al., 1990; Dodge et al., 1990; Widom, 1989a; 1989b; 1991). Evidence is more suggestive that maltreatment increases the risk of alcohol and drug problems (National Research Council, 1993).

Ystgaard, Hestetun, Loeb and Mehlum (2004) report that physical and sexual abuse are significantly and independently associated with repeated suicide attempts. In other words, physical and sexual abuse increase the risk of suicide attempts, even when controlling for other adverse events and situations children experience.

Research on the consequences of sexual abuse finds that inappropriate sexual behavior, such as frequent and overt sexual stimulation and inappropriate sexual overtures to other children, are commonly found among victims of sexual abuse (Kendall-Tackett et al., 1993). Roberts and his colleagues (Roberts, O'Connor, Dunn, Golding et. al., 2004) conducted a longitudinal study of 8,292 families and found that sexual abuse experienced before age 13 was associated with poorer psychological well-being, teenage pregnancy and adjustment problems in the victim's own children. Widom (1995) has found that people who were sexually abused during childhood are at higher risk of arrest for committing crimes as adults, including sex crimes, compared to people who did not suffer sexual abuse. However, this risk is no greater than the risk of arrest for victims of other childhood maltreatment, with one exception: Victims of sexual abuse are more likely to be arrested for prostitution than other victims of maltreatment.

As noted in the discussion of the extent of child maltreatment, child neglect is by far the most common form of maltreatment. While the more dramatic forms of maltreatment—physical abuse and sexual abuse—receive considerable attention in terms of the impact on children, there is far less research, and even concern, for the impact of the chronic form of maltreatment: child neglect. Hildyard and Wolfe (2002) reviewed the research on the impact of child neglect and find considerable support for the conclusion that child neglect produces significant developmental problems for child victims. Neglect has a deleterious effect on children's cognitive, socioemotional and behavioral development. The earlier in life a child is neglected, the more comprised the child's development. The impact of neglect is somewhat unique, producing more severe cognitive and academic deficits, social withdrawal and limited peer interactions. Victims of neglect tend to internalize the impact of that neglect as opposed to externalizing through aggressive and violent behavior (Hildyard and Wolfe, 2002).

As severe and significant as the consequences of child abuse and neglect are, it is also important to point out that the majority of children who are abused and neglected do not show signs of extreme disturbance. Despite having been physically, psychologically or sexually abused, many children have effective coping abilities and thus are able to deal with their problems better than other maltreated children. There are a number of protective factors that insulate children from the effects of maltreatment. These include: high intelligence and good scholastic attainment; temperament; cognitive appraisal of events—how the child views the maltreatment; having a healthy relationship with a significant person; and the type of interventions, including placement outside of the home (National Research Council, 1993).

Witnessing Domestic Violence

Children who witness domestic violence are a unique population warranting research and clinical attention (Rosenberg and Rossman, 1990). Witnessing is at the intersection of child abuse and neglect and domestic violence. Researchers and clinicians report that children who witness acts of domestic violence experience negative behavioral and developmental outcomes, independent of any direct abuse or neglect that they may also experience from their caretakers (Jaffe, Wolfe and Wilson, 1990; Osofsky, 1995; Rosenberg and Rossman, 1990). Estimates from the two National Family Violence Surveys are that between 1.5 million and 3.3 million children three to 17 years of age are exposed to domestic violence each year (Gelles and Straus, 1988; Straus, Gelles and Steinmetz, 1980).

Prevention and Treatment

As noted earlier, all 50 states had enacted mandatory reporting laws for child abuse and neglect by the late 1960s. These laws require certain professionals (or in some states, all adults) to report cases of suspected abuse or neglect. When a report comes in, state or local protective service workers

investigate to determine if the child is in need of protection and if the family is in need of help or assistance. Although a wide array of options are available to child protection workers, they typically have two basic ways to protect a victim of child abuse: (a) removing the child and placing him or her in a foster home or institution; or (b) providing the family with social support, such as counseling, food stamps, day care services, etc.

Neither solution is ideal, and there are risks in both. For instance, a child may not understand why he or she is being removed from the home. Children who are removed from abusive homes may be protected from physical damage, although some children are abused and killed in foster homes and residential placements. Abused children frequently require special medical and/or psychological care and it is difficult to find a suitable placement for them. They could well become a burden for foster parents or institutions that have to care for them. Therefore, the risk of abuse might even be greater in a foster home or institution than in the home of the natural parents. In addition, removal may cause emotional harm. The emotional harm arises from the fact that abused children still love and have strong feelings for their parents and do not understand why they have been removed from their parents and homes. Often, abused children feel that they are responsible for their own abuse.

Leaving children in an abusive home and providing social services involves another type of risk. Most protective service workers are overworked, undertrained and underpaid. Family services, such as substance abuse treatment, crisis day care, financial assistance and suitable housing and transportation services, are limited. This can lead to cases where children who were reported as abused, investigated and supervised by state agencies are killed during the period when the family was supposedly being monitored. Half of all children who are killed by caretakers are killed *after* they have been reported to child welfare agencies (Gelles, 1996).

Only a handful of evaluations have been made of prevention and treatment programs for child maltreatment. In Elmira, New York, Olds and his colleagues (1986) evaluated the effectiveness of a family support program during pregnancy and for the first two years after birth for low-income, unmarried, teenage first-time mothers. Nineteen percent of a sample of poor unmarried teenage girls who received no services during their pregnancy period was reported for subsequent child maltreatment. Of those children of poor, unmarried, teenage mothers who were provided with the full compliment of nurse home visits during the mother's pregnancy and for the first two years after birth, 4% had confirmed cases of child abuse and neglect reported to the state child protection agency. Subsequent follow-ups by the home health visiting intervention worker demonstrated the long-term effectiveness of this intervention. However, the effectiveness varied depending on the populations receiving the service, the community context and who made the visits (nurses or others) (Olds, Henderson, Kitzman, Eckenrode, Cole and Tatelbaum, 1999).

Daro and Cohn (1988) reviewed evaluations of 88 child maltreatment programs that were funded by the federal government between 1974 and 1982. They found that there was no noticeable correlation between a given set of services and the likelihood of further maltreatment of children. In fact, the more services a family received, the worse the family got and the more likely children were to be maltreated. Lay counseling, group counseling and parent education classes resulted in more positive treatment outcomes. The optimal treatment period appeared to be between seven and 18 months. The projects that were successful in reducing abuse accomplished this by separating children from abusive parents, either by placing them in foster homes or requiring the maltreating adult to move out of the house.

The National Academy of Sciences panel on "Assessing Family Violence Interventions" identified 78 evaluations of child maltreatment intervention programs that met the panel's criteria for methodologically sound evaluation research. The one commonality of the 78 evaluations of child abuse and neglect prevention and treatment programs was, in scientific terms, a failure to reject the null hypothesis. While it may be too harsh a judgment to say these programs have not and do not work as intended, the National Research Council report did come to the following conclusion regarding social service interventions:

> Social service interventions designed to improve parenting practices and provide family support have not yet demonstrated that they have the capacity to reduce or prevent abusive or neglectful behaviors significantly over time for the majority of families who have been reported for child maltreatment (National Research Council, 1998, p. 118).

Thus, while we have made great strides in identifying child abuse and neglect as a social problem, and we have developed numerous programs to attempt to treat and prevent abuse and neglect, we still have much to learn about what causes parents and caretakers to abuse their children and what steps society must take to prevent the maltreatment of children.

—Richard J. Gelles, Ph. D.,
Dean
Joanne and Raymond Welsh Chair of Child Welfare and Family Violence
Director, Center Research on Youth and Social Policy
Director, Ortner-Unity Program on Family Violence
Codirector, Field Center for Children's Policy, Practice, and Research, School of Social Policy & Practice
University of Pennsylvania, Philadelphia

References

Aber, J. L., J. P. Alien, V. Carlson, and D. Cicchetti. "The effects of maltreatment on development during early childhood: Recent studies and their theoretical, clinical, and policy implications." In D. Cicchetti and V. Carlson, eds. *Child Maltreatment: Theory and Research on Causes and Consequences.* New York: Cambridge University Press, 1990, pp. 579–619.

Azar, S. T., T. Y. Povilaitis, A. F. Lauretti, and C. L. Pouquette. "The current status of etiological theories in intrafamilial child maltreatment." In J. R. Lutzker, eds. *Handbook of Child Abuse Research and Treatment.* New York: Plenum Press, 1998, pp. 3–30.

Bakan, D. *The Slaughter of the Innocents.* Boston: Beacon Press, 1971.

Belsky, J. "Child maltreatment: An ecological integration." *American Psychologist* 35 (1980): 320–335.

————. "Etiology of child maltreatment: A developmental-ecological approach." *Psychological Bulletin* 114 (1993): 413–434.

Bennie, E. H., and A. B. Sclare. "The battered child syndrome." *American Journal of Psychiatry* 125 (1969): 975–978.

Bowlby, J. *Attachment and Loss.* Vol. 2, *Separation.* London: Hogarth Press, 1973.

————. *A Secure Base.* London: Hongarth Press, 1988.

Burgdorf, K. *Recognition and Reporting of Child Maltreatment.* Rockville, Md.: Westat, 1980.

Burgess, R. L. "Family violence: Some implications from evolutionary biology." Paper presented at Annual Meeting of the American Society of Criminology, Philadelphia, 1979.

Burgess, R. L., and J. Garbarino. "Doing what comes naturally? An evolutionary perspective on child abuse." In D. Finkelhor, R. Gelles, M. Straus, and G. Hotaling, eds. *The Dark Side of the Families: Current Family Violence Research.* Beverly Hills, Calif.: Sage, 1983, pp. 88–101.

Burrell, B., Thompson, B., and D. Sexton. "Predicting and child abuse potential across family types." *Child Abuse & Neglect* 18 (1994): 1,039–1,049.

Caffey, J. "Multiple fractures in the long bones of infants suffering from chronic subdural hematoma." *American Journal of Roentgenology, Radium Therapy, and Nuclear Medicine* 58 (1946): 163–173.

Daly, M., and M. Wilson. "Discriminative parental solicitude: A biosocial perspective." *Journal of Marriage and the Family* 42 (1980): 277–288.

————. "Child abuse and other risks of not living with both parents." *Ethology and Sociobiology* 6 (1985): 197–210.

————. *Homicide.* New York: Aldine DeGruyter, 1988.

Daro, D. "Current trends in child abuse reporting and fatalities: NCPCA's 1995 annual fifty state survey." *APSAC Advisor* 9 (1996): 21–24.

Dodge, K. A., J. E. Bates, and G. S. Pettit. "Mechanisms in the cycle of violence." *Science* 250 (1990): 1,678–1,683.

Egeland, B., and B. Vaughan. "Failure of 'bond formation' as a cause of abuse, neglect, and maltreatment." *American Journal of Orthopsychiatry* 51 (1981): 78–84.

Egeland, B., and L. A. Sroufe. "Attachment and early child maltreatment." *Child Development* 52 (1981): 44–52.

Egeland, B., D. Jacobvitz, and K. Papatola. "Intergenerational continuity of abuse." In R. J. Gelles and J. B. Lancaster, eds. *Child Abuse and Neglect: Biosocial Dimensions.* Hawthorne, N.Y.: Aldine de Gruyter, 1987, pp. 255–276.

Elmer, E. *Children in Jeopardy: A Study of Abused Minors and Their Families.* Pittsburgh, Pa.: University of Pittsburgh Press, 1967.

Fergusson, D. M., J. Fleming, and D. O'Neil. *Child Abuse in New Zealand.* Wellington, New Zealand: Research Division, Department of Social Work, 1972.

Finkelhor, D. *Child Sexual Abuse: New Theory and Research.* New York: Free Press, 1984.

Finkelhor, D., and J. Korbin. "Child abuse as an international issue." *Child Abuse and Neglect: The International Journal* 12 (1988): 3–23.

Friederich, W. N., and J. A. Boriskin. "The role of the child in abuse: A review of literature." *American Journal of Orthopsychiatry* 46 (1976): 580–590.

Galdston, R. "Observations of children who have been physically abused by their parents." *American Journal of Psychiatry* 122 (1965): 440–443.

Garbarino, J. "The human ecology of child maltreatment." *Journal of Marriage and the Family* 39 (1977): 721–735.

Gelles, R. J. "Violence in the family. A review of research in the seventies." *Journal of Marriage and the Family* 42 (1980): 873–885.

————. "An exchange/social control theory." In D. Finkelhor, R. Gelles, M. Straus, and G. Hotaling, eds. *The Dark Side of Families: Current Family Violence Research.* Beverly Hills, Calif.: Sage, 1983, pp. 151–165.

————. "Child abuse and violence in single parent families: Parent-absence and economic deprivation." *American Journal of Orthopsychiatry* 59 (1989): 492–501.

Gelles, R. J., and M. A. Straus. "Is violence towards children increasing? A comparison of 1975 and 1985 national survey rates." *Journal of Interpersonal Violence* 2 (1987): 212–222.

————. *Intimate Violence.* New York: Simon and Schuster, 1988.

Gil, D. *Violence against Children: Physical Child Abuse in the United States.* Cambridge, Mass.: Harvard University Press, 1970.

Greven, P. *Spare the Child: The Religious Roots of Punishment and the Psychological Impact of Physical Abuse.* New York: Knopf, 1990.

Hildyard, K. L., and P. A. Wolfe. "Child Neglect: Developmental Issues and Outcomes." *Mental Child Abuse and Neglect* 26 (2002): 679–695.

Hrdy, S. B. "Infanticide among animals: A review classification, and examination of the implications for reproductive strategies of females." *Ethology and Sociobiology* 1 (1979): 13–40.

Johnson, C. *Child Abuse in the Southeast: An Analysis of 1172 Reported Cases.* Athens, Ga.: Welfare Research, 1974.

Kaufman, J., and E. Zigler. "Do abused children become abusive parents?" *American Journal of Orthopsychiatry* 57 (1987): 186–192.

Kempe, C. H., F. N. Silverman, B. F. Steele, W. Droegemueller, and H. K. Silver. "The battered child syndrome." *Journal of the American Medical Association* 181 (1962): 107–112.

Kendall-Tackett, K. A., L. Williams, and D. Finkelhor. "The impact of sexual abuse on children: A review and synthesis of recent empirical literature." *Psychological Bulletin* 113 (1993): 164–180.

Korbin, J., ed. *Child Abuse and Neglect: Cross-cultural Perspectives.* Berkeley: University of California Press, 1981.

National Center on Child Abuse and Neglect. *Study findings: Study of national incidence and prevalence of child abuse and neglect: 1988.* Washington, D.C.: U.S. Department of Health and Human Services, 1988.

———. *Study findings: Study of national incidence and prevalence of child abuse and neglect: 1993.* Washington, D.C.: U.S. Department of Health and Human Services, 1996.

National Research Council. *Understanding Child Abuse and Neglect.* Washington, D.C.: National Academy Press, 1993.

———. *Violence in families: Assessing prevention and treatment programs.* Washington, D.C.: National Academy Press, 1998.

Nelson, B. J. *Making an Issue of Child Abuse: Political Agenda Setting for Social Problems.* Chicago: University of Chicago Press, 1984.

Newberger, E., R. Reed, J. H. Daniel, J. Hyde, and M. Kotelchuck. "Pediatric social illness: Toward an etiologic classification." *Pediatrics* 60 (1977): 178–185.

Olds, D. L., C. R. Henderson Jr., R. Tatelbaum, and R. Chamberlin. "Preventing child abuse and neglect: A randomized trial of nurse home visitation." *Pediatrics* 77 (1986): 65–78.

Olds, D. L., C. R. Henderson, H. J. Kitzman, J. J. Eckenrode, R. E. Cole, and R. C. Tatelbaum. "Prenatal and infancy home visitation by nurses: Recent findings." *The Future of Children* 9 (1999): 44–65.

Parke, R. D., and C. W. Collmer. "Child abuse: An interdisciplinary analysis." In M. Hetherington, ed. *Review of Child Development Research.* Vol. 5. Chicago: University of Chicago Press, pp. 1–102.

Pelton, L. The role of material factors in child abuse and neglect. In G. B. Melton and F. D. Barry, eds. *Protecting Children from Abuse and Neglect: Foundations for a New National Strategy.* New York: Guilford Press, 1994, pp. 131–181.

Peters, S. D., G. E. Wyatt, and D. Finkelhor. "Prevalence." In D. Finkelhor, ed. *A Sourcebook on Child Sexual Abuse.* Beverly Hills, Calif.: Sage, 1986, pp. 15–59.

Quinsey, V. L. "Sexual aggression: Studies of offenders against women." In D. N. Weisstub, ed. *Law and Mental Health: International Perspectives.* Volume 1. New York: Pergamon Press, 1984, pp. 84–121.

Radbill, S. "Children in a world of violence: A history of child abuse." In C. H. Kempe and R. Heifer, eds. *The Battered Child.* 3rd ed. Chicago: University of Chicago Press, 1980, pp. 3–20.

Roberts, R., T. O'Connor, J. Dunn, J. Golding et. al. "The effects of child sexual abuse in later family life: Mental health, parenting and adjustment of offspring." *Child Abuse & Neglect* 28 (2004): 525–545.

Robin, M. "Historical introduction: Sheltering arms: The roots of child protection." In E. Newberger, ed. *Child Abuse.* Boston: Little, Brown, 1980, pp. 1–41.

Starr, R. H., Jr., K. N. Dietrich, J. Fischoff, B. Schumann, and M. Demorest. "The contribution of handicapping conditions to child abuse." *Topics in Early Childhood Special Education* 4 (1984): 55–69.

Starr, R. H., Jr. "Physical abuse of children." In V. B. Van Hasselt, R. L. Morrison, A. S. Bellack, and M. Hersen, eds. *Handbook of Family Violence.* New York: Plenum, 1988, pp. 119–155.

Steele, B. F., and C. Pollock. "A psychiatric study of parents who abuse infants and small children." In R. Heifer and C. H. Kempe, eds. *The Battered Child.* Chicago: University of Chicago Press, 1968, pp. 103–137.

Steele, B. F., and C. Pollock. "A psychiatric study of parents who abuse infants and small children." In R. Heifer and C. Kempe, eds. *The Battered Child.* 2nd ed. Chicago: University of Chicago Press, pp. 89–134.

Steinmetz, S. K, "Violence between family members." *Marriage and Family Review* 1 (1978): 1–16.

Straus, M. A. *Beating the Devil out of Them: Corporal Punishment in American Families.* New York: Lexington Books, 1994.

Straus, M. A., and R. J. Gelles. "Societal change and change in family violence from 1975 to 1985 as revealed in two national surveys." *Journal of Marriage and the Family* 48 (1986): 465–479.

Straus, M. A., R. J. Gelles, and S. K. Steinmetz. *Behind Closed Doors: Violence in the American Family*. New York: Doubleday/Anchor, 1980.

Ten Bensel, R. L., M. Rheinberger, and S. X. Radbill. "Children in a world of violence: The roots of child maltreatment." In M. E. Heifer, R. S. Kempe, and R. D. Krugman, eds. *The Battered Child*. 4th ed. Chicago: University of Chicago Press, 1997, pp. 3–28.

U.S. Advisory Board on Child Abuse and Neglect. *A Nation's Shame: Fatal Child Abuse and Neglect in the United States*. Washington, D.C.: U.S. Department of Health and Human Services, 1995.

U.S. Department of Health and Human Services, Administration on Children, Youth and Families. *Child Maltreatment 1996: Reports from the States to the National Child Abuse and Neglect Data System*. Washington, D.C.: U.S. Government Printing Office, 1998.

Waldfogel, J. *The Future of Child Protection: How to Break the Cycle of Abuse and Neglect*. Cambridge, Mass: Harvard University Press, 1998.

Widom, C. S. *The Cycle of Violence*. Science 244 (1989a): 160–166.

———. "Child abuse, neglect, and violent criminal behavior." *Criminology* 27 (1989b): 251–271.

———. *Victims of Childhood Sexual Abuse—Later Criminal Consequences*. National Institute of Justice research in brief. Washington, D.C.: U.S. Department of Justice Office of Justice Programs, 1995.

Wolfe, D. A., and St. Pierre, J. "Child abuse and neglect." In T. H. Ollendick and M. Hersen, eds. *Handbook of Child Psychotherapy*. 2nd ed. New York: Plenum Press, 1989, pp. 377–398.

Wooley, P., and W. Evans. "Significance of skeletal lesions resembling those of traumatic origin." *Journal of the American Medical Association* 158 (1955): 539–543.

Wulczyn, F., R. P. Barth, Y. Y. Yuan, B. J. Harden, and J. Landsverk. *Beyond Common Sense: Child Welfare, Child Well-being and the Evidence for Policy Reform*. New Brunswick, N.J.: Aldine/Transaction, 2005.

Ystgaard, M., Hestetun, I., Loeb, M., and Mehlum, L. "Is there a specific relationship between childhood sexual and physical abuse and repeated suicide behavior?" *Child Abuse & Neglect* 28 (2004): 863–875.

ENTRIES A to Z

abandonment Leaving a minor child alone for an extended period, depending on the definitions of the laws of the state or area. Criminal abandonment generally means that the caregiver, usually a parent, made no provisions for another adult to care for the child during an absence, particularly an infant or young child. Infants may be abandoned in hospitals or, much worse, in Dumpsters or deserted areas where they are likely to die.

In the United States and other Western countries, parents who abandon the child can, in some cases, be charged with neglect. Each state has its own, different statute with regard to the legal definition of abandonment; these statutes apply not only to infants and small children but to adolescents as well. There are legal precedents for abandonment charges to be brought against parents who lock their teenage children out of the house.

Most states have statutes regarding criminal neglect and abandonment, although the laws and the penalties for violating such laws vary greatly.

Abandonment is a felony offense in some states and a misdemeanor in others. The age of the child who was abandoned is also addressed in some statutes; for example, it being a crime to abandon a child under 10, 12 or some other age. The federal ADOPTION AND SAFE FAMILIES ACT allows states to terminate the parental rights of parents of abandoned children after a hearing is held.

In non-Western countries, parents sometimes abandon their children (usually infants) at orphanages or in hospitals or churches because they are unable to care for them. They may hope that another family will adopt the child.

As of this writing, this practice is relatively common in China, where there is a state-imposed limit of one child per family. Most families want male children, and as a result, if a female child is born, she may be abandoned. Children are also abandoned in other countries, such as in Latin America, because the biological mother cannot care for her child but is too ashamed, in large part because of social stigma against unmarried mothers, to come forth and express her desire for the child to have another family. It may also be illegal or extremely difficult for her to openly arrange an adoption, depending on the laws of the country. Thus, abandonment may be seen as the only option.

abdominal injuries Abdominal trauma is a common but often overlooked result of physical abuse. Such trauma includes damage to kidneys, blood vessels, stomach, duodenum, small bowel, colon, pancreas, liver or spleen. Frequently more than one organ is affected. Because there are few outward signs of abdominal injuries, they may go untreated for extended periods of time, subjecting the child to a great deal of pain and sometimes resulting in death.

Injuries to the abdomen are usually caused by one of three forces: compression, crushing or acceleration. A blow to the midsection can compress organs filled with fluid or gas, causing them to rupture. Compression injuries most often affect the stomach and colon. Crushing of internal organs can occur when a blow to the front of the abdomen presses the organ against a hard structure such as the spinal column or rib cage. Rupture of the kidneys, pancreas, spleen or liver may result from such crushing. Rapid acceleration, such as when a child is thrown or struck so forcefully that he or she is knocked down, can tear connective tissue, resulting in hemorrhage or perforation of the small intestines.

A thorough screening for abdominal trauma is recommended when children show evidence of having been physically abused or when abuse is suspected.

abduction   See CHILD STEALING.

abuse, adolescent   See ADOLESCENT ABUSE.

abuse, cycle of   See INTERGENERATIONAL CYCLE OF ABUSE.

abuse, drug   See SUBSTANCE ABUSE.

abuse, emotional   See PSYCHOLOGICAL/EMOTIONAL MALTREATMENT.

abuse, institutional   See INSTITUTIONAL ABUSE AND NEGLECT.

abuse, neurological manifestations   See NEUROLOGIC MANIFESTATIONS OF ABUSE AND NEGLECT.

abuse, passive   See PASSIVE ABUSER.

abuse, physical   See PHYSICAL ABUSE.

abuse, prediction of   See PREDICTION OF ABUSE AND NEGLECT.

abuse, psychological   See PSYCHOLOGICAL/EMOTIONAL MALTREATMENT.

abuse, psychopathological   See PSYCHOPATHOLOGY.

abuse, sexual   See SEXUAL ABUSE.

abuse, sibling   See SIBLING ABUSE.

abuse, situational   See SITUATIONAL ABUSE AND NEGLECT.

abuse, social   See SOCIAL ABUSE.

abuse, spouse   See SPOUSE ABUSE.

abuse, substance   See SUBSTANCE ABUSE.

abuse, verbal   See VERBAL ABUSE.

abused children, placement   See PLACEMENT OF ABUSED CHILDREN.

abusers   Individuals who abuse and/or neglect children. Although each case of child maltreatment is unique, and there is no one specific type of parent or other individual who abuses or neglects a child, there *are* some observable patterns among abusers. For example, among parents who abuse or neglect their children, factors such as substance abuse, mental or physical illness and other factors play a role in some cases of child abuse. Also, some individuals who have been abused during their childhood will later abuse their own children; however, at least half of individuals abused in childhood do *not* grow up to abuse their own children.

The patterns found among many child abusers do *not* mean that everyone who fits the category of one or more of these factors will abuse their children. However, the risk is greater. As a result, generalizations can be made about the primary perpetrators of child maltreatment, based on research done in the field of child abuse, and a synopsis of this information follows.

Note that the statistical information on child abuse in the United States is primarily based on data provided by the states to the federal government and is included in the report *Child Mal-*

TABLE I
PERPETRATORS BY RELATIONSHIP TO VICTIMS AND TYPES OF MALTREATMENT, UNITED STATES, 2003

Maltreatment type	Parent		Other relative		Foster parent	
	Number	%	Number	%	Number	%
Physical abuse only	60,565	11.0	4,577	10.4	524	16.9
Neglect only	341,167	62.0	16,509	37.5	1,552	50.0
Sexual abuse only	14,850	2.7	13,159	29.9	197	6.3
Psychological maltreatment only, other only or unknown only	49,835	9.1	2,568	5.8	226	7.3
Multiple maltreatment	83,598	15.2	7,197	16.4	608	19.6
Total	550,015		44,010		3,107	
		100.0		100.0		100.0

Source: Adapted from Administration on Children, Youth and Families, *Child Maltreatment 2003*. Children's Bureau, U.S. Department of Health and Human Services, Washington, D.C., 2005, page 68.

treatment 2003, published in 2005 by the U.S. Department of Health and Human Services. In contrast, observations about the psychological mindset of abusers, patterns among abusers and other issues related to child abuse are offered through research studies.

Although most child abuse is committed by parents or relatives, in some cases abusers come from outside the family; for example, it is commonly known that sometimes people in a position of trust, such as teachers, members of the clergy and other individuals in environments where children congregate, sometimes abuse children.

See CLERGY, SEXUAL ABUSE BY; TRUSTED PROFESSIONALS, CHILD ABUSE BY.

Types of Abuse

As can be seen from Table I, among the categories of physical abuse only, neglect only, sexual abuse only and other categories, of the parents who abuse or neglect their children, the largest percentage (62%) fits the category of "neglect only." This category is also the greatest percentage of all forms of abuse among foster parents who maltreat children (50%) as well as among other relatives (37.5%). The next most prominent form of maltreatment for parents is "multiple maltreatment" (15.2%), which is also the next greatest form of maltreatment among foster parents (19.6%); however, among other relatives who maltreat children, after the category of

neglect only, the next greatest category is sexual abuse only (29.9%).

Statistical Patterns among People Who Maltreat Children

There are many statistical generalizations about child abusers that can be made, such as that, in most cases of child abuse (with the exception of SEXUAL ABUSE), the perpetrator is a parent (75%). Both males and females abuse children, but females (58.2%) are more likely to be abusive.

Sometimes siblings abuse each other, with the abuse going far beyond the normal teasing and some minor pushing and shoving in which brothers and sisters may engage; instead, it is actual physical abuse or sexual abuse.

See SIBLING ABUSE.

Age of Perpetrators

The majority of known perpetrators of child maltreatment (about 80%) are under age 40, and the largest single group of perpetrators, including both males and females (about 42%) is 30–39 years old. Individuals who are age 19 or younger represent only about 5% of the abusers. About 5% of child maltreatment perpetrators are age 50 or older. (See Table II.)

Male Perpetrators

In 2005, the Department of Health and Human Services released a report on male perpetrators of

TABLE II
AGE AND SEX OF PERPETRATORS OF CHILD ABUSE IN THE UNITED STATES, 2003

Age	Men		Women		Total	
	Number	%	Number	%	Number	%
Less than 20	18,630	6.2	17,463	4.2	36,093	5.1
20–29	80,269	26.9	164,398	39.6	244,667	34.3
30–39	114,032	38.2	161,748	39.0	275,780	38.6
40–49	64,368	21.5	56,278	13.6	120,646	16.9
50+	21,402	7.2	15,220	3.7	36,622	5.1
Total	298,701	100.0	415,107	100.0	713,808	100.0

Source: Administration on Children, Youth and Families. *Child Maltreatment 2003.* Children's Bureau, U.S. Department of Health and Human Services, Washington, D.C., 2005, page 65.

child maltreatment, based on data from 18 states. Of these male perpetrators, about half were biological fathers (51%), and about 20% were men who filled another parental role (stepfather, adoptive father or mother's boyfriend).

The balance of the male perpetrators was individuals in nonparental roles, such as relatives, foster parents, day-care providers or friends. Of the men who were not biological parents but were acting in a parental role, boyfriends accounted for 10% of all perpetrators, followed by stepfathers (8%) and adoptive fathers (1%).

Biological fathers were more likely than the other categories of males to maltreat young children and to be involved in neglect cases. They were, however, much *less* likely to be sexual abusers. Instead, nonparental male perpetrators were the most likely to be involved in sexual abuse.

In considering recidivism (re-abuse) rates among male perpetrators, the rates were highest among biological fathers, mother's boyfriends and nonparents and lowest among adoptive fathers and stepfathers.

Table III delineates child maltreatment by males that is either committed alone or in concert with the child's mother. For example, in considering physical abuse only, males acting alone represented a greater percentage than males acting with the child's mother. In the category of physical abuse, both father surrogates (42%) and biological fathers (40%) acting alone had the highest rates of abuse. In considering sexual abuse only, however, non-parents acting alone had the highest rate of abuse (78%), much higher than the 35% found among

surrogate fathers alone or the 11% among biological fathers acting alone.

In considering the category of multiple maltreatment, male perpetrators acting *with* the child's mother were most prominent; for example, nonparent males acting alone had a multiple maltreatment rate of 6%, compared to the rate for abusive nonparents who were acting with mothers, or 24%.

With the abuse category of neglect or medical neglect only, biological fathers acting *with* mothers had the highest rates of abuse: biological fathers with mothers represented 70%, while father surrogates and mothers accounted for 46% and nonparents for 37%.

Live-in boyfriends Experts report that violence against children may be committed by the live-in boyfriend or girlfriend of the parent. In one study in North Carolina of 220 child abuse homicides, 28% of the perpetrators were the mothers' boyfriends. Mothers' boyfriends were the third most likely perpetrators, after the children's fathers and then their mothers.

Wilson and Daly used research from Canada and the United States; for example, they studied police department homicide records in Chicago for 1965–90 and found that 115 children under age five were killed by their fathers, "while 63 were killed by stepfathers or (more or less co-resident) mothers' boyfriends. Most of these children were less than 2 years old, and because very few babies reside with substitute fathers, the numbers imply greatly elevated risk to such children."

TABLE III
ACTIONS AND CATEGORIES OF MALE PERPETRATORS BY TYPE OF MALTREATMENT

Type of maltreatment	Acting alone				Acting with mother				Total
	Biological father	Father surrogate	Non-parent	Total	Biological father	Father surrogate	Non-parent	Total	
Physical abuse only	9,982 (40%)	3,854 (42%)	1,947 (12%)	15,783 (31%)	1,686 (9%)	1,172 (18%)	294 (11%)	3,152 (11%)	18,935 (24%)
Neglect or medical neglect only	8,587 (34%)	1,079 (12%)	1,027 (6%)	10,693 (21%)	13,201 (70%)	2,944 (46%)	1,032 (37%)	17,177 (62%)	27,870 (35%)
Sexual abuse only	2,698 (11%)	3,198 (35%)	13,055 (78%)	18,951 (37%)	340 (2%)	575 (9%)	700 (25%)	1,615 (6%)	20,566 (26%)
Other or emotional abuse only	2,001 (8%)	484 (5%)	234 (1%)	2,718 (5%)	874 (5%)	297 (5%)	64 (2%)	1,235 (4%)	3,953 (5%)
Multiple maltreatment	1,913 (8%)	583 (6%)	535 (3%)	3,031 (6%)	2,626 (14%)	1,383 (22%)	666 (24%)	4,675 (17%)	7,706 (10%)
Total	25,181 (100%)	9,198 (100%)	16,798 (100%)	51,176 (100%)	18,727 (100%)	6,371 (100%)	2,756 (100%)	27,854 (100%)	79,031 (100%)

Source: Schusterman, G. R., J. D. Fluke, and Y. T. Yuan. *Male Perpetrators of Child Maltreatment: Findings from NCANDS.* U.S. Department of Health and Human Services, Office of the Assistant Secretary for Planning and Evaluation, 2005, page 20.

Wilson and Daly found a much higher rate of abuse among some categories of nonbiological fathers; for example, stepfathers were 120 times more likely to beat a child to death than were their genetic fathers.

It is important to point out, however, that these researchers specifically studied homicide, and most fathers and stepfathers are not child murderers.

Type of Household

An earlier federal report on child abuse, *The Third National Incidence Study of Child Abuse and Neglect,* published in 1996, looked at types of households, including households with both parents, mother only, father only and other arrangements. This information continues to be useful. A striking difference was noted in some households; for example, in households with fathers only, children were about 1.7 times more likely to be abused than when living with their mother only.

In the category of neglect, single fathers were at a greater risk than single mothers of perpetrating neglect, with a rate of 21.9 per 100,000 perpetrators for single fathers and the rate of 16.7 per 100,000 for single mothers. Married parents were the least neglectful, at 7.9 per 1,000. In the category of emotional abuse, single mothers showed a lower rate than married parents or single fathers: the single mothers' rate was only 2.1 per 100,000 single mothers versus 2.6 for married parents and 5.7 for single fathers.

Race

In considering race alone, the prevalence of abuse depends on the type of abuse. For example, in terms of physical abuse only, the highest percentage of victims who were physically abused in 2003, in terms of race, were Asian (16.6%). It should be noted that this statistic was derived by considering all Asian child victims (3,933) in the United States and then taking into account the percentage of Asian children who were abused according to different categories.

In terms of neglect only, the highest percentage of victims within their race were American Indians or Alaska Natives (this is one category). There were 7,469 American Indian or Alaska Native victims, and of these victims, 67.8% experienced neglect only.

With regard to sexual abuse, the greatest percentage of victims among their race were whites. There were 29,411 victims, and of these, 8.8% were sexually abused. (See Table IV for more information.)

Family Size

Another impact on child maltreatment found in the National Incidence Study was family size, and families with four or more children were at greatest risk. Interestingly, families with two or three children were at the lower risk in some categories of abuse (sexual abuse, emotional abuse and neglect) than families with only one child. Perhaps when there are two or three children, there is some protective factor. If so, this factor disappears when there are four or more children in the household. Table V illustrates the differences.

Childhood Abuse Experienced by Parents

Most experts agree that if a person is abused as a child, that person is more likely to become abusive when he or she becomes a parent. (As mentioned earlier, however, future abuse by an abused child is not a certainty; it is only a higher probability than if the person had not been abused.)

One study compared formerly abused women who were now mothers and a control group of non-abused women who were mothers. In this study, 25 mothers known to child protective services (CPS) as abusers in 1987 (referred to as CPS mothers) and a control group of 25 non-abusive mothers were studied by researchers in 1994–95 and reported on in a 1999 issue of the *Journal of Interpersonal Violence*. The goal was to look for predictive patterns and also to determine if women who were abused as children were more likely to become abusive parents than were non-abused individuals.

Case files revealed that about a third of the CPS mothers had abused and neglected their children. The researchers found that the key predictor of abuse was whether or not the mothers' social problems continued. Having been abusive in the past was an indicator of future abuse; however, it

TABLE IV
VICTIMS BY RACE AND MALTREATMENT TYPE, 2003

Race	Number of victims	Physical abuse only		Neglect only		Sexual abuse only		Psychological maltreatment, other only or unknown only		Multiple maltreatment	
		Number	%	Number	%	Number	%	Number	%	Number	%
African American	159,361	24,354	15.3	81,651	51.2	8,451	5.3	23,711	14.9	21,194	13.3
American Indian or Alaska Native	7,469	728	9.7	5,061	67.8	296	4.0	398	5.3	986	13.2
Asian	3,933	653	16.6	1,873	47.6	210	5.3	548	13.9	649	16.5
Pacific Islander	1,390	119	8.6	329	23.7	69	5.0	580	41.7	293	21.1
White	334,965	40,956	12.2	161,703	48.3	29,411	8.8	49,586	14.8	53,309	15.9
Multiple races	10,133	1,124	11.1	5,669	55.9	440	4.3	1,223	12.1	1,677	16.5
Hispanic	78,207	10,383	13.3	39,740	50.8	5,792	7.4	10,318	13.2	11,974	15.3
Unknown or missing	34,224	4,898	14.3	18,236	53.3	2,586	7.6	3,226	9.4	5,278	15.4
Total	629,682	83,215		314,262		47,255		89,590		95,360	

Source: Adapted from Administration on Children, Youth and Families, *Child Maltreatment 2003*. Children's Bureau, U.S. Department of Health and Human Services, Washington, D.C., 2005, page 48.

TABLE V
MALTREATMENT INCIDENCE RATES
PER 100,000 CHILDREN FOR DIFFERENT FAMILY SIZES

	1 child	2–3 children	4+ children
All maltreatment	22.0	17.7	34.5
Physical abuse	5.1	5.2	6.4
Sexual abuse	3.2	2.5	5.8
Emotional abuse	3.2	2.8	3.4
Neglect (all forms)	12.6	8.8	21.5

Source: Adapted from The Third National Incidence Study of Child Abuse and Neglect. NIS 3, Administration on Children, Youth and Families, 1996.

was not as significant as the continuing existence of substance abuse, mental illness and/or criminal behavior.

See ADULTS ABUSED AS CHILDREN, EFFECTS OF.

Characteristic Patterns among Maltreating Parents

Although abusive parents differ from each other, there are some characteristic patterns, according to social work professor and author David Howe in *Child Abuse and Neglect: Attachment, Development and Intervention.* Howe said that abusive parents often find it far more difficult to cope with the needs of their children than do other parents. Said Howe, "Faced with a needy, vulnerable or distressed child, the maltreating parent feels disorganized, out of control, and without a strategy to deal with his or her own emotional arousal, or that of his or her child. The result is abuse, neglect, or both."

Howe explained that caring for children is a very emotionally demanding role for everyone, but maltreating parents find it far more difficult. This care, said Howe, "appears to activate old unresolved attachment issues from their own childhood having to do with fear and danger, loss and rejection, causing them such difficulties in the caregiving role. Research has established that maltreating parents are vulnerable to stress (cognitively they are not good problem solvers), and poor at relationships, tending towards withdrawal and/or conflict whenever faced with the emotional demands of others."

Significant Risk Factors Toward Abuse and Protective Factors Away from Abuse

Research has revealed that some situational risk factors increase the probability of child abuse, while protective factors decrease the probability. The National Center for Injury Prevention and Control has discussed both risk factors and protective factors related to child abuse.

According to this organization, risk factors include the following circumstances, which increase the likelihood of committing abuse:

- Disabilities or mental retardation in children
- Social isolation of families
- Parents' lack of or inadequate understanding of child development and the needs of children
- A history of domestic abuse in parents
- Poverty and/or unemployment
- Family violence
- Substance abuse in the family
- Parental stress
- Community violence

Protective factors, on the other hand, reduce the risk of child abuse. Some protective factors against child abuse include the following factors:

- Stable family relationships
- A supportive family environment
- Nurturing parents
- Adequate housing
- Access to health care and social services
- Caring adults outside the family who can serve as role models or mentors
- Household rules and monitoring of the child

Mental Health of Parents

Some studies have clearly shown that the mental health status of parents is a predictive factor for child abuse. For example, in a study of the mothers' child abuse potential and their current mental health symptoms, reported in a 2005 issue of the *Journal of Behavioral Health Services & Research,* the researchers examined data from sites in Colorado and Florida of women whose children were born when the women were younger than age 18. The data were drawn from the national Women Co-occurring Disorders and Violence Study (WCDVS). The researchers considered current mental health symptoms, alcohol and drug use severity and trauma and found that the mothers' current mental health symptoms were the strongest predictors of child abuse.

The women were recruited from residential treatment programs in Colorado and mental health and substance abuse treatment outpatient centers in central Florida. This is a high-risk population because of the presence of both mental illness and substance abuse issues, also known as a "dual diagnosis."

Six factors in the Child Abuse Potential Inventory (CAP) were evaluated, including the women's distress, unhappiness, rigidity and problems with their children, themselves, their families and others. The researchers found that 65% of the women in Colorado and 66% of the woman in Florida had elevated CAP scores. The authors concluded that "The primary recommendation from this study is that mothers who are experiencing current mental health symptoms should be further screened for potential to abuse their child and linked to parenting support services when needed."

In another study of women who killed their babies, discussed in a 2004 issue of the *American Journal of Psychiatry,* Dr. Spinelli argued that mental illness, particularly postpartum psychosis, may play a major role in the deaths of some infants.

See INFANTICIDE.

Assessing Abusers with Substance Abuse Issues

Many abusive and neglectful parents are also substance abusers, and most states identify substance abuse as a key risk factor for child maltreatment. (See SUBSTANCE ABUSE.) According to the National Center on Child Abuse and Neglect, in their manual on protecting children in substance-abusing families, protective service workers can gain important assessment information about substance abuse from parents by asking the following questions:

- How often do you drink beer, wine, liquor?
- How many drinks do you generally have when you are drinking?
- How old were you when you had your first drink?

- When do you tend to want a drink? When alone or with others? If you drink with others, with whom? When bored or when you want to party? When you are angry, frustrated or stressed?
- What drugs have you tried?
- How often do you use?
- How do/did you use/take it?
- How long have you been using? How long did you use?
- How much do you smoke?
- When do you usually want a cigarette?
- When you were pregnant, what was your drinking/drug use like?
- How does your behavior change when you drink/use?
- How do you feel when you drink/use?
- What impact has alcohol and/or any other drug use had on your own health?
- What legal problems have you encountered as a result of your alcohol and/or drug use?
- How has the use of alcohol and/or other drugs affected your employment?
- How has your use of alcohol and/or other drugs affected your social relationships?
- Has the use of alcohol and/or other drugs resulted in violence or abuse in the home?
- What concerns do you have about your use of alcohol and/or other drugs?

In addition, it is also recommended that questions be asked about the impact of substance abuse on other members of the family, including such questions as

- How do family members view alcohol and/or other drug use?
- Do family members deny use and/or its impact?
- Do family members express worry about the user?
- Do family members feel tense, anxious or overly responsible?
- Are family members angry with the user?
- Do children in the family exhibit adult behaviors or assume adult parenting roles?

Protective service workers should also evaluate the parents' awareness of the relationship of their substance abuse and their children's care. Professionals need to consider the following issues:

- If the parents were under the influence when the suspected child abuse or neglect occurred, and this was a contributing factor, do the parents acknowledge this relationship, and are they willing to make the changes necessary to avoid repeated injury or neglect?

- How have the parents provided for their children's needs in situations of relapse? It is helpful to determine whether parents have exercised the judgment to leave their children in the care of responsible relatives or friends, or whether the children have been left with strangers or brought along with the parents into dangerous situations.

- In cases of prenatal substance abuse (that affects the child after birth), how do the parents view the infant's symptoms? Initially, parents may deny that symptoms or developmental problems exist. Although this initial denial can serve as a protective coping mechanism for parents, continual denial may interfere with the parents' obtaining needed services for their children.

In the 2004 government manual *Understanding Substance Abuse and Facilitating Recovery,* it is suggested that when substance abuse is suspected by protective service workers performing a maltreatment investigation, the following in-home signs of substance abuse should be considered by the worker:

- Paraphernalia is found in the home (syringe kit [and the parent is not a diabetic], or there are pipes, charred spoon, foils, large number of liquor or beer bottles.

- The home or the parent may smell of alcohol, marijuana or drugs.

- A child reports alcohol and/or other drug use by parent(s) or other adults in the home.

- A parent appears to be actively under the influence of alcohol or drugs (slurred speech, inability to mentally focus, physical balance is affected, extremely lethargic or hyperactive).

- A parent shows signs of addiction (needle tracks, skin abscesses, burns on inside of lips).

- A parent shows or reports experiencing physical effects of addiction or being under the influence, including withdrawal (nausea, euphoria, slowed thinking, hallucinations or other symptoms).

Cognitive Patterns

The way that people perceive a situation directly affects how they react to it. According to Howe in *Child Abuse and Neglect: Attachment, Development and Intervention,* there are four basic cognitive areas that are problematic for most maltreating parents. First, in the area of perceptions, they may only see the negative behaviors of their children; these parents do not notice when the child behaves well. In addition, they often entirely misinterpret their children's emotional expressions; for example, the child may express surprise, which the parent misinterprets as dissatisfaction. The parent then acts on his or her own distorted perception rather than on the child's actual behavior.

Second, parents at high risk for maltreatment are more likely to exaggerate their children's negative behavior than are low-risk parents, often seeing these behaviors as deliberate and willful. Third, parents who maltreat their children are less likely to consider the particular situation when interpreting the child's behavior. If the dog knocks over a child's drink, the maltreating parent is likely to criticize the child, rather than accepting that the child was not to blame.

Last, maltreating parents are inflexible and rigid, and they do not adapt to changes in the environment as readily as non-abusive parents. Says Howe, "An injured child, an ill child, and a tired child might all be seen as conditions demanding a response, the effect of which is to annoy the parent. The distressed child is immediately told off and disciplined."

Patterns of Family Violence and Child Abuse

In their landmark studies of family violence in 1975 and 1985, Murray Straus and Richard Gelles found patterns between FAMILY VIOLENCE and child abuse. For example, they found that blue-collar workers were about one-third more likely to abuse their children than were white-collar workers. In addition, wives of blue-collar workers were also more likely to abuse their children than were wives of white-collar workers.

Parents who were verbally aggressive to their children were also more likely to be physically abusive than nonverbally aggressive parents: verbally aggressive parents had a six times greater probability of abusing their children. If it was the mother who was verbally abusive, she was almost 10 times more likely to be physically abusive as well. In addition, parents who were verbally aggressive to each other were more likely to abuse their children than parents who did not exhibit verbal aggression to each other.

There are some general characteristics among abusive parents that may indicate that a parent is abusive. The lists that follow were developed from information obtained from a large number of cases. Observation of one or more indicators does not prove that a parent is abusive. The presence of such characteristics simply suggests that further investigation by a trained child protection worker should be considered. In general, the following characteristics apply to abusive or neglectful parents.

Abusive parents

- Seem unconcerned about the child
- Offer illogical, unconvincing, contradictory explanations or have no explanation of the child's injury
- Attempt to conceal the child's injury or protect the identity of person(s) responsible
- Routinely employ harsh, unreasonable discipline that is inappropriate to the child's age, transgressions and condition
- Were often abused as children
- Were expected to meet high standards of their own parents
- Were unable to depend on their parents for love and nurturance
- Cannot provide emotionally for themselves as adults
- Expect their children to fill the parent's emotional void
- Have poor impulse control

- Expect rejection
- Have low self-esteem
- Are emotionally immature
- Are isolated; have no support system
- Marry a nonemotionally supporting spouse, and the spouse passively supports the abuse

Neglectful parents

- May have a chaotic home life
- May live in unsafe conditions (no food; garbage and excrement in living areas; exposed wiring; drugs and poisons kept within the reach of children)
- May abuse drugs or alcohol
- May be mentally retarded, have a low IQ or have a flat personality
- May be impulsive individuals who seek immediate gratification without regard to long-term consequences
- May be motivated and employed but are unable to find or afford child care
- Generally have not experienced success
- Had emotional needs that were not met by their parents
- Have little motivation or skill to effect changes in their lives
- Tend to be passive

Some behavioral indicators of child abuse in the caretaker's behavior are as follows:

- Uses harsh discipline inappropriate to the child's age, transgression or condition
- Offers illogical, unconvincing, contradictory or no explanation for a child's injury
- Seems unconcerned about the injured child
- Significantly misperceives the child (as bad, evil, a monster and so forth)
- Is a psychotic or psychopathic parent
- Is a substance abuser
- Attempts to conceal the child's injury or the person responsible for the injury

- Maintains a chaotic home life
- Shows evidence of apathy or futility
- Is mentally ill or of diminished intelligence
- Encourages the child to engage in acts of prostitution or sexual acts in the presence of the caretaker
- Is experiencing marital difficulties
- Was sexually abused as a child
- Is frequently absent from the home
- Blames or belittles the child
- Is cold and rejecting
- Treats siblings unequally
- Seems unconcerned about the child's problems

Abusive parents who are untreatable Although with effort and professional assistance, many parents are able to overcome their problems that led them to abuse their children (such as substance abuse or emotional illness), social work dean and author Richard Gelles, who wrote a chapter in *Treatment of Child Abuse: Common Ground for Mental Health, Medical, and Legal Practitioners*, argued that some parents are essentially untreatable. Gelles estimated that between 10% and 15% of parents and other abusive caretakers are treatment-resistant individuals who will not consider changing their behavior and who also have social and psychological attributes that cause them to be treatment-resistant.

Some patterns among abusive parents who may be untreatable are as follows:

- Violent behavior at an early age
- Substance abuse
- Social isolation
- Poverty
- Antisocial personality disorder

These parents may be highly resistant to change, and they are also likely to be dangerous to their children.

Said Gelles, "Caretakers who do not recognize or admit to the harm they have inflicted on their children, by acts of either omission or commission, are not going to respond to an action-oriented intervention such as intensive family preservation, a parenting class, additional social resources, or even psychotherapy."

Gelles said officials should also take the abused children's needs into account, and says, "Decisions about treatment of intervention should be made with a child's sense of time and a child's need for permanence as the main criteria for choice of intervention. For treatment-resistant families, the intervention of choice would be to terminate parental rights and seek a permanent placement for the child or children."

Abusers outside the Family

Sometimes children are abused by people they barely know, particularly in the case of sexual abuse. For example, of the women abused before age 18 by males not in their family, 15% were sexually abused by strangers and 40% by acquaintances.

In considering abusers outside the family, such as day-care providers, legal guardians, other professionals and friends and neighbors by category of abuse, researchers have found that "neglect only" is the most prominent form of abuse among all of these categories, including day-care providers (48.4%), legal guardians (55.7%) and other professionals (31.7%). However, within the category of friends and neighbors, the most prominent form of abuse is sexual abuse (75.9%).

According to Cynthia Crosson-Tower in her book *Understanding Child Abuse and Neglect* (Boston: Allyn & Bacon), in some cases parents may not perceive the risk to their children from people outside the family for several key reasons:

- Parents may have formed an emotional bond with the abuser (a trusted babysitter, a family friend and so forth).
- Parents may not supervise their children, thinking that is all right to leave younger children unsupervised.
- Parents may be unaware of the risks of the Internet, where the child may meet abusers.
- Parents may leave children at home alone, increasing their risk for abuse.

TABLE VI
NONPARENT PERPETRATORS BY RELATIONSHIP TO VICTIMS AND TYPES OF ABUSE

Maltreatment type	Day-care provider		Legal guardian		Other professionals		Friends or neighbors	
	Number	%	Number	%	Number	%	Number	%
Physical abuse only	679	12.9	165	14.0	241	23.9	54	3.4
Neglect only	2,544	48.4	655	55.7	313	31.1	153	9.7
Sexual abuse only	1,209	23.0	49	4.2	270	26.8	1,192	75.9
Psychological maltreatment only, other only, or unknown only	130	2.5	69	5.9	73	7.2	42	2.7
Multiple maltreatments	689	13.1	238	20.2	110	10.9	130	8.3
Total	5,251		1,176		1,007		1,571	
Total %		100.0		100.0		100.0		100.0

Source: Adapted from Administration on Children, Youth and Families, *Child Maltreatment 2003,* Children's Bureau, U.S. Department of Health and Human Services, Washington, D.C., 2005, page 68.

See also ATTACHMENT DISORDER; INFANTICIDE; NEGLECT; PARENTAL SUBSTANCE ABUSE; PHYSICAL ABUSE; SEX OFFENDERS, CONVICTED; SEXUAL ABUSE; SHAKEN INFANT SYNDROME; SIBLING ABUSE; SUDDEN INFANT DEATH SYNDROME.

Administration on Children, Youth, and Families. *Child Maltreatment 2003.* Children's Bureau, U.S. Department of Health and Human Services, Washington, D.C., 2005.

Breshears, E. M., S. Yeh, and N. K. Young. *Understanding Substance Abuse and Facilitating Recovery: A Guide for Child Welfare Workers.* Rockville, Md.: U.S. Department of Health and Human Services, Substance Abuse and Mental Health Services Administration, 2004.

Crosson-Tower, Cynthia. *Understanding Child Abuse and Neglect.* Boston: Allyn & Bacon, 2004.

Daly, Martin, and Margo I. Wilson. "Some Differential Attributes of Lethal Assaults on Small Children by Stepfathers versus Genetic Fathers." *Ethnology and Sociobiology* 15 (1994): 207–217.

Gelles, Richard. "Treatment-Resistant Families." In *Treatment of Child Abuse: Common Ground for Mental Health, Medical, and Legal Practitioners.* Baltimore: Johns Hopkins University Press, 2000, pp. 304–312.

Haapasalo, Jaana, and Terhi Aaltonen. "Child Abuse, Potential: How Persistent?" *Journal of Interpersonal Violence* 14, no. 6 (June 1999): 571–585.

Howe, David. *Child Abuse and Neglect: Attachment, Development and Intervention.* New York: Palgrave Macmillan, 2005.

Kropenske, Vickie, and Judy Howard. *Protecting Children in Substance-Abusing Families.* U.S. Department of Health and Human Services, Administration for Children and Families, National Center on Child Abuse and Neglect, 1994.

National Center for Injury Prevention and Control. "Child Maltreatment Fact Sheet." Available online. URL: http://www.cdc.gov/ncipc/factsheets/cmfacts. htm. Downloaded November 4, 2005.

Rinehart, Deborah J., et al. "The Relationship between Mothers' Child Abuse Potential and Current Mental Health Symptoms." *Journal of Behavioral Health Services & Research* 32, no. 2 (2005): 155–166.

Schusterman, G. R., J. D. Fluke, and Y. T. Yuan. *Male Perpetrators of Child Maltreatment: Findings from NCANDS,* U.S. Department of Health and Human Services, Office of the Assistant Secretary for Planning and Evaluation, 2005.

Spinelli, Margaret G., M.D. "Maternal Infanticide Associated with Mental Illness: Prevention and the Promise of Saved Lives." *American Journal of Psychiatry* 161, no. 9 (September 2004): 1,548–1,557.

Straus, Murray A., and Richard E. Gelles. *Physical Violence in American Families: Risk Factors and Adaptation in 8,115 Families.* New Brunswick, N.J.: Transaction Publishers, 1995.

acting out The term *acting out* is often used to refer to aggressive or socially undesirable behavior displayed by children or adults. Some mental health professionals see such behavior as an outward manifestation of internal (intrapsychic) conflict. According to psychodynamic theory, individuals may act out feelings that, because of their highly sensitive emotional content, are difficult to discuss directly. In some cases, these feelings may be unconscious.

Psychodynamic theorists and practitioners often attribute the abusive behavior exhibited by parents to the expression of repressed or unconscious feelings. Abusive behavior directed toward a child may be traced to internal conflicts that have little direct connection with the child. Based on this theoretical model, treatment of abusers focuses on helping the patient to become aware of internal conflicts and to address these problems in a more effective and socially acceptable manner.

Acting out may partially explain the behavior of abusers. When displayed by a child, however, it may help to identify him or her as a possible victim of abuse. Though antisocial behavior is a feature of normal child development some behaviors are associated with maltreatment.

Sexually abused children may display sexual knowledge and aggressiveness beyond that expected for their age. Conversely, some child victims may display fear and/or aggression toward all males. Behaviors that have no apparent rational basis may lead the trained child protection worker to question the child further.

In adolescents, running away from home and sexual promiscuity are often connected to abuse. Studies of runaways show a high incidence of incest and other forms of abuse.

Physically abused children sometimes display extreme aggression toward other children. This behavior may be seen as an attempt by the child to gain control over his or her life. A child, defenseless against physical attacks by an adult, may become abusive toward other children as a way of acting out aggressive feelings that cannot be expressed safely in the presence of the abuser.

Most child development experts agree that a certain amount of acting out is to be expected of children. These experts caution, however, that such behavior should be examined closely when it is persistent and extreme.

addiction, infantile Infants born to drug-addicted mothers are at great risk of being addicted at birth. Withdrawal symptoms usually appear during the first 24 hours following birth. The severity of the infant's symptoms is proportional to the quantity of any drug used on a daily or frequent basis by the mother. Symptoms frequently observed in infants experiencing narcotic withdrawal are listed in the following table.

While most acute symptoms of infantile addiction disappear within 10 days of birth, follow-up studies have shown that these infants continue to appear irritable, restless and unresponsive for up to a year. They may need frequent feeding, tend to regurgitate often and require almost constant attention. These characteristics would challenge even a non-addicted mother and this may increase the likelihood that the infant will be physically abused or neglected by the primary caretaker if or when she continues to use drugs.

See "AT RISK" CHILDREN.

Laws on Drug-Exposed Infants

Some states have enacted laws that require physicians to report the presence of drugs in a newborn infant. (See Appendix V) Laws may also require the

---

NEONATAL WITHDRAWAL SYMPTOMS

Tremors
Irritability
Tachypnea (unusually rapid respiration)
Muscular rigidity
Diarrhea
Watery stools
Vomiting
Shrill crying
Excessive perspiration
Sneezing
Yawning
Fever
Myoclonic jerks (erratic muscular spasms)
Convulsions

---

state social services department or another organization to monitor a drug-addicted infant and his or her mother shortly after birth.

In some states, in the case of the child of a drug-addicted mother or a child with FETAL ALCOHOL SYNDROME, the state may offer rehabilitative services to the mother; if she declines this opportunity, she may lose her parental rights to the child.

See also PARENTAL SUBSTANCE ABUSE.

addiction, maternal See MATERNAL DRUG DEPENDENCE.

adjudicatory hearing Once charges of abuse or neglect have been filed, a court hearing is held to determine the extent to which these charges are supported by admissible evidence. If insufficient evidence is presented, a judge may decide not to proceed with a trial. A trial may be scheduled if, in the judge's opinion, there is sufficient evidence to warrant further consideration of the charges. An adjudicatory hearing may also be called a "factfinding" hearing.

See also EVIDENCE.

adolescent abuse Abuse of adolescents has attracted less public attention than maltreatment of younger children. Many assume that the age of the child is relatively unimportant or that adolescents are better able to defend themselves and thus adolescent abuse is less serious. Yet, the abuse of adolescents can have profound and lifelong impacts on the adolescents, their peers and others with whom they interact.

Available data indicate that adolescent abuse is, in many ways, significantly different from abuse of children under the age of 12. Psychological and sexual abuse levels are higher among adolescents. Adolescents receive less serious injuries as a result of abuse, reflecting both fewer physical assaults and a greater ability to protect themselves.

Boys are at greatest risk of abuse during early childhood, becoming less susceptible as they grow older. Conversely, girls are more likely to be abused as they grow older, particularly in the case of SEXUAL ABUSE.

Some abuse of adolescents is a continuation of an abusive pattern that began in early childhood. In other cases abuse of adolescents is a new phenomenon brought on by a complex set of factors. Children may outgrow methods of parental control that relied heavily on use of physical force, indulgence or intrusion. Abusive families may be less able to adapt to these changes, thereby increasing the level of conflict.

Adolescents at high risk of abuse often have more poorly developed social skills and display more negative behavior than their peers. The combination of an aggressive or defiant adolescent with a parent who uses a harsh or inappropriate parenting style greatly increases the likelihood of abuse.

Abuse and Runaways

A disproportionate number of adolescents who run away from home are victims of abuse. Studies show that abused adolescents tend to run farther from home and stay away longer than those with no history of maltreatment. Further, the act of running away greatly increases the likelihood of sexual abuse for both boys and girls. Runaways, particularly those who have been sexually abused, often fall into prostitution as a means of supporting themselves. One study found that 60% of runaways involved in prostitution had been sexually abused at home. Another study of adolescents housed in a Canadian runaway shelter found that 38% of boys and 73% of girls had been sexually molested.

Not all adolescent runaways leave home by choice. Statistics show that 10% to 25% of adolescents housed in runaway programs had been put out of their homes by their parents. These adolescents are considered victims of parental neglect, just as infants are abandoned by their parents.

See ABANDONMENT.

Sexual Abuse and Psychological Maltreatment and Consequences

Adolescent sexual abuse is predictive of serious problems among adolescents in middle school and high school. Many studies have demonstrated that sexually abused adolescents are at risk for depressive disorders as well as for the abuse of drugs and/or alcohol. They also have an increased risk for SUICIDE.

In one study of sexual victimization among adolescent women, reported in a 2004 issue of *Perspectives on Sexual and Reproductive Health,* the researchers studied adolescents in 1995 and again in 1996. They found that 7% of their sample (of more than 7,000 adolescent women) was forced into sexual intercourse. Some predictive factors for sexual victimization were alcohol use in the past year, marijuana use in the past 30 days and having been exposed to violence in the past year. Other risk factors for sexual victimization were parental heavy drinking and/or drug use, living away from both parents before age 16, the permanent physical disability of the adolescent and living in poverty.

Of the sexually abused females, 8% were revictimized within the next year. Some predictors of revictimization were alcohol use, recent cocaine use and increasing levels of emotional distress.

A study reported in the *American Journal of Public Health* in 2005 studied adults who injected illegal drugs. These subjects had a higher rate of childhood or adolescent sexual abuse (14.3%) than among subjects in the general population (about 8%). The researchers found that childhood and adolescent sexual abuse was significantly associated with an early initiation of injection drug use.

The researchers found that among those sexually abused before age 13, the average age of starting injection drug use was 17.4 years. Of those who were sexually abused between the ages of 13 and 17 years, the average age of starting injection drug use was 18 years. (Of the subjects who injected drugs but were *not* sexually abused, the average age when they started injecting illegal drugs was 19.1 years.)

The researchers also found that women were more likely to have been sexually abused *before* they began injecting illegal drugs.

Said the researchers,

> Although further investigation is needed to fully elucidate the association between sexual abuse and the initiation of substance use, we can conclude that childhood sexual abuse is strongly associated with early initiation of injection drug

use and vulnerability to HIV infection among those young injection drug users. Furthermore, we observed, as have other researchers, that sexual abuse is associated with higher rates of trading sex for money or drugs. Whether or not the relation between sexual abuse and the initiation of injection drug use is causal, childhood sexual abuse can be considered a valuable marker of risk for behaviors that comprise the health of young adults. The integration of substance abuse interventions with postvictimization and protective services for children and adolescents is warranted.

In another study reported in the *Journal of American Academy of Child & Adolescent Psychiatry,* the researchers sampled students from 27 high schools in Australia. They found that sexual abuse was linked to the risk for suicide as a result of feelings of hopelessness and/or depressive symptoms. Feelings of hopelessness correlated with a high suicide risk, while depression was associated with both a high suicide risk and suicide attempts.

The researchers found that hopelessness was more strongly associated with the sexual abuse of boys than among girls, while depressive symptoms were more prominent among sexually abused girls. Said the researchers about childhood and adolescent sexual abuse (CSA), "CSA should be considered a risk factor for suicidal behavior even in the apparent absence of other psychopathology, although depressive symptoms may further increase its likelihood." In addition, they stated, "Sexually abused adolescents may also be more likely to make more frequent and more severe [suicide] attempts, requiring prompt interventions and persistent follow-up."

A Canadian study reported in a 1997 issue of *Development and Psychopathology* looked at the impact of perceived and actual abuse among adolescents and the victims' subsequent adjustment. Researchers studied 160 children (70 boys and 90 girls) ages 11–17, with a mean age of about 14 years. Most (96%) were white, with a small percentage of blacks and Native Canadians. Most of the children (68%) came from families receiving public assistance and most (about 69%) had been in child services custody more than once.

All the children had experienced abuse, as documented by child protective services. About one-third had been sexually abused and about two-thirds had experienced physical abuse. Most (87%) had also experienced neglect or psychological maltreatment (92%). The researchers interviewed and tested the children, reviewed the child protective service records and also interviewed and tested caretakers.

The researchers found that PSYCHOLOGICAL MALTREATMENT had the most significant impact on the negative behavior of the adolescents studied, and it also seemed to make the effects of physical or sexual abuse worse.

One interesting finding was that when there was a discrepancy between the adolescent's perception of sexual abuse and documented abuse in social service records, greater maladjustment then occurred. For example, the best adjustment occurred when both the adolescent and the record reflected no sexual abuse. However, the next best level of adjustment occurred when the adolescent and the record reflected that sexual abuse *did* occur. In contrast, the poorest levels of adjustment occurred when sexual abuse was documented in the record but it was denied by the adolescent OR when abuse was not documented in the record but it was reported by the adolescent.

Interestingly, these findings for sexual abuse did not also hold in the case of psychological maltreatment. Instead, as the perception of actual psychological maltreatment increased, so did the stress and maladjustment of the adolescent. Thus, learning about and accepting psychological maltreatment caused greater maladjustment than learning about and accepting sexual abuse.

Said the researchers, "One might speculate that as youths' 'eyes are opened' to a harsh emotional family climate, their attachment system comes under new strain—the resulting conflict produces acute inner pain. If this finding is borne out in future research, one implication is that clinicians must tread carefully when helping youth recognize ongoing psychological maltreatment."

Why did stress and acting-out behavior decrease with the acceptance of previous sexual abuse but increase with acceptance of psychological abuse? The researchers said, "One might speculate that a psychical experience such as sexual abuse is more difficult to deny or minimize, and that such denial would result in more serious affective and behavioral distortion."

The researchers also found gender differences, in that females were more likely to exhibit behavior problems than were males in response to psychological maltreatment, and they speculated that females might have a "developmentally greater vulnerability to parental criticism and hostility."

Abuse and Antisocial Behavior

In another study of abuse and adolescents, researchers used questionnaires on 4,790 public school children in grades 8, 10 and 12 in the state of Washington. The goal was to determine if abuse was linked to antisocial and suicidal behavior.

Students were asked "Have you ever been abused or mistreated by an adult?" (which researchers considered "abuse") and "Has anyone ever touched you in a sexual place, or made you touch them, when you did not want them to?" (which researchers considered "molestation").

Antisocial behavior among students was determined by responses to questions on whether the student had ever carried a handgun, sold illegal drugs, stolen a motor vehicle, been arrested or taken a handgun to school. Questions about suicidal behavior ranged from questions about having suicidal thoughts to making a suicide plan through taking an actual suicide attempt.

Most students (about 74%) did not report abuse. With regard to antisocial behavior, about 18% reported one or more such acts. About 7% reported a suicide attempt.

The researchers found a positive correlation between mild and severe antisocial behavior and abuse and molestation. They also found a significant correlation between abuse or molestation and suicidal thoughts and behavior. They noted that "[t]he associations were especially strong for the more severe forms of the behaviors (such as injurious suicide attempts) and for the combination of antisocial and suicidal behaviors,"

Although not all children who exhibit antisocial or suicidal behavior are abuse victims, it is possible that abuse could be an underlying factor for some children.

Sometimes It Is Their Own Peers Who Torment Adolescents

In a Canadian study of abused adolescents, researchers found a significant correlation between sexual harassment of female adolescents and their subsequent attempts at suicide. Females who experienced more sexual harassment by their male peers were more likely to be emotionally disturbed and more likely to make suicide attempts.

Abuse Affects Relationships

Abuse also can have a profound impact on the way the adolescent interacts with peers in friendship and dating relationships. In a study reported in a 1998 issue of *Development and Psychopathology,* researchers studied 132 abused teenagers and compared them to 227 non-abused teens. The average age of the teens was about 15 years. Researchers found significant differences between the maltreated adolescents and the non-abused teens.

For example, the abused adolescents had more hostility and problems related to closeness and trust in intimate relationships. Abused adolescents were significantly more negative and hostile toward dates or friends of the opposite sex than were non-abused teens. The authors said, "Adolescents who were abused as children appear to choose partners who continue to act abusively toward them (and to whom they can act abusively as well)."

See also ADOLESCENT PERPETRATORS OF SEXUAL ABUSE.

Bensley, Lillian Southwick, et al. "Self-Reported Abuse History and Adolescent Problem Behaviors, I. Antisocial and Suicidal Behaviors." *Journal of Adolescent Health* 24, no. 3 (1999): 163–172.

Bergen, Helen A., et al. "Sexual Abuse and Suicidal Behavior: A Model Constructed from a Large Community Sample of Adolescents." *Journal of American Academy of Child & Adolescent Psychiatry* 42, no. 11 (November 2003): 1,301–1,309.

McGee, Robin A., et al. "Multiple Maltreatment Experiences and Adolescent Behavior Problems: Adolescents' Perspectives." *Development and Psychopathology* 9, no. 1 (1977): 131–149.

Ompad, Danielle C., et al. "Childhood Sexual Abuse and Age at Initiation of Injection Drug Use." *American Journal of Public Health* 95 (2005): 703–709.

Raghavan, Ramesh, et al. "Sexual Victimization among a National Probability Sample of Adolescent Women." *Perspectives on Sexual and Reproductive Health* 36, no. 6 (2004): 225–232.

Wolfe, David A., et al. "Factors Associated with Abusive Relationships among Maltreated and Nonmaltreated Youth." *Development and Psychopathology* 10, no. 1 (1998): 61–85.

adolescent perpetrators of sexual abuse The extent of SEXUAL ABUSE perpetrated by adolescents is unknown; however, many who work with adult sex offenders believe it to be a serious problem. Adolescent perpetrators may engage in sexually abusive or exploitative behavior toward dates or friends or while employed as babysitters. Like adult child molesters, adolescent offenders are predominantly male and usually known to their victims.

The amount of sibling-to-sibling abuse is thought to be greatly underreported. Parents may view it as harmless sexual play or may be embarrassed to talk about it with others outside the family. In some cases, sexual abuse by a sibling can have more harmful effects on the victim than an incident involving an extrafamilial offender, especially if allowed to continue over an extended period of time. Sexual abuse by a sibling often involves a high degree of coercion. As with other forms of INCEST this type of exploitation may make it difficult for the victim to form trusting relationships and may result in marital difficulty and a sexual dysfunction later in life.

Sexual abuse by adolescents is often passed off as experimentation or diagnosed as an adolescent adjustment reaction. Many professionals who work with adolescents are reluctant to label them as sex offenders. Adolescents who sexually molest children or other adolescents are seldom brought to court.

Recent evidence indicates that many incarcerated adult sex offenders began their sexually abusive behavior as adolescents. Some professionals who work with sex offenders believe that the seriousness of adolescent sexual assault has been minimized. Some argue that the failure of court- and youth-serving institutions to intervene effectively in such behavior has prevented young offenders from receiving treatment at a critical period. Repeat adult offenders have proven to be especially resistant to treatment. Treatment providers believe that these adult offenders may have been more amenable to intervention at an earlier age.

Another problem associated with the failure to recognize the seriousness of sexual abuse perpetrated by adolescents is that offenses often go undocumented. In the absence of a record of past assaults, each offense may be treated as an isolated incident. Young offenders can sometimes engage in a number of assaults before being charged with a criminal offense.

A large number of adolescent sexual offenders are themselves victims of sexual abuse. This fact suggests that, like PHYSICAL ABUSE, there may be a cyclical pattern to sexual abuse. Most psychotherapists believe early intervention with victims as well as offenders is an effective way to break the cycle of abuse.

Though relatively little research has been done on the problem of adolescent sex offenders, most treatment providers agree that it is important for them to be held accountable for their behavior. Further, most providers believe treatment should be specific to the problem and should combine individual treatment with peer group and family counseling. Court involvement can be helpful in making sure offenders follow through with treatment recommendations.

adopting abused or neglected children The assumption of permanent parental rights and obligations over a child who was abused and/or neglected. The family may be aware of the abuse and/or neglect before the adoption; however, in some cases social workers are unaware of some cases of past abuse or neglect unless it was egregious.

Abused and Neglected Children in the United States and Other Countries

Most children in the FOSTER-CARE system in the United States were abused and/or neglected; few parents or other caretakers willingly place their children in foster care. It is also true that many children in foreign orphanages also suffer from neglect and/or abuse, particularly older children. Some children were placed in an orphanage because they were

abused or neglected, while some children experienced neglect or abuse during their orphanage stay. Children may also have experienced maltreatment both before arriving in an orphanage and during their stay. Of course, orphanages vary depending on their location and many other factors, and some orphanages provide much better care than others.

Some people adopt older children from other countries because they say that they do not want to adopt a child who was abused or neglected, not realizing that neglect and abuse are common problems in many orphanages worldwide.

Some people will adopt a child who is five years old or older from an orphanage and assume that a five-year-old child who is adopted from another country will—with the exception of needing to learn a new language—behave essentially the same as a child reared in the United States (or Canada) from birth. This is an unrealistic expectation that cannot be met in the short term, although many older adopted children eventually adapt well to their new country. However, older children adopted from other countries (as well as infants) may suffer from malnutrition and other health problems as well as past abuse.

Note that most adoption agencies insist that prospective adoptive parents be informed about the risks involved in adopting foster children or children from other countries, sometimes even having them sign disclaimers that they understand these risks, yet some adoptive parents are fixated on their idea that *all* any child needs is love. Love is vitally important to every child, but sometimes abused children (whether from the foster-care system or from an overseas orphanage) also need therapy, careful discipline and strong parenting skills.

Experts say that there are many similarities between children adopted from the foster-care system and older children who are adopted from orphanages in other countries, including health problems, emotional disorders and adjustment difficulties. In both cases, children adopted at earlier ages (younger than age three or four years) generally tend to adapt the most successfully to their new families. However, foster children are often not freed for adoption until they are older; according to data for 2003, the average age of children adopted that year was seven years old. Yet some children are adopted from foster care as infants or very young children, particularly infants who were abandoned.

The Process of Adopting

If the abused and/or neglected child is adopted from the foster care system, the prospective parent(s) (many single people, primarily females, adopt children from foster care) will undergo scrutiny by the state or county social services department. The hopeful parents will receive a home study, which is a thorough background investigation to determine important screening information about the prospective parents. (Adoptive parents who adopt children from other countries also must be screened by a licensed adoption agency.)

The department will verify that the individuals have no criminal record and are not on a state child abuse registry. The agency will also check that the individuals have sufficient income to support the child (they need not be wealthy) and that they are healthy enough to rear a child, by having their health status verified through a medical examination screening.

The prospective parents will be interviewed personally, and their home will be checked to ensure that it is a safe environment for a child. The agency social worker will have numerous questions for the prospective parent(s), to ensure that they understand the type of children the agency has, the age of the child the parent wishes to adopt and so forth. Some agencies require prospective parents to take classes that the agency or another organization offers.

Once approved for adoption, the prospective parents will wait until the agency identifies a child or children (there are many sibling groups in foster care) who they believe might fit well in the family. When that happens, they will describe the children to the prospective parents. If the family is interested in the child or children, the social worker will often arrange for a visit. If the family and child get along well, the agency may then arrange for a weekend visit if the child is in foster care. If the family decides to adopt the child(ren), and the agency concurs, the children are placed with the family, and the adoption is finalized about six months later, depending on state law.

Tax Credits and Subsidies to Adopt Foster Children

It should be noted that because the federal government seeks to encourage the adoption of foster children in the United States, a tax credit of about $10,000 is offered for the adoption of children from foster care, even when little or no money was expended by the adoptive parents. Tax credits are also available to families who adopt their children *not* in foster care, but in such cases, the parents must have expended the money credited, and they also must meet certain income limitations. Read IRS Publication 968 for the most recent information on adoption tax credits.

Adoption tax credits of about $1,600 are also available to Canadian families who adopt, according to the Adoption Council of Canada.

Adoption subsidies are available to many families who adopt children from foster care in the United States. These subsidies usually include monthly payments as well as Medicaid coverage for the child. In most cases, the family must apply for the subsidy before the adoption is finalized. These subsidies are not available to families who adopt abused and/or neglected children from other countries.

The Newly Adopted Child

It takes time for an older child to adjust to a new family, particularly when he or she was abused or neglected in the past. Said Andrew Adesman, M.D., in his book, *Parenting the Adopted Child,* "If your child has been abused or neglected in the past, it can take time before he can learn to trust you as someone who doesn't hit or hurt, as well as someone who pays attention and provides food and clothes." Adesman advises that parents should work on projects together, such as creating a garden, and going places as a family, such as to picnics, movies and other events.

Other books offer good advice on how to help the newly adopted child who has suffered from past abuse and/or neglect, such as *Parenting the Hurt Child: Helping Adoptive Families Heal and Grow,* by Gregory C. Keck and Regina M. Kupecky (Pinon Press, 2002), and *Attaching in Adoption: Practical Tools for Today's Parents,* by Deborah Gray (Perspective Press, 2002). Laurie C. Miller, M.D., discussed neglected and abused children in her book on international adoption: *The Handbook of International Adoption: A Guide for Physicians, Parents, and Providers* (Oxford University Press, 2005).

Past Abuse and/or Neglect May Be Problematic for Many Families

Some researchers have studied children to determine which children have the most difficulty adapting to their new families. In one study of 1,343 foster children who were adopted, described in *After Adoption: The Needs of Adopted Youth,* the researchers found the major risk factor for predicting a behavioral problem with children was the prenatal substance abuse of the birth mother. Prenatal substance abuse is a problem among children in the United States and other countries.

They also discovered that many of the children adopted from foster care had trouble in school, and 40% of the children had been placed in special classes in school. Many of the children had problems with paying attention. The overwhelming majority of the parents were glad that they had adopted their children, and 93% said that, knowing what they now knew about the child, they would definitely or probably adopt again.

It should be noted, however, that some children have been so severely damaged by past abuse and neglect that it is difficult or even impossible for them to develop normal relationships with their adoptive parents and others. At the same time, some children who were severely abused or neglected are more resilient and do respond well to the love and care of their adoptive parents.

Researchers continue to seek to determine predictive patterns for which children are more likely to recover from past abuse than others. One common thread appears to be whether the child developed a past strong bond with a caring person; however, it may be difficult or impossible to determine whether such a bond had occurred prior to the adoption.

Past Sexual Abuse

Children who have experienced past SEXUAL ABUSE often have the most difficulty with adjusting to their new families, and many adoptive parents find it difficult to cope with children who were sexually abused. These children are the most at risk for suffering from an adoption disruption or the failure of the adoption. If an adoption fails, the child is either returned to foster care or he or she may be placed with another family by an adoption agency. In some cases, children must be placed in institutional care, such as a residential treatment center.

Children who were sexually abused may behave in a provocative and even overtly sexual manner with their new parents, because this behavior was learned and was acceptable in their past families. Such behavior can be managed by the new parents, but it is especially difficult for those adoptive parents who did not realize that the child was sexually abused in the past. In most cases in the study, social workers did not withhold this information from the parents, but it was not documented in the records.

A foster child may have been removed from parents or other caretakers because of physical abuse and the sexual abuse was unknown. In some cases, foster children are sexually abused after they were placed into foster care.

"Testing" Adoptive Parents

Often after an older child is adopted, after weeks or even months, the child will purposely misbehave to see if they will be rejected by their new parents. Adoptive parents should be prepared for this common behavior, having a plan ready to react to misbehavior with appropriate discipline.

At the same time, however, it is important to keep in mind that the discipline should be tailored to the needs of the individual child; for example, children who have suffered hunger in the past should not be sent to bed without their supper, because such a punishment is far more frightening and distressing to a child with past experiences of starvation than to a child who has never known hunger. If the parents do not know about such past experiences, but the child seems to overreact, this may be because of such deprivation in the past.

Some parents may react to misbehavior exhibited by their newly adopted child by ignoring the behavior and/or failing to use any discipline, such as mild admonishments or other forms of effective discipline. They may believe that the child has "suffered enough" in the past and should not be punished in the present for minor infractions. However, all children need some form of discipline to help them shape their behavior, so that they can learn to differentiate appropriate behaviors from those that are less appropriate in society.

Comprehensive Preparation/Information Is a Protective Factor

Study after study has revealed that adoptive parents who were told ahead of time and before the adoption about the problems of abuse that the children experienced in the past are also the most successful at establishing successful parent-child relationships. This is true no matter what type of problem the child experienced or what type of abuse he or she encountered in the past.

If there is little or no information available on an older child who is to be adopted, parents should not assume that there is no important information to be discovered about the child. Prospective adoptive parents should request that the agency provide medical records and social information on each child. If there is little or no written information, parents should ask the agency to contact the most recent caregivers (whether they were foster parents or orphanage supervisors) to obtain information on the past experiences of the child.

Despite the best efforts of the agency, however, parents may learn about past physical or sexual abuse of a child months or even years later. For example, in one case, a new adoptive father was distressed because he was shunned by the little girl he and his wife had adopted. He later discovered that the girl had been physically and sexually abused by her father and that she associated all men as victimizers. Patience, gentle kindness and paying attention to the cues sent by the child eventually enabled the father to attain a successful and happy relationship with his daughter.

See also ABUSERS; CHILD ABUSE; FOSTER CARE; NEGLECT; PHYSICAL ABUSE; RESILIENCE OF ABUSED CHILDREN; SEXUAL ABUSE.

Adamec, Christine, and Laurie C. Miller, M.D. *The Encyclopedia of Adoption.* 3rd ed. New York: Facts On File, 2007.

Adesman, Andrew, M.D. *Parenting Your Adopted Child: A Positive Approach to Building a Strong Family.* New York: McGraw-Hill, 2004.

Adoption and Foster Care Analysis and Reporting System (AFCARS). "The AFCARS Report: Preliminary FY 2003 Estimates as of April 2005." U.S. Department of Health and Human Services, Administration for Children and Families, Administration on Children, Youth and Families, Children's Bureau. Available online. URL: http://www.acf.hhs.gov/programs/cb/publications/afcars/report10.pdf. Downloaded July 17, 2005.

Hilborn, Robin. "Adoption Tax Credit of up to $1,600." Adoption Council of Canada. Available online. URL: http://www.adoption.ca/news/050223.tax.htm. Downloaded May 20, 2005.

Howard, Jeanne A., and Susan Livingston Smith. *After Adoption: The Needs of Adopted Youth.* Washington, D.C.: CWLA Press, 2003.

Livingston Smith, Susan and Jeanne A. Howard. "The Impact of Previous Sexual Abuse on Children's Adjustment in Adoptive Placement." *Social Work* 39, no. 5 (1994): 491–501.

Adoption and Safe Families Act of 1997 (ASFA)

The federal law that directs states in the United States on actions to take regarding children in foster care. The law, commonly known as ASFA, was primarily an effort to correct the problems that largely stemmed from the interpretation of the Adoption Assistance and Child Welfare Act of 1980 (AACWA), the most recent child welfare law prior to ASFA.

Although the primary goal of the Adoption Assistance and Child Welfare Act of 1980 was to decrease the number of children in foster care, the law itself, along with other societal factors (for example, the increased use of illegal drugs such as cocaine), ultimately had the opposite effect: the number of children in foster care increased to as many as 500,000 by 1996, nearly double the number in foster care in 1982. By the time state and county social workers began efforts to terminate parental rights so that children who could not be reunited with their families could be adopted, many children had been in foster care continuously for years (or in and out of care) and were adolescents. In addition, many children "aged out" of the system, and there were never any attempts to terminate parental rights, including among children who entered the foster care system as infants or toddlers.

Some of the key problems underlying the foster-care system, the old law and ASFA solutions are described below.

"Reasonable Efforts" Undefined

The 1980 act caused confusion in its requirement for states to make "reasonable efforts" to reunite children with their biological families. Because the states had to follow the law in order to obtain federal funds, it was extremely important to states. In many cases, the law was strictly interpreted to mean that children should *always* be returned to parents. In some states, social workers returned children to parents who had tortured, sexually abused or chronically abused them in the recent past.

In some cases, even though one child was severely abused, if a sibling had *not* been abused, social workers either did not remove the non-abused child or they quickly returned the child to the family, keeping only the abused child in the foster care system for some period. However, the risk with removing one child is that the remaining sibling(s) may become targets for the abusive parent.

Despite that risk, unless and until an individual child experienced abuse, he or she was usually not placed in foster care. In addition, common sense often seemed to take a backseat to the primary goal of reunifying all families. In some cases, children were placed back (or simply not removed from the home) even when parents had murdered or tortured other children. Some experts termed children who had been returned to their parents and then killed by them *reunification murders.*

In effect, children remained in or were forcibly sent back to situations that adults would never agree to—nor would they have to. For example, a battered woman may choose to leave an abusive husband, as difficult as it may be for her to make this decision. But state "protective services" staff compelled children to return to abusive parents.

The old law equalized all abusive parents by the underlying assumption that with sufficient effort by social services personnel, all families could recover from the problem(s) that led to the abuse (often alcoholism, drug abuse/addiction and/or mental illness). Once social workers had somehow "fixed" the families, it was assumed that the parents could and should be reunited with the children. However, resolving serious issues in families proved far more difficult than was anticipated. For example, although some parents entered a rehabilitative facility to recover from alcoholism or drug abuse, many relapsed from treatment and began abusing alcohol and drugs again and returned to abusing their children.

In addition, although recovery from mental illness is possible, some mentally ill patients refuse to take the psychiatric medications that could help them. In one case, discussed in the first edition of *The Encyclopedia of Adoption,* an attorney argued in favor of a woman who was raising her child as a cat, saying that it was not her fault that she was mentally ill.

Although it was true that it was not the woman's fault that she was mentally ill, most people would argue that a child should not suffer because of the severe mental health problems of the parents. After the story appeared in a newspaper, the woman decided to voluntarily relinquish her rights so that her child could be adopted. It is unknown what would have happened had she refused to do so, but this extreme example illustrated the strength of parental rights over children's rights.

In a 1999 article for the *University of Illinois Law Review,* Cristine Kim said,

> In some cases, no amount of effort could help rehabilitate a parent, but state agencies assumed that they must try anyway. When children were returned to abusive parents, they were often reabused and came back to foster care. Worse yet, some were killed by their abusive parents. Sadly, abuse and neglect is the number one killer of children age four and under. Of those killed, almost half had been previously investigated by state child welfare agendas.

In contrast, ASFA does not require that efforts be made to reunite children with their families in cases where the child was abandoned or would be in danger of sexual abuse, chronic physical abuse or torture or when another sibling was murdered or tortured. In those cases, a permanency hearing would he held within 30 days. Said Kim,

> The rationale behind the reasonable efforts requirement under AACWA was that children are always better off with their natural parents. This has been

shown to be untrue, for adoptive or other substitute parents can be just as loving, if not more so, than a child's natural parents. Under ASFA, the message is clear: the "rights" of parents to their children are not so great as to justify jeopardizing children's health and safety.

ASFA provided guidance on what constituted "reasonable efforts" and also in what cases mandatory reasonable efforts need not be made, such as in the case of a child who had been tortured or a sibling who had been severely abused or murdered, among other circumstances.

Children Remained in Foster Care for Years

ASFA requires that a permanency plan be made within 12 months of a child's entry into foster care and also sets rules on the TERMINATION OF PARENTAL RIGHTS. For example, it requires a plan for termination of parental rights if the child has been in foster care for 15 of the past 22 months.

There are several exceptions to the 15-month requirement, such as when the child is in KINSHIP CARE (living with a relative) or when there is a "compelling reason" that termination of parental rights would not be in the child's best interest.

The law requires a formal permanency plan, which must be created at the one-year point; however, a problem in the past, and one that continues, is that it is often very difficult to successfully treat people with drug or alcohol abuse problems within one year. Experts say that such individuals make up as much as two-thirds of all the biological parents of foster children. They are also more likely to re-abuse and neglect their children, and they are a key reason why so many children are in care, as social workers seek to resolve family problems.

Congress decided that the child's safety and the child's "timeline" were paramount, which is another reason for the time limitations in ASFA. To a child, a month or a year is much longer than to an adult. For example, a year to a five-year-old is almost unfathomably long. For this reason, it is important to make permanency plans in a timely manner.

Financial Incentives Kept Children in Foster Care

Under the old law, states received funds for family preservation and for the children in foster care. Thus, in effect, the 1980 act provided financial incentives for states to keep children in foster care, incentives that would be lost if a child were adopted. ASFA instituted financial incentives that favored adoption, while at the same time funds were also provided to assist families in recovering from the problems that had led to children being placed in foster care, when possible. Thus, with the old law, there was a financial disincentive for states and for social service offices to move foster children into adoption.

In contrast, in addition to continuing family preservation funds, ASFA provides for "adoption incentive payments" to states for children adopted from foster care.

Delayed Switching from Foster Care to an Adoption Plan

Another reason why foster children remained in care for so many years was that once the decision was made to terminate parental rights, the adoption unit of social services would need to make an adoption plan. This involved a paradigm shift from family reunification to adoption, and it also caused practical problems. The foster-care worker had to turn the case over to the adoption worker. The foster-care worker might not have provided the documentation needed to terminate parental rights. As a result, that documentation had to be gathered. It also took time to decide what kind of family the child needed and to locate such a family.

To address this problem, ASFA allowed for "concurrent planning," which means that states can work toward reunifying a family, but at the same time, they can also make a plan to find an adoptive family for the child in care should the reunification not work out.

Another key provision of ASFA was that it listed specific circumstances under which states could require the termination of parental rights. Because the termination of parental rights is such a serious step, forever severing the parental rights of a parent to a child, states do not take this provision lightly.

See also FOSTER CARE.

Adamec, Christine, and Laurie C. Miller, M.D. *The Encyclopedia of Adoption.* 3rd ed. New York: Facts On File, Inc., 2007.

Kim, Cristine H. "Putting Reason Back into the Reasonable Efforts Requirement in Child Abuse and Neglect Cases." *University of Illinois Law Review* 1999, no. 1 (1999): 287–325.

Printz Winterfeld, Amy. "An Overview of the Major Provisions of the Adoption and Safe Families Act of 1997." *Protecting Children* 14, no. 3 (1998): 4–8.

Adoption Assistance and Child Welfare Act of 1980   A federal law that once largely governed foster-care placements. Concerned about large numbers of children living in foster care, the United States Congress amended the Social Security Act in 1980 to include specific guidelines for out-of-home placements and ostensibly to remove barriers to adoption. The act made special provisions for medical assistance and other payments (adoption subsidies) to families who adopted such children. The act placed a heavy emphasis on the importance of FAMILY PRESERVATION and on the reunification of a child with his or her family members.

The ADOPTION AND SAFE FAMILIES ACT OF 1997 (ASFA) has largely supplanted the former requirements of the older federal law, in terms of the provisions of removal from a family and the provisions of involuntary termination of parental rights. The key impetus behind the passage of the newer federal law was that there were recognizable but originally unforeseen negative consequences of the Adoption Assistance and Child Welfare Reform Act. These consequences were that children often remained in foster care for long periods (sometimes their entire childhoods) and also that the termination of parental rights was extremely difficult.

Children were often in a "revolving door" situation in which they entered foster care, were eventually returned to their parents and later reentered the foster-care system because they were abused or neglected yet again. Many children "aged out" of the foster-care system at age 18, never having had a chance to develop a relationship with one family. Foster parents were urged to avoid getting attached to their foster children and, in some cases, if social workers felt the children and their foster parents were becoming too attached to each other, the children were removed and placed in another foster home.

Most parents were given repeated and extended chances to resolve the problems that led to the abuse or neglect which necessitated the child entering foster care, whether it was drug abuse, alcoholism or other problems.

It was also true that states received federal funds for children in foster care under the earlier law, and there was little or no financial incentive to terminate parental rights and place the children with adoptive families.

Congress ultimately decided that the primary emphasis should be placed on the needs of the child rather than on the needs of the parents. In some cases, termination of parental rights and adoption of a child by the foster parents, a relative or by unrelated individuals appears to be the best plan, as with parents who cannot (or will not) resolve their serious problems. ASFA authorized bonus payments to states that increased the numbers of their adoptions, and many states responded to these financial incentives.

Congress passed ASFA in 1997, and since that time, the numbers of children adopted from foster care have doubled to more than 50,000 children nationwide each year.

adults abused as children, effects of   Childhood and/or adolescent abuse that often leads to lifelong and seriously negative effects in adulthood, as proven in study after study. Childhood abuse is linked to major psychiatric and health problems in adulthood as well as other problematic and harmful behaviors, such as drug addiction, alcoholism and eating disorders. In addition, adults who were abused as children are at a greater risk than others for suffering from re-victimization by others in adulthood.

Types of Problems Experienced by Adults Abused as Children

Not all adults who were abused as children experience every problem that may occur to this population, but they are at a greater risk for some or many serious problems in adulthood because of the past abuse they have suffered.

Some key problems for which adults with childhood abuse in their background have an increased risk include

- Substance abuse
- Chronic pain and chronic illness
- Abuse of their own children
- Depression and other psychiatric problems
- Domestic violence
- Marital problems
- Eating disorders (and extreme obesity)
- Suicide
- Prostitution
- Physical assaults and other victimizations in adulthood
- Homelessness
- Smoking

Substance abuse   A common problem among adults abused as children is the abuse of alcohol and/or drugs in adulthood. This may be learned behavior (from those who had abused them), an attempt to alleviate the pain of the past or it may be caused by a combination of both reasons or other reasons altogether; for example, adults abused as children may have inherited a genetic predisposition to the abuse of alcohol or drugs.

Adults abused as children have an increased risk for alcoholism and/or drug dependence (addiction) compared to adults who did not suffer from childhood abuse. For example, women who were sexually abused during childhood are especially at risk for drug dependence in adulthood, and they have nearly three times the risk of drug addiction in adulthood as those women who were *not* abused as children.

In a study by the National Institute on Drug Abuse, researchers found that childhood sexual abuse was associated more strongly with drug addiction than with the development of any psychiatric disorders, although women abused as children were also at risk for psychiatric disorders.

Chronic pain and chronic illness   Some studies have looked solely at childhood abuse and chronic illness in adults and found a link between the two factors. A meta-analysis of chronic pain studies was reported by Debra David et al. in the *Clinical Journal of Pain* in 2005. These researchers found that adults who reported being abused or neglected in childhood also had a greater risk of experiencing chronic pain in adulthood.

In a different study reported in the *Clinical Journal of Pain* in 2005 by Jocelyn Brown et al., the researchers evaluated adults with chronic pain, and they found a correlation between self-reported childhood sexual abuse and chronic pain in adulthood.

B. A. Arnow reported in 2004 in the *Journal of Clinical Psychiatry* that childhood sexual abuse is particularly linked to adults with chronic pain that is associated with depression, and these individuals are also high utilizers of both medical care and emergency services.

Chronic painful conditions are common among adults abused as children. According to Kathleen A. Kendall-Tackett in her chapter on chronic pain syndromes that were related to childhood abuse in *Childhood Maltreatment*, women with a history of childhood abuse are more likely to experience headaches as adults, particularly chronic headaches.

Other chronic pain syndromes have a greater prevalence among women who were abused as children, such as fibromyalgia, irritable bowel syndrome and pelvic pain. In many cases, women with a childhood abuse history have two or more chronic pain conditions.

Researchers disagree among themselves on whether the chronic pain of those adults who were abused as children is an imaginary "somatic" type of pain or if these individuals are more highly sensitive to pain than those who were not abused as children. Other issues may be at play as well; for example, some preliminary studies indicate that childhood abuse may affect the brain.

Said Kendall-Tackett, "There is increasing evidence that past abuse is related to chronic pain. In the wake of traumatic events, the body learns to hyperrespond to stimuli, increasing pain."

She said that treatment can help the body to "unlearn" this response to daily stressors and that "Relaxation techniques and biofeedback are examples of helping the body unlearn its dysfunctional patterns. Both of these techniques teach patients to be more aware of their bodies, how they work, and what some of the early warning signs of impending pain are." Cognitive therapy can also help adults whose chronic pain stems from childhood abuse, according to Kendall-Tackett.

Abuse of their own children   Although most adults who were abused as children do *not* abuse their own children, it is also true that such individuals have a greater risk of committing child abuse than adults who were not abused as children. Experts say that about one-third to as many as 40% of adults who were abused as children will repeat this behavior pattern among their own children later in life.

Abusive adults may have a low frustration tolerance or may think that their abusive behavior is normal, since this is how they were brought up themselves. (As a result, this may perpetuate a pattern, because often their own abusive parents were also abused by *their* parents, and the abuse may have occurred for generations.)

Psychiatric problems   Studies have shown that childhood abuse nearly triples the risk of an individual suffering from an anxiety disorder or mood disorder in adulthood, and more than doubles the risk of phobias in adulthood. In addition, adults abused as children have four times the risk of having an antisocial personality disorder and 10 times the risk of suffering from a panic disorder in adulthood.

Researchers have also discovered that childhood emotional abuse in women nearly triples the risk for depression in adulthood.

Some adults who were abused as children suffer from severe psychotic disorders, such as dissociative identity disorder, formerly known as multiple personality disorder. Some researchers believe that bipolar disorder or schizophrenia may be induced by severe childhood abuse, although this belief is controversial.

Domestic violence   Domestic violence encompasses the abuse of adult victims within the household and may often also include the abuse of children as well. Many abused children have witnessed the abuse of a parent (often a mother) as well as of other siblings in the household. Because of this FAMILY VIOLENCE, the child may have incorporated feelings of guilt (because of the child could not stop the abuse), and he or she may also have angry feelings toward the abusing parent. These feelings may continue unabated into adulthood and may be at the root of the expression of maladaptive behaviors.

Marital/relationship problems   Adults abused as children often have difficulty in their adult relationships, such as with marital relationships or live-in relationships. They may choose husbands or partners who are similar to their abusive parents, perpetuating the abuse they have known as children. These adults may have trouble with trust issues and with the necessary give and take of most intimate relationships.

Studies of adults revealed that those who reported childhood sexual abuse had a 40% greater risk of marrying an alcoholic than adults who were not sexually abused as children. In addition, they also experienced a 40–50% greater risk of having current marital problems.

Eating disorders and obesity   Some studies have shown that childhood abuse, including physical abuse and sexual abuse, increases a woman's risk for exhibiting eating disorders in adulthood. In a study reported in a 2004 issue of *Epidemiology,* the researchers found that women who reported both physical and sexual abuse in childhood had three times the risk of developing eating-disorder symptoms during adulthood, compared to women who were *not* abused during childhood.

Some studies have shown that childhood abuse is associated with a risk for obesity, and verbal abuse in childhood is associated with an 88% increased risk for severe obesity.

As a result, women abused in childhood are also more likely to be obese than women who were not abused. (This does not mean that all obese women were abused in childhood. There are many reasons for obesity in adulthood.)

In an earlier analysis of studies, reported in 1997 in the *Journal of the American Academy of Child & Adolescent Psychiatry,* the authors concluded that childhood sexual abuse was a risk factor for the development of bulimia nervosa, a binging and purging type of eating disorder.

Suicide   According to Shanta Dube et al., in a report in a 2005 issue of the *American Journal of Preventive Medicine,* men and women with a history of childhood sexual abuse had twice the risk of attempting suicide compared to the risk of individuals who were not abused as children.

In a study reported in the *Journal of the American Medical Association* in 2001, researchers Shanta Dube et al., found that among subjects who experienced no emotional abuse as a child, 2.5% had attempted suicide; however, among subjects who had suffered childhood emotional abuse, 14.3% had attempted suicide, nearly a seven times greater risk. Among those subjects who did *not* suffer from physical abuse in childhood, 2.2% had attempted suicide, while among those who *did* suffer from childhood physical abuse, 7.8% of these individuals had attempted suicide.

Other significant findings were identified by these researchers; for example, among those subjects who were not sexually abused in childhood, 2.4% had attempted suicide, while among those who were sexually abused, the percent who had attempted suicide was 9.1%. Among those whose parents were not substance abusers in the home, 2.6% had attempted suicide, while among those whose parents were substance abusers in the home, 7.0% had attempted suicide. Clearly, childhood abuse has a major impact on the risk for suicide in adulthood.

Prostitution   In one study reported in *Psychiatric Services* on the pathways leading to prostitution, the researchers found that more than one-third of the prostitutes (35.3%) reported being sexually abused as children. The researchers found that childhood sexual abuse nearly doubled the probability of a female becoming a prostitute as an adult. Another risk factor the researchers found was being a childhood RUNAWAY.

Interestingly, drug abuse was not linked to causing adult prostitution, although some prostitutes do abuse drugs.

Research has also shown that females who were sexually abused before the age of 15 years were found to be more likely than others to become prostitutes.

Assaults and victimizations in adulthood   Some studies have indicated that victims of physical abuse in childhood have twice the risk of suffering from physical abuse as adults. This may be due at least in part because victims of childhood abuse have a greater risk of marrying or continuing to associate with an adult with a substance abuse problem.

According to the National Violence Against Women study reported by the National Institute of Justice in 2000, of the nearly 18% of those women who said they were victimized by attempted rape or rape, 22% were younger than 12 at the time of the rape, and 32% were ages 12–17 years. Women who were raped before the age of 18 years were twice as likely to be raped again as adults. The researchers also found that women who were physically assaulted as a child were twice as likely to be physically assaulted in adulthood. In addition, women who reported being stalked before age 18 were seven times more likely to be stalked again as an adult.

Most violence against adult women is at the hands of those they know. According to the National Violence Against Women study, 64% of the women who were raped, assaulted or stalked were victimized by a former or current husband, cohabiting partner, boyfriend or date. The risk of injury is also increased when the assailant is known to the woman, and about a third of these women who were injured by rape and physical assault required medical treatment.

Homelessness   Some studies have indicated that 87% of homeless women experienced severe physical and/or sexual abuse during childhood and adulthood. Childhood abuse alone does not cause homelessness, yet it is common among those who are homeless individuals.

Smoking   Adults with a history of childhood sexual abuse have about four times the risk for smoking and twice the risk for smoking by the age of 14.

The Adverse Childhood Experiences Study

Some researchers have chosen to study the impact of a variety of different childhood events, particularly adverse events, comparing these self-reported childhood events to behavior that occurs in adulthood. The findings of this study are reported separately, since not all adverse events were specific forms of child abuse.

Based on Adverse Childhood Experiences (ACEs), a study of thousands of subjects drawn from a population of individuals receiving medical care at the Health Appraisal Clinic in San Diego, California, part of Kaiser Permanente's health maintenance organization, the researchers found that 64% of the sample reported one or more ACEs. Common ACEs were physical abuse in childhood (28%) and alcohol or substance abuse by a family member during the individual's childhood (about 27%).

Researchers using data drawn from the ACE study have discovered that those adults who suffered from childhood abuse and/or other severe adverse childhood events are more likely to suffer as adults.

The eight categories of ACEs that were considered are as follows:

- Individuals who experienced recurrent childhood emotional abuse
- Those who suffered from childhood physical abuse
- Those who experienced sexual abuse
- Individuals who witnessed violence against their mothers in childhood
- Those who lost a biological parent in childhood for any reason
- Those who lived with someone in the household with mental illness (depression, suicide or other mental illness)
- Those who lived with someone who abused drugs or alcohol
- Those who lived in a household in which a member was incarcerated for crimes

Females v. males For all ACEs except physical abuse, female respondents reported a higher prevalence of ACEs. For example, 25% of the women reported experiencing sexual abuse in childhood, compared to 16% of the men. About 30 percent of the women reported household alcohol/drug abuse in childhood, compared to 24% of the men. Of the women, 13% reported childhood emotional abuse, compared to 8% of the men. In the case of physical abuse, however, 30% of the men reported experiencing this form of childhood abuse, compared to 27% of the women.

Women were also more likely to report a greater number of ACEs; for example, 2% of the male subjects reported four or more ACEs, compared to 4% of the women. As a result, women were at a greater risk than men for suffering from the negative health and behavioral consequences in adulthood that stem from experiencing more ACEs in childhood.

Researchers have found that adults with a past history of ACEs were more likely than those with no ACEs to

- Become substance abusers of drugs and/or alcohol
- Abuse their own children
- Suffer from psychiatric emotional disorders, such as DEPRESSION or ANXIETY DISORDERS
- Commit SUICIDE (the suicide rate for women was about three times higher than for men)
- Have unintended pregnancies
- Contract sexually transmitted diseases
- Have marital problems
- Smoke heavily (more than a pack a day)
- Become obese or severely obese

It is also true that the ACE risk factors have been found to have a multiplier effect, which means that the greater the number of the adverse experiences in childhood, the higher the probability of problems in adulthood. For example, according to a study reported in *Pediatrics* in 2003, when comparing people with no adverse childhood experiences to those individuals with five or more ACEs, the individuals with the five ACEs had a seven to 10 times greater risk of using illegal drugs or being addicted to illicit drugs, as well as injecting drugs.

Said the researchers, "Because ACEs seem to account for one half to two thirds of serious problems with drug use, progress in meeting the national goals for reducing drug use will necessitate serious attention to these types of stressful and disturbing childhood experiences."

Health risks Adverse childhood experiences are also linked to health risks. As pointed out by Valerie Edwards in her chapter in *Child Maltreatment* on the wide-ranging health outcomes of ACEs, adults with four or more ACEs were about twice as likely to report having cancer, as well as more than twice as likely to have ischemic heart disease. In addition, adults with four or more ACEs were more than twice as likely to describe their own health as poor.

Sexual risk behaviors Researchers have found that women with four or more ACEs were nearly six times more likely to have initiated sexual activity by the age of 15 years and 5.5 times more likely than others to report 30 or more lifetime sexual partners. They were also more than twice as likely to describe themselves as at risk for developing acquired immunodeficiency syndrome (AIDS).

Psychosocial problems Edwards said that the risk of psychosocial problems increased with a greater number of ACEs: "For instance, women with five or more ACEs were 3.3 times more likely to report that they were presently having serious family problems, 2.9 times more likely to report job problems, and 4.5 times more likely to report uncontrollable anger."

Psychiatric problems The risk of suffering from depression as well as alcoholism in adulthood was found to be greater among those with ACEs, according to a 2002 study reported in *Psychiatric Services* by Robert F. Anda, M.D., et al. The researchers found that the risk for experiencing all ACEs was significantly greater among the 20% of the respondents who reported parental alcohol abuse.

The researchers concluded, "Depression among adult children of alcoholics appears to be largely, if not solely, due to the greater likelihood of having had adverse childhood experiences in a home with alcohol-abusing parents."

They also said that "Improved recognition and treatment of alcoholism in adults and tandem family interventions to reduce the burden of adverse childhood experience in alcoholic households would probably decrease the long-term risk of alcoholism, depression, and other adverse effects of trauma observed among adult children of alcoholics."

Suicide In a study reported in the *Journal of the American Medical Association* in 2001, researchers Shanta Dube et al. compared and contrasted the prevalence of individuals who had experienced various adverse events in their childhoods to their lifetime risk of an attempted suicide. Childhood abuse was one of the adverse events that increased the risk for suicide in adulthood. Researchers have found that for every increase in ACE score (each ACE is scored as one point), the risk of a suicide attempt by an individual increases by 60%.

The incarceration of a family member was also a risk factor for suicide. Among those who did not have incarcerated family members in childhood, 3.5% had attempted suicide, while among those who did have an incarcerated family member in childhood, the suicide prevalence was 10.8%.

Said the researchers, "In conclusion, we found that adverse childhood experiences dramatically increase the risk of attempting suicide." They added, "Thus, recognition that adverse childhood experiences are common and frequently take place as multiple events may be the first step in preventing their occurrence; identifying and treating persons who have been affected by such experiences may have substantial value in our evolving efforts to prevent suicide."

Smoking and ACEs Individuals with five or more ACEs have nearly three times the risk for becoming heavy smokers (more than one pack per day) in adulthood. They are also more than five times more likely to start smoking by age 14. Sexual abuse that occurred by the age of 14 years is associated with a four times greater risk of initiating smoking.

Resilience in adulthood Many studies have been performed on the long-term effects of child abuse, and these studies have demonstrated again and again that many abused children have difficulties in adulthood. However, some abused children have developed an inner RESILIENCE that apparently allows them to rise above the abuse and to develop normally.

In many cases, this resilience is most likely to occur among abused children who had a close and positive relationship with an adult during their youth, a person who believed in and emotionally supported him or her. Researchers continue to evaluate other factors that may be related to resilience.

In one study of resilience among adults who were abused or neglected as children, reported in a 2001 issue of *Development and Psychopathology* by Jean Marie McGloin and Cathy Spatz Widom, the researchers studied 676 formerly abused and neglected subjects, along with 520 control subjects who were not abused or neglected. The researchers considered success (resilience) in factors including education, employment, homelessness, social activity, psychiatric disorder, substance abuse, official arrests and self-reported violence.

They found that 22% of the abused and neglected women met their criteria for resilience, and females were more likely to be resilient than males. They stated that more research needed to be performed to determine protective factors and processes that led to greater resilience among abused and neglected children and that aided them into adulthood.

Treatment for adults abused as children Many adults who were abused as children may benefit from therapy and from membership in self-help groups that include others who were abused or neglected in a similar manner. If the adult victim of childhood abuse suffers from chronic pain, treatment may help alleviate or at least improve this problem.

See also ABUSERS; CHILD ABUSE; INCEST; NEGLECT; PARENTAL SUBSTANCE ABUSE; PHYSICAL ABUSE; SEXUAL ABUSE.

Anda, Robert F., M.D., et al. "Adverse Childhood Experiences, Alcoholic Parents, and Later Risk of Alcoholism and Depression." *Psychiatric Services* 53, no. 8 (August 2002): 1,001–1,009.

Arnow, B. A. "Relationship between Childhood Maltreatment, Adult Health and Psychiatric Outcomes, and Medical Utilization." *Journal of Clinical Psychiatry* 6, supplement 12 (2004): 10–15.

Brown, Jocelyn, M.D., Kathy Berenson, and Patricia Cohen. "Documented and Self-Reported Child Abuse and Adult Pain in a Community Sample." *Clinical Journal of Pain* 21, no. 5 (2005): 374–377.

David, Debra, et al. "Are Reports of Childhood Abuse Related to the Experience of Chronic Pain in Adulthood?: A Meta-analytic Review of the Literature." *Clinical Journal of Pain* 21, no. 5 (2005): 398–405.

Dube, Shanta R., et al. "Childhood Abuse, Household Dysfunction, and the Risk of Attempted Suicide throughout the Life Span: Findings from the Adverse Childhood Experiences Study." *Journal of the American Medical Association* 286, no. 24 (December 26, 2001): 3,089–3,096.

———. "Childhood Abuse, Neglect, and Household Dysfunction and the Risk of Illicit Drug Use: The Adverse Childhood Experiences Study." *Pediatrics* 111, no. 3 (March 2003): 564–572.

———. "Long-Term Consequences of Childhood Sexual Abuse by Gender of Victim." *American Journal of Preventive Medicine* 28, no. 5 (2005): 430–438.

Edwards, Valerie J., et al. "Relationship between Multiple Forms of Childhood Maltreatment and Adult Mental Health in Community Respondents: Results from the Adverse Childhood Experiences Study." *American Journal of Psychiatry* 160, no. 8 (August 2003): 1,453–1,460.

———. "The Wide-Ranging Health Outcomes of Adverse Childhood Experiences." In *Child Maltreatment.* Kingston, N.J.: Civic Research Institute, 2005.

Kendall-Tackett, Kathleen A. "Chronic Pain Syndromes as Sequelae of Childhood Abuse." In *Child Maltreatment.* Kingston, N.J.: Civic Research Institute, 2005.

McClanahan, Susan F., et al. "Pathways into Prostitution among Female Jail Detainees and Their Implications for Mental Health Services." *Psychiatric Services* 50, no. 12 (1999): 1,606–1,613.

McGloin, Jean Marie, and Cathy Spatz Widom. "Resilience among Abused and Neglected Children Grown Up." *Development and Psychopathology* 13 (2001): 1,021–1,038.

National Institute on Drug Abuse. "Childhood Sexual Abuse Increases Risk for Drug Dependence in Adult Women." Available online. URL: http://www.nida.nih.gov/NIDA_Notes/NNVol17N1/childhood.html. Downloaded December 29, 2005.

Office of Justice Programs. *Full Report of the Prevalence, Incidence and Consequences of Violence against Women: Findings from the National Violence Against Women Study.* Washington, D.C.: United States Department of Justice, November 2000. Available online. URL: http://www.ncjrs.org/pdffiles1/nij/183781.pdf. Downloaded December 29, 2005.

Rayworth, Beth. "Childhood Abuse and Risk of Eating Disorders in Women." *Epidemiology* 15, no. 3 (May 2004): 271–278.

Wonderlich, Stephen A., et al. "Relationship of Childhood Sexual Abuse and Eating Disorders." *Journal of the American Academy of Child & Adolescent Psychiatry* 36, no. 8 (August 1997): 1,107–1,115.

advisement After arguments of both sides are presented in a court of law the judge or jury takes evidence under advisement. Advisement takes place before rendering of an opinion and includes consideration of evidence presented and consultation among jurors.

advocacy For most children, a parent acts as an advocate. Various needs, including physical, psychological, educational and emotional, are met by the parent or parents so that children are nurtured and protected until they are able to care for themselves. For children who are the victims of neglect or abuse, however, advocacy extends to institutions, groups and individuals in society who are best able to provide for children whose needs are not met by their parent(s).

In the United States at different times, a variety of efforts have constituted child advocacy. Among these, the report in 1969 from the Joint Commission on the Mental Health of Children recommended that a child advocacy system be put in place in order to guarantee that children be represented adequately no matter what their family situations. Some decades earlier, in 1909, as a result of the first White House Conference on Children, the Children's Bureau was established by the federal government to meet this goal of advocacy for children.

According to some experts, there are certain factors that characterize effective child advocacy. These include: (1) the making of connections among the different units (family, society etc.) of a child's life; (2) addressing child development; (3) conflict resolution; (4) fact-finding; (5) interdisciplinary teamwork; and (6) legal protection for CHILDREN'S RIGHTS. Ideally, combinations of all these exist when a group or individual works on behalf of the needs of children.

In legal proceedings where a child's welfare is concerned, an advocate is often appointed by the court. Recognizing that the child's interests may differ from those of the parents and the state, the court seeks to have the child represented by a competent adult who functions independently of other parties to the case. This advocate may represent the child in other proceedings as well (i.e., case conferences, administrative hearings etc.).

See also COURT-APPOINTED SPECIAL ADVOCATE; GUARDIAN AD LITEM.

affidavit   In legal proceedings, a written, sworn statement known as an affidavit is sometimes introduced as evidence. The document must bear the seal of a notary public who has administered a legal oath to the signer. False statements contained in an affidavit are subject to penalties for perjury. Affidavits are frequently used in juvenile court hearings.

aggressor, identification with   See IDENTIFICATION WITH THE AGGRESSOR.

aid, categorical   See CATEGORICAL AID.

AIDS   See HUMAN IMMUNODEFICIENCY VIRUS.

alcoholism   See SUBSTANCE ABUSE.

allegation   Legal proceedings related to child abuse or neglect are initiated by statements, called allegations, of what a particular party seeks to prove. These allegations are usually contained in a petition that outlines specific charges of maltreatment against the defendant. Both parties may introduce evidence to support or disprove allegations.

alopecia, traumatic   Alopecia refers to hair loss in both children and adults, usually as a result of disease. Traumatic alopecia is a term used to describe hair lost as a result of pulling. While traumatic alopecia may occur by accident as well as by deliberate abuse, it is a symptom that generally calls for further investigation. Close examination by a trained physician can generally determine the cause of hair loss.

anatomically correct dolls   See NATURAL DOLLS.

animal abuse in relation to child abuse   The purposeful abuse or murder of a family pet or the family pet of someone known to the abuser may be a precursor of maltreatment of a family member. It may also be an indicator of ongoing abuse to both humans and animals in the household; for example, an adult who abuses family pets may be abusive to other adults and/or children in the household.

Sometimes children exhibit abusive behavior toward animals. When the cruel and abusive actions of a child result in the torture or death of an animal, this is a clear sign that the child has a serious problem. Experts advise that the child should receive psychological assistance so that the pattern of violence can be interrupted before it escalates.

Sometimes abuse of an animal can occur in a group setting outside the family, in which one or more children slowly torture or kill an animal to impress or shock other children. Such behavior is abnormal and the children involved should receive psychological treatment, again, to halt the cycle of violence before it advances further. Experts may also find a pattern of violence and abuse within the families of those children who severely abuse animals. It may be necessary for state or county social workers to intervene.

When animal abuse or murder is perpetrated by an adult family member, the offender is usually a male. In some cases, the abusing adult uses torture or murder of a pet—or the threat of torturing and murdering a pet—as a means of punishment or a way to control or harm children. Experts have found that if a child genuinely fears the death of a pet, that child may actually murder the pet himself, to provide a more merciful death that the one the child fears would be inflicted by the adult abuser. However, that act in itself causes psychological trauma and can perpetuate the cycle of abuse into adulthood.

In an essay in *Child Abuse, Domestic Violence, and Animal Abuse: Linking the Circles of Compassion for Prevention and Intervention*, Barbara Boat said,

> The evidence continues to mount that where animals are abused people are abused and vice versa. . . . Higher rates of animal abuse by parental figures have been found in substantial cases of child physical abuse than in the general population. . . . Abused animals were found in 88% of the homes of 57 families with pets where child physical abuse had been substantiated. Two-thirds of the pets were abused by fathers; a disconcerting one-third of pet abuse was perpetrated by the children.

Ascione, Frank R., and Phil Arkov, eds. *Child Abuse, Domestic Violence, and Animal Abuse: Linking the Circles of Compassion for Prevention and Intervention.* West Lafayette, Ind.: Purdue University Press, 1999.

anxiety disorders Crippling, chronic emotional problems that cause overwhelming anxiety and

fear that may become progressively worse. Physically abused children are about four times more likely to develop anxiety disorders than nonabused children. These disorders can be devastating to those who suffer from them unless treatment is provided. Children and adolescents may develop anxiety disorders that usually continue into adulthood. Some examples of anxiety disorders include generalized anxiety disorder (GAD), panic disorder, obsessive-compulsive disorder (OCD), post-traumatic stress disorder and phobias.

Generalized Anxiety Disorder (GAD)

Generalized anxiety disorder refers to the state of constantly ruminating and worrying about everyday events over which most people do not worry or even think about at all. The person with GAD inevitably expects the worst to happen, even when there is little or no reason to take this attitude. Terrible consequences are always likely, in the world of the person with generalized anxiety disorder. According to the National Institute of Mental Health, the onset of GAD usually occurs in childhood or middle age.

Panic Disorder

The person with panic disorder is extremely fearful when there is no actual threat that is present. Physical symptoms may be present with panic disorder, including chest pain, abdominal pain, dizziness, and also a fear of imminent death. When it occurs, panic disorder often develops in late adolescence or early adulthood.

Obsessive-Compulsive Disorder (OCD)

The patient with OCD has repeated and unwanted thoughts or compulsive behaviors that the individual feels compelled to perform, such as repeatedly washing hands or counting items. OCD often first presents in childhood or adolescence.

Post-traumatic Stress Disorder (PTSD)

Post-traumatic stress disorder causes symptoms in some people who actually have suffered an extremely traumatic event, such as experiencing (or seeing) child abuse or witnessing extreme violence during a war or a natural disaster. The person with PTSD may suffer from flashback memories of the distressing events. He or she may also experience DEPRESSION, anger, distractibility and easy startling, such as jumping at a minor touch or sound.

Phobias

Phobias are irrational and persistent fears. There are many different types of phobias; for example, social phobia, which usually develops during childhood or adolescence and can cause extreme avoidance of social activities.

Treatments for Anxiety Disorders

Antidepressants and medications called antianxiety medications or benzodiazepines are often used to treat patients with anxiety disorders. Some examples of benzodiazepine medications are alprazolam (Xanax), lorazepam (Ativan), clonazepam (Klonopin) and diazepam (Valium). Some patients may need several medications to treat their anxiety disorder effectively. Often antidepressants are used as the primary treatment for anxiety disorders, and benzodiazepines are used as adjunct or temporary treatments until the antidepressants take effect.

Cognitive behavioral therapy has been proven to be helpful in the treatment of many anxiety disorders, as have hypnosis, relaxation exercises and biofeedback. Exposure therapy, or desensitization to the thing that is feared, is used for specific phobias. With exposure therapy, the individual is gradually exposed to the feared object or experience until he or she builds up the ability to face it without experiencing feelings of panic or excessive fear.

apathy-futility syndrome Based on studies of families in southern Appalachia and Philadelphia, Norman Polansky, a professor of social work at the University of Georgia, developed a diagnostic description of mothers who tended to be most neglectful. These mothers appeared passive, withdrawn and lacking in expression. In his description of the apathy-futility syndrome, Polansky de-emphasizes the role of poverty, pointing to the majority of poor families in which there is no abuse or neglect. Extreme apathy exhibited by some mothers is compared to the sense of futility

displayed by individuals suffering from characterological disorders or schizophrenia.

Major features of the apathy-futility syndrome include the following traits:

- A feeling that nothing is worth doing (futility)
- Emotional numbness similar to deep psychological depression
- Development of superficial, clinging interpersonal relationships, often accompanied by intense loneliness
- Unreasonable fear of failure resulting in an unwillingness to attempt new tasks and leading to a lack of competence in many tasks of daily living
- Passive-aggressive expression of anger
- Stubborn negativism
- Limited verbal communication, making it difficult to engage in meaningful dialogue and limiting problem-solving capability
- An uncanny skill in bringing to consciousness the same feelings of futility in others—a trait interpreted as a defense against change, which appears very threatening to the parent

Though mothers suffering from the apathy-futility syndrome are severely and chronically neglectful of their children, they are unlikely to abandon them outright. Little information is available concerning the father/husband's role in the family. They are described as typically "the first or second man who showed interest in [the mother] and . . . ill equipped in education and in vocational skills."

Often limited in intellectual ability, these mothers tend to be lacking in basic knowledge of child rearing. Polansky cites the mother's own deprived childhood as evidence for an INTERGENERATIONAL CYCLE OF ABUSE.

Polansky, Norman A., Mary Ann Chalmers, Elizabeth Buttenwieser, and David P. Williams. *Damaged Parents.* Chicago: University of Chicago Press, 1981.

appeal Any party to a child abuse or neglect case has the right to request that the procedures followed and decision reached be reviewed by a higher court. In cases where accurate records are not available (e.g., some juvenile courts) the appeal may involve a rehearing of all evidence, including testimony. At the second hearing a record is kept from which an appeal can be filed.

Upon reviewing court transcripts, the court to which the appeal was made may: (1) uphold the lower court's decision; (2) reverse the decision and return the case to the lower court; or (3) in the event of a procedural or DUE PROCESS violation, order a new trial.

assault   Any violent act, physical or verbal, may be called assault. The term assault is sometimes used as a euphemism for sexual molestation or rape.

Legally, assault is defined as "an intentional or reckless threat of physical injury." Aggravated assault implies an intent to carry out the threat. Simple assault refers to a threat without intent actually to commit the act. If an act is not attempted the threat is considered a simple assault.

Assault and BATTERY often appear together in legal charges related to PHYSICAL ABUSE or SEXUAL ABUSE of children.

assessment   Following an initial INVESTIGATION to verify that a child has been abused or neglected, an assessment is conducted. The primary function of this process is to determine why abuse occurred and identify specific areas where intervention is needed. Assessment is the basis for development of a SERVICE PLAN. While assessment serves a purpose separate from investigation the two terms are sometimes used interchangeably. In practice, gathering of information for assessment often begins during an initial investigation to determine the validity of a report of suspected abuse. The investigatory process includes an assessment of immediate risk to the child. This initial evaluation serves as the basis for emergency intervention on behalf of the child and is followed by a more thorough social assessment.

The social assessment is based on the child protection worker's direct observation of the child's home environment and family interaction patterns. Important information is also obtained from inter-

views with the family, teachers, physicians, neighbors and others who have special knowledge of the child's living situation. Under certain circumstances a psychological, psychiatric or medical examination may be required for a thorough assessment.

The following information may be included in a social assessment:

- Factual information on the family—names, ages occupations of members of the immediate family, and existence of extended family
- A brief summary of the family's contact with other agencies, as part of the investigation
- The family's perceptions of the incidence of abuse and neglect, the worker's perceptions and notations of any discrepancies between the two
- Strengths and weaknesses in the family
- Ways in which the family interacts
- Significant historical data about the parents' upbringing that describe events that formed their ideas of child rearing, parent-child relations, appropriate behavior for children etc.
- A listing of the family's needs that should be met to assure the health and safety of the child

The result will be a report summarizing family problems related to abuse and neglect, family strengths and the type of help families will need. Information is usually gathered by a single social worker; however, a MULTIDISCIPLINARY TEAM often assists in reviewing and interpreting data gathered.

U.S. Department of Health, Education and Welfare, Office of Human Development Services, Administration on Children, Youth and Families, Children's Bureau, National Center on Child Abuse and Neglect, *Child Protective Services: A Guide for Workers*. Washington, D.C.: 1979; (OHDS) 79-30203.

"at-risk" children   A variety of personal, familial and environmental factors serve to place some children at greater risk of abuse or neglect than others. Even prenatal occurrences such as parental substance abuse or an unwanted pregnancy can predispose a child to maltreatment.

Usually the presence or absence of a particular trait in a child is less important than the perception by the parent or other caregiver that it exists; however, perpetrators of abuse may attempt to explain their behavior as a response to a characteristic or behavior of the child. For example, an infant may be colicky and cry more than other children, and parents may justify their abuse or neglect by saying the child's behavior drove them to the abuse. However, it should also be noted that even infants who cry at about the same rate as most other infants may be perceived by some caregivers as behaving badly or purposely, whether it is because the caregiver does not have experience in childrearing, is affected by drugs or alcohol or for another reason.

Infants born prematurely have been shown to have a significantly greater chance of subsequent abuse than those carried to full term. Studies of abused children have identified from 12% to 33% as prematurely born. These children tend to have a low birth weight and may be more restless, distractible, unresponsive and demanding than the average child. Child-specific factors when combined with a parent who is inexperienced or easily frustrated greatly increase the risk of abuse.

Age is also an important characteristic in determining the likelihood and type of maltreatment. In general, younger children and particularly babies and children under age four, are at greater risk than their older peers. Young children are also especially likely to experience neglect. Reports of sexual and emotional maltreatment, however, increase as children get older. And, while abused children of all ages show high rates of physical injury, older children are the most frequently reported victims.

Mentally retarded, physically handicapped, mentally ill and emotionally impaired children all have an increased chance of being singled out for abuse by parents or other caregivers. Developmentally delayed children require more attention from caregivers and often do not respond to parental direction and affection as quickly as others. Parents may become frustrated or embarrassed by these behaviors. In such cases, the risk of abuse is increased, especially if the parent is inadequately prepared or under a great deal of stress.

A child or adolescent's gender is a contributing factor in some forms of abuse; for example, girls are significantly more likely to experience sexual abuse than boys.

Characteristics of parents play an important role in determining the likelihood of abuse. A child whose primary caregiver is younger than 18 years old is more likely to be abused or neglected. Children of parents who were themselves abused as children are at risk for abusing their own children, although it should not be assumed that all adults who were abused as children will, when they grow up to adulthood, also abuse their children. Social isolation and marital discord are also associated with child abuse and neglect.

Divorce increases the likelihood that girls will be abused. This phenomenon is often attributed to an increased contact with unrelated adult males as a result of the mother dating. Statistics also show that stepfathers are more likely than natural fathers to assault the daughter sexually.

Other environmental stresses can increase the risk of abuse or neglect. Many abuse and neglect cases involve families receiving public assistance. Many researchers and clinicians have noted the role of POVERTY in child maltreatment. In some cases, poverty may prevent a parent from providing for basic needs of food, shelter, clothing, medical and educational care. More often poverty is seen as a source of family stress that is conducive to maltreatment.

Any child may be at risk of abuse from time to time. No one factor or combination of factors makes abuse or neglect inevitable. Most low-income families are free of abuse; many disabled children receive adequate and loving care. The majority of stepfathers are not child molesters. Nevertheless, the presence of these and other factors do place children at greater risk of maltreatment.

In evaluating the potential for abuse, it is important to consider the number of risk factors present, the severity of each factor and the length of time the child is at risk. To date, there is no foolproof method for evaluating the level of risk.

See also ABUSERS; INFANTICIDE.

attachment disorder An inability of an infant or small child to form a healthy emotional attachment with a parent or parental figure, which experts believe impedes future relationships. The term *bonding* refers to the process by which the attachment is formed. An attachment disorder may result from physical and/or psychological harm caused by a parent or other primary caregiver. It may also result from neglect; for example, infants and children reared in orphanages with constantly changing caregivers may not have an opportunity to develop an attachment to one or two individuals.

Some experts say that even when parents exhibit normal and healthy responses to their children, sometimes children will fail to develop an attachment to the parent, for unknown reasons.

Said Klaus Minde in his article on attachment disorders in *Attachment & Human Development* in 2003, "In my personal clinical experience with some 150 biologically and cognitively fragile small premature infants I have observed at least three children who had bewildered yet 'good enough' parents but nevertheless showed the signs of 'disordered attachment,' i.e., they displayed significant and pervasive role reversal and/or excessive clinging at age 4."

Bonding and the Age of the Child

Most children form an emotional attachment to their parents or other caregivers during infancy or their toddler years. Psychoanalyst John Bowlby first wrote about bonding and attachment in 1951, based on his research with institutionalized children. Bowlby believed that children needed to form a close attachment to a parent by the age of about two and a half, and if attachment did not occur by that time, then the child's future character was in jeopardy.

British researcher and psychiatrist Michael Rutter has said that although the concept of "sensitive periods" when environmental factors are critical to bonding has some validity, the upper age limits of sensitive periods may be older than believed in the past. Rutter has studied adoptive parents and their children, and he found that children adopted before the age of four bonded well with their parents, while children adopted when they were older than four experienced many of the same problems as orphaned children who had remained in an institution. Despite this finding, Rutter said that it was

possible for children adopted after the age of four years to bond with their adoptive parents.

Reactive Attachment Disorder

The sole type of attachment disorder that is recognized by the American Psychiatric Association is reactive attachment disorder. This attachment disorder occurs as a result of receiving pathological care before the child is five years old. There are several types of this disorder, including the inhibited and disinhibited types. If the child has the inhibited type of reactive attachment disorder, he or she is resistant to being comforted and also exhibits hypervigilance. If the child has the disinhibited type, then he or she is extremely sociable and is equally friendly to total strangers as to their parents.

According to authors Gregory Keck and Regina Kupecky in their book *Parenting the Hurt Child: Helping Adoptive Parents Heal and Grow*, it can be difficult for caregivers to help children with reactive attachment disorder, but therapy can help. Said the authors, "Therapy with hurt children needs to include high energy and intense focus, close physical proximity, frequent touch, confrontation, movement, much nurturing and love, almost constant eye contact, and fast-moving verbal exchanges."

Other Forms of Attachment Disorders

Some therapists believe that there are other forms of attachment disorders beyond reactive attachment disorder. For example, clinical social worker Deborah Gray wrote about attachments in *Attaching in Adoption: Practical Tools for Today's Parents*. Gray believed that attachments could be secure (normal) or insecure, and she further subdivided insecure attachments into avoidant, ambivalent and disorganized attachments. According to Gray, children with avoidant attachments feel a connection with their caregiver, but they are insecure about how the caregiver will react to them, not knowing whether their behavior will elicit hugs or hits.

Children with ambivalent attachments may alternate between clinging to their parents and then pushing them away—behavior that is usually very frustrating and confusing to the parents.

Children with disorganized attachments may exhibit fear or rage. According to Gray, the original caregivers of such children had "set the child up for overwhelming situations and then responded in a rejecting, frightening, or abandoning manner. Children with disorganized attachments tend to have a sense of helplessness about their relationship with parents."

Symptoms and Diagnostic Path

Some symptoms of attachment disorders may include the following behaviors:

- Self-destructive behavior
- Stealing from parents
- Cruelty to animals
- Sleep disorders
- Intense rage, especially toward female caregivers
- Above or below-average response to pain
- Little or no eye contact with others
- Inappropriate emotional responses, such as laughing when someone is hurt

Children with possible attachment disorder should be screened for attention-deficit/hyperactivity disorder, autism spectrum disorders and social phobias, among other possible diagnoses.

Treatment Options and Outlook

There are no known consistent and validated treatments for attachment disorders, although therapy is available, according to experts such as O'Connor and Zeanah. Parents can often be trained to identify and respond to the subtle indications of a developing attachment in children with attachment disorders.

In addition, new caregivers need to appreciate that disciplinary measures that may be effective in healthy children may be very counterproductive when it is used with children who have attachment disorders. For example, according to experts such as Lieberman, the use of "time outs" is inappropriate among children with attachment disorders, because they are perceived as a form of rejection. Few experts recommend spanking as a form of discipline for any children, but spanking is particularly harmful for children who have attachment disorders, especially among children who have been abused in the past.

Lieberman also stated that parents of children with attachment disorders may help children to understand the emotional responses of others by exaggerating their own responses to the child, such as showing an exaggerated joy when the parent and child are reunited or exhibiting simulated excessive sadness when they must be separated.

Risk Factors and Preventive Measures

Abuse and neglect are risk factors for the development of attachment disorders in children. Although abuse and neglect cannot always be prevented, the next best preventive measure to avoid any continuing or further psychological damage is to help children be placed with loving, caring and secure adults, whether the adults are related to the child or not. Whenever possible, the placement should be made before the child is five or six years old, to increase the chances for a successful attachment. This action is more possible today in the United States, because of passage of the ADOPTION AND SAFE FAMILIES ACT, which is meant to prevent children from remaining in foster care from infancy until they age out at 18 years.

Adamec, Christine, and Laurie C. Miller, M.D. *The Encyclopedia of Adoption.* 3rd ed. New York: Facts On File, 2007.

American Psychiatric Association. *Diagnostic and Statistical Manual of Mental Disorders. Fourth Edition, Text Revision. (DSM-IV-R).* Washington, D.C.: American Psychiatric Association, 2000.

Bowlby, John. *Maternal Care and Mental Health.* Geneva, Switzerland: World Health Organization, 1951.

Gray, Deborah D. *Attaching in Adoption: Practical Tools for Today's Parents.* Indianapolis, Ind.: Perspective Press, 2002.

Keck, Gregory C., and Regina M. Kupecky. *Parenting the Hurt Child: Helping Adoptive Parents Heal and Grow.* Colorado Springs, Colo.: Pinon Press, 2002.

Lieberman, Alicia F. "The Treatment of Attachment Disorder in Infancy and Early Childhood: Reflections from Clinical Intervention with Later-adopted Foster Care Children." *Attachment & Human Development* 5, no. 3 (September 2003): 279–282.

Minde, Klaus. "Attachment Problems as a Spectrum Disorder: Implications for Diagnosis and Treatment." *Attachment & Human Development* 5, no. 3 (September 2003): 289–296.

O'Connor, Thomas G., and Charles H. Zeanah. "Attachment Disorders. Assessment Strategies and Treatment Approaches." *Attachment & Human Development* 5, no. 3 (September 2003): 223–244.

Rutter, Michael. "Family and School Influences on Behavioural Development." *Journal of Child Psychology and Psychiatry* 26, no. 3 (1985): 349–368.

Australia   According to a report from the Bureau of Democracy, Human Rights, and Labor, released in 2005, state and territorial governmental agencies in Australia investigate and prosecute cases of child abuse and neglect, while the federal government primarily collects data and provides education. According to the Federal Department of Family and Community Services, substantiated cases of child abuse and neglect increased by about 43% over the period 1992 to 2002.

Laws in Australia make it a crime to trade in or possess CHILD PORNOGRAPHY. In addition, suspected pedophiles may be tried even if the crime was committed by an Australian while in another country. The Child Sex Tourism Act bans tourists to Australia from using children for sex, and the maximum sentence for this crime is 17 years.

One problem that continues in Australia is the illegal sterilization of children with disabilities. As a result, doctors who sterilize children without receiving an authorization from the federal family court are subject to both civil and criminal action. However, anecdotal reports indicate that the practice of illegal sterilizations continues.

It is also illegal in Australia for children to be placed elsewhere out of the jurisdiction of their families for the purpose of receiving female genital mutilation.

See also SEXUAL TRAFFICKING.

Bureau of Democracy, Human Rights, and Labor. *Country Reports on Human Rights Practices, 2004: Australia.* United States State Department. Available online. URL: http://www.state.gov/g/drl/rls/hrrpt/2004/41635.htm. Downloaded September 1, 2005.

autopsy   Postmortem examination by a forensic pathologist is recommended whenever abuse or neglect is the suspected cause of a child's death. The forensic medical specialist often works with a team of law enforcement and social work personnel in investigating circumstances surrounding the death.

A careful autopsy includes information gained from an examination of the child's environment. Assessment of the cleanliness and adequacy of the child's physical surroundings and interviews with family members, neighbors and others to learn more about family relationships, discipline patterns etc. often provide useful information.

The autopsy begins with a thorough external medical examination. Items such as the child's clothing, cleanliness, height, weight and apparent nutritional state are noted. A careful inspection of the skin for evidence of trauma or neglect includes a search for bruises, cuts, scars, swelling, untreated or infected lesions, parasitic infestation and severe diaper rash. Physical evidence that might lead to identification of the assailant is carefully labeled and preserved.

The medical examiner is also alert to attempts to conceal abuse. Appearance of severe diaper rash on a freshly washed, carefully scrubbed body may suggest an attempt to conceal previous neglect. Close inspection of the soles of the child's feet sometimes yields evidence of abuse, such as cigarette burns or bruises, at the hands of a caretaker attempting to avoid detection.

Internal examination includes a thorough examination and description of all organ systems, with careful photographic documentation of pathology. When neglect is the suspected cause of death the examiner is alert for evidence of chronic disease that might provide an alternative explanation of starvation or nutritional deficiency. Careful attention is given to determining when the trauma occurred. Dating of injuries may be helpful in establishing evidence of long-standing abuse and may help identify the perpetrator. Toxicological screens are also used to identify any poisons or medication that might have contributed to death. A thorough SKELETAL SURVEY is always conducted to detect fractures and separations of the bones.

An autopsy may reveal evidence of serious internal injury such as liver or spleen damage when there is scant external evidence of trauma. Examination of the galea (area between the scalp and the cranium) sometimes shows well-defined hemorrhages that reflect the outline of the weapon used to strike the child.

Comparison of evidence obtained from an autopsy with the caretaker's explanation often serves as the basis for criminal charges. By carefully establishing and documenting the probable cause of death an autopsy can support or call into question such an explanation. In combination with other evidence, medical evidence can help convict a child abuser and possibly protect other children from abuse or neglect by the same perpetrator.

Weston, James T. "The Pathology of Child Abuse and Neglect." In C. Henry Kempe and Ray E. Helfer, eds., *The Battered Child*, 3rd ed. Chicago: University of Chicago Press, 1980.

autoptic evidence   See EVIDENCE.

aversive conditioning   Painful measures such as spanking or electric shock have been used in the treatment of certain psychiatric disorders as a way of controlling behavior considered dangerous or socially undesirable. This mode of treatment has often been abused and is the subject of continuing debate among advocates, practitioners and lawyers.

avitaminosis   A condition caused by a deficiency of one or more essential vitamins. This condition may occur in children suffering from nutritional neglect. Also called hypovitaminosis.

Some examples include children whose diets contain insufficient levels of vitamin C. These children are at risk of developing SCURVY, a disease that is characterized by multiple hemorrhages. Also, children with vitamin D-deficient diets may develop RICKETS, in which stunted growth and skeletal deformities are common. Vitamin A deficiency often denotes a general malnourished state. Children who lack sufficient intake of vitamin A are at risk for a range of eye problems, including, in cases of severe vitamin A deficiency, blindness.

B

Baby Doe A controversial court case in the United States illustrates the difficulty in defining child abuse. In October of 1983, a baby, known simply as Baby Jane Doe, was born in a New York hospital. In addition to an exposed spine (spina bifida), Baby Doe suffered from excess fluid on the brain and an abnormally small head. Corrective surgery could add several years to her life but could not correct her severe mental and physical retardation. After consulting with several physicians, the parents decided not to give permission for an operation to enclose the spine. Baby Doe was treated with nonsurgical techniques, including antibiotics and measures to encourage natural enclosure of the spine.

The U.S. Department of Health and Human Services, reeling from public criticism for failure to intervene in a similar case in Indiana, filed a child abuse complaint with the New York Child Protection Services. When NYCPS did not substantiate the complaint, a private citizen from Vermont filed suit to force the parents to give permission for surgery. Again the parents' decision was upheld. HHS then attempted to enforce newly developed regulations that forbade withholding medical treatment or nutrition on the basis of an infant's impairment. The Department appealed the case to the U.S. Supreme Court, arguing that disabled infants were entitled to protection from discrimination under the Rehabilitation Act of 1973. In 1986, the Supreme Court ruled the new regulations unconstitutional. Baby Doe continued to receive nonsurgical medical treatment.

Concern over this and similar cases led the U.S. Congress to amend the CHILD ABUSE PREVENTION AND TREATMENT ACT to include withholding of medically indicated treatment as a form of abuse. Subsequent regulations allowed parents to deny permission for treatment if it is judged ineffective in improv-ing or correcting a life-threatening condition, if it only prolongs dying, or if the infant is irreversibly comatose. This expanded definition of child abuse is similar in content to the regulations struck down by the U.S. Supreme Court.

baby farms The practice of nursing or rearing children in exchange for money was widespread in 19th-century England. Working mothers often entrusted infants to a caretaker for a lump sum payment. Unscrupulous "nurses" were known to accept large numbers of infants at prices far lower than what was necessary to provide adequate care. Needless to say, these "baby farms" provided substandard care and were often filthy.

In 1868, Ernest Hart, editor of the *British Medical Journal* decried the practice, saying ". . . many of these women carried on the business with a deliberate knowledge that the children would die very quickly and evidently with a deliberate intention that they should die." Hart's attempts to regulate baby farms were largely unsuccessful until a celebrated case known as the "Brixton Horrors" was brought to light in 1870.

While investigating a large number of abandoned infant corpses found in various parts of the city, police discovered a baby farm run by a Margaret Waters and her sister, Sarah Ellis. Evidence found at the Waters home showed that infants were fed only limewater and that many had been drugged, poisoned or starved to death.

Subsequent investigations of other baby farms uncovered additional horror stories. It was estimated that 80% to 90% of the infants entrusted to the care of "professional nurses" perished.

Public outrage stimulated the passage of the INFANT LIFE PROTECTION ACT in 1872. Though it was

40

an important first step, the act was largely ineffectual in curbing the abuses found in baby farms.

Baker v. Owen, 1975 The issue of schools' use of CORPORAL PUNISHMENT has been the subject of a great deal of litigation and public debate in recent years. United States courts have consistently ruled in favor of a school's right to use physical punishment as a means of discipline as long as certain safety precautions are followed.

In the case of *Baker v. Owen*, the United States Supreme Court upheld a teacher's right to punish a child physically in spite of a parent's wishes to the contrary. The case involved a sixth-grade student in a North Carolina school. A school official punished the child after his mother had submitted a note forbidding the official to do so.

battered child syndrome The late C. Henry Kempe, a professor of pediatrics at the University of Colorado School of Medicine, is credited with coining the term "battered child syndrome." Concerned by the number of abused infants and children receiving medical care who were misdiagnosed or improperly treated, Dr. Kempe sought to bring the problem of child abuse to the attention of physicians. Using his position as president of the American Academy of Pediatrics, he organized a symposium on the subject in 1961. The name battered child syndrome was chosen, in part to create public interest in a phenomenon many people considered repugnant. The symposium generated a great deal of interest and was followed a year later by a much-quoted article of the same name published in *The Journal of the American Medical Association.* In the article, Kempe and others outlined the basic features of the syndrome. Though many of the symptoms had been outlined previously by John Caffey, Frederick Silverman and other pediatric radiologists, the Kempe article was the first to bring together information on clinical/radiologic manifestations, psychiatric factors, evaluation and incidence.

The battered child syndrome as originally described included a range of physical abuse suffered by children primarily under age three. Later definitions have expanded the age to five years and even older. Specific symptoms may include:

general poor health, evidence of neglect, poor skin hygiene, multiple soft tissue injuries, malnutrition, a history suggesting parental neglect or abuse, marked discrepancy between clinical evidence and information supplied by the caretaker, subdural hematoma and multiple fractures in various stages of healing. Symptoms can be present in different combinations but the last two were particularly important to physicians. Due to advances in pediatric radiology, physicians were able to verify the presence of subdural hematomas and, more importantly, to distinguish between bone fractures caused by accidental injury and those typical of inflicted abuse. Kempe wrote: "To the informed physician, the bones tell a story the child is too young or too frightened to tell."

Linking verifiable clinical/radiological phenomena to child abuse was a particularly important step in encouraging physicians to pursue adequate measures for protecting children from further abuse. Indeed the general reluctance on the part of physicians, social workers and others to acknowledge child abuse is still a cause for concern. However, willingness to identify and report child abuse has increased somewhat as a result of mandatory reporting laws in many areas.

Though not widely used today, the term battered child syndrome played an important role in refocusing public attention on child abuse. By making child abuse a medical phenomenon, the considerable influence of physicians was brought to bear on a problem that many had chosen to ignore. Increasing concern over abuse has shifted the focus from protection of parents and caretakers to an emphasis on the rights and welfare of the child. This approach attributes most child abuse to a poorly functioning family system or to individual pathology on the part of parents or caretakers.

Kempe, Henry C., N. Frederick Silverman, Brandt F. Steele, William Droegemueller, and Henry K. Silver. "The Battered-Child Syndrome." *Journal of the American Medical Association* 181 (1962): 17–24.

battering child Attacks from other children represent a small percentage of reported child abuse. These attacks may range from relatively harmless sibling rivalry (see SIBLING ABUSE) to attempted murder.

Abuse by a child outside the family is more likely to be reported to authorities than sibling abuse. Parents are often reluctant to report abuse that occurs at the hands of an older brother or sister. In such cases, parents may be afraid to acknowledge that a child's behavior is beyond their control. Rather than taking steps to protect the victimized sibling, parents attempt to placate the aggressor and downplay the extent of the abuse.

A parent or caretaker's failure to protect children from harmful assaults by another child constitutes, at a minimum, neglect. In particularly serious cases, caretakers may be considered coconspirators in the abuse.

Ironically, mental health professionals, like parents, have tended to focus more attention on the treatment needs of the abuser than on those of the abused child. Victims of sibling attacks, lacking parental support or fearing further abuse, are reluctant to participate in psychotherapy. This being the case, they frequently require extended treatment before improvement is seen.

Battering children attack others for a variety of reasons. These include jealousy, emotional disturbance or a history of being abused themselves. Abusive children are sometimes acting out a parent's wishes. Older children are sometimes given too much responsibility in caring for younger brothers and sisters. Rarely, children may misunderstand a parent's idle threats to strangle a crying child and actually attempt to carry out such a punishment.

battery   Illegal contact, especially physical violence, with a person is known as battery. The term is most often used in reference to beating.

For contact to be considered illegal, it must take place without the consent of the victim. Since a minor cannot give legal consent, any offensive or violent contact with a child can be considered battery. Acts of battery may be classified as either aggravated or simple. Aggravated battery refers to intentional acts of violence. Unintentional acts or acts that do not cause severe harm may be called simple battery.

See also ASSAULT.

bed-wetting   See ENURESIS.

behavior   See SEDUCTIVE BEHAVIOR; SELF-DESTRUCTIVE BEHAVIOR.

best interests of the child   It has long been held that parents usually act in the best interests of children. In cases of child abuse or neglect, however, this benevolent parental action is found lacking and judicial intervention on behalf of the children is necessary.

The legal standard of a child's best interest was developed in response to a need to establish guidelines in safeguarding children's rights. The standard of best interest of the child takes into consideration the many variables of a child's life, including the fitness of parent(s) or legal guardian. Aside from abuse and neglect cases, it is a standard invoked most frequently in cases of custody or placement, when a court is obliged to determine with whom a child should make his or her home.

In recent years, the best interest standard has been challenged on the grounds that it places too much emphasis on an unattainable ideal. A suggested substitute, the "least detrimental alternative," holds that a court's determination should be based on careful weighing of many alternatives open to discussion. According to proponents of the least detrimental alternative standard, placement made on the basis of best interest generally seeks to find a solution without negative ramifications for the child. It is against this ideal of "best" interest that critics argue.

Goldstein, Joseph. *The Best Interests of the Child: The Least Detrimental Alternative.* New York: Free Press, 1996.

beyond a reasonable doubt   This is a legal standard of proof required in criminal trials and, frequently, for termination of parental rights.

See also EVIDENTIARY STANDARDS.

biting   Human bites leave distinctive, crescent-shaped bruises containing tooth marks. In some cases, the bruise marks may join to form a ring. Bite marks on children may be self-inflicted or the result of an attack by a playmate or caretaker. Careful measurements of the space between the canine teeth can determine whether the perpetrator has permanent teeth (greater than 3 cm) or not (fewer than 3 cm). Location of bite marks in areas that would be difficult for the child to reach is also an indicator of suspicious origin. Since bite marks usually leave a distinct impression, they can sometimes be traced to the abusers by comparing them to wax dental impressions taken from suspected perpetrators. The attacker's blood type can sometimes be identified from small amounts of saliva surrounding the wound.

blaming the victim   A common rationalization of child maltreatment is that the victim of the abuse is in some way responsible for the abuse. Abusive parents often have unrealistic expectations of their children and punish them for behavior that may be natural for children of a given age. Punishing children for behavior over which they have little control is not only ineffective but may cause further negative behavior. Thinking the child has not learned his or her lesson, immature parents may increase punishment to the point of physical or emotional injury. Frustrated caretakers often label the child sick or bad and use these judgments as excuses for further abuse.

Blaming the child for the parent's abusive behavior is a form of denial that prevents parents from accepting responsibility for their own actions. Sometimes abusers are able to convince others that a child's extreme behavior justifies severe punishment. Family members and friends may engage in a conspiracy of denial to avoid acknowledging abuse. In such instances perceptions of the child as the initiator of abuse are reinforced, increasing the likelihood of further abuse. Often parents choose particular traits of the child as justification for abuse. Low birth weight infants may cry incessantly, developmentally disabled children may not respond to parents' demands or children may simply be defiant. These and other characteristics of children may make parenting more difficult. They do not, however, justify abuse. Responsibility for abuse rests with the abuser's own inability to manage his or her actions.

Children often come to believe that they are indeed responsible for their own abuse. Even when abuse is unprovoked a child may feel that he or she must have done something to deserve punishment. Internalized feelings of guilt and negative self-worth become deeply ingrained in the child's psyche and respond slowly to treatment. Often, long-term psychotherapy is recommended to help abuse victims overcome self-blame.

Abusers must learn to accept responsibility for their own actions before they can make full use of treatment services. Repeat sexual offenders can be particularly persistent in blaming children for being seductive or for initiating sexual contact. Their inability to acknowledge the child's vulnerability and to accept their own responsibility as adults makes them particularly slow to respond to treatment.

bruises   Easily recognizable as discolored patches of skin, bruises are caused by bleeding beneath the skin. They are perhaps the most common observable indicator of child battering. For purposes of easier description, bruises are divided into three categories.

Petechiae: Very small bruises caused by broken capillaries. These lesions may be caused by trauma such as bumps or blows or may be the result of a clotting disorder. Clotting factor tests are sometimes conducted to determine the origin of bruises.

Purpura: The term *purpura* may refer to a group of petechiae or a small bruise up to one centimeter in diameter.

Ecchymosis: Refers to any bruise larger than one centimeter in diameter.

bullying   The use of force and/or verbal threats to compel a child or adolescent to do something that he or she does not wish to do and/or to humiliate the victim, usually in front of others of about the same age. Some experts have estimated that nearly 30% of schoolchildren have either been bullied or have acted as bullies. In the case of male bullies, they are usually considerably larger and stronger than the victim and are also usually older. Female bullying is different from male bullying, in that girls are more likely to use words alone to torment their chosen victims, rather than threatening physical injury as well as using verbal threats. Girls may bully other girls with name-calling or by spreading vicious and untrue rumors about the female victims to others.

In some cases, bullying is a temporary and minor annoyance; in other cases, children are so traumatized that they develop a "learned helplessness," believing that they cannot do anything and even that they deserve to be bullied. This negative attitude may continue into adulthood if no intervention occurs in childhood or adolescence.

According to the Substance Abuse and Mental Health Administration (SAMHSA) booklet *Take Action against Bullying,* bullying may include hitting, name-calling, threatening, intimidating, kicking, spreading rumors, teasing, pushing, tripping and destroying another person's property. Note that bullies may also steal the victim's property, such as money, bicycles or other items of value to the victim.

The SAMHSA booklet offers key reasons for stopping bullying, including the following:

- Bullying interferes with learning in school and may increase absenteeism and school dropout rates.
- Bullying children may later become bullying adults, and they are also more likely to become child abusers and spouse abusers as adults.
- The longer that the bullying lasts, the harder it is for the child bully to change this behavior.
- Bullying may be linked to other delinquent behaviors or gang activities, such as vandalism, drug abuse and shoplifting.
- The victims of bullies often become socially insecure and anxious, with decreased self-esteem and increased depression that may last into adulthood.

State Laws on Bullying

At least 15 states have laws against bullying; for example, Colorado's law defines bullying as, "Any written or verbal expression, or physical act or gesture, or a pattern thereof, that is intended to cause distress upon one or more children." In Georgia, bullying is defined as, "Any willful attempt or threat to inflict injury on another person . . . or any intentional display of force such as would give the victim reason to fear or expect immediate bodily harm."

Most state laws require school boards to create a policy prohibiting bullying; for example, Louisiana law requires a policy banning the harassment, intimidation and bullying of one student by another student. In some states, such as Connecticut, New Hampshire, New Jersey, New York, Washington and West Virginia, state laws either require or urge that school bullying be reported to authorities.

Victims of Bullying

In *Adult Bullying,* a book that also provides information on bullying among children, author Peter Randall said that victims are often ostracized by other children who are not bullies, yet they attribute negative traits to victims, taking the attitude that the victim deserved his or her fate. Note that other children may also avoid the victim, fearing that any association with the victim could lead to the bully transferring his or her abusive attentions to them.

Characteristics of Victims

In general, bullies choose other children who are smaller in size than they are and appear unlikely to retaliate. The victims may have no or few friends and may be physically immature compared to others in the same age group. In general, bullied girls are more likely to become depressed than boys who are victimized.

Victims of bullies tend to have low self-esteem, and they are more cautious and withdrawn than their peers. They may seek to avoid school, where they would encounter the bully, and they may have suicidal thoughts. They may also experience anxiety and/or depression. They may complain of many headaches, stomachaches and other body pains that have a psychological basis rather than a physical one.

Some victims, however, are hyperactive and hot-tempered, and they fight back, although usually ineffectually. Said Watson et al., "Sadly, children in this group are among the most rejected of all children and show the most severe psychopathological outcomes."

Victims with Disabilities

In general, disabled children or those with special needs are more likely than others to be victimized with bullying. Such children include

- Those with learning disabilities
- Those with attention-deficit/hyperactivity disorder (children with ADHD may also *become* bullies)
- Those with medical conditions affecting their appearance, such as cerebral palsy, spina bifida and so forth
- Those who are obese
- Those with diabetes who are insulin-dependent
- Those who stutter

The bullying of children who are disabled may be considered "disability harassment," which is illegal under Section 504 of the Rehabilitation Act of 1973 and Title II of the Americans with Disabilities Act of 1990. Schools should immediately investigate all allegations of the bullying of disabled children or children with special needs.

In addition, if bullying continues, parents should ask the school to convene a special meeting of the Individualized Education Program (IEP) team to discuss the harassment and ensure the school is taking (or will take) steps to stop harassment. If the school refuses to take appropriate actions to end the bullying or harassment, it may be in violation of federal, state or local laws. The parent may then wish to contact the superintendent of schools or the school board. If no action is taken subsequent to that contact, organizations such as the U.S. Department of Education Office for Civil Rights (800-421-3481) or the U.S. Department of Education Office of Special Education Programs (202-245-7468) should be contacted.

Behavioral Indicators of Bullying among Victims

According to SAMHSA, there are some warning signs that a child may be experiencing bullying. These include children who

- Evidence social withdrawal; they have few or no friends
- Frequently complain of illness

- Bring home damaged possessions or report them as "lost"
- Talk about running away and/or suicide
- Have changes in sleeping or eating patterns
- Take or attempt to take items of protection to school, such as a knife, stick, gun or other weapons
- Display "victim" body language, such as hunching of the shoulders, avoiding eye contact and hanging the head down
- Cry easily, display mood swings and talk about hopelessness
- Threaten violence to themselves or others

In addition, victims may resort to stealing from their parents and others, in order to pay off the bully.

Aggressive Children/Bullies

According to Watson et al. in their chapter in *Child Maltreatment,* children and adolescents who behave in a bullying manner are usually males who are of a larger size than their victims. Contrary to popular belief, research has shown that bullies often have very high self-esteem, with little or no empathy for their peers. They see violence as an acceptable goal for achieving their ends.

Unlike their victims, who are usually alone when attacked, bullies travel in groups, and they rarely attack others physically when they are alone with the victim. Bullies want and need an audience.

Bullies often interpret the behavior of others in a negative manner. Said Watson et al., "Although bullies will usually report that they are victims, and thus that their aggression is justified, they in fact are not usually victimized by peers. Instead they tend to possess a hostile attribution bias in reading aggressive intent into the ambiguous behaviors of those around them and their solutions to social dilemmas are thus aggressive responses to their biased perceptions of being targeted by others or simply instrumental aggressive acts to achieve their needs and goals."

According to Randall, up to about age seven, bullies may harass almost anyone, but after that age, they tend to narrow down their victims, singling one person to torment psychologically and physically.

According to SAMHSA in their booklet on taking action against bullying, some warning signs of a bully are when the following behaviors occur often. The child who may be a bully

- Seeks to dominate and/or manipulate others
- Enjoys feeling powerful and in control (whether these feelings are valid or not)
- Is both a poor winner (boastful and arrogant) and a poor loser
- Seems to derive satisfaction from other's fears, discomfort or pain
- Is good at hiding behaviors or doing them where adults cannot notice
- Is excited by conflicts between others
- Blames others for his/her problems
- Displays uncontrolled anger
- Has a history of discipline problems
- Displays a pattern of impulsive and chronic hitting, intimidating and aggressive behaviors
- Displays intolerance and prejudice toward others
- Lacks empathy toward others

The Health Resources and Services Administration, a division of the U.S. Department of Health and Human Services has a list of the characteristics of children who bully, which include tendencies to

- Be impulsive, hot-headed, dominant
- Be easily frustrated
- Lack empathy
- Have difficulty following rules
- View violence in a positive way

Family risk factors for children who become bullies are as follows:

- A lack of warmth and involvement on the part of parents
- Overly permissive parenting (including a lack of limits for children's behavior)
- A lack of parental supervision
- Harsh physical discipline

Children who bully others are more likely to

- Get into frequent fights
- Be injured in a fight
- Vandalize property
- Steal property
- Drink alcohol
- Smoke
- Be truant from school
- Drop out of school
- Carry a weapon

Female Bullies

Girls are bullied by both girls and boys, while most boys are bullied by other boys. According to Randall in *Adult Bullying,* female children and adolescents manipulate other girls by using social exclusion or telling others that they should not like a girl, often for a perceived slight. Said Randall, "It is believed that bullying girls choose these forms of aggression because they are aware that other girls are particularly dependent upon having good relationships. The easiest way to hurt such girls is to threaten those relationships and exclude the victim from them. Girls who become relational bullies in this way increasingly put themselves at risk of being rejected. Other children become bored with their behaviour and increasingly irritated with being manipulated."

Randall says girl bullies usually chose as their friends girls who are easily manipulated and non-aggressive.

As with boys, female bullies may exhibit their negative behavior because of real, but often imagined, slights. They may also be jealous of their female victims. Often it takes little (or nothing) to incur the wrath of the child who is a female bully.

When the Bullied Victim Reacts Violently

Most victims of bullies do not act against them and instead remain passive. However, sometimes victims do become violent. In a study of school-associated violent deaths from 1994 to 1999, reported in the *Journal of the American Medical Association* in 2001, the researchers identified 172 deaths of students in school. Most of the victims were male (120 students). In addition, most victims were white non-Hispanic (66 students) or black non-Hispanic (59 students). The largest numbers of deaths (129) occurred in senior high, followed by middle school/junior high (26 deaths). The largest numbers of deaths (75) occurred in urban areas followed by suburban areas (63).

About 20 percent of the murders were committed by students who had previously been bullied and who later became homicidal.

According to Watson et al. in their chapter on bullying in *Child Victimization,* these children who turn violent "have a history of being victimized, harassed, and humiliated by peers and feel strongly rejected. Perhaps for this reason, though they are withdrawn, they may be quick to take offense and overreact to a threat, be it real or perceived."

The authors also reported that such children who were formerly bullied and who later become violent may have both aggressive and suicidal fantasies. In addition, they have access to and interest in weapons, such as guns and explosives. These "reactive aggressors" or "victim aggressors" are usually quiet and not impulsive. They may have experienced harsh punishments from their parents.

Parents of Bullied Children

Parents of children who are bullied may be insensitive to the child's problem. Boys may be told to "act like a man" or "stand and fight." If they follow this advice, however, negative results usually occur, since the male bully is much bigger and stronger than the victim. Parents may also not recognize when the bullying has become severe and traumatic for the child, whether it is because the child tries to hide the effects of bullying and/or the parents are diverted by their own problems or issues.

Adults who would never tolerate physical abuse from other adults may expect that learning to deal with bullies is a rite of passage through which children must pass. As a result, they may fail to react in a protective and helpful manner when their own child is bullied.

SAMHSA has offered do and don't suggestions for parents whose child may be experiencing bullying. According to SAMHSA, parents should

- Make sure the child knows that being bullied is not his or her fault.
- Let the child know that he or she does not have to face being bullied alone.
- Discuss ways of responding to bullies and consult with the school for assistance on how to help your child.
- Teach the child to be assertive.
- Tell the child not to react, but to walk away and get help if pursued.
- Tell the child to report bullying immediately to a trusted adult.
- Contact the school/teachers.

In contrast, SAMHSA recommended the following "don'ts" for parents:

- Do not ask children to solve a bullying problem between themselves (the bully and the victim)—because of the differences in power, the child who has been bullied will suffer further. Bullying problems require adult intervention.
- Do not advise the bullied child to fight the bully—fighting is in violation of the school conduct code, and the child might be seriously injured.
- Do not try to mediate a bullying situation yourself. Bringing together children who are bullied and those who do the bullying, in order to "work out" the problems between them, generally is not a good idea. It may further victimize a child who is being bullied, and it sends the wrong message to both parties.
- Do not blame either the victim or the bully. Instead, gather as much information as possible. Look at your own child's behavior and style of interaction and consider how you might help him/her to handle these types of situations in the future. Contact the school for assistance.

Parents of Bullies

SAMHSA also offers the following advice for parents who think that their child is a bully:

- Be sure that your child knows that bullying is NOT acceptable behavior.

- Tell your child the penalties for bullying and be sure that you enforce them fairly and consistently.

- Help your child learn alternative ways to deal with anger and frustration.

- Teach and reward more appropriate behavior.

- Work out a way for your child to make amends for acts of bullying.

- Help your child develop an understanding of the impact of bullying on the target.

- Seek help or counseling if the behavior continues.

- If contacting the school, stay calm and avoid becoming angry and defensive. Make yourself really listen. This is ultimately about the well-being of your child.

See also PHYSICAL ABUSE; PSYCHOLOGICAL/EMOTIONAL MALTREATMENT.

Anderson, Mark, M.D., et al. "School-Associated Violent Deaths in the United States, 1994–1999." *Journal of the American Medical Association* 286, no. 21 (December 5, 2001): 2,695–2,702.

Finkelhor, David, et al. "The Victimization of Children and Youth: A Comprehensive, National Survey." *Child Maltreatment* 10, no. 1 (February 2005): 5–25.

Health Resources and Services Administration. "Bullying among Children and Youth with Disabilities and Special Needs." Available online. URL: http://stopbullyingnow. hrsa.gov/HHS-PSA/pdfs/SBN_Tip_24.pdf. Downloaded December 8, 2005.

———. "Children Who Bully." Available online. URL: http://stopbullyingnow.hrsa.gov/HHS_PSA/pdfs/ SBN_Tip_1.pdf. Downloaded December 8, 2005.

———. "State Laws Related to Bullying among Children and Youth." Available online. URL: http://stopbullying now.hrsa.gov?HHS_PSA/pdfs/SBN_Tip_6.pdf.

Randall, Peter. *Adult Bullying: Perpetrators and Victims.* London: Routledge, 1997.

Substance Abuse and Mental Health Services Administration. *Take Action against Bullying.* Washington, D.C.: U.S. Department of Health and Human Services, 2003.

Watson, Malcolm W., et al. "Patterns of Risk Factors Leading to Victimization and Aggression in Children and Adolescents." In *Child Victimization.* Kingston, N.J.: Civic Research Institute, 2005.

burden of proof   In a court of law the petitioner or plaintiff is responsible for producing evidence establishing the truth of allegations made against the defendant. This duty is referred to as the burden of proof or, in Latin, *onus probandi.* The burden of proof in child abuse and neglect cases rests with the governmental unit charged with enforcing such laws, usually the state. Depending on the nature of the charges different standards of proof may be required.

Burden of proof can also refer to the "burden of going forward with the evidence," which may shift back and forth between the two parties. Under this meaning of the term either party may be required to raise a reasonable doubt concerning the existence or nonexistence of a particular fact.

See also EVIDENTIARY STANDARDS.

burnout   Staff burnout is a frequent problem among child protection services (CPS) workers. The work is demanding and the benefits of staff efforts often cannot immediately be seen by the staff. Typically, CPS workers carry caseloads that are too large to permit satisfactory attention to each case. Time pressures, hostile reactions of parents and children and inadequate support from supervisors also take their toll on workers.

Frustration with working conditions has led to a high rate of turnover among CPS staff. Some workers who do not leave their jobs may become apathetic or angry. In addition to the obviously negative consequences of burnout for workers, frequent turnover and worker apathy also diminish the effectiveness of the child protection system.

Apathy and frustration associated with burnout can be reduced and in some cases prevented. Thorough, ongoing training plays an important role in reducing burnout. Well-trained workers feel more confident and are better prepared to handle the inevitable stresses they encounter in their work.

Competent and accessible supervision is essential. Regular feedback and emotional support from the supervisor is especially important for CPS workers. Peer support and consultation from specialists may also help reduce stress when workers must make difficult decisions concerning a child's well-being. Many child protection agencies have found that regularly scheduled meetings of workers are important ways of encouraging peer support and exchanging professional information.

Finally, the CPS worker must be careful to set limits between his or her personal and professional activities. The intense nature of child abuse investigation and the dedication of many workers often cause them to bring job-related problems home. Workers who have a variety of interests outside of work are often better able to avoid burnout than those who have few outside supports.

burns One of the leading causes of accidental death to children, burns are also a frequent method of abuse. Treatment of a child's burns is painful, and permanent scarring may result from full thickness (third-degree) burns. Young children have thinner skin than older children or adults, and, consequently, a child's skin may be damaged or destroyed more quickly and with a lower heat temperature.

According to Moore and Smith in their chapter on child abuse by burns, in *Understanding the Medical Diagnosis of Child Maltreatment: A Guide for Nonmedical Professionals,* an estimated 10% of all burns suffered by children are caused by child abuse, and the most frequent victims are boys ages two to three years old.

Burns that are suspicious of abuse are those which are not compatible with the doctor's physical findings or with the developmental age of the child. In addition, burns that appear older than the information that is provided by the child's caretaker are suspicious. If the burned child has not been brought in for treatment until after 24 hours or more have passed, this is an indication of abuse, as is a prior history of burns. Most caretakers seek immediate and emergency attention when a child is seriously burned. If the child is also bruised, lacerated or scarred in addition to the burns, this is an indication of abuse, as is X-ray evidence of bone fractures.

Levels of Severity of Burns

There are three levels of severity of burns, including superficial burns, partial thickness burns and full thickness burns. Superficial burns (formerly called first-degree burns) are burns that occur on the outer layer of the skin. The skin is red, but the redness disappears under pressure. A sunburn is one example of a superficial burn. In most cases, these burns are not serious unless they cover a large part of the body.

Partial thickness burns (formerly called second-degree burns) are worse burns than superficial burns, and they extend into the second layer of the skin and cause pain and weeping blisters. If no infection occurs, these wounds take about two to three weeks to heal, although some severe wounds require surgery.

The most severe level of burns is the full thickness burn, formerly called third- and fourth-degree burns.

With full thickness burns, said Moore and Smith, "The area looks white or charred and is not sensitive to touch or a pinprick because the blood vessels and nerve endings are destroyed. If bone or muscle is involved, the burn is equivalent to the formerly classified fourth-degree burn. These injuries require hospitalization and usually require skin grafting. These burns heal with scarring, creating a change in color and a 'parchment' type of skin."

Burns are also evaluated by the extent of the body covered, as well as by the age of the child. For example, according to Moore and Smith, a burn is severe when it covers greater than 10% of the body of a child who is younger than age two. If the child is between two and 12 years old, the burn is considered severe when more than 15% of the body is burned. However, a child of any age is considered severely burned when more than 20% of the body is burned or the genitals, face or hands are burned.

Common Types of Burns

The most common types of abuse burns are immersion burns, splash burns and contact burns. Other types of burns of abuse are chemical, electrical and microwave burns. Scalding burns are the most common of all burns, and they may occur with immersion burns or splash burns. Most scalding burns that are caused intentionally are caused by extremely hot tap water.

Immersion burns Immersion burns are burns in which the child is placed in or under very hot liquid, usually water. The depth of the burn is usually uniform on the body when the immersion was made deliberately and abusively. Deep immersion burns on the buttocks or between the anus and genitals are usually caused by the deliberate immersion of the child, often involving punishment for a problem related to toilet training, such as the child soiling him or herself.

A clear line on the lower back indicates that the child was forcibly held in the water, whereas a child who fell into the water would splash about trying to get out and would show irregular burn patterns on the body.

With immersion burns, a parent who claims to have tested the bathwater ahead of time is usually lying, since adults are uncomfortable at water temperatures greater than 109 degrees Fahrenheit, while full thickness burns are caused by 130 degrees or greater over a 10-second period.

Immersion burns may occur during toilet training, when the child's hands are immersed in scalding water for punishment and/or cleaning, often for not learning toilet training quickly enough or having an "accident." (Note that some parents and other caretakers are unaware of the normal development stages of children and may expect a child to be toilet trained before it is possible for him or her to do so, such as when the child is 18 months old or younger.)

The child's hands may be immersed in a hot pot on the stove as a punishment for touching the stove, for playing nearby or for aggravating the caretaker (in his or her mind). It is a terrifying image, but some people will place a child in a hot oven, as a punishment or to murder the child.

Splash burns   Splash burns are burns in which the liquid traveled through the air before making contact with the child. With abusive splash burns, the liquid is either poured on or thrown at the child, usually as a punishment. Splash burns may be serious, but they usually do not cause as deep a burn as an immersion burn, since the liquid is cooled somewhat by the air before skin contact occurs. However, if the liquid is a chemical, the chemicals continue to act on the skin and thus are more dangerous to the child than a water-based liquid.

If a splash burn is accidental, the physician can usually determine this by considering the part of the body which is burned. In general, if a child spills hot liquid or causes it to fall upon himself or

herself, the back of the body is rarely affected. In addition, if a parent or other person accidentally spills coffee or tea on the child, this burn should not affect a large part of the child's body since an average cup cannot hold enough fluid to cover a large body surface.

Contact burns   Contact burns are burns made directly to the skin. The most common abusive contact burns are made by cigarettes and irons, according to *Burn Injuries in Child Abuse*. Intentional cigarette burns are easily distinguished from accidental burns; for example, if a child brushed against a lighted cigarette, he or she is unlikely to sustain a burn on the back or the buttocks. Multiple cigarette burns are clearly indicative of abuse.

"Branding" injuries, such as with a cigarette lighter or a curling iron, cause a much deeper burn than when the child accidentally touches these items. In most cases, an accidental injury with a hot item is caused by the child either grasping the item and/or the item falling on the child.

Children may also receive contact burns with hot plates, curling irons, hair dryers, radiators, irons and so forth. Physicians can usually determine whether the burn was intended or accidental. For example, a hair dryer is usually moved around and not held against the body for a fixed period.

If the contact burn caused by an object is accidental, the burns are usually irregular, because in most cases, the child will have reflexively moved away from the hot object.

Moore and Smith concluded in their chapter that "Encountering burns resulting from child abuse is perhaps one of the more difficult injuries for CPS [child protective services] workers to deal with in the course of conducting casework. The potential for scarring and other long-term damage does create an emotional reaction by all persons involved in the case. Thus, it is even more important that CPS workers objectively understand the injuries and work collaboratively with medical providers to ensure proper treatment for the child."

Skin conditions that may mimic abusive burns Some skin conditions may appear to be inflicted by abuse, but upon further investigation, the child was not abused. For example, the child may have a skin infection that resembles a scald injury. In other cases, the child may have an allergic reaction to a substance, such as a citrus fruit, that causes a skin condition that may resemble a splash burn. Some topical antiseptics may cause a burn-like appearance.

In investigating suspicious cases of burns, criminal investigators may wish to use the following checklist provided by the Office of Juvenile Justice and Delinquency Prevention:

- Have you contacted the emergency response team?
- Have you contacted the child protective services team?
- Have you reviewed the medical findings with the appropriate medical staff?
- Have you carefully considered the suspicion index findings?
- Where was the primary-care provider at the time of the incident?
- Where is the burn injury located on the child's body?
- How serious is the burn?
- Is the burn a wet contact burn or a dry contact burn?
- If the burn appears to have been caused by a dry source of heat, what is the shape of the burn and what object does it resemble?
- Have you completed the Evidence Worksheet for Immersion Burns?
- If the burn was produced by a hot liquid, was the child dipped or fully immersed?
- What does the line of demarcation look like?
- Are there any splash burns present?

- How symmetrical are the lines of immersion if stocking or glove patterns are present?
- Is toilet training, soiling or wetting an issue?
- Have you recorded information concerning the child's age, height, degree of development and coordination; location of fixtures; temperature and depth of water; weight of burn object, etc.?
- Have you compared the burn injury with the area of sparing?
- Was the child in a state of flexion (tensing of the body parts in reaction to what was happening) indicating resistance? Examples of flexion on a child's body include:
  - Folds in the stomach
  - Calf against back of thigh
  - Arms tightened and held firmly against body or folded against body
  - Thighs against abdomen
  - Head against shoulder
  - Legs crossed, held tightly together

See also ABUSERS; PHYSICAL ABUSE.

Moore, Joyce K., and Jean C. Smith. "Abuse by Burns." In *Understanding the Medical Diagnosis of Child Maltreatment: A Guide for Nonmedical Professionals.* New York: Oxford University Press, 2006, pp. 37–48.

Office of Juvenile Justice and Delinquency Prevention. *Burn Injuries in Child Abuse.* Washington, D.C.: U.S. Department of Justice, Office of Justice Programs, June 2001, p. 11.

callus A meshwork of new bone tissue develops (usually beneath the periosteum) as a result of a fracture. The new tissue, called callus, forms along the pattern of the original clot caused by the injury. Callus shows up as a hazy, undifferentiated mass on X-rays. Presence of callus sometimes provides confirmation of battering injuries not immediately observable at the time of occurrence. Later in the healing process, the new bone tissue thickens and is incorporated into the cortex or shaft of the damaged bone.

Canada, child abuse in According to the *Canadian Incidence Study of Reported Child Abuse and Neglect, 2003: Major Findings,* published in 2005, about 217,319 child maltreatment investigations were held in 2003 among all Canadian jurisdictions except Quebec. Of these cases, 47% were substantiated, while in 13% of cases, there was insufficient evidence to substantiate the abuse or neglect. About 40% of the cases were unsubstantiated.

Types of Child Maltreatment

As in the United States, neglect was the largest category of substantiated maltreatment, and in 30% of all cases, neglect was the main category of maltreatment. Other types of maltreatment were exposure to domestic violence (28%), PHYSICAL ABUSE (24%), emotional maltreatment (15%) and SEXUAL ABUSE (3%). In about 81% of the cases of substantiated maltreatment, one category alone was identified, while in the other cases, multiple maltreatment forms were present.

When only one category was identified, 25% of the 81% of cases involved neglect only, 25% involved allegations of domestic violence only, 18% of the cases involved physical abuse only, and 11% involved emotional maltreatment only. (Two percent involved sexual abuse only.)

Physical Abuse Definitions and Incidence

The Canadians identified physical abuse as including one or more of five forms of physical abuse, including the following:

- Pulling, dragging or shaking or throwing a child
- Slapping or hitting a child
- Biting, punching or kicking a child
- Hitting a child with an object or throwing an object at a child
- Abusing a child in another way, such as stabbing, burning, poisoning, shooting, choking, strangling and so forth

In 2003, there were 25,257 substantiated investigations of physical abuse nationwide in Canada. Physical abuse represented 24% of all substantiated forms of child maltreatment. Male children were victimized in 54% of the cases of physical abuse, and females were victimized in 46% of the cases.

Sexual Abuse Definitions and Incidence

The Canadians defined several separate forms of sexual abuse, including

- Penile, anal, digital or object penetration of the vagina or anus
- Attempted penetration of the vagina or anus
- Oral sex
- Fondling of the genitals
- Sex talk in person, on the phone, in writing or over the INTERNET

There were 2,935 substantiated investigations of sexual abuse in Canada in 2003. Sexual abuse represented 3% of the cases of all forms of substantiated child maltreatment. Girls were victims in 63% of the cases, and boys were involved in 37% of the cases.

Neglect Definitions and Incidence

The Canadian researchers identified eight different forms of neglect, including

- Failure to supervise the child—physical harm (The parent or caretaker failed to protect the child adequately, such as with drunk driving with a child in the car or performing criminal activities in the presence of a child.)
- Failure to supervise—sexual abuse
- Physical neglect (insufficient or inadequate nutrition or clothing or dangerous living conditions)
- Medical neglect
- Failure to provide psychological/psychiatric treatment to a child
- Permitting criminal behavior
- Abandonment
- Educational neglect

In 2003, neglect cases represented 24% of all substantiated forms of child abuse. Fifty-two percent of the cases involved boys and 48% involved girls.

Emotional Maltreatment Definitions and Incidence

The Canadian researchers defined emotional maltreatment as the following:

- Emotional abuse (emotional, mental or developmental problems caused by extreme verbal abuse and overt hostility)
- Nonorganic FAILURE TO THRIVE (For example, if a child under age three has ceased growing or has marked retardation due to inadequate nutrition caused by physical neglect.)
- Emotional neglect (emotional, developmental or mental problems caused by inadequate nurturance)
- Exposure to non-intimate violence exclusive of domestic violence (such as violence occurring between adults within the home setting, i.e.,

between the child's father and an acquaintance of the father)

In 2003, emotional maltreatment represented 15% of all substantiated forms of child maltreatment. Fifty-four percent of the cases involved girls and 46% involved boys.

Domestic Violence and Incidence

In most areas of Canada, exposure to domestic violence (such as between two parents or a parent and a live-in partner) is considered a separate category of abuse. In 2003, there were 35,116 substantiated investigations of domestic violence in the presence of children in Canada.

Exposure to domestic violence represented 28% of all cases of substantiated child maltreatment in 2003. Fifty-two percent of the cases involved boys and 48% involved girls.

Child Abuse Laws Vary by Province or Territory

Child maltreatment laws in Canada are written at the provincial or territorial level, and they vary considerably. Some areas investigate allegations of abuse only for children younger than ages 16 (Newfoundland and Labrador, Nova Scotia, Ontario, Saskatchewan, the Northwest Territories and Nunavut), while others will investigate allegations for individuals younger than age 18 or 19 years (Quebec, Manitoba, Alberta and the Yukon Territory). Some areas will investigate allegations up to age 18 or 19 only if the youths are disabled, such as Prince Edward Island and New Brunswick.

Characteristics of Maltreated Children in Canada

The *Canadian Incidence Study of Reported Child Abuse and Neglect, 2003* also revealed information about maltreated children. For example, girls represented 49% of victims of all maltreatment, but they represented a greater percentage of those who suffered SEXUAL ABUSE (63%) and emotional maltreatment (54%) than boys. In contrast, boys were more frequently victims of physical abuse (54%), neglect (52%) and exposure to domestic violence (52%).

In considering age, children ages seven and younger were more likely to be exposed to domestic violence (60%) than older children. However, older children, ages eight to 15 years, were more likely to be physically abused (70%) or sexually abused (67%) than younger children.

Household Characteristics of Abused Children

The *Canadian Incidence Study of Reported Child Abuse and Neglect, 2003* also revealed characteristics of the households of maltreated children. For example, about a third (32%) of the abused children lived with both biological parents, while 16% lived in families in which one caregiver was either a step-parent, common law partner or adoptive parent. In 39% of the cases, the abused child or children lived with the mother only, while in 4% of the cases, the child or children lived with the father only.

Perpetrators of Child Abuse

According to the Canadian report, the largest numbers of the perpetrators of neglect, physical abuse, emotional maltreatment and exposure were biological mothers and fathers; however, the largest numbers of perpetrators of sexual abuse were other relatives.

In considering nonrelative perpetrators of abuse, there were few perpetrators for most forms of abuse; however, the largest number of cases of sexual abuse was perpetrated by a peer of the child, followed by an acquaintance.

See also SUBSTANTIATION.

Trocmé, Nico, et al. *Canadian Incidence Study of Reported Child Abuse and Neglect, 2003: Major Findings.* Ontario, Canada: Minister of Public Works and Government Services Canada, 2005. Available online. URL: http://www.phac-aspc.gc.ca/ncfv-cnivf/familyviolence/pdfs/childabuse_final_e.pdf. Downloaded December 15, 2005.

caning   Until recently, as part of an established disciplinary tradition, teachers have, for centuries, caned students. To implement this CORPORAL PUN-ISHMENT, adults most generally use a flexible rod made of rattan or bamboo, which is usually about three feet long and 0.5 inch in diameter.

Caning in British public schools (the equivalent of U.S. private, independent schools) has long been an accepted practice; masters and students alike proclaim its efficacy both as a deterrent and as a disciplinary technique. In 18th- and 19th-century

America, teachers widely employed caning as a means of maintaining classroom order.

Numerous accounts by educators and pupils attest to the fear and injury resulting from caning. Currently, caning is merely one of the many legal forms of corporal punishment that continue to be carried out in the 21st century.

See also INGRAHAM V. WRIGHT; PADDLING.

Hyman, Irwin A., and James D. Wise, eds. *Corporal Punishment in American Education.* Philadelphia: Temple University Press, 1979.

Cao Gio   Often, practices considered therapeutic in one culture are considered abusive in another. *Cao Gio*—a Vietnamese folk medicine practice believed to cure fever, chills and headaches—is an example of this phenomenon. Meaning literally, "scratch the wind," *Cao Gio* is thought to rid the body of "bad winds." The procedure involves rubbing hot oil on the skin of the afflicted child, then stroking the area with a heated metal object, usually a coin. BRUISES may result from this procedure and cause it to be reported as suspected child abuse.

It is not clear how painful this practice is or whether it presents a significant health risk to the child. The cultural origins and practices of the family generally must be taken into consideration in evaluating suspected abuse and neglect.

CASA   See COURT-APPOINTED SPECIAL ADVOCATE.

case plan   See SERVICE PLAN.

castration   Usually refers to a bilateral orchiectomy, or the surgical removal of male gonads. Surgical castration makes it difficult (or very unlikely) for a man to have erections.

In some rare cases, males voluntarily consent to surgical castration. They may be male sex offenders who wish to suppress their sex drive and consequently decrease their risk of reoffending and thus returning to prison.

Rather than surgical castration, some sex offenders willingly take drugs that suppress their sexual drive, which is often referred to as "chemical castration." The effects of the drugs are not permanent, and they are reversible if the man stops taking the drugs. Men suffering from some forms of cancer, such as prostate cancer, may also take drugs that decrease their sex drive as a necessary part of their treatment. Assuming that their sex drive and erectile ability were normal before treatment, it should return to normal within a month or so after the treatment ends.

Although often condemned, the castration of young boys was widely practiced in earlier times. In the Middle and Far East, castration produced eunuchs to serve in harems, so that they could not seduce the females. Castration was also used by the military and used on individuals employed as servants. In some Western cultures, boys were routinely castrated as a way of preserving their high-pitched singing voices until Pope Clement XIV (pontificate: 1769–74) effectively ended the practice by forbidding these "castrati" from singing in church. Castration has also been used as a punishment in the past for men who have raped or sexually abused others.

Voluntary Surgical Castration of Sex Offenders

In more modern times, some experts view surgical castration as a means of treatment for sexually violent predatory offenders who are likely to repeat their crimes without this treatment. Although studies are mixed, in most cases, studies of men incarcerated for sexual offenses who were subsequently surgically castrated compared to those who were not castrated show that the castrated men have a significantly lower rate of reoffending.

In considering the recidivism (reoffending) rates of sex offenses committed by surgically castrated men in studies performed in the United States and Europe, the rates range from zero to about 10%. For example, in one study in Switzerland in 1973, of castrated sex offenders compared to non-castrated sex offenders, with a follow-up period ranging from five to 35 years, the castrated offenders had a recidivism rate of about 7%. The comparison group of male sex offenders who were *not* castrated had a recidivism rate of 52%, or more than seven times greater.

Of course, most men greatly dislike the idea of being surgically castrated, but some sex offenders willingly choose the option of castration because they believe that they are more likely to be let out of jail, less likely to be required to receive psychological counseling or to be ordered into a civil commitment program and also less likely to reoffend.

Studies on sexual predators from the 1930s to the modern times were discussed in a 2005 article in the *Journal of the American Academy of Psychiatry Law*. These studies indicated that a bilateral orchiectomy greatly reduced the ability for men to have an erection, although it did not eliminate erections and/or sexual desire in some men exposed to sexually stimulating material.

Chemical Castration

It is also possible to achieve a "chemical castration" with drugs that suppress testosterone, such as Depo-Provera (medroxyprogesterone acetate) or Depo-Lupron (leuprolide acetate), and some studies have shown that Trelstar (triptorelin), a drug used outside the United States, is effective at suppressing testosterone levels; however, in order for any form of chemical castration treatment to be effective, the individual must be monitored to ensure that he is actually taking his medication. Some men thwart their treatment by obtaining drugs that counteract the effects of suppressive drugs, thus restoring their sexual potency. These individuals have an increased risk of reoffending.

According to an article on pedophilia in the *Journal of the American Medical Association* in 2002, "Although these drugs suppress the intensity of libidinal drive, they generally allow erectile function, thereby making intercourse with an age-appropriate partner possible. Persons receiving testosterone-lowering medication should be maintained on a treatment protocol that includes a complete medical examination with appropriate laboratory testing yearly."

They also added that "The primary goal of sex drive–lowering medications in pedophilia is to enhance the capacity to exercise appropriate self-control. These medications should not be denied to persons who fear losing control or who appear to be at risk of failing a more conservative treatment approach. Incarcerated persons with this disorder may also benefit from such care to the extent that they can be relieved of intrusive pedophilic sexual preoccupations and urges."

See also CIVIL COMMITMENT LAWS; PEDOPHILIA; SEX OFFENDERS, CONVICTED.

Fagan, Peter J., et al. "Pedophilia." *Journal of the American Medical Association* 288, no. 19 (November 20, 2002): 2,458–2,465.

Weinberger, Linda E., et al. "The Impact of Surgical Castration on Sexual Recidivism Risk among Sexually Violent Predatory Offenders." *Journal of the American Academy of Psychiatry Law* 33, no. 1 (2005): 16–36.

categorical aid Government financial aid provided to individuals in different categories, e.g., children in low-income families or disabled individuals, is known as categorical aid. Categorical aid is one response to societal child abuse and neglect.

In the United States, most categorical aid available to children and their families is authorized under the Social Security Act. Title IV of the act provides for payments to low-income families with children. This program, known as Temporary Aid to Needy Families (TANF), is designed to allow single parents to care adequately for children in their own homes.

celiac syndrome A condition in which gluten, a protein found in grains, is incompletely absorbed by the intestines. Symptoms of celiac syndrome can include diarrhea, GROWTH FAILURE, anorexia, irritability and a distended abdomen. Celiac disease is one of several malabsorption problems that can cause organic FAILURE-TO-THRIVE SYNDROME in infants.

central registry, abuse A central place within the state where records are kept regarding individuals accused of child abuse or neglect and/or those with substantiated charges of child abuse or neglect. Child protection agencies and law enforcement authorities in many states maintain a central registry that is usually located in the central social services office headquarters of the state capital.

Information maintained in the registry varies from state to state, but it usually includes the names of children who have been the subject of child protection reports, the names of suspected or verified perpetrators of maltreatment and the results of past investigations and interventions.

Central registries serve several different purposes. One of the most important purposes is the documentation of past allegations of abuse and the results of previous investigations. Parents found guilty of child abuse and/or neglect often seek to avoid detection by moving frequently, bringing the child to different hospitals or physicians for the treatment of injuries (see HOSPITAL HOPPING) and providing inaccurate or misleading information to investigators if the child is re-abused in the new location and another investigation occurs. By checking a state central registry, a child protection worker can identify patterns of maltreatment that may otherwise have gone undetected. Of course, the parent may leave the state altogether, making verification of past offenses more difficult.

Central registries also allow employers to check on whether those whom they are considering hiring for jobs that are related to children, such as teachers, day-care center workers, school bus drivers, and other jobs, are *not* listed on the registry as a child abuser. Other uses of a central registry include improving the coordination of treatment and prevention efforts, monitoring the performance of child protection agencies and providing data for research and planning.

Some critics have opposed central registries because of their potential for misuse. They fear that the reputations of persons who have been wrongfully accused of child abuse may be damaged if such information is carelessly or maliciously revealed to others.

See also ABUSERS; CIVIL COMMITMENT LAWS; PARENTAL SUBSTANCE ABUSE; PEDOPHILIA; PHYSICAL ABUSE; SEX OFFENDERS, CONVICTED; SEXUAL ABUSE; SUBSTANTIATION.

central reporting agency Most areas designate one agency to receive all reports of suspected abuse or neglect. A central reporting agency is responsible for conducting an investigation of alleged abuse or assigning that duty to another appropriate agency.

In the United States each state and territory has designated an agency to receive reports of child abuse. Most jurisdictions designate a social service department; however, some have designated juvenile courts or law enforcement agencies.

cerebral palsy A number of brain syndromes that interfere with motor function are grouped under the inclusive name cerebral palsy. These syndromes may be the result of genetic traits or may be acquired through trauma, illness or nutritional deficiency. Conditions that give rise to cerebral palsy can occur before or during birth or in infancy. Low birth weight and premature birth are often contributing factors.

In addition, cerebral palsy may be induced through head injuries caused by battering or shaking. Extreme nutritional deficiency caused by neglect can also damage brain tissue, causing cerebral palsy. Victims of cerebral palsy frequently become targets for abuse by caretakers because of adults' reactions to symptomatic muscular control problems, feeding difficulty and need for additional care.

characteristics of abusing and neglectful parents See ABUSERS.

chicken hawk A slang expression for men who seek young boys as sexual partners. The boys on whom these pederasts prey are known as "chickens."

Chicken hawks represent a broad cross section of society, including both professional and working-class men. Their boy victims often come from poor families and are lured by money or gifts; some work for prostitution rings.

Organizations such as the North American Man/Boy Love Association (NAMBLA) and Great Britain's Pedofile Information Exchange have sought to legalize sex between men and boys, claiming children have a civil right to such activities.

Several newsletters with names such as *Hermes* and *Straight to Hell* help match chicken hawks with groups through which they can meet boys. In some Asian and Middle Eastern countries, boys as well as girls are openly sold into white slavery. Boys are commonplace in the brothels of these countries.

Prepubic boys who are feminine in appearance are usually preferred; however, many adolescent boys also serve as prostitutes.

See also CHILD PROSTITUTION; PEDERASTY.

chickens A slang name for boys used by pederasts. The term usually refers to boys who have not yet reached puberty.

See also CHICKEN HAWK.

child The term *child* is used generally to refer to a person, from birth to the legal age of maturity. Age of legal maturity varies from state to state and from country to country. Some states consider anyone who has a developmental disability—regardless of age—as a child. In the United States, the CHILD ABUSE PREVENTION AND TREATMENT ACT OF 1974 defines a child as anyone under age 18.

child, battering See BATTERING CHILD.

child, best interest of See BEST INTERESTS OF THE CHILD.

child, removal of See DISPOSITION; PLACEMENT OF ABUSED CHILDREN.

child abuse Refers to the maltreatment of a child and may include physical, sexual or emotional abuse as well as child neglect.

In the United States, under the CHILD ABUSE PREVENTION AND TREATMENT ACT (CAPTA), an encompassing definition of both abuse and neglect was used subsequent to 1998: "Any recent act or failure to act on the part of a parent or caretaker, which results in death, serious physical or emotional harm, sexual abuse, or exploitation, or an act or failure to act which presents an imminent risk of serious harm." CAPTA was reauthorized with the Keeping Children and Families Safe Act in 2003.

Each state in the United States has its own definition of what constitutes abuse (See Appendix VI), and all states must have a plan for reporting child abuse statistics to state authorities.

Worldwide, there is no universally agreed upon definition of what constitutes child abuse (or child maltreatment), although each country has its own definition of child abuse. In its broadest sense, the term *child abuse* refers to any harm, physical or emotional, that is done intentionally to a child. Abuse may include physical assault, sexual exploitation and verbal or emotional assault. Some states include the presence of controlled substances in a child at birth or in the child's home as a form of child abuse. No state bans CORPORAL PUNISHMENT as of this writing, although some states prohibit extreme corporal punishment.

Child abuse also encompasses child neglect, which is the most common form of child maltreatment, and which can lead to severe injuries or even fatalities among infants and young children.

Traditionally, child abuse has been limited to the actions of a parent/guardian or other person responsible for a child's welfare. Crimes committed against children by strangers or by other children were not, strictly speaking, known as child abuse. More recently, however, child abuse statutes in many states have expanded their state laws to encompass teachers, day-care workers and others who are responsible for the out-of-home care of children.

Types of Child Maltreatment

The key types of child maltreatment are NEGLECT, PHYSICAL ABUSE, SEXUAL ABUSE and PSYCHOLOGICAL/EMOTIONAL MALTREATMENT. Most maltreated children in the United States (about 63%) suffer from neglect, followed by physical abuse (19%), sexual abuse (10%) and psychological or emotional maltreatment (5%) as well as other forms of abuse as defined by state laws. Children may also suffer from multiple forms of abuse.

Neglect

The neglect of children may be as extreme as depriving infants and young children of food, water and basic care. It also may include many other types of behaviors, such as withholding medical treatment (medical neglect) or preventing or discouraging a child from obtaining an education (educational neglect). Neglect is the most common form of child maltreatment among nearly all categories of abusers, with the one exception of abusive friends or neighbors, who are much more likely to commit sexual abuse than to neglect a child. (See Table I.)

Physical Abuse

Physical abuse of a child may be extreme—encompassing severe beatings or torture that result in fractures, disfigurement or even death—or lead to injuries that are harmful but less severe, such as beatings that cause bruising over most or all of

TABLE I
PHYSICAL ABUSE, NEGLECT AND SEXUAL ABUSE OF CHILD VICTIMS OF MALTREATMENT, 2003, BY PERCENTAGE AMONG DIFFERENT CATEGORIES OF CHILD ABUSERS

	Parent	Other relative	Foster parent	Residential facility staff	Child day-care provider	Unmarried partner of parent	Friends or neighbors
Physical abuse only	11.0	10.4	16.9	19.0	12.9	16.6	3.4
Neglect only	62.0	37.5	50.0	46.3	48.4	37.0	9.7
Sexual abuse only	2.7	29.9	6.3	11.5	23.0	11.5	75.9
Psychological maltreatment only, other only or unknown only	9.1	5.8	7.3	8.4	2.5	14.4	2.7
Multiple maltreatments	15.2	16.4	19.6	14.7	13.1	19.6	8.3
Total percent	100.0	100.0	100.0	100.0	100.0	100.0	100.0

Source: Adapted from Administration on Children, Youth and Families, *Child Maltreatment 2003.* Children's Bureau, U.S. Department of Health and Human Services, Washington, D.C., 2005, page 68.

the child's body. Repeated physical abuse is usually more harmful than a single incident; however, one severe incident of physical abuse may be sufficient to disable or kill a child. Corporal punishment is not considered a form of physical abuse by states unless it is extreme. (Each state determines what constitutes extreme corporal punishment.)

Sexual Abuse

Some children are sexually abused by others, usually those outside the family. As can be seen from Table I, of all abusive parents, less than 3% (2.7%) are sexual abusers.

Sexual abuse may include sexual intercourse, sexual touching, exposure of the genitals by the perpetrator or the child and many other examples. Some states are explicit in their definitions of sexual abuse, while others provide a general definition.

An increasing number of states now include the photographing or depicting of a child in a sexual situation for the arousal of others as a form of sexual abuse. With the popularity of the INTERNET, there are increasing opportunities for pedophiles, as well as those seeking to profit from their lust, to maltreat children sexually, whether by creating CHILD PORNOGRAPHY, exhibiting sexual photographs of minor children or even using live webcam depictions of minors engaging in sexual acts. Some adults engage in the SEXUAL TRAFFICKING of children and adolescents, in the United States and in other countries.

Psychological/Emotional Maltreatment

Psychological maltreatment (also known as emotional maltreatment) is much more difficult to define than other forms of abuse, and most state laws are vague on what constitutes this form of maltreatment. Frequently screaming at a child that she is evil and has always been an unwanted child may be one form of maltreatment. However, children are not usually removed from their homes for psychological maltreatment only. Instead this form of abuse usually accompanies another form of abuse, such as physical abuse or sexual abuse.

Some states look at the child's current outcome; for example, in the case that the child appears developmentally delayed, depressed or excessively anxious because of the parent's behavior toward the child. Compelling an abused child to lie by saying that he was *not* abused is considered emotional maltreatment in some states.

Multiple Maltreatments

Many abused children suffer from two or more forms of child maltreatment. For example, they may be both physically abused and sexually abused or both physically abused and psychologically abused. After neglect, multiple maltreatment is the most common category of abuse among parental abusers, or 15.2%. (See Table I.)

Other Forms of Abuse

Because each state defines what constitutes abuse, some states include additional categories of abuse that they incorporate under the definition of physical abuse or neglect. For example, increasing numbers of states have laws that have made the presence of alcohol or controlled drugs in a newborn infant an automatic offense of either neglect or physical abuse. In some states, if the children are in the presence of others using illegal drugs, this behavior constitutes abuse. Some states list specific drugs, such as methamphetamine, that children may not be around, and if they *are* in the presence of these drugs, that action constitutes a child abuse offense.

Fatalities among Children Who Were Abused or Neglected

In 2003, an estimated 1,500 children died of neglect or abuse in the United States, up from 1,400 children who died of maltreatment in 2002. About 79% were from zero to three years old, followed by 10% who were from four to seven years old. The other children who died were about evenly split between those who were eight to 11 years old and 12–17 years old.

Most were white (43%) or African American (31%). Infant boys younger than age one were at greatest risk, with a fatality rate of 17.7 deaths per 100,000 boys of the same age. Infant girls were also at risk, with a fatality rate of 14.1 deaths per 100,000 infant girls.

Neglect only (36%) was the primary cause of the child fatalities, followed by multiple maltreatment (29%) and physical abuse only (28%). The remaining children died from psychological maltreatment or unknown causes, as well as a small percentage (less than 1%) who died from sexual abuse.

In considering children who died and whose families had received FAMILY PRESERVATION services in the past five years, this category represented about 11% of all the child deaths. Children who had been returned to their families from the foster-care system represented about 3% of all the child deaths. As a result, about 14% of the children were known to child protective services authorities before their deaths.

Most of the children were killed by their mother only (31%) or their mother and father together (20%), followed by their father only (18%).

Victimized Children

According to statistics for 2003 (reported in 2005) by the Administration on Children, Youth, and Families, the rate of child victimization dropped from 13.4 children per 1,000 in 1990 to 12.4 children per 1,000 in 2003, a 7.5% decrease. (The reason for this decrease is unknown.)

Most child victims in 2003 were neglected (60.9%), followed by those who were physically abused (18.9%), sexually abused (9.9%), emotionally or psychologically maltreated (4.9%) or medically neglected (2.3%). Some children suffered from other or multiple forms of maltreatment as defined by state law.

Age of the Maltreated Child

Children of all ages, including adolescents, are abused; however, according to U.S. statistics on child maltreatment in 2003, infants comprised the largest single age group of all victims, and children younger than age one represented nearly 10% of all child victims. Infants and young children are also the most likely to die from abuse and/or neglectful treatment.

Gender of Abused Children

The incidence of abuse and neglect is about the same between boys (48.3%) and girls (51.7%), although girls are more likely to be sexually abused than boys.

Race of Abused Children

According to U.S. statistics in 2003, most child victims were white (53.6%), followed by African-American children (25.5%). Hispanic children rep-resented 11.5% of victims. American Indian/Alaska Native children represented about 1.7% of all victims. Asian children and Asian/Pacific Islander children represented less than 1% each of all victimized children. In considering the types of disability, however, of all victimized children, they have the greatest risk for physical abuse. (See Table I.)

In contrast, of neglected children who are Native American/Alaska Native, this group has the highest percentage of neglect (See Table III.)

Disability of the Child

Some states report on disabled children who are abused and/or neglected, and in 2003, 34 states reported on this information. Among these states, disabled children represented 6.5% of all victims. Experts believe this is most likely to be an undercount, since not every child receives a diagnostic assessment from child protective services.

Of the information that is available for states on child abuse, disabled children who were victimized included children with the following disabilities:

- Mental retardation
- Emotional disturbance
- Visual impairment
- Learning disability
- Physical disability
- Behavioral problems
- Other medical problems

Perpetrators of Child Abuse

Most child abusers are parents, with the exception of perpetrators of sexual abuse, who are usually individuals outside the family; less than 3% of parental abusers are also sexual abusers. The most common form of child maltreatment among all categories of abuse is neglect despite who the perpetrator is, with the one exception of neighbors and friends who are abusive. In that case, the most common form of abuse is sexual abuse, which represents 75.9% of all forms of abuse perpetrated by friends and neighbors. (See Table II.)

Often abusers are substance abusers of alcohol and/or illegal drugs, while others are mentally or emotionally ill or developmentally delayed (such

TABLE II
VICTIMS OF PHYSICAL ABUSE BY RACE, NUMBERS AND PERCENTAGES, 2003

Race	Number of all abuse victims	Number of physical abuse–only victims	Percentage of physical abuse–only victims
African-American	159,361	24,354	15.3
American Indian or Alaska Native	7,469	728	9.7
Asian	3,933	653	16.6
Pacific Islander	1,390	119	8.6
White	334,965	40,956	12.2
Multiple race	10,133	1,124	11.1
Hispanic	78,207	10,383	13.3
Unknown or missing	34,224	4,898	14.3
Total	629,682	83,215	13.2

Source: Adapted from Administration on Children, Youth and Families, *Child Maltreatment 2003.* Children's Bureau, U.S. Department of Health and Human Services, Washington, D.C., 2005, page 48.

TABLE III
VICTIMS OF NEGLECT ONLY BY RACE, 2003

Race	All victims	Number	Percentage
African-American	159,361	81,651	51.2
American Indian or Alaska Native	7,469	5,061	67.8
Asian	3,933	1,873	47.6
Pacific Islander	1,390	329	23.7
White	334,965	161,703	48.3
Multiple race	10,133	5,669	55.9
Hispanic	78,207	39,740	50.8
Unknown or missing	34,224	18,236	53.3
Total	629,682	314,262	

Source: Adapted from Administration on Children, Youth and Families, *Child Maltreatment 2003.* Children's Bureau, U.S. Department of Health and Human Services, Washington, D.C., 2005, page 48.

as those who are intellectually below normal and proven to be incapable of caring for a child).

About two-thirds of all perpetrators are adults in their 20s and 30s, and a few are age 50 or older. (See Table IV.)

How Children Are Maltreated

Children are maltreated in many different ways, and the means that are used to abuse the child can vary greatly, from physical force using the hands (which can cause death or permanent injury in an infant or small child) to the use of clubs, belts, irons, paddles and many other items that are used as weapons.

Even a substance as innocuous as water can cause death; a June 1999 article in *Pediatrics* reported on the deaths of three children who were forced to drink more than six liters of water as punishment, causing the children to suffer from water intoxication and then death. Because the forced water intoxication was not revealed to emergency room staff, nurses or physicians, the children were not treated for the actual cause of their medical distress, and they subsequently died.

Politics of Child Abuse

Many experts say that political issues inevitably enter into what (if anything) is done about the

TABLE IV
AGE AND SEX OF PERPETRATORS OF CHILD ABUSE IN THE UNITED STATES, 2003

Age	Men		Women		Total	
	Number	%	Number	%	Number	%
Less than 20	18,630	6.2	17,463	4.2	36,093	5.1
20–29	80,269	26.9	164,398	39.6	244,667	34.3
30–39	114,032	38.2	161,748	39.0	275,780	38.6
40–49	64,368	21.5	56,278	13.6	120,646	16.9
50+	21,402	7.2	15,220	3.7	36,622	5.1
Total	298,701	100.0	415,107	100.0	713,808	100.0

Source: Administration on Children, Youth and Families. *Child Maltreatment 2003.* Children's Bureau, U.S. Department of Health and Human Services, Washington, D.C., 2005, page 65.

problem of child abuse. Creating a program for abused children or reworking existing programs uses up money and assets that a country or a state may wish to use to resolve other problems.

In *The Politics of Child Abuse*, the authors wrote that child abuse laws are often vague and that child protective services workers are inexperienced because of a large turnover of personnel in this field. In addition, it may take weeks or months for a case to be heard by a judge.

They concluded, "Caught in this crossfire are the innocent victims of child abuse, who find themselves enmeshed in a complex web of money, power, politics and ideology that they neither understand nor care about. These children are the ones who never make it into show trials, television news shows, or tabloids—their deaths often rate only one column in the back page of a metropolitan newspaper."

See also ABUSERS; ADOLESCENT ABUSE; ADOPTING ABUSED AND NEGLECTED CHILDREN; ADULTS ABUSED AS CHILDREN; BATTERED CHILD SYNDROME; FATALITIES, CHILD ABUSE; INCEST; MEDICAL NEGLECT; MUNCHAUSEN SYNDROME BY PROXY; PSYCHOLOGICAL/EMOTIONAL MALTREATMENT; SHAKEN INFANT SYNDROME; SIBLING ABUSE.

ADMINISTRATION ON CHILDREN, YOUTH AND FAMILIES. *Child Maltreatment 2003.* Children's Bureau, U.S. Department of Health and Human Services, Washington, D.C., 2005.

Besharov, Douglas J. *Recognizing Child Abuse: A Guide for the Concerned.* New York: Free Press, 1990.

Costin, Lela B., et al. *The Politics of Child Abuse in America.* New York: Oxford University Press, 1996.

Gilbert, Neil, ed. *Combating Child Abuse: International Perspectives and Trends.* New York: Oxford University Press, 1997.

Kempe, C. Henry, and Ray F. Heifer, eds. *The Battered Child.* 3rd ed. Chicago: University of Chicago Press, 1980.

child abuse, continuum model of   See CONTINUUM MODEL OF CHILD ABUSE.

child abuse, media coverage   See MEDIA COVERAGE OF CHILD ABUSE.

Child Abuse Prevention and Treatment Act of 1974   This act, originally introduced into Congress by Sen. Walter F. Mondale, was signed into law on January 31, 1974. Its purpose was to establish the National Center on Child Abuse and Neglect (NCCAN) as part of the federal Children's Bureau and to appropriate annual funding for NCCAN.

The act was amended in 1996 (P.L. 235) by the Child Abuse Prevention and Treatment Act Amendments of 1996. As part of the amendments, the National Center on Child Abuse and Neglect ceased to be a separate agency. Instead, child abuse and neglect functions were consolidated under the Children's Bureau, which was divided into five divisions, including the Office on Child Abuse and Neglect, the Division of Policy, the Division of Program Implementation, the Division of Data, Research and Innovation and the Division of Child Welfare Capacity Building.

The federal monies provided by this act support research into the causes and consequences of child abuse and neglect, and also provide a clearinghouse for information on the incidence of child abuse in the United States. Training materials are used in prevention programs, and various technical assistance, as well as some direct support, is given to state programs. The act was most recently amended and reauthorized by the Keeping Children and Families Safe Act of 2003.

Childhood Level of Living Scale   Unlike some forms of PHYSICAL ABUSE that are easily recognized, child neglect is difficult to define. Though various statutes have attempted to define neglect, such legal definitions are often vague and too broadly defined to be of use to the average person. One reason for the difficulty in defining neglect is the absence of agreed-upon standards for child rearing. In an attempt to measure the quality of child care more accurately Norman Polansky, a professor of social work at the University of Georgia, and others have developed a scale for assessing child care.

The Childhood Level of Living Scale (CLL) was adopted for use in urban areas. It is divided into two parts, which focus on physical care and emotional/cognitive care. Part A, physical care, consists of 47 items broken down into five subcategories: general positive child care, state of repair of house, negligence, quality of household maintenance and quality of health care and grooming. Emotional/cognitive questions, part B, focus on: encouraging competence, inconsistency of discipline and coldness, encouraging superego development and material giving (to the child). Part B contains 52 items.

Families are evaluated on each item by an independent scorer. Maximum possible score on the CLL is 99. A score of 62 or less is considered indicative of neglect. Acceptable child care begins at 77. A score of 88 or higher is judged as good.

In addition to its use as a research tool, the CLL has been used by protective service workers in several areas to assess the quality of child care in a family where neglect is suspected.

For the full text of the CLL, see: Carolyn Hally, Nancy F. Polansky, and Norman A. Polansky, *Child Neglect: Mobilizing Services* (Washington, D.C.: Government Printing Office, 1980; DHHS, OHDS 80-30257).

Polansky, Norman A., Mary Ann Chalmers, Elizabeth Buttenwieser, and David P. Williams. *Damaged Parents.* Chicago: University of Chicago Press, 1981.

childhood, loss of See PARENTIFIED CHILD.

child maltreatment A general term that encompasses both the abuse and neglect of children. Federal law defines child maltreatment as a serious harm (NEGLECT, PHYSICAL ABUSE, SEXUAL ABUSE or EMOTIONAL ABUSE) that is usually caused by parents or other primary caregivers, such as baby-sitters or extended family members. In addition, child maltreatment includes harm that a caregiver did not directly inflict but that the person allowed or did not prevent from happening. In most cases, harm that is caused by acquaintances or strangers is not investigated by child protective services but is instead referred directly to law enforcement agencies.

child molester A child molester is any adult who engages in sexual activity with a child. Most molesters are male. The molester may be a stranger or may be known to the victim, as in the case of intrafamilial SEXUAL ABUSE.

The term *child molester* encompasses a wide spectrum of offenders and types of sexual exploitation. Molestation can range from verbal sexual stimulation or EXHIBITIONISM to forced rape. Contrary to the popular image of the child molester as a "dirty old man" obsessed with PEDOPHILIA, the term applies equally to customers of child prostitutes, single and repeat offenders, male and female perpetrators. Though many child molesters are pedophiles a significant number are not. Some child molesters actually prefer sex with adults and prey on children only because they are more readily available or more vulnerable.

Mental health professionals may differ from law enforcement officials in their application of this term. The former sometimes make a distinction between the child molester who attempts to coax or lure the child into sexual activity and rapists who use violence or physical force. Law enforcement officials are more likely to refer to a child molester as anyone who engages in legally prohibited sexual activity with children. In the case of convicted child sex offenders, federal law requires the registration of sex offenders with state officials. (See WETTERLING ACT.) In addition, in most states a community must be notified if a previously convicted child sex offender is moving to their community. (See MEGAN'S LAW.) The purpose of such laws is to enable parents to be more protective of their children in residential areas and to refuse contact between them and the molester. Since many molesters are repeat offenders, this seems like a logical step. Others have argued that it is a violation of the rights of the individual (the offender) in that once he has served his term, he has met his debt to society and should be allowed the life of a private citizen.

See also CIVIL COMMITMENT LAWS; PRISONS, CHILD VICTIMIZERS IN.

child pornography Material that depicts children or adolescents under age 18 engaged in explicit sexual acts or posed nude in a provocatively sexual manner. Also known as "kiddie porn." Child pornography may include written materials, photographs, drawings, films, videos, cartoons or computer graphics of children who are engaged in sexual acts or posed provocatively. Law enforcement and other experts consider child pornography to be directly linked to sexual molestation and CHILD PROSTITUTION.

Because of the ubiquity of the INTERNET and the fact that it is much more difficult to track, monitor and control than with other means of purveying child pornography (such as by mail or with a direct purchase from another person), the Internet has become a popular means to obtain such material. However, it is also illegal to purchase child pornography over the Internet, and individuals who obtain child pornography over the Internet can be prosecuted as well.

Said Finkelhor and Ormrod in their article for *Juvenile Justice Bulletin* in 2004, "Pornography that depicts actual juveniles has a very different status under the law than other types of pornography. It is not subject to first amendment protection and the more contentious standards that apply to other types of pornography. It is also regarded as having victims—the children who are depicted."

One potentially new concern is that increasing numbers of children and adolescents use cellular phones, and many phones can access Internet sites remotely, including pornographic sites. Thus, parents and other caregivers who believe that they are carefully monitoring their children's use of the Internet at home may be unaware of the potential impact of the cell phone in both the transmission and viewing of child and/or adult pornography.

Possessing Child Pornography Is Illegal

The possession of child pornography is illegal under federal law as well as under all state laws. For example, federal law prohibits sexually explicit conduct that involves a minor and also bans the depiction of children engaged in acts of sexual intercourse, bestiality and masturbation. It is illegal to purchase child pornography through the United States Postal Service, and the buyers of such material are prosecuted by law enforcement officials.

It is also illegal to take sexual photographs of children, and if the film is given to photography developers in some states, child protective services must be contacted. However, the increasing prevalence of digital cameras may enable users to skip the need for film processing because digital images can be immediately viewed as well as sent to others by cellular phone or computer.

Victimized Children

Often children are unwilling or even unknowing players in the production of child pornography. Children may be given alcohol or drugs to increase their susceptibility to victimization.

If children or adolescents know or discover that they have been used to create pornographic images or videos, they may initially believe that these images or videos made in private will remain private; they are subsequently horrified to discover that these materials are sold (or the child victims are threatened that they will be sold unless the child agrees to whatever terms that the adult victimizer demands) to others who may view them on the Internet. Children who know or suspect that there are images of themselves engaging in sexually explicit acts will often fear that others, such as family members and friends, will discover these images. As a result, they are more easily controlled by a sexual predator.

Said John Carr in his report on child abuse and child pornography in the United Kingdom,

> While rapes and sexual assaults that resulted from initial contacts in a chatroom [on the Internet] are perhaps the most extreme forms of contact-based predation, they are by no means the only forms. No reliable numbers are yet available, but we know, for example, that children have been persuaded to perform and photograph or take videos of sexual acts that they have undertaken either alone or with friends, and these images have then been sent to the abuser. Such images might later be published on the internet and become part of the stock of child abuse images that are traded between collectors or sold commercially. They can also give the abuser a greater hold over the child because they can be used to blackmail the child into per-

forming other sexual acts and into keeping the relationship a secret.

Children have also been persuaded to perform or witness sexual acts live via web cams, to watch videos online or to listen to audio files with sexual content. Sexual predators have inveigled children into abusive, sexually explicit conversations either online in chatrooms or via email or directly by voice, and these can be psychologically very damaging for the child.

Types of Offenders

According to experts Ormrod and Finkelhor in *Child Victimization,* child pornography users, as with most other users of any form of pornography, are primarily adult males. When adult females view child pornography, in nearly half of these cases (45%), the pornography was used along with a male viewer.

A study of nearly 400 state, county and law enforcement agencies in the United States was performed by Mitchell, Wolak and Finkelhor over a one-year period starting on July 1, 2000. Their research results, known as the National Juvenile Online Victimization Study, were published by the National Center for Missing & Exploited Children in 2005 and also described in the 2005 book *Child Victimization.*

In considering the demographic characteristics of the possessors of child pornography, the researchers found that most were employed full time (73%), and the largest group had incomes between $20,000 and $50,000 (41%), followed by those with incomes of less than $20,000 (18%). Most did *not* have a diagnosed mental illness (89%) or a diagnosed sexual disorder (87%). Most did *not* have known problems with drug or alcohol abuse (75%). Most had *not* been arrested for prior sexual offenses with minors (87%). As a result, the general perception that purchasers of child pornography are always or nearly always convicted SEX OFFENDERS is inaccurate.

This study revealed that most child pornography possessors were male (91%), and 86% were older than 25 years. A minority of 3% were younger than age 18.

About one-third (34%) of the arrested individuals had minor children living in their homes at the time when their crimes were committed. A total of 46% had direct access to children, either because they lived with them or because they interacted with them at work or in an organized youth activity.

Most of the child pornography that was possessed by the arrested individuals involved children ages six to 12 years old (83%), while 75% of the possessors of child pornography had images of children ages 13 to 17 years old; 39% had pornographic images of children ages three to five years old; and 19% had images of children younger than age three. (Many arrestees had pornographic images of children in more than one age group.)

The majority of offenders had mostly pictures of girls (62%), while 14% had mostly pictures of boys. In 15% of the cases, the offenders had about an equal number of pictures of girls and boys. (In 9% of the cases, the gender was unknown.)

Some offenders had a large number of images; for example, about half (48%) had more than 100 graphic images, while 14% possessed 1,000 or more such images.

Most of the offenders (91%) had downloaded child pornography using a home computer. About 18% of the arrested offenders accessed child pornography in more than one location, primarily home and work.

In most cases (57%), complaints by other individuals brought the possessors of child pornography to the attention of law enforcement, while in 43% of the cases, law enforcement investigations identified the possessors.

Possessors of child pornography appear to have a variety of motivations for their behaviors in addition to their sexual attraction to children. In an article published in Australia on the individuals who possess child pornography obtained over the Internet, published in *Psychiatry, Psychology and Law,* the authors provided some "cognitive distortions" that are often seen with these individuals.

An example of justifying behavior is seen with a statement such as, "Some children are married and having babies before they turn 16." An example of blaming others is seen with a comment such as, "The guys at work showed me where to find it. I wouldn't have gone looking for it on my own." Some users blame external factors, making such statements as "I was trying to make a point against unfair censorship and went too far" or "I was under pressure and just wanted a distraction." Some individuals state that they believe fantasy is acceptable and make a statement such as, "Just because I'm thinking about it doesn't mean I'd ever do it."

Yet according to the authors, some of their clients have contacted children. Said the authors,

> When discussing their cycle of offending behaviour, some clients have described an escalation in the severity or frequency of their behaviour. Reports have included spending increased time accessing child pornography, progressing from viewing child pornography to seeking children for sexual conversations in chat rooms, and attempting to telephone children met online. Clients have also described experiencing child fantasies more frequently or beginning to fantasise about children they know or encounter in everyday life.

Apparently in some cases, viewing child pornography online may lower the threshold of some individuals and lead them to contact children and engage in acts that they might not otherwise have considered.

Graphic Sexual Abuse Is Common

It has been speculated that some individuals are arrested for innocuous and innocent images of children who are nude but who are not portrayed in a sexual way. This appears to be incorrect based on research by Mitchell, Wolak and Finkelhor that appears in the National Juvenile Online Victimization Study, which was published by the National Center for Missing & Exploited Children in 2005 and also in the 2005 book *Child Victimization*.

The researchers found that 83% of the child pornographic images for which people were arrested were of graphic sexual abuse involving children. In the 1,713 cases of the arrested possessors of child pornography, 92% owned images that depicted the child's genitals or explicit sexual activity, while 80% owned images that showed the sexual penetration of a minor. In 71% of the cases, the images showed sexual contact between a minor and an adult, and in 21% of the cases, violence was depicted, such as rape, bondage or torture.

Said the researchers, "This suggests that offenders are not being arrested for possessing marginal or ambiguous sexual images of minors, such as images

where it is hard to ascertain whether the subject is a minor or where the context was casual nudity without sexual abuse to the child." They added, however, that "Researchers cannot extrapolate from these cases to the topic of child-pornography possession in general, however, because it is likely that more serious images would predominate among cases ending in arrests."

It should also be noted that, contrary to the belief of some, most possessors of child pornography acquired over the Internet did not have morphed pictures, or photographs that were altered using computer graphics or digital photography. Only 3% of the arrested child pornography possessors used such "morphed" images.

Child Pornography Fulfills Several Goals among Users

Child pornography serves a number of functions for the purchaser in addition to the obvious goal of sexual gratification. It may be used as a fantasy aid in pedophiles that serves as a reassurance to the pedophile that he or she is not alone in his preoccupation.

In addition, photographs of children engaged in sexual acts are often employed as a means of convincing a particular child to pose and/or engage in a sexual act with the adult. (This is known as "grooming" the child, or preparing the child to agree to engage in sexual acts.)

The molester hopes to convince the child that it is all right to engage in these acts because other children do it too. Later, photographs taken by the molester may be used as blackmail to prevent the child from telling others about the exploitation. As the child grows older and is no longer attractive to the pedophile, photographs may be exchanged with others as a means of gaining access to other children.

Some Wish to Legalize Child Pornography

Arguments for the legalization of child pornography put forth by some organizations assert that pornographic material in itself is harmless when used privately. Some have argued that depictions of adult-child and child-child relations are not harmful as long as prophylactics (condoms) are used.

Most law enforcement officers and mental health professionals strongly disagree with this assertion. Almost all pornographic material requires that children engage in or simulate an illegal act. Even artistic renderings that do not use real children as models are considered dangerous by experts who are opposed to child pornography because such drawings can be used to seduce children.

Harmful Effects of Child Pornography

Many studies have documented the harmful effects, both immediate and long term, of SEXUAL ABUSE. Sexual exploitation is, by definition, an abuse of power on the part of the adult. Though some children may appear to participate willingly, they are usually not in a position to evaluate the possible future consequences of their actions or in a position of power in which they can say "no" with ease.

See also PEDOPHILIA.

Burke, et al. "Child Pornography and the Internet: Policing and Treatment Issues." *Psychiatry, Psychology and Law* 9, no. 1 (2002): 79–84.

Carr, John. *Child Abuse, Child Pornography and the Internet.* London: NCH. Available online. URL: http://image.guardian.co.uk/sysfiles/Society/documents/2004/01/12/pornographyreport.pdf. Downloaded September 23, 2005.

Finkelhor, David, and Richard Ormrod. "Child Pornography: Patterns from NIBRS." *Juvenile Justice Bulletin.* Office of Juvenile Justice and Delinquency Prevention, Office of Justice Programs, U.S. Department of Justice, December 2004, pp. 1–8.

Mitchell, Kimberly J., Janis Wolak, and David Finkelhor. "Internet Sex Crimes against Minors." In *Child Victimization.* Kingston, N.J.: Civic Research Institute, 2005.

Ormrod, Richard K., and David Finkelhor. "Using New Crime Statistics to Understand Crimes against Children—Child Pornography, Juvenile Prostitution, and Hate Crimes against Youth." In *Child Victimization.* Kingston, N.J.: Civic Research Institute, 2005.

Wolak, Janis, David Finkelhor, and Kimberly H. Mitchell. *Child Pornography Possessors Arrested in Internet-Related Crimes: Findings from the National Juvenile Online Victimization Study.* Alexandria, Va.: National Center for Missing & Exploited Children, 2005. Available online. URL: http://www.missingkids.com/en_US/publications/NC144.pdf. Downloaded September 25, 2005.

child prostitution   Refers to children and adolescents receiving money or other items of value in exchange for engaging in sexual acts or allowing sexual acts to be performed on them. Child prostitution is a form of SEXUAL ABUSE. According to *Child Maltreatment 2003,* published in 2005, sexual abuse is defined as a type of maltreatment that refers to the involvement of the child in sexual activity to provide sexual benefit or financial benefit to the perpetrator, including contacts for sexual purposes, molestation, STATUTORY RAPE, (child) prostitution, (child) pornography, exposure, INCEST or other sexually exploitative activities.

Both girls and boys may be prostituted. Some children have had hundreds of sex partners. They usually continue a life of prostitution into adulthood.

Federal laws in the United States, as well as laws in every state, ban child prostitution. In the United States, any person who knowingly transports any child under the age of 18 years in interstate or foreign commerce or in any commonwealth, territory or possession of the United States, with the intent that the individual engage in prostitution or in any sexual activity for which any person can be charged with a criminal offense, or attempts to do so, may be fined or imprisoned. In some states, such as Maine and Wisconsin, prostituting one's child is specific grounds for the TERMINATION OF PARENTAL RIGHTS. (In other states, parental rights may be terminated for sexual abuse, abandonment and other crimes; thus, in effect, it is likely that parents in every state could lose their parental rights for prostituting their children.)

Internationally, the United Nations Convention on the Rights of the Child prohibits child prostitution. (The United States is not yet a signatory to this UN Convention.) Organizations such as End Child Prostitution, Child Pornography and Trafficking of Children for Sexual Purposes (EPCAT), formed in Stockholm, Sweden in 1996, work to end child prostitution and the sexual exploitation of children.

Said Queen Silvia of Sweden in a United Nations UNICEF report published in 2004, "Trafficking is made possible by a breakdown in the protective environment. When social, political or economic conflicts are accompanied by poor legal and justice systems, deepening poverty as well as a lack of education or economic opportunities for children and their families—not to mention the growing demand from the industrialized world for exploitive sex—children are left much more vulnerable to the prey of traffickers." Queen Silvia recommended raising awareness of child trafficking rings, enforcing existing laws and reintegrating victims of child prostitution and trafficking.

According to Willis and Levy in their 2002 article for the *Lancet*, the numbers of prostituted children worldwide may be as high as 10 million.

Child prostitutes may also be involved with CHILD PORNOGRAPHY and are more vulnerable to being exploited in this manner because they have already experienced sexual exploitation.

Some children are sexually exploited through the INTERNET, where they may be advertised for sale or for phone sex.

Child Sex Tourism

Other children are exploited by tourists who travel to countries such as Cambodia, Costa Rica, the Dominican Republic, the Philippines and Thailand, where they use and abuse adolescent and prepubescent children. Some parents advertise and prostitute their own children. In most countries (including the United States), child prostitution is illegal.

Said O'Connell Davidson in 2004 in her article on child sex tourism for the *Journal of Contemporary European Studies*, "'Ordinary' tourists who visit brothels or use street prostitutes, like 'ordinary' clients in other settings, do not necessarily care very much whether the prostitute they use is fifteen or sixteen or twenty or older, providing they fancy the look of her. The same point holds good for those tourists who find sexual partners in the informal tourist-related prostitution sector, where the bulk of child prostitution often takes place." O'Connell Davidson said the main goal of sex tourists is to enjoy themselves, and if a young teenager offers her sexual favors, they will often accept. However, it is also known that some individuals specifically seek out underage children in other countries in order to have sex with them.

Child prostitutes may work on their own or under the control of pimps or gang members. Organized crime members may be involved in the trafficking of children for sex.

The Path to Prostitution

There is little evidence to support the popular myth of the happy prostitute, particularly among children. Child prostitutes often see the selling of sexual favors as the only way that they can survive in the adult world; this is also known as "survival sex." Children addicted to drugs may be forced into prostitution in exchange for receiving drugs. Some gangs have an initiation practice requiring new members to engage in sex for money. In developing countries, impoverished children may be lured into prostitution by promises of marriage to a wealthy foreigner. In some cases, children are sold into prostitution by their own parents, who may be impoverished and see no other means of survival. Children who are runaways may perceive prostitution as their only means to stay alive.

Health and Emotional Problems

Though some may be lured into prostitution with promises of money and an exciting lifestyle, most young prostitutes suffer a great deal of abuse, unhappiness and poor health. Drug addiction, violence and suicide claim the lives of many who are prostituted as children, either during their childhood or into their adulthood.

Children and adolescents who are prostituted have a high risk of contracting the human immunodeficiency virus (HIV). In some areas, the majority of child "sex workers" are infected with HIV. Prostituted children are also at an increased risk for contracting tuberculosis as well as SEXUALLY TRANSMITTED DISEASE such as GONORRHEA, HERPES and SYPHILIS.

Child prostitutes may suffer from rapes and beatings, as with adult prostitutes. Those who manage to avoid serious physical harm are likely to bear significant psychological scars, including DEPRESSION, POST-TRAUMATIC STRESS DISORDER, extreme feelings of worthlessness and difficulty forming close relationships.

Historical Background

Throughout history, children have been sought as prostitutes. In ancient Rome and Greece, prepubescent boys were especially popular in brothels. Captain Cook, the British explorer, forbade sexual relations between members of his crew and young Polynesian women when the trading of iron nails for sexual favors threatened to destroy his ship. A sensational scandal involving child prostitution in England during the late 19th century caused Parliament to raise the legal age of sexual consent.

In the early 20th century, citizens of the United States became very disturbed over reports of unscrupulous traders who kidnapped young girls and shipped them to foreign countries where they were in great demand as prostitutes. Newspaper accounts estimated 60,000 girls were lost to "white slavery" each year. Today youthful prostitutes are still in the greatest demand, and SEXUAL TRAFFICKING of children continues worldwide, despite the efforts of private organizations and governmental entities to end this form of abuse.

Child Prostitution around the Globe

Some countries prohibit prostitution in any form, while others attempt to regulate it by imposing minimum age limits on prostitutes and requiring their registration. Both practices have resulted in various attempts to circumvent laws, including creating false identifications for young prostitutes to make them appear to be of legal age, as well as the transporting of children across governmental boundaries for purposes of their sexual exploitation in other countries.

Users of Child Prostitutes

Customers of child prostitutes are most often adult men between the ages of 40 and 65. Some are pedophiles (see PEDOPHILIA) who have an exclusive desire for sex with children. These men may go to great lengths and take significant risks to engage in sex with children. However, others are not pedophiles but instead may see the use of child prostitutes, especially while they are tourists in another country, as exotic and exciting. They may rationalize their abuse of children, assuming that the children need the money. They may have racist views that the native children are more highly sexed than children in their own country and that child prostitutes in other countries enjoy engaging in sex.

Male users of child prostitutes may also believe that children are less likely to have sexually transmitted diseases, which is an erroneous assumption, since some children engage in "raw sex" (sex without condoms) because their handlers know that such practices will earn greater fees.

Children Who Become Child Prostitutes

Many children who are not part of organized sex rings may prostitute themselves in exchange for small amounts of money, gifts, drugs, alcohol or simply companionship. Contrary to the popular image of prostitutes as exclusively female, child prostitution claims approximately equal numbers of boys and girls.

Runaways are particularly at risk of involvement in prostitution. Unable to obtain legal employment and often lonely and hungry, runaways are easy targets for recruitment by pimps and sexual traffickers. In addition, some studies of runaways show that a high percentage of them were previously sexually victimized at home. Ironically, these children may actually be running from one sexually exploitative situation to another.

Orphaned children in impoverished countries are also at risk for child prostitution; for example, according to the UNICEF report on children worldwide, of child prostitutes in Zambia, about half (47%) were orphans.

Some child prostitutes have children themselves, although little is known about what happens to these children. It is believed that in many cases, when their children reach puberty (or before then), these children are also prostituted, continuing the cycle of abuse.

See also CHILD ABUSE.

Administration on Children, Youth and Families. *Child Maltreatment 2003.* Children's Bureau, U.S. Department of Health and Human Services, Washington, D.C., 2005.

Bellamy, Carol. *The State of the World's Children 2005.* New York: United Nations Children's Fund (UNICEF), 2004.

Finkelhor, David, and Richard Ormrod. "Prostitution of Juveniles: Patterns from NIBRS." Office of Juvenile Justice and Delinquency Prevention, Office of Justice Programs, U.S. Department of Justice. Available online. URL: http://www.ncjrs.org/pdffilesl/ojjdp/203946.pdf. Downloaded September 1, 2005.

O'Connell Davidson, Julia. "Child Sex Tourism": An Anomalous Form of Movement?" *Journal of Contemporary European Studies* 12, no. 1 (April 2004): 31–46.

Ormrod, Richard K., and David Finkelhor. "Using New Crime Statistics to Understand Crimes against Children—Child Pornography, Juvenile Prostitution, and Hate Crimes against Youth." In *Child Victimization.* Kingston, N.J.: Civic Research Institute, 2005.

Willis, Brian M., and Barry S. Levy. "Child Prostitution: Global Health Burden, Research Needs, and Interventions." *Lancet* 359 (2002): 1,417–1,422.

child protection team   See MULTIDISCIPLINARY TEAM.

Children and Young Persons Acts (Britain)   Between 1908 and 1969, the passage of several parliamentary acts evolved a range of policies, procedures and agencies to meet the needs of children and youth. The first, the Children and Young Persons Act of 1908, set up a juvenile court system. The Children and Young Persons Act of 1933 brought closer together the provisions for care and treatment of delinquent as well as deprived, abused or neglected children, since delinquent children and youth had previously been viewed as a separate group with entirely separate problems. The 1933 act also established a system of alternative living arrangements for children in need of care and protection.

In 1948, the Children and Young Persons Act made it possible for the court to order specific placement for children, i.e., send a child to an approved school, place a child with a local authority or other fit person, place a child in the care of a probation officer or order a child's parent or guardian to promise proper care. The act also empowered local authorities to set up Children's Departments, which now are part of the local Social Services Department. These Children's Departments were made responsible for homes, hostels, remand homes, reception centers and special schools into which children in need of different categories of care were placed. The act shifted the courts' focus away from the punishment of abusive parents and toward enhancing the welfare of the child.

It allowed voluntary placement of children by parents and guardians as a preventative measure for "at risk" children. This eliminated the need to convict parents of a criminal act in order for children to be placed out of the home. Social workers became more active in working with families of abused children as a result of expanded roles granted them under this act.

In recognition of the importance of family in a child's life, the Children and Young Persons Act of 1963 enabled local authorities to take steps to prevent the breakdown of families, such as providing financial assistance when needed. Several years later, the Children and Young Persons Act of 1969 eliminated the approved school orders and fit person orders laid down by the 1948 act. By so doing, it placed care orders in the hands of the local authorities, leaving the court with the power to remove a child from the home but relinquishing the power to determine under whose care the child should be placed. This act also helped develop a system of community homes and facilities to replace the schools and homes designated under the 1948 act.

The Children and Young Persons Act of 1975 was an outgrowth of the much publicized inquiry into the death of Maria Colwell, a seven-year-old Brighton girl who, despite protective intervention, was beaten to death by her stepfather. It made sweeping changes in the way children under the care of the government were treated. Parliament placed increased emphasis on the use of community (foster) care and gave greater control to local authorities. By emphasizing the needs of the child over those of the parent, the act made it easier to sever parental ties and also made it less difficult for abused children to be adopted. As a result of this act, children received separate representation in court proceedings for the first time.

children as property   Traditionally, the law has treated children not as individuals with legal standing equal to that of adults but as the property of their parents or the state. When viewed as property, children have no rights to self-determination.

In earlier times, children were viewed as an economic asset. Families often depended upon their children's labor for survival. In 19th-century England and in North America children were treated in much the same way as farm animals. They could be placed in servitude, beaten and, if they consistently disobeyed, even killed by their parents. Though communities did occasionally condemn parents for cruel treatment of their children, the children themselves had no legal standing to complain about maltreatment. Indeed, some of the first child protection cases in both England and America were brought by societies organized to prevent cruelty to animals. No child protection societies existed in the U.S. or in Britain before the latter half of the 19th century.

Abused and neglected children still cannot directly petition the court for protection. Child protection agencies and the courts typically make decisions in what they believe to be the BEST INTERESTS OF THE CHILD. The child is often consulted but has little recourse if he or she disagrees with a decision.

Recent decisions by the United States Supreme Court have established that children do have some legal standing under the Constitution. *Tinker v. Des Moines,* for example, held that children have a right to free speech under the First Amendment. Still, the relationship between children under the age of legal majority and their parents is heavily tilted in favor of parents.

Some child advocates favor treating children and adults equally under the law. Others believe parents need legal power in order to protect children adequately from their own immature judgments. In the United States, courts and lawmakers have attempted to give children a status above that of property but below that of parents.

See also CHILDREN'S RIGHTS; PARENS PATRIAE; PARENTS' RIGHTS.

Children's Petition of 1669 (Britain) This appeal to the British Parliament was the first formal attempt in Britain to place legal limitations on CORPORAL PUNISHMENT of children in schools. A sequel to the petition came in 1698–1699, and it contains the passage, "There is nothing but an Act of Parliament about the education of children can deliver the nation from this evil."

children's rights When speaking of children's rights, advocates often combine the concepts of legal and moral rights. Claims for children's moral rights are usually broad statements of principle such as "All children have a right to develop to their full potential." Moral rights often are not enforceable under existing laws. Rather, they are principles whose existence is often debated. Legal rights are entitlements under existing law. The right to vote is an example of a legal right.

Children's legal rights vary from state to state and from country to country. In the United States the ages at which children may marry, obtain a driver's license, purchase alcohol or quit school differ according to locale.

In Scotland, legal rights and responsibilities of children are spelled out very specifically, including such items as when the child may go to the cinema (age seven), when he or she may be given alcohol at home (age five) and when the child is considered capable of committing a criminal offense (age eight). A legal distinction is made between prepubescent children, called "pupils," and adolescents, who are known as minors. Girls obtain minority at age 12 while boys must wait until they are 14 to be termed minors. Different treatment of girls and boys is apparently based on differences in physical maturation, although both males and females attain legal adulthood at 18 years of age.

In many countries, children are treated as the property of their parents and, as such, have no legal rights. Not until the 1960s did courts in the United States begin to consider children as individuals having constitutional rights of their own.

The first Supreme Court case to clearly establish constitutional protections for children was in IN RE GAULT.

In this 1967 ruling involving a delinquency hearing for an Arizona youth, the high court ruled that children are entitled to procedural due process under the Fourteenth Amendment. Specific due process protections include proper notice of charges, the right to counsel, the right to confront and cross-examine witnesses, privilege against self-incrimination, the right to a transcript of the proceedings and the right to an appellate review of the case.

The right to political expression was affirmed two years later in *TINKER V. DES MOINES.* Subsequent rulings in some states have invoked due process protections for dependent children who are committed to a mental institution against their wishes. Some states now allow children to sue parents for willful acts of physical violence that go beyond the limits of reasonable discipline.

Despite these protections, children are far from having legal status equal to that of adults. In *Ginsberg v. New York,* the Supreme Court affirmed that children's rights can be restricted in some instances.

Internationally, the United Nations issued a Declaration on the Rights of the Child in 1959. This document spells out 10 basic rights and freedoms of children throughout the world. Among the rights claimed for children by the United Nations declaration are the right to grow and develop in a healthy manner and freedom from abuse and neglect. Though the declaration as well as the U.N. CONVENTION ON THE RIGHTS OF THE CHILD, which was proposed in 1978, represent important philosophical and political statements, neither document affords children specific legal status or protection.

See also CHILDREN AS PROPERTY; PARENTS' RIGHTS; UNITED NATIONS DECLARATION OF THE RIGHTS OF THE CHILD, 1959.

Franklin, Bob. *The Rights of Children.* Oxford: Basil Blackwell, 1986.
Wringe, C. A. *Children's Rights.* London: Routledge & Kegan Paul, 1981.

Children's Trust Funds   Beginning in 1980, the National Committee for Prevention of Child Abuse spearheaded an effort to establish trust or prevention funds in each state. The United States Congress authorized a challenge grant program in 1985 to encourage states to establish and maintain trust funds. By 1988, 44 states had established such trusts.

The goal of the effort is to make available to community-based child abuse services a dependable source of funding. Money placed in the trust fund is usually earmarked specifically for child abuse prevention and cannot be used for other purposes. Though sources of revenue for trust funds vary, many states generate income for these projects by increasing fees for marriage licenses or divorce decrees. Since funds are held in trust, they are less susceptible to changes in government funding policy.

child slavery   See SEXUAL TRAFFICKING.

child stealing   Primarily as a result of child custody disputes, large numbers of children are victims each year of parental abduction. This phenomenon is known as child stealing or, less accurately, child snatching, to differentiate it from third-party abduction or kidnapping. The International Parental Kidnapping Crime Act of 1993, as well as similar state laws, make it a crime for a noncustodial parent to abduct a child. The Federal Bureau of Investigation is the primary agency that pursues parents who have abducted their children.

In addition to U.S. laws, the 1980 HAGUE CONVENTION ON THE CIVIL ASPECTS OF INTERNATIONAL CHILD ABDUCTION is an agreement between 48 countries, including the U.S. It established the procedures in locating or returning abducted children. About half of the abductions of children from the U.S. are to member countries. The State Department is the central authority for the United States.

In 1983, Richard J. Gelles, a sociologist who specializes in family violence, published survey results indicating the probability that between 459,000 and 751,000 such abductions per year occurred among American families. Further, Gelles's research suggested that large numbers of child stealing cases involve more than one child per family. He also indicated that households other than that of the child and the parent are often involved. These other households typically include grandparents, uncles, aunts and other relatives and may include professionals such as lawyers, teachers, police officers and private detectives.

As a result, separate states adopted the UNIFORM CHILD CUSTODY JURISDICTION ACT, and the U.S. Congress worked to support individual states' efforts at cutting down on parental child stealing by passing the Federal Parental Kidnapping Prevention Act and the International Parental Kidnapping Crime

Act of 1993. This law makes parental abduction a federal felony.

In 1994, the Justice Department created a Missing and Exploited Children's Task Force to help state and local authorities with difficult cases. In 1997, the task force established the Subcommittee on International Child Abduction. In 1998, the U.S. Attorney General created the Policy Group on International Parental Kidnapping.

Experts have identified some problems with the statutes. In a statement before the Committee on International Relations of the U.S. House of Representatives on October 14, 1999, Jess T. Ford, associate director of international relations and trade issues, national security and international affairs, pointed out several major problems including:

- Gaps in federal services to the left-behind parents, thus making it difficult for them to recover their abducted children. One parent told the General Accounting Office he spent more than $200,000 pursuing the return of his abducted child while the foreign government where his child was taken to paid the abducting parent's full legal expenses.

- Weaknesses within the State Department's case-tracking process which impair case coordination

- Lack of aggressive diplomatic efforts to improve international responses to parental child abductions

- Limited use of the International Parental Kidnapping Crime Act of 1993 in pursuing abducting parents. State attorneys general may be reluctant to use the federal law. Only 62 abducting parents were indicted as of 1999 and of these, 13 parents were convicted of felony parental kidnapping.

The disruption in a child's life that results from abduction by a parent or other family member is considered by most experts to be quite serious and to have a long-term, negative effect. Besides a child's home life, his or her school life and general social development are seriously affected by the abrupt and invariably confusing incidents surrounding parental abduction. Some children who are taken from, but subsequently retrieved by, the custodial parent are described as hostile, frightened and physically unhealthy following their return to the custodial home.

Agopian, Michael W. *Parental Child Stealing.* Lexington Mass.: Lexington Books, D.C. Heath, 1981.

Chesler, Phyllis. *Mothers on Trial: The Battle for Custody and Children.* New York: McGraw-Hill, 1986.

Gelles, Richard J. "Parental Child Snatching: A Preliminary Estimate of the National Incidence." *Journal of Marriage and the Family* (August 1984): 735–739.

Katz, Sanford N. *Child Snatching: The Legal Response to the Abduction of the Children.* Chicago: ABA Press, 1981.

Lawrence, Bobbi, and Olivia Taylor-Young. *The Child Snatchers.* Boston: Charles River Books, 1983.

China, People's Republic of The *Country Reports on Human Rights Practices*, released by the United States State Department in 2005 on behavior that occurred in 2003 and 2004, reported on child abuse and other human rights problems in China. According to the China Society for Human Rights, cited in the report, two-thirds of Chinese children are victims of family violence during their lives.

The Population and Family Planning Law regulates population control. Most married couples are limited to having one child only, and it is illegal for single women to bear children in most provinces. One province, Jilan Province, passed a law in 2002 making it permissible for a single woman to bear a child if she intended to remain single for life.

If a married couple has a second child in a province that limits children to one child per family, they may be given heavy financial penalties, such as one-half to 10 times the annual income of the average worker. In some cases, there is strong pressure, or it may be mandatory, to abort the second pregnancy.

Because sons are much more highly valued than daughters, female fetuses are often aborted once identified as females, and many females who are born are abandoned at birth. This has resulted in a skewed population of male children and adolescents, and as a result, there are insufficient numbers of Chinese females for Chinese men to marry. Some consequences of the shortage of Chinese females are that some female children, adolescents and young women are kidnapped and sold to Chinese men for marriage. Some infants are even sold as future laborers or as future wives.

Some Chinese children are adopted by families in other countries; for example, 7,044 children from China were adopted by citizens of the United States in 2004, representing nearly a third of all international adoptions worldwide. Most children adopted from China are females. The few males who are adopted by individuals in other countries usually have disabilities or medical problems.

There is reportedly a high rate of SUICIDE among Chinese girls and women. According to the *Country Report,* "Many observers believed that violence against women and girls, discrimination in education and employment, the traditional preference for male children, the country's birth limitation policies, and other societal factors contributed to the especially high female suicide rate."

Abuse and Abandonment of Children

The mistreatment or abandonment of children is illegal in China under the Law on the Protection of Juveniles; however, it was estimated in 1994, the latest figures available in 2004, that 1.7 million children are abandoned each year. The numbers of abandoned children may have increased since then.

Many Chinese children reside in orphanages, and most are girls or ill or disabled boys. The government denies that children in orphanages are mistreated but acknowledges that it is often not possible to provide medical care to all the children, especially those with serious health problems. In 1997, a revision of the adoption law made it possible for Chinese citizens to adopt a child, but the adopted child was counted toward the one-child-per-family limitation, which may have discouraged some Chinese families from adopting a child.

In some cases, the needs of children are ignored. For example, in 2003, a three-year-old girl starved to death when her mother was arrested and detained for stealing two bottles of shampoo, despite the mother's pleas for someone to check on her child. Two police officers were arrested and sentenced with two to three years in prison.

In 2004, two cities, Guangzhou and Chengdu, established China's first juvenile courts. An estimated 69,780 juveniles were arrested in 2003, and about 19,000 children were imprisoned.

Homeless children are a problem in China, and an estimated 150,000 children live on the streets. Most survive by begging.

Some Chinese children are forced into CHILD PROSTITUTION, especially in urban areas, while other children are sold into forced labor.

The Law on the Protection of Juveniles bans INFANTICIDE in China; however, few doctors are charged, and there are indications that this practice is a continuing problem, primarily because of the strong preference for healthy boys.

Trafficking in Children

According to the *Country Report,* trafficking in women and children is against the law; however, China is both a source country and an interim country for trafficked humans, primarily females. Most trafficking is internal and often done for the purposes of providing brides or sons to lower-middle-income farmers. Because of betrothal fees, it is financially more attractive for some men to buy a bride (often without her consent and knowledge beforehand).

In some cases, crime gangs kidnap girls and women or trick them by telling them that they will provide them with jobs, after which the gang members then sell the females to the buyers. Once in their new area, adolescents and women are forcibly married and then raped.

The Ministry of Public Security estimates that 1,000 children are kidnapped and sold per year. In one case that occurred in 2003, officials discovered 28 female infants placed in suitcases, where they were to be sold to become child brides or to work when they were older. The oldest infant was five months old. One child died. Two of the leaders of the baby-selling scheme were given a death sentence.

Traffickers also sometimes purchase children directly from their parents, lying to them that the children eventually will be able to send money to their poor parents.

Trafficking of girls and women from other countries into China, from Burma, Laos, North Korea, Vietnam and Russia, occurs. Often North Korean girls and women who are sold are forced to become prostitutes or brides. North Korean brides were reportedly sold for $38 to $150 each in 2003.

See also SEX TRAFFICKING.

Bureau of Democracy, Human Rights, and Labor. *Country Reports on Human Rights Practices, 2004: China.* United States State Department, released on February 28, 2005. Available online. URL: http://www.state.gov/g/drl/rls/hrrpt/2004/41640.htm. Downloaded September 1, 2005.

chylous ascites When chyle, a milky substance normally absorbed during the process of digestion, accumulates in the peritoneal cavity, the resulting condition is known as chylous ascites. This condition can occur as a result of physical anomalies, obstruction of the thoracic duct or injury. It is sometimes observed in children who have experienced abdominal trauma as a result of battering.

circumstantial evidence See EVIDENCE.

civil commitment laws Laws that provide for sexually violent predators (SVPs) to be involuntarily and civilly committed to an institution subsequent to serving their jail sentences. In some states, the institution is the prison itself, while in other states, the sexually violent predator is treated in a mental hospital or other secure facility. In Texas, the civilly committed person is treated on an outpatient basis, and the offender is monitored electronically; in all other states, the individual remains in the facility.

Civil commitments are made because these individuals are deemed to be a serious threat to society, in that it is believed that they will recommit the sexually violent acts if they are freed from prison. Many of these individuals are pedophiliacs, while others have sexually assaulted adults. All are expected to commit these crimes again upon their release from prison without a civil commitment.

According to Miller et al. in their 2005 article in *Law and Human Behavior,* more than 2,500 sexually violent predators have been civilly committed since the late 20th century, and an additional several thousand more have been evaluated for possible commitment.

The first civil commitment laws were passed in the late 1930s and were used at that time to treat sexually violent predators instead of incarcerating

them. It was believed that such individuals were too sick to be rehabilitated in a prison system, and consequently, they needed psychiatric hospitalization instead. By 1960, 25 states had enacted similar civil commitment laws for sex offenders; however, after that time, states began to abandon these laws, largely because psychiatric commitment alone had proved to be ineffective in treating sexually violent predators.

Civil commitment laws became of interest again in the latter part of the 20th century, when the offenses of some individuals who had committed sexually violent acts became widely known to the public. Rather than concentrating on attempts to treat the sexual offender, the new laws were created to protect the public from him. (All or nearly all individuals who are civilly committed as sexual offenders are males.)

Washington was the first state to pass a new type of civil commitment law, which required the continued incarceration of convicted sexually violent predators in an institution *after* the serving of their sentences, under the 1990 Community Protection Act. This law was passed after public horror over several extremely violent crimes. For example, Earl Shriner, a retarded man, was released from prison in 1987. Shriner had a long history of sexual assault, kidnapping and murder. While in prison, Shriner described his plan to cage and sexually torture children. Two years after his release, Shriner kidnapped a seven-year-old boy whom he raped, strangled, sexually mutilated and left to die. In another case, an adult female was kidnapped and killed by Gene Raymond Kane, a man who was on a work release from his 13-year sentence for attacking two women.

These cases mobilized the public to seek changes in the laws and led to the passage of a civil commitment statute, which enabled the state to retain and treat repeat sex offenders indefinitely.

Sixteen states have civil commitment laws as of this writing, including Arizona, California, Florida, Illinois, Iowa, Kansas, Massachusetts, Minnesota, Missouri, New Jersey, North Dakota, South Carolina, Texas, Virginia, Washington and Wisconsin.

The Kansas U.S. Supreme Court Cases
As mentioned, the first sex-offender civil commitment law that required continued incarceration of offenders was passed in the state of Washington

in 1990. However, it was the state of Kansas whose civil commitment law was challenged in the courts. This law was subsequently upheld by the U.S. Supreme Court in 1997, and, consequently, it is considered a very important law by experts.

In *Kansas v. Hendricks,* 117 S.Ct. 2072 (1997), Leroy Hendricks, the offender, challenged the civil commitment law. According to Dr. Grinage in his article in 2003 for the *Journal of Forensic Science,* Hendricks had been previously convicted of indecent exposure, lewdness, molestation of young boys and the sexual assault of a young boy and girl. The jury decided that Hendricks, who had also been diagnosed with pedophilia, met the criteria for a sexually violent predator. Hendricks appealed and the Supreme Court of Kansas reversed the lower court. The case was further appealed by the state to the U.S. Supreme Court.

Hendricks had stated that the only way that he could control his pedophiliac impulses was to die. The Supreme Court ruled that, "This admitted lack of volitional control, coupled with a prediction of future dangerousness, adequately distinguishes Hendricks from other dangerous persons who are perhaps more properly dealt with exclusively through criminal proceedings."

The Supreme Court found that the Kansas law was a civil proceeding rather than a criminal one and thus was not equivalent to double jeopardy (being punished twice for the same crime), nor was it a violation of due process. As a result, the Kansas civil commitment law was upheld.

In a subsequent case, *Kansas v. Crane,* heard by the U.S. Supreme Court in 2002, the Kansas civil commitment law was again challenged. Michael Crane argued that the statute mandated a complete lack of control on the offender's part and that he had some control. The Supreme Court established that a total lack of control was not necessary but rather only "serious difficulty" in maintaining control was sufficient to civilly commit the violent sex offender. As a result, the civil commitment law was again upheld.

In Miller et al., the authors added further:

With respect to the civil commitment of dangerous sexual offenders under the statute, the Federal Constitution required the state to prove that such offenders have serious difficulty in controlling their behavior. Such required proof—when viewed in light of such features of the case as the nature of the psychiatric diagnosis and the severity of the mental abnormality itself—had to be sufficient to distinguish the dangerous sexual offender whose serious mental illness, abnormality, or disorder subjected the offender to civil commitment from the dangerous but typical recidivist convicted in an ordinary criminal case.

States Have Used Kansas Law as a Model

Most states have modeled their laws on the Kansas statutes that relate to civil commitment. Said Jackson and her colleagues in her 2004 article in the *International Journal of Forensic Mental Health,* "Most SVP statutes are similar to the Kansas statute and share four common elements: (a) a past act of sexually harmful conduct, (b) a current mental disorder or abnormality, (c) a finding of risk of future sexually harmful conduct, and (d) some connection between the mental abnormality and the potential sexual harm." In addition, most state laws require that the individual has already been convicted or at least charged with a sexually violent crime.

Evaluating Potential Reoffenders

It can be difficult for mental health professionals to determine which offenders will reoffend. Some experts believe that *all* individuals who are diagnosed with pedophilia will inevitably reoffend, and thus they should all be civilly committed. Others believe that some form of evaluation instrument should be developed to differentiate likely reoffenders from those who may recover.

The presence of a psychiatric diagnosis is crucial, said Jackson et al., who stated, "The importance of the legal mental abnormality requirement in SVP statutes cannot be understated as it is the fundamental principle upon which civil commitment laws rest."

It is important to note that both a diagnosed psychiatric disorder and a lack of control are together not sufficient to justify civil commitment in most states. According to Jackson et al., the "key element is that the abnormality *causes* the lack of control."

One indication of an increased risk of reoffending is if the sexually violent predator is diagnosed as psychopathic. Psychopathic individuals are usually considered untreatable, as they do not experience regret or guilt for their behavior. According to Edens et al. in the *International Journal of Forensic Mental* Health in 2002, "Emotionally, psychopaths lack empathy for others or guilt for their misdeeds, and they have difficulty forming strong affective bonds. Behaviorally, psychopaths tend to be irresponsible and prone to criminality. Interpersonally, psychopaths are grandiose, callous, and deceitful."

In their retrospective study of incarcerated male sex offenders, Edens et al. included 55 incarcerated male sex offenders and 37 males who were being considered for civil commitment. The researchers found that the men who were psychopathic sex offenders had an increased risk for reoffending.

However, it is important to note that psychopathy is not a necessary condition among pedophiles and that pedophiles who are *not* psychopathic may commit their crimes again. In many cases, individuals who have been civilly committed were diagnosed with pedophilia rather than psychopathic behavior.

Jackson et al. pointed out that it is not sufficient to identify offenders who are likely to commit any form of violence, but rather it must be sexual violence that they are most likely to commit.

Pros and Cons of Civil Commitment Laws

Proponents of civil commitment laws say that they are needed to protect children (and adults) from repeat violent offenders, some of whom are quite open about stating that they will "do it again." Supporters believe that such individuals are a serious danger to society and specifically to the children living in society.

Those who are skeptical of such laws believe that they exemplify double jeopardy, despite the finding of the U.S. Supreme Court, and some have also stated their fear that involuntary civil commitment laws might be expanded to other crimes at some time in the future. In addition, opponents point to the high cost of civil commitments to the taxpayers. For example, according to Beyer Kendall and Cheung, "Alabama anticipates spending between $10 and $12 million for new construction at a cost of $70,000 per offender per year. Florida estimated costs of $27 million during the third year of its program. These examples provide insight into the cost/

benefit factors that may contribute to or hinder the success of civil commitment programs."

See also CASTRATION; IMPULSE CONTROL; MEGAN'S LAW; PEDOPHILIA.

Beyer Kendall, Wanda D., and Monit Cheung. "Sexually Violent Predators and Civil Commitment Laws." *Journal of Child Sexual Abuse* 13, no. 3 (2004): 41–57.

Edens, et al. "Psychopathy and Institutional Misbehavior among Incarcerated Sex Offenders: A Comparison of the Psychopathy Checklist-Revised and the Personality Assessment Inventory." *International Journal of Forensic Mental Health* 1, no. 1 (2002): 49–58.

Falk, Adam J. "Sex Offenders, Mental Illness and Criminal Responsibility: The Constitutional Boundaries of Civil Commitment." *American Journal of Law & Medicine* 25, no. 1 (Spring 1999): 117–147.

Grinage, Bradley D., M.D. "Volitional Impairment and the Sexually Violent Predator." *Journal of Forensic Science* 48, no. 4 (July 2003): 1–8.

Jackson, Rebecca L., Richard Rogers, and Daniel W. Shuman. "The Adequacy and Accuracy of Sexually Violent Predator Evaluations: Contextualized Risk Assessment in Clinical Practice." *International Journal of Forensic Mental Health* 3, no. 2 (2004): 115–129.

Kennedy Bailey, Rahn, M.D. "The Civil Commitment of Sexually Violent Predators: A Unique Texas Approach." *Journal of the American Academy of Psychiatry Law* 30 (2002): 525–532.

Miller, Holly A., Amy E. Amenta, and Mary Alice Conroy. "Sexually Violent Predator Evaluations: Empirical Evidence, Strategies for Professionals, and Research Directions." *Law and Human Behavior* 29, no. 1 (February 2005): 29–54.

"What Are States Doing to Confine Dangerous Sex Offenders?" *State Legislatures* 25, no. 3 (March 1999): 52.

civil court   See COURT.

civil proceeding   Sometimes referred to as a civil action, this term describes any lawsuit that is not a criminal prosecution. Juvenile court cases and family court (or domestic relations court) cases fall under the general description of civil proceedings, as do probate court cases. Child abuse and neglect cases can be civil or criminal proceedings. Criminal proceedings concern punishment of abusers while civil proceedings usually focus on matters pertaining to the child's well-being. Each state handles abuse and neglect cases differently, assigning a case to a court depending on a variety of judicial factors or criteria.

See also COURT.

clear and convincing evidence   See EVIDENTIARY STANDARDS.

clergy, sexual abuse by   Members of the clergy who sexually abused children in their parish. Clergymen primarily abused adolescent males, but some abused both male and female children. This problem first became known to the general public in the 1980s, and extensive media reports of cleric child abuse continued into the 1990s; sporadic reports still appear. Many lawsuits were filed by adults who alleged abuse in their childhood. For example, in 2003 in California alone, 800 lawsuits were filed by individuals alleging cleric sexual abuse. Expert estimates of the percent of all Catholic priests who had sexually abused children from the 1950s to 2002 range from 2 to 4% of all priests. (Note that the converse is true, or that 96 to 98% of priests did *not* sexually abuse children.)

Experts estimate that 4,392 priests abused children from the 1950s to 2002, and of these, about 149 priests were alleged to have victimized 10 or more children each. These serial abuser priests were responsible for nearly one-third of all the allegations of child sexual abuse incidents in the United States. It is estimated by experts that 10,667 children and adolescents alleged having been abused by priests from 1950 to 2002. About 10% of these allegations were not substantiated. (This does not mean that the allegations were untrue, but rather that it was not determined whether they were true or false.) Also, in about 20% of the allegations, the priest was either inactive or dead, so no investigation occurred, an outcome which distressed the alleged victims.

In some cases in the past, if it became known that a priest was alleged to have molested a child or children, he was simply moved by his bishop to another parish, where the sexual abuse usually continued unabated. Some abusers were moved repeatedly, but often with the same effect: continued child sexual abuse.

Some abusers were sent to treatment centers, but the "cure" rate for child SEX OFFENDERS is generally low.

It should also be noted that not all members of the clergy who are also sexual offenders are Catholic priests, and some were members of other religious denominations; however, most information on members of the clergy who have committed child sex abuse is based on cases of abusers who were Catholic priests. In addition, the sexual abuse perpetrated by Catholic priests occurred for so many years and on such a large scale, often with the knowledge of the church hierarchy, that this scandal was particularly shocking to many people.

Some Examples of Serial Abusers

Recent research has revealed that most priest abusers did not abuse large numbers of children. However, there were some serial abusers who were flagrant. In 2002, it was revealed by the media that Father John Geoghan, a serial pedophile in the Boston archdiocese, had been transferred from parish to parish, although there were many complaints of child molestation against him. One hundred and fifty adults complained that Geoghan had fondled or raped them.

The first complaint about Geoghan's sexual abuse of a child had been received in 1979, and additional reports were received in the 1980s and the 1990s. Yet he was not suspended from priestly duties until 1998. In 2002, Geoghan was arrested for molesting a boy in a swimming pool. He was convicted of molestation and sent to prison for nine to 10 years. In 2003, Geoghan was murdered in prison.

Another flagrant abuser was James R. Porter, a priest who reportedly abused about 200–300 children over 20 years, including about 100 boys and girls in three parishes where he served. He was sent to a treatment center in 1967, but the sexual abuse of boys continued after he left treatment. In 1993, Porter received a prison sentence of 18–20 years for his abuse offenses.

Cardinal Law publicly acknowledged in Boston in 1984 that he had relocated priests accused of sexual abuse to new parishes. In 2002, amid the wake of continued reports of priests who had committed child sexual abuse and the public outcry that continued, Cardinal Law resigned from his position as archbishop of Boston.

Of course, it should be noted that not all cleric abusers were in Boston, and there were complaints from dioceses nationwide from alleged victims of past child sexual abuse by priests.

There were so many lawsuits in the diocese of Boston that the church filed for Chapter 11 protection, according to Thomas Plante in his 2004 article for *Ethics & Behavior*. Plante said that in 2002, an estimated 350 priests in the United States were charged with child sexual abuse accusations that were credible.

The Response of Church Leaders

In 2001, Pope John Paul II e-mailed a public apology for the cleric perpetrators of child sexual abuse and said, "Sexual abuse by some clergy has caused great suffering and spiritual harm to the victims. . . . Sexual abuse within the church is a profound contradiction of the teaching and witness of Jesus Christ. . . . The synod fathers wish to apologize unreservedly to the victims for the pain and disillusionment caused to them."

As Cynthia Crosson-Tower said in her book *Understanding Child Abuse and Neglect,* "The hierarchy so central to the administration of this denomination is encumbered with numerous layers of authority amidst which reports of clergy misconduct can be lost. Instead of being answerable to their parishes, as is the case in many denominations, Catholic priests work for their bishops. If a bishop does not know what is transpiring at the parish level, or if he chooses not to respond, an abusive priest may be allowed to continue his perpetration. And, traditionally, priests were seen as representatives of God and therefore not subject to public scrutiny."

Plante agreed that the ethical obligations of the superiors of abusive priests is an important issue to consider, and said, "The lesson that may be especially important to grasp is that church leaders, such as bishops and other religious superiors, have not adequately managed clergy sexual abuse issues when it has come to their attention."

He also added, "Certainly religious superiors are culpable if they were aware of problematic abusive behavior among priests under their supervision and failed to responsibly manage the wayward priest to minimize additional harm. Many have complained that bishops and other religious superiors were too focused on preventing scandals from receiving press or legal attention or were too willing to minimize and deny the impact of clergy sexual abuse behavior."

Motivations of Clergy Abusers

Some experts say that the clergy offers some benefits that are uniquely suited to perpetrators who are also sex offenders.

For example, members of the clergy receive the respect of their community, while at the same time, they often receive unquestioned acceptance. They are often held apart from the community in the minds of many people, which also offers the perpetrator the benefit of social isolation. (See the table for a comparison of what is offered in the priesthood and ministry compared to the potential benefits for abusive members of the clergy.)

Some priests may have felt "safe," knowing that unless their ordination was in some way deficient, within the Catholic Church a priest is a priest for life. However, this does mean that church leaders had no way to act. They could withdraw the abusive priest from a public ministry. This is more difficult with a diocesan priest, who typically has a parish, but it is possible.

Impact of Sex Abuse Perpetrated by Priests on the Victims

The impact of sexual victimization by a priest or other member of the clergy is often profound. Many victims said that they lost their faith and their interest in spiritual matters. Some of the incidents of abuse occurred during confession or in relation to other religious rituals, making some victims feel that they could not hold any religious belief, because of the traumatic association with the sexual abuse perpetrated by the priest, who may have been considered an intermediary to God. Some victims wondered why God was "punishing" them.

Some male victims questioned their sexuality, reporting that they felt they must be homosexual because of the abuse, even if their sexual inclinations were heterosexual. Females also may have developed long-lasting sexual dysfunction, in part

TABLE I
COMPARISON OF THE OFFERINGS OF AN ECCLESIASTICAL CAREER AND THE NEEDS OF PERPETRATORS

What is offered by the priesthood/ministry	What an offender searches for
Respected as priest or a member of clergy	Unquestioned acceptance/respect
Due to faith of parishioners, usually unquestioned	
Due to profession, is elevated in status	Respect in the community
Held apart from general community in minds of most	Some isolation from general community
Authority based on a higher power, an association that makes him powerful	Power
Head of the congregation	Control
Contact with youths in a variety of ways, often unsupervised, with the trust of both parents and youths	Opportunity with children
Under the protection of the "Mother Church," also nurtured by parishioners	An all-loving parent or nurturance
Provided with housing and structure in daily tasks	Limited self-care responsibility
Celibacy in some denominations. Ethical concern for not becoming romantically involved with congregation in others	Threatened by adult relationships and prefers not to have them on an intimate level

Source: Crosson-Tower, Cynthia. *Understanding Child Abuse and Neglect.* 6th ed. Boston: Allyn and Bacon. Copyright © 2005 by Pearson Education. Reprinted by permission of the publisher.

because they had perceived the priest as a father figure, even calling him "Father." Victims also suffered from some or all of the many effects of sexual abuse in childhood, such as depression, substance abuse, eating disorders and so forth. Some victims of clergy abuse have committed suicide.

Often in past years, if sexually abused victims reported the abuse to their parents or others, they were not believed, since it seemed impossible to others, including their parents, that a trusted member of the clergy could perform such behavior. Some of these individuals were pathologized by others, who believed and may have stated that the child or adolescent must be emotionally disturbed to have made such a charge of sexual abuse against their priest. If the children were believed, some were blamed for the abuse themselves. These reactions were very painful to already victimized children.

Reaction of the Catholic Church

When the massive scale of the child sexual abuse perpetrated by some priests was evident to the general public, the church took action, albeit much

slower than many people would have preferred. They studied the extent of the problem before taking major action in about 2002; for example, in 2002, it was reported that 700 priests were removed from the ministry, which was about 2% of all priests at that time.

In 2002, the United States Conference of Catholic Bishops voted for the Charter for the Protection of Children and Young People, which acknowledged the crisis caused by both the abuse of children by priests and the past response of bishops.

Seminaries began actively screening prospective priests, in contrast to past years, to attempt to ensure that seminarians could and would maintain a celibate lifestyle. In 2002, the church adopted a "zero-tolerance" policy, in that no priest who had sexually abused a minor could continue as a priest. Bishops were to consult with lay review boards to evaluate abuse allegations and determine whether the priest could remain in the ministry.

According to *A Report on the Crisis in the Catholic Church in the United States* from the National Review Board for the Protection of Children and Young People, most dioceses adopted policies that taught adults how to recognize the signs of child abuse and also taught parents to instruct their children to report if they were abused.

This report also stated that the sexual abuse of a minor is both a "serious canonical crime and a grievous sin." They noted that in long past years, such behavior was condemned. For example, in A.D. 1178, according to the report, clerics who "engaged in pederasty or sodomy were to be 'dismissed from the clerical state or else confined to monasteries to do penance.'" In 1566, a papal decree ordered that any cleric guilty of "crimes against nature" was to be given over to the secular authorities for punishment by them. In both the 1917 version of the Code of Canon Law and the 1983 version (Canon 1395), any cleric who committed an act of sexual abuse against a minor was to be dismissed. However, Canon 1395 was rarely enforced in the United States.

In 1992, a policy statement called the Five Principles, was issued that stipulated that allegations of abuse should be promptly investigated if it was reasonable that abuse could have occurred. If the investigation determined that the abuse was likely, the cleric would be removed from all ministerial duties.

The obligations and requirements of civil law were to be obeyed and any abuse reported to the authorities. Victims and their families were to be contacted. However, these Five Principles were not binding, and only an estimated half of all dioceses implemented a policy regarding sexual abuse.

The Issue of Homosexuality

Some experts have blamed homosexuality as the cause for the abusive incidents, while others have stated that homosexuals have been scapegoated for the clergy abuse problem. *A Report on the Crisis in the Catholic Church in the United States* addressed this issue, and largely blamed homosexuality for the abuse, disbelieving that celibacy was a problem related to the abuse.

According to the report,

> There are, no doubt, many outstanding priests of a homosexual orientation who live chaste, celibate lives, but any evaluation of the causes and context of the current crisis must be cognizant of the fact that more than eighty percent of the abuse at issue

was of a homosexual nature. Likewise, celibacy does not cause sexual abuse; but the Church did an inadequate job both of screening out those individuals who were destined to fail in meeting the demands of the priesthood, and of forming others to meet those demands, including the rigors of a celibate life.

The report also blamed a past gay subculture in seminaries that may have also hindered the recruitment of male heterosexuals to the priesthood, and which the authors apparently believed contributed to the extent of the sexual abuse of boys. According to the report,

> In the 1970s and 1980s, in particular, there developed at certain seminaries a 'gay subculture,' and at these seminaries, according to several witnesses, homosexual liaisons occurred among students or between students and teachers. Such subcultures existed or exist in certain diocese or orders as well. The Board believes that the failure to take disciplinary action against such conduct contributed to an atmosphere in which sexual abuse of adolescent boys was more likely. In light of this background, it is vital that bishops, provincials, and seminary rectors ensure that seminaries create a climate and a culture conducive to chastity.

Both of these issues are actively disputed by experts who say that such contentions are examples of homophobia. Some point to the fact that some heterosexuals with an underlying PEDO-PHILIA who have no access to sex with females or who feel insecure will resort to the sexual abuse of children. (Note that some priests did have sex with adult females; however, it is much harder to conceal sex with an adult than sex with a child who can be easily cowed into submission by an adult predator.)

Possible Key Reasons Why the Church Failed to Act

A Report on the Crisis in the Catholic Church in the United States discussed why church leaders failed to act on allegations of child sexual abuse perpetrated by priests, discussing several key reasons why the abuse and its magnitude were not addressed. One reason was that the bishops and other church leaders did not treat the problem as a major issue but rather as one that was "sporadic and isolated," not realizing the magnitude of the problem. Other reasons were that the bishops' fear of litigation caused them to "adopt an adversarial stance not worthy of the Church," while other bishops put the interests of individual priests above those of victims. Some church leaders were wary of seeking information from alleged victims or outside authorities, instead relying on the information provided by the alleged perpetrator or other priests.

It was also stated that it was very difficult for church leaders to remove a predatory priest, although some bishops failed to use the authority that they did have to respond to this problem.

Many lawsuits held the church to blame for knowing that there was a problem, yet failing to act; for example, in 1993, the Diocese of Bridgeport and Bishop Egan were sued, based on the allegation that the church had known since 1982 that some priests were abusive. One priest, Father Charles Carr, reportedly had abused young boys for years. Despite the lawsuit, Carr was not suspended until 1995. He was then reinstated to the church in 1999, working as a chaplain in a nursing home until Bishop Lori, who followed Bishop Egan, removed him in late 2002. Bishop Egan had recently become archbishop of New York.

John Jay College of Criminal Justice Study

Several key studies have provided important information on clergy sexual abuse, most prominently *The Nature and Scope of the Problem of Sexual Abuse of Minors by Catholic Priests and Deacons in the United States,* published by the John Jay College of Criminal Justice in 2004. The John Jay College study was commissioned by the National Review Board of the United States Conference of Catholic Bishops. The study was a comprehensive look at clergy sexual abuse in the Catholic Church, from the 1950s to 2002, based on self-reported survey results from dioceses and Catholic religious organizations nationwide.

The researchers of the John Jay College report found that there were credible claims of abuse against 4,392 priests or deacons between 1950 and 2002. They also found that the clergy abuse problem was endemic and that more than 95% of the dioceses in the United States reported acts of clergy abuse.

They also found that the great numbers of alleged sexual acts for the entire period occurred in the 1970s, or 35%, followed by the 1960s, with 26%. Abuse in the 1980s was down to 22% and fell thereafter, with about 5% in the 1990s and less than 1% over the period 2000–02.

Most of the priests who were alleged abusers were associate pastors (42%) or pastors (25%). The location of the abuse was primarily in the priest's home or parish residence (41%), followed by in the church (16%). In 29% of the incidents, the victim's siblings were also abused.

Most of the victims were male (81%), and two-thirds of the victims were ages 12 and older when the first incident of abuse occurred. The majority of the priest abusers (54%) committed one offense, and 27% committed two to three offenses. Fifteen percent committed four to nine offenses, and 4% committed 10 or more offenses.

In about 13% of the cases, penile penetration occurred. In 15% of the cases, the cleric performed oral sex, while in 10% of the cases, the victim performed oral sex on the priest. Sexual touching occurred under the victim's clothes in 42% of the cases and over the clothes in 37%. (Note that multiple types of sex acts may have been performed by or to the victim.)

In most of the cases of past alleged abuse (91%), the priests were not charged with any crime. In many cases (77%), the abuse allegation was not investigated by police. When abuse *was* reported to the police, in 75% of the cases there was no police report made.

With regard to the age of the priest at the time of the first instance of alleged abuse, the largest percentage were ages 30–34 (23%), followed by ages 25–29 (19%), and ages 35–39 (17%). Thus 59% were 25 to 39 years old at the time of the first alleged incident.

About 53% of the victims were abused numerous times, 29% were abused once and 18% were abused more than once. Fifteen percent of the victims reported being threatened by the cleric. Of those who were threatened, 22% of the victims received verbal threats of harm. Four percent were threatened with a weapon. There were also threats of spiritual manipulation (21%) or threats to the family (4%).

Of cleric sex offenders who received treatment, 42% received individual psychological counseling, and 41% were treated in a specialized program for clergy sex offenders.

Priest Sex Offenders v. Other Offenders

In a study reported in 2000 in *Child Abuse & Neglect,* the researchers compared 23 priests accused of sex offenses to 24 non-priest sex offenders, and both groups were compared to a third group of sex offenders. The priest offenders were similar to the subjects in the other two groups, except that the priests were older and better educated; however, the clerics were less likely to have antisocial personality disorders, and they were more likely to have used force when they sexually offended. The clerics also had a longer delay than the subjects in the other two groups before they were arrested, or they were not arrested at all.

Fees to Settle Abuse Cases

It is estimated that by 2006, the Catholic Church in the United States paid more than $1.5 billion to settle multiple child sex-abuse cases, and this settlement figure may increase considerably over time. Some churches and their assets have been sold to provide the funds to cover the expenses of settling these cases. According to a 2005 article in the *Wall Street Journal,* "The Boston Archdiocese has closed 62 parishes in the past two years, netting about $90 million in property sales. The archdiocese, which has paid $99.3 million in abuse claims and fees disclosed so far, sold off the archbishop's residence—to Boston College—to help pay for the settlements."

Some parishes have fought the sale of their churches, but the church and all assets are owned by the Catholic Church, and these lawsuits are likely to fail, according to experts.

See also ABUSERS; ADULTS ABUSED AS CHILDREN; CHILD ABUSE; SEXUAL ABUSE.

Crosson-Tower, Cynthia. *Understanding Child Abuse and Neglect.* Boston: Allyn & Bacon, 2005.

John Jay College of Criminal Justice. *The Nature and Scope of the Problem of Sexual Abuse of Minors by Catholic Priests and Deacons in the United States, 2004.* Available online. URL: http://www.usccb.org/nrb/johnjaystudy. Downloaded December 31, 2005.

Langevin, R., S. Curnoe, and J. Bain. "A Study of Clerics Who Commit Sexual Offenses: Are They Different from Other Sex Offenders?" *Child Abuse & Neglect* 24, no. 4 (April 2000): 35–545.

The National Review Board for the Protection of Children and Young People. *A Report on the Crisis in the Catholic Church in the United States.* Washington, D.C.: United States Conference of Catholic Bishops, February 27, 2004. Available online. URL: http://www.priestsofdarkness.com.johnjayreport.pdf. Downloaded December 26, 2005.

Plante, Thomas G. "Bishops Behaving Badly: Ethical Considerations Regarding the Clergy Abuse Crisis in the Roman Catholic Church." *Ethics & Behavior* 14, no. 1 (2004): 67–73.

Pope's Web apology about child sex abuse, 2001. Available online. URL: http://www.cnn.com/world/eurpoe/11/22/pople.apology. Downloaded December 31, 2005.

Sataline, Suzanne. "Catholic Parish Pays High Price for Independence." *Wall Street Journal* CCXLVI, 134 (December 20, 2005): A1, A9.

clitoridectomy Sexual mutilation of females is practiced in many countries throughout the world. Clitoridectomy is one form of painful mutilation widely practiced in African countries. Specifically, this ritual involves removal of the clitoris and accompanying labia minora. Among the Gusii, an African tribe, young girls have their clitoris removed in a brutal ceremony, which also includes other extremely painful and humiliating rituals. Originally performed in late adolescence, victims now average eight to 10 years of age. Young girls who wish may postpone participation in the ritual. However, due to the great cultural significance attached to it, virtually all females eventually submit to the practice. To refuse is to be denied status as an adult member of the tribe.

The procedure is typically performed by older women on children, beginning as early as age three. In some areas, removal of the clitoris is performed, ostensibly as a medical procedure, in hospitals. Wherever it takes place, it is an extremely painful and dangerous procedure. Children often die from shock, excessive bleeding or infection following such operations. Survivors may experience a number of painful complications later.

Origins of this practice are unclear. Though some explain it as a religious rite, there is little evidence that any religion specifically requires such a procedure. All major religions are represented in groups that practice clitoridectomy. Other explanations include custom, prevention of female promiscuity and a host of "health" reasons. As recently as the 1940s, clitoridectomy was practiced in the United States and Great Britain as a cure for child masturbation, insomnia and other ills.

Although approved of within many subcultures the practice of clitoridectomy is widely condemned around the world as a cruel and abusive practice. Many groups that formerly engaged in this painful ritual have now abandoned it.

See also FEMALE GENITAL MUTILATION; INITIATION RITES; INFIBULATION.

clotting factor   When child battering is expected, one of the laboratory tests sometimes used by physicians is a test for clotting factor. Clotting factor refers to the length of time it takes for the blood to clot. Children with the hereditary condition known as hemophilia have a very low clotting factor. These children tend to bruise easily and may appear to have been subjected to battering when in fact their bruises are the result of normal daily activities.

Colwell, Maria   The unfortunate death of Maria Colwell and the resulting inquiry into the handling of her case had far-reaching effects on the protective service system in Great Britain. Maria, born on March 25, 1965, was one of nine children. Authorities placed her in foster care with an aunt for more than five years. Shortly before her seventh birthday, Maria was returned home to live with her mother and her stepfather, Mr. Kepple, in Brighton, England. Despite concerns expressed by a schoolteacher and neighbors over the ill-treatment she received, Maria was allowed to remain at home until she was beaten to death by her stepfather early in January of 1973. Maria had achieved only about 75% of the expected normal height and weight for a child her age.

Maria Colwell's stepfather, Mr. Kepple, was sentenced to eight years in prison on manslaughter charges and the case sparked a public inquiry that ultimately revealed numerous faults in Britain's existing child protection system. This inquiry eventually resulted in parliament's passage of the Children Act of 1975.

Parton, Nigel. *The Politics of Child Abuse.* New York: St. Martin's Press, 1985.

community education   Education is an important tool in the prevention of child abuse. Efforts to educate citizens about child abuse often focus on identification and reporting of abuse. However, parent education programs also play an important role in preventing abuse.

Community education efforts that heighten public awareness of the nature and extent of child abuse lay the groundwork for future efforts to treat and prevent maltreatment. Recent surveys indicate that, in the United States, public knowledge about child abuse has risen dramatically over the past two decades. Heightened awareness of child abuse has contributed to increased reporting of suspected abuse and to expansion of services to families.

See also MEDIA COVERAGE OF CHILD ABUSE.

community neglect   The term *community neglect* assumes that members of a community, and the government that represents them, have a collective responsibility to provide an environment that promotes healthy growth and development for the community's children. Communities that fail to provide adequate support for families and children are considered neglectful of their responsibility to children. Examples of community neglect include: condoning or failing to control activities that are illegal or discriminatory, failure to provide adequate social services for the support of children and families and failure to provide adequate educational opportunities for all children. Unlike individuals, communities cannot be legally prosecuted for neglect. The absence of widely accepted standards for social support services hampers efforts to eliminate community neglect.

community team   A community team consists of three components. The first is a multidisciplinary team of professionals responsible for diagnosis, crisis intervention and initial treatment planning for all child abuse and neglect cases. The second or long-term treatment component is made up of representatives of all programs involved in the treatment of children or their families, of child advocacy groups and supportive services. This group reviews the treatment progress of cases on a regular basis. A third component, also known as the community council, is responsible for education, training and public relations.

complaint   This is a legal term that is used, variously, in reference to a written or oral assertion. It can describe a statement made orally when charging criminal, abusive or neglectful conduct toward a child. The term may be used in describing a document employed by a district attorney to begin a criminal prosecution. Further, it is employed when referring to a document that begins a civil proceeding, although it is generally referred to as a PETITION in either juvenile or family court. Less often, the term complaint is used in some jurisdictions instead of the term report, in cases of suspected abuse or neglect.

compliance   When state legislation conforms to the requirements detailed in the CHILD ABUSE PREVENTION AND TREATMENT ACT OF 1974, as well as certain Department of Health and Human Services regulations, it is said to be in compliance. This compliance therefore allows for federal funding of state-sponsored child abuse and neglect activities.

The term is also used to describe the behavior of children who are anxious to please an abusive or neglectful parent. Compliant children are more than ordinarily yielding and biddable in the face of demands made by the abusing or neglectful adult.

comprehensive emergency services (CES)   In order to respond effectively to a variety of child protection emergencies some communities have developed a comprehensive system of services. Such services are usually available around the clock and can be reached by telephone. Compo-

nents of these systems may include availability of a child protection worker at all times, homemaker services, crisis nurseries, family shelters and emergency foster care.

See also EMERGENCIES.

conciliation, court of   See COURT.

conditioning, aversive   See AVERSIVE CONDITIONING.

confidentiality   Reports of suspected child abuse or neglect as well as the results of investigations are usually considered confidential and specifically protected by law. In the United States, the confidentiality of child protection records is required under the CHILD ABUSE PREVENTION AND TREATMENT ACT. In most states, unauthorized disclosure of such information is a misdemeanor.

Many areas specifically restrict access to child protection records to the agency legally mandated to investigate cases of suspected maltreatment. Some states allow all MANDATED REPORTERS access to the central register, a practice that has been criticized by some as compromising the right to privacy.

The confidentiality of communications between certain professionals and religious leaders is specifically protected by law. A breach of confidentiality by a professional can result in legal action on behalf of the client, patient or communicant. Laws requiring these parties to report suspected child abuse and neglect supersede laws that provide for privileged communication. Not only are mandated reporters allowed to share with child protection workers information that is normally considered confidential, they are also subject to legal action if they fail to do so.

continuum model of child abuse   Some experts suggest there is no fundamental difference between abusive and non-abusive parents. In contrast to others who view abuse as evidence of psychopathology, proponents of this model see parental behavior on a continuum from affectionate, loving interactions at one end to extreme abuse or murder at the other. The specific point at which behavior becomes abusive is hard to determine and is often interpreted differently. All parents are seen as potential abusers. Whether or not a parent actually batters or otherwise abuses a child depends on environmental and familial factors.

Based on this model, treatment of abusive parents focuses on management of stress and development of a sense of which behaviors are appropriate and which are not. Behavioral therapy and educational techniques are sometimes used. The continuum model eliminates some of the stigma that attaches to abusers under a psychopathological approach.

See also ABUSERS.

contusion   See BRUISES.

Convention on the Rights of the Child (U.N.)   In order to address more completely the rights of all children under international law, in 1978 the government of Poland submitted a draft Convention on the Rights of the Child to the United Nations General Assembly. This draft was one of many contributions made by various national governments in conjunction with observances of the International Year of the Child.

Previously, children's rights had been encompassed most principally by adoption in 1959 of the U.N. DECLARATION ON THE RIGHTS OF THE CHILD. The 1978 draft is different from other U.N. conventions because it specifies not only social and economic rights of children but their political and civil rights as well. It has yet to be determined which of the many children's rights detailed in the convention are mandatory on the part of states/parties affected by the convention when it is made part of international law.

In 1979, the draft Convention on the Rights of the Child was referred for consideration by a group that is part of the U.N. Center on Human Rights. This group has been meeting annually to work on the provisions included in the convention. The group has also been discussing means of implementing the convention. Currently, most members of the working group favor establishment of a formal committee on the rights of

the child to review the convention on a periodic basis and to report to the General Assembly on compliance etc., once the convention is made law.

The General Assembly adopted the convention in 1990. The U.S. has not ratified the convention as of 2005.

cord injuries   The use of electric cords as instruments for punishing children is particularly dangerous due to the high potential for severe laceration and permanent scarring. In one study, 95% of all children who had been struck with electric cords had visible lacerations or scarring. In the remaining 5%, the skin was marked but unbroken. Particularly distressing is the finding, in the same study, that 96% of the parents who used electric cords to strike their children saw nothing wrong with the practice.

Electric cords leave easily recognizable linear or hook-shaped lacerations, bruises and scars. Children between the ages of six and 13 consistently appear most likely to be victims of this method of abuse.

corporal punishment   Inflicting bodily pain on a child as a response to misbehavior, with the goal of immediately stopping the behavior and preventing a repetition of the behavior in the future. Some examples of corporal punishment are spanking, slapping and paddling. In most cases, corporal punishment is not regarded as abuse, unless the child is severely harmed. Those who oppose corporal punishment see it as ineffective and even cruel, with serious potential problems stemming from its use. Those who support it believe that it would be wrong for the government to take away a form of discipline that many parents use and support. Some parents continue to use corporal punishment as a method of discipline. In some states, schools may use corporal punishment.

One problem with corporal punishment is that in the process of inflicting corporal punishment, some parents become increasingly angry as they discipline the child, and corporal punishment may become physical abuse, as when harm beyond minor bruising occurs.

Countries that ban parental use of corporal punishment include Austria, Croatia, Cyprus, Denmark,

Finland, Germany, Israel, Italy, Latvia and Norway. In the United States, no states ban corporal punishment by parents outright, although excessive corporal punishment is explicitly illegal in most states. In general, physical punishment that results in serious injury to the child beyond minor bruising is considered beyond the realm of corporal punishment.

Corporal Punishment and Babies

Corporal punishment should never be used with infants because it could lead to SHAKEN INFANT SYNDROME or INFANTICIDE. Despite this risk, some inexperienced and young mothers use corporal punishment with their infants. It is never appropriate to spank a two-month-old baby for crying.

Perceived Problems with Corporal Punishment

Many experts in childrearing are fervently opposed to corporal punishment. Murray Straus, in his chapter in *Current Controversies about Family Violence,* said children should never be spanked. Yet according to Straus, many parents rely on this form of discipline. In one of his studies, 94% of the parents said they used corporal punishment with their toddlers.

Straus said that some parents and even some experts (such as pediatricians), although they were opposed to corporal punishment in general, viewed it as a last resort solution when other methods of discipline appeared to have failed. However, Straus said studies have shown that *all* methods of discipline, including spanking, have a very high failure rate among toddlers and that about 80% of toddlers will repeat the same act for which they were earlier disciplined.

He contended that spanking is problematic for two reasons: It interferes with cognitive functioning, causing the child to experience such negative emotions as stress and fear. Second, small children who are spanked usually do not understand why they are being spanked, and they do not equate the spanking with throwing food on the floor or other behavior that has annoyed the parent.

Said Straus, "Spanking teaches a child to avoid misbehavior if a parent is watching, or will learn about it, rather than avoiding misbehavior because the parents have explained why some things are right and others wrong. When parents explain, children gradually understand and accept these standards, and they are likely to remain in effect in

situations when no parent is present, and probably also for life." Even when the spanking is given by a loving parent, Straus said it is still a negative act and perceived as such by the child.

A Meta-Analysis of Corporal Punishment Studies

In an extensive meta-analysis of the association between parental corporal punishment and child behaviors, encompassing over 100 studies and described in a 2002 issue of *Psychological Bulletin,* researcher Gershoff found many negative effects of corporal punishment; for example, some studies found a correlation between harsh parental discipline and arrest rates of males from ages 17 to 45.

In addition, some studies showed a correlation between corporal punishment in childhood and later abuse of a spouse and children. Gershoff said several studies indicated that

> A tendency toward intergenerational transmission of aggression in close relationship is evident in a strong tendency for parents who were corporally punished to continue the practice with their own children. Similarly, experience with both average (e.g., spanking) and extreme (e.g., kicking, biting, burning, and beating up) forms of corporal punishment by parents are associated with increases in an individual's likelihood of acting violently with an adult romantic partner.

Problems with Some Studies

Gershoff also noted some distinct problems with the overall studies. She found that the frequency and severity of corporal punishment among parents varied considerably, and some parents punished their children several times a week, while others punished far less frequently. Among some parents, a spanking was a slap across the child's buttocks, while for others, repeated slaps were used. Unfortunately, few of the studies that she analyzed (only about 5%) asked parents about both the frequency and severity of their corporal punishment, and most concentrated on frequency only. Some studies asked only if patients had ever used corporal punishment.

Another problem with research studies identified by Gershoff was that most researchers failed to recognize that corporal punishment is rarely used in isolation, and instead, in most cases, the punishment is combined with other forms of discipline, such as time-outs, withdrawal of privileges or other punitive techniques. In addition, some parents who use corporal punishment frequently also use verbal abuse, such as swearing at, insulting or threatening the child, which may magnify the effect of the corporal punishment.

Key Characteristics of Corporally Punished Children

Gershoff's meta-analysis of studies on corporal punishment also identified key characteristics of children who received corporal punishment. For example, most parents who used corporal punishment believed that this form of discipline was most appropriate for children under age five, with the exception of infants. The severity of corporal punishment also increased with the child's age; for example, slaps, pinches or hitting the child on the bottom with an object were more commonly used with children ages five to eight than for children either ages zero to four or nine to 17.

Parental Characteristics of Users of Corporal Punishment

In considering the parental characteristics of those using corporal punishment, Gershoff's analysis of studies found that younger mothers were more likely to use corporal punishment; for example, in one study, more than 90% of the low-income adolescent mothers of toddlers said that they used corporal punishment. Some studies have found that mothers are more likely to rely upon corporal punishment than fathers. In addition, parents with aggressive and antisocial behaviors are more likely to use corporal punishment on their children. Some studies have shown that depressed parents are more likely to use corporal punishment on their children.

Gershoff identified other factors among the studies she analyzed. For example, a mitigating factor toward the use of corporal punishment was family size, and some studies showed that as family size increased, the use of corporal punishment also increased. In addition, parents in unhappy marriages appeared more likely to use corporal punishment than those in happy relationships. Some studies showed that single, separated or divorced parents were more likely to use corporal punishment. The part of the country where the family lived also apparently played a role in whether corporal punishment was used: corporal punishment was more likely to occur in families who lived in the south of the United States and least likely to be used in the northeast.

State Laws on Corporal Punishment

Each state in the United States has its own laws on corporal punishment. Many states rely upon such words as *reasonable* (which means a form of corporal punishment that is allowable) and *excessive* (not allowable). For example, in Wyoming, under the physical abuse statutes, the minor bruising of "reasonable" corporal punishment is not considered physical abuse.

In Indiana, a parent has the right to use reasonable corporal punishment to discipline a child. In South Carolina, excessive corporal punishment is considered physical abuse, as it is in Illinois, New Jersey, North Dakota, Rhode Island and other states. In New York, "the infliction of excessive corporal punishment" is considered a form of neglect rather than physical abuse.

What is "reasonable" or "excessive" in these states is unclear and may be open to interpretation by protective services workers; however, the point is that states do not ban corporal punishment. In many states, if there is an allegation of spanking, the child protective services worker may not bother to investigate unless there is also an allegation that severe harm to the child has also occurred.

History of Corporal Punishment in Schools from Ancient Times to the Present

In ancient Greece and Rome, as well as in Egypt, students were regularly beaten for a variety of infractions. Medieval Europe saw a continuation of this practice, which also has biblical precedents. The books of Proverbs, Chronicles, Joshua and Kings in the Old Testament positively sanction violence against children and have provided moral defenses for those accused of being too harsh with children.

One of the more significant references to corporal punishment in modern times came in 1669 with the Children's Petition in Britain. This appeal to the British Parliament was the first formal attempt to place legal limitations on corporal punishment of children in schools. A sequel to the petition came in 1698–99, although neither effected any change in the practice of corporal punishment.

Corporal punishment was not limited to European schools. As a means of keeping order in the classroom, corporal punishment was widely employed in colonial America. There exist specific references to various types of corporal punishment used by parents and community officials as well as by educators, in the interest of maintaining social order. In fact, obedience was so prized by the Puritans that laws governing corporal punishment made provision for capital punishment as well. According to the 1642 records of the Massachusetts Bay Colony,

> If a man have a stubborn or rebellious son, of sufficient years and understanding, viz, 16, who will not obey . . . then shall his father and mother bring him to the magistrate assembled in Court, and testify unto them . . . that this son is stubborn and rebellious, and will not obey their voice and chastisement, but lives in sundry notorious crimes, such a son shall be put to death.

Thus from its inception, American law viewed corporal punishment as an effective and acceptable means of maintaining order, in and out of the classroom.

Educators, parents and civil authorities in the United States and elsewhere have long debated the ultimate effectiveness of corporal punishment. Its inherent morality (or immorality) and the long-term effects on the child victim have been the focus of discussion among many social scientists and researchers. But not until the mid-19th century was any legal action taken against perpetrators of corporal punishment in American schools.

In 1867, New Jersey banned corporal punishment in public school classrooms. More than 100 years passed before another state, Massachusetts, made corporal punishment illegal in schools.

In 1977, legal challenges to policies of corporal punishment resulted in a clear message to children and adults alike. In that year, the United States Supreme Court upheld the constitutionality of corporal punishment in *Ingraham v Wright,* a case involving a student whose physical injuries resulted from paddling by school authorities and who required hospitalization for treatment of these injuries.

The Court determined in this ruling that corporal punishment remained an acceptable means of maintaining discipline in the schools. In a related case, *Baker v. Owen,* the United States Supreme Court ruled that the school had authority over parents in issues involving discipline. This case upheld the constitutional authority of schools over parents, despite a parent's objection to the corporal punishment of a child. These two cases, as well as others, clearly establish the acceptability of corporal punishment with children in institutional settings in the United States.

However, despite this ruling, more than half the states have laws banning corporal punishment in schools as of 2006, including the following states. (The year of the enactment of the law is included in parentheses.)

Alaska (1989)
California (1986)
Connecticut (1989)
Delaware (2003)
Hawaii (1973)
Illinois (1993)
Iowa (1989)
Maine (1975)
Maryland (1993)
Massachusetts (1971)
Michigan (1989)
Minnesota (1989)
Montana (1991)
Nebraska (1988)
Nevada (1993)
New Hampshire (1993)
New Jersey (1867)
New York (1985)
North Dakota (1989)
Oregon (1989)
Pennsylvania (2005)
Rhode Island (1977)
South Dakota (1990)
Vermont (1985)
Virginia (1989)
Washington (1993)
West Virginia (1994)
Wisconsin (1988)

See also CHILD ABUSE; PHYSICAL ABUSE.

Gershoff, Elizabeth Thompson. "Corporal Punishment by Parents and Associated Child Behaviors and Experiences: A Meta-Analytic and Theoretical Review." *Psychological Bulletin* 128, no. 4 (2002): 539–579.

Straus, Murray A. "Children Should Never, Ever, Be Spanked No Matter What the Circumstances." In *Current Controversies about Family Violence.* 2nd ed. Thousand Oaks, Calif.: Sage, 2004.

Wolraich, Mark L., et al. "Guidance for Effective Discipline." *Pediatrics* 101, no. 4 (April 1998): 723–728.

cot death   See SUDDEN INFANT DEATH SYNDROME.

court   Most child abuse and neglect cases are handled outside the court system. When legal action is necessary child abuse cases may appear in different types of courts depending on the purpose of the hearing. Alleged perpetrators of child abuse or neglect may be tried in a *criminal court.* The purpose of criminal courts is to determine guilt or innocence and, if guilty, assign appropriate punishment. *Civil court* proceedings focus primarily on the child's welfare.

Criminal Proceedings

Perpetrators of abuse or neglect are often prosecuted under criminal codes that apply to a wide range of behavior such as ASSAULT, BATTERY and homicide. Some states have separate laws dealing with criminal aspects of child maltreatment. Criminal courts typically operate in a more formal manner than civil courts and require a higher standard of proof (i.e., BEYOND A REASONABLE DOUBT).

The defendant in a criminal hearing is entitled to: trial by jury, strict adherence to EVIDENTIARY STANDARDS, cross-examination of WITNESSES, appointed legal representation if necessary and a speedy and public trial. Evidence that may be admissible in a civil court proceeding may not meet stricter evidentiary standards imposed in criminal courts. Criminal courts can sentence those convicted of child abuse or neglect to penalties ranging from probation and counseling to incarceration or, in some areas, death.

Child victims are often called on to testify in criminal court, but such courts deal only with punishment and rehabilitation of the offender. Issues related to the child's welfare are handled through a variety of noncriminal courts.

Civil Proceedings

Legal questions related directly to a child's welfare are decided through a civil court process. States vary in the names they assign to civil courts as well as the jurisdiction assigned to each court. Cases related to child abuse may be tried in any of the following courts:

Domestic Relations—Hears divorce and custody cases.

Court of Conciliation—A division of domestic relations court that seeks to promote reconciliation in divorce and custody disputes.

Juvenile Court—Often handles issues such as protective custody, adjudicatory hearings to establish that a child has been abused and is therefore "dependent" (i.e., in need of state care of protection), dispositional hearings related to the family's ability to care for the child and recommendations for treatment and/or placement, periodic review of dependency cases and termination of parental rights for the purpose of freeing the child for adoption. Juvenile courts also hear cases involving alleged delinquent behavior of minors and children or families in need of court-supervised services for reasons other than child abuse and neglect.

Family Court—May combine domestic relations, juvenile and probate functions into one court. In some areas family courts hear criminal cases involving family relations.

Probate Court—Processes adoption and guardianship cases and handles matters related to the estates of deceased persons.

The largest number of child abuse-related cases are heard in family or juvenile courts. Civil courts are usually more informal than criminal courts and require less stringent standards of proof (evidentiary standards). In some situations a case may be the subject of both criminal proceedings against the alleged abuser and civil proceedings related to the child's welfare. Recently the number of child abuse cases heard in United States criminal courts has increased substantially.

court, civil   See COURT.

court, criminal   See COURT.

court, family See COURT.

court, juvenile See COURT.

court, probate See COURT.

court-appointed special advocate (CASA) Judges often appoint an adult to represent a child's interests. The advocate should be someone who has no personal stake (i.e., is independent of parents and state), knows the legal and child welfare systems, is sympathetic to the child and has the time necessary to research and present the child's interests. CASAs are usually volunteers with special training. Court-appointed advocates need not be lawyers but should have access to independent legal counsel.

See also GUARDIAN AD LITEM.

court of conciliation See COURT.

crib death See SUDDEN INFANT DEATH SYNDROME.

criminal court See COURT.

criminal prosecution Persons who abuse or neglect children may be subject to criminal as well as civil charges. Alleged child abusers are often prosecuted under statues that deal with contributing to the delinquency of a minor, ASSAULT, BATTERY, homicide or RAPE. Some jurisdictions have separate criminal laws written specifically for child abuse.

Criminal proceedings are conducted for the sole purpose of determining the guilt or innocence of the alleged perpetrator. Convicted abusers are subject to a range of penalties including probation and incarceration. Legal questions concerning the victim of child abuse or neglect are decided in civil court.

Typically, criminal proceedings afford defendants far greater legal protection than civil trials. In the United States defendants have rights to trial by jury, to cross-examine witnesses, to free legal counsel and to a speedy public trial. Criminal courts adhere more closely to rules of evidence than civil courts. The highest standard of evidence, proof beyond a reasonable doubt, is required to convict someone of a criminal offense.

Prosecution of child abusers is often made more difficult by the absence of credible evidence. Young children may not be allowed to testify or may have their credibility challenged by the defendant. Testifying in court can be a traumatic experience for a child, particularly when the defendant is a family member.

Despite the difficulty of successfully prosecuting child abusers, the number of criminal cases brought to trial in the United States has risen substantially. Many states have enacted laws that permit children to testify in the judge's chambers, on videotape or closed circuit television.

See also COURT; EVIDENTIARY STANDARDS; TESTIMONY.

crisis intervention A speedy response may be necessary to protect a child who is being abused. In other cases prompt intervention may prevent abuse or neglect. For further discussion of crisis intervention, see EMERGENCIES.

crisis nursery In some areas specialized nurseries are available to relieve parental stress that might lead to abuse. Crisis nurseries provide short-term child care for parents temporarily unable or unwilling to care for their children. A child may attend a crisis nursery for periods ranging from a few hours to several days. Parents who have requested the service or who have been identified as likely to abuse their children are encouraged to seek child care relief as a preventative measure. Such services are particularly important for parents who are isolated from friends and relatives.

cruelty, mental See MENTAL CRUELTY.

cunnilingus Oral stimulation of the female genitals. In the case of SEXUAL ABUSE, the child may be the subject of the stimulation or may be forced to perform the act on an adult or another child.

custody Primary responsibility for the care of a child usually rests with the biological parents. If both parents die, become incapacitated or otherwise unable to discharge adequately their parental responsibility, the court may award custody to another person or persons. In cases of abuse and neglect, a state protective services agency or juvenile probation department usually assumes custody. Court-awarded custody may be temporary, for example, while the parent seeks psychological treatment, or permanent, upon formal TERMINATION OF PARENTAL RIGHTS. Temporary custody places control of the child in the hands of the state but does not relieve parents of the duty to provide financial support.

The state's right to assume custody of an abused or neglected child stems from the doctrine of PARENS PATRIAE. During the late 19th and early 20th centuries, removal of maltreated children from parents was the primary intervention used by child protection workers. More recently, concern over inadequate treatment of children in institutions and by foster families has caused child advocates to be more cautious. Many experts now believe even temporary removal of children from the home may have long-term psychological consequences that must be weighed carefully against the risk to the child of staying at home.

See also BEST INTERESTS OF THE CHILD; DETENTION; EMERGENCIES; EMERGENCY CUSTODY; PROTECTIVE CUSTODY.

custody, emergency See EMERGENCY CUSTODY.

custody, protective See PROTECTIVE CUSTODY.

cycle of abuse See INTERGENERATIONAL CYCLE OF ABUSE.

defect model of child abuse A great number of treatment, prevention and research efforts are guided by the belief that child abuse is the result of a defect inside the perpetrator. This approach has also influenced thinking about differences in educational achievement, mental illness and poverty. The tendency to abuse children may be seen as genetic or biological inferiority, a malformed personality structure or moral weakness. Repeated efforts to identify a particular trait or defect that makes an individual more likely to abuse children have been unsuccessful.

The defect model leads practitioners and policymakers to focus on individual problems, often at the cost of ignoring larger societal factors that may be related to abuse and neglect. This approach represents one extreme in a long-standing debate over the origins of child abuse and other forms of deviance. An opposing view seeks to explain social problems wholly in terms of societal forces. Most experts now agree that abuse and neglect are the result of many different factors, some individually based, others not.

See also ABUSERS.

de homine replegando This legal proceeding is an English writ invoked in the 1874 case in the United States involving Mary Ellen Wilson, an eight-year-old New York girl abused by her stepparents (see WILSON, MARY ELLEN). The proceeding was unique for this type of case at that time. It provided a means by which a child could be removed from the custody of the home without prior parental consent. Initially, an injury into Mary Ellen Wilson's situation was brought to the attention of Henry Bergh, founder of the American Society for the Prevention of Cruelty to Animals. Later, in the courtroom,

Mary Ellen Wilson's lawyer, Elbridge Gerry, successfully argued that a child deserved protection in the same way that animals required protection from cruel owners. The landmark case eventually led to Gerry's helping to establish the New York Society for the Prevention of Cruelty to Children. This New York group was the first charitable group of its kind in the United States and was a forerunner of the American Humane Association.

De homine replegando, a judicial order delivering a person out of prison or out of the custody of another person, has been superseded by a writ of habeas corpus but is still used in an amended or altered form in some areas of the United States.

See also EMERGENCY CUSTODY.

demonstrative evidence See EVIDENCE.

denial Failure to acknowledge reality plays an important role in the psychodynamics of abuse and neglect. Parents who neglect their children may unconsciously deny their existence. Such parents cut themselves off from their children emotionally and sometimes physically. Denial of children is often seen in parents who have a great deal of difficulty naming a child.

The psychological process of PROJECTION may contribute to denial. The parent, seeing the child as the personification of his or her own negative self-image, wishes to avoid or deny existence of the child. When confronted with their own neglect, parents may blame the child for rejecting them. In this case, denial represents a defense mechanism protecting parents against their own unconscious desires.

Abusive families also practice denial. Incest is often referred to as "the family secret." Frequently, several nonparticipating family members are aware of sexual abuse but deny its existence to outsiders. Denial may reflect embarrassment or a feeling that "things like this should not be discussed outside the family." Also, other family members may derive secondary benefits from the abuse and therefore wish it to continue. Mothers are sometimes accused of being silent partners to father-daughter incest in order to avoid sexual relations with their own husbands or to protect themselves from abandonment or abuse.

Finally, BLAMING THE VICTIM is a form of denial in which abusers try to avoid responsibility for their actions by accusing the child of provoking the abuse. Children may be portrayed as seductive or evil. By investing the child with negative intentions, abusers hope to convince others that maltreatment is excusable or even necessary. Many self-help and treatment groups place a great deal of emphasis on cutting through denial and getting abusers to accept responsibility for their own actions.

Denmark According to the *Country Reports on Human Rights Practices, 2004* on Denmark, there was no societal pattern of child abuse in Denmark in 2003. However, domestic violence was a problem that affected an estimated 30,000 children in Denmark. Some immigrant groups sought to impose forced marriages on young women, and the government set up crisis centers to help adolescents and young women who had been victimized by a forced marriage or for whom such a marriage was imminent.

There were some problems with Denmark as both a transition point and a final destination for children and women who were trafficked illegally for sexual exploitive purposes. Many of these children and women emigrated from the former Soviet Union, eastern Europe, Thailand and Africa, lured by promises of employment. SEXUAL TRAFFICKING in women and children is illegal in Denmark.

Prostitution among adults is lawful in Denmark, but soliciting a minor for CHILD PROSTITUTION is a crime.

See also SWEDEN.

Bureau of Democracy, Human Rights, and Labor. *Country Reports on Human Rights Practices, 2004: Denmark.* United States State Department, released on February 28, 2005. Available online. URL: http://www.state.gov/g/drl/rls/hrrpt/2004/41678.htm. Downloaded September 1, 2005.

depression Clinical depression is marked by sustained deep feelings of hopelessness and profound sadness. Many people will say that they feel "depressed" when they are sad; however, depression is *not* a transient mood of sadness that lifts within days or weeks without treatment. Many people experience depression at some point in their lives. Individuals who are ABUSERS may suffer from depression, both before and after the abusive acts they commit, as may the children who are their victims.

Men and women who were abused as children have an increased risk for both depression and suicide in adulthood compared to non-abused children in later adulthood. They also have an increased risk of abusing their own children, although the majority of adults who are abused as children do not abuse their children.

Depression is often cited as a factor contributing to child maltreatment, including both the abuse and neglect of children. Postpartum depression is another form of depression, and it is a severe and sometimes even psychotic depression that is experienced by some mothers who have recently given birth to a child. Postpartum depression may be hormonally based, although further research is needed. A woman who has had postpartum depression in the past may reexperience the condition if she becomes pregnant again.

The depressed parent often lacks sufficient ego strength to cope with the inevitable stresses of child-rearing, and as a result, he or she may impulsively lash out at the child in anger or frustration. The depressed parent may also act apathetically, failing to meet the child's basic needs and, as a result, neglecting the child. Some depressed parents turn to SUBSTANCE ABUSE. Poor IMPULSE CONTROL is sometimes linked to depression. Depressed parents may also suffer from ANXIETY DISORDERS.

Some people have psychotic depression, in which case they cannot distinguish reality from what they fear or believe. In the worst case, the depressed parent may feel that life is not worth living for himself or herself, as well as for the children. They may attempt and succeed at SUICIDE. In addition, before their own planned suicide attempt, some individuals may choose to murder their children, believing that they are relieving them from the extreme sadness and hopelessness that life would inevitably bring. They also usually believe that others could not care for their children or bring them any happiness.

Abused children also often experience depression, because the individuals whom they have counted upon to provide for them cannot or will not do so. Even infants may suffer from depression when they are severely neglected by their parents or other caretakers.

The depression of child abuse and neglect victims is well documented in many studies. Depression is sometimes attributed to a sense of "learned helplessness" that is acquired by a child or adult who feels trapped in a painful situation and with no apparent hope of escape. The sense of being unable to control one's situation is a pervasive characteristic of those with depression.

Symptoms and Diagnostic Path

Depressed individuals may exhibit a wide variety of symptoms, such as

- Changes in appetite (overeating or undereating)
- Changes in sleep patterns (insomnia or sleeping too much)
- Frequent or constant crying
- Lack of interest in work or hobbies
- Physical symptoms, such as headaches or stomachaches
- Talking about suicide (such words should be taken seriously in children and adults)

The depressed person may be diagnosed by a psychiatrist, psychologist or other mental health professional, as well as by family practitioners or general internists. If medication is needed, it must be prescribed by a physician.

Treatment Options and Outlook

Individuals suffering from depression may be treated with both psychotherapy and medication, which has proven to be the best combination of treatment for most people with depression. The outlook is good for most depressed people, and depression is generally considered very amenable to treatment. Without treatment, however, the outlook is not good. Although some individuals rebound without treatment, most people with depression need professional help.

Risk Factors and Preventive Measures

Depression appears to have both a genetic and environmental component. For example, a depressed parent may have been born into a family with depressed parents and siblings, as well as an environment of abuse and/or neglect. Researchers continue to argue over which factor is more important: heredity or environment. However, most experts agree that both environment and genetics are important, and it is often difficult to impossible to determine which factor is dominant in a given case.

There are no known preventive measures against depression, but the illness can be readily identified by most mental health professionals and treated effectively.

Concurrent Psychiatric Problems

It should also be noted that many people with depression also have other psychiatric diagnoses that should also be treated, such as ATTENTION-DEFICIT/HYPERACTIVITY DISORDER, an eating disorder, an anxiety disorder, PARENTAL SUBSTANCE ABUSE or other serious emotional disorders. Most of these other disorders can be treated with medication and therapy.

See also ADULTS ABUSED AS CHILDREN; FAILURE-TO-THRIVE SYNDROME.

deprivation See EMOTIONAL NEGLECT; SLEEP DEPRIVATION.

deprivation/failure-to-thrive syndrome See FAILURE-TO-THRIVE SYNDROME.

detention A public authority may take a child into temporary custody pending a hearing to determine whether it is safe for him or her to return home.

Children may be detained in an emergency shelter, foster home or hospital.

See also EMERGENCY CUSTODY.

diagnostic team   See MULTIDISCIPLINARY TEAM.

disabilities, children with   A disability is a physical or mental impairment that significantly impairs an individual in one or more major life activities. Studies indicate that children with disabilities compared to nondisabled children are about 1.7 times more likely to be abused, 1.8 times more likely to be neglected and 2.2 times more likely to be sexually abused. In addition, some disabled children are disabled as a direct result of abuse; as many as 16% of disabled children are estimated to have a physical disability or a learning disability stemming from previous abuse.

"Abuse and Neglect of Children with Disabilities: Report and Recommendations." The National Symposium on Abuse and Neglect of Children with Disabilities, November 1994.

Westcott, Helen L. and David P. H. Jones. "Annotation: The Abuse of Disabled Children." *Journal of Child Psychology and Psychiatry and Allied Disciplines* 40, no. 4 (May 1999): 497–506.

direct evidence   See EVIDENCE.

discipline   The means of behavior correction or punishment utilized by parents and/or other adults to control the behavior of children; the means are usually employed subsequent to actual or perceived misbehavior. The methods of child discipline have varied widely over the centuries and across cultures, but, in general, their purposes have been aimed at the proper socialization of children. Discipline may range from sending a child to stand in a corner to taking away privileges or using physical punishment. Debate continues as to the best means of achieving discipline.

In some cases, parents (especially those who are young and inexperienced) who are unaware of normal growth milestones and the cognitive abilities of children may use CORPORAL PUNISHMENT against infants and small children, assuming that they are using good disciplinary means. Such action constitutes PHYSICAL ABUSE and may lead to SHAKEN INFANT SYNDROME or even to INFANTICIDE.

Most child advocates have been encouraged by the growing international trend to condemn violent forms of discipline in favor of methods that teach children to identify inappropriate behavior and to prevent it from happening in the first place.

However, there are still supporters of harsh disciplinary measures, and conversely, there are educators, parents and others who draw correlations between aberrant behavior in later life and excessive discipline in childhood. Most experts agree that parents who resort to disciplinary measures such as spanking, yelling, humiliation or restricting a child's freedom of action do so as a way of asserting their own power over the child.

Power-assertive parents who vigorously act out through punishment differ from non-power-assertive parents, who use the withholding of affection and turning away from a child as a means of discipline. The latter group may refuse to speak to a disobedient child as a way of punishment. Experts tend to agree that neither method is in the best interests of the child's health development. However, no matter which disciplinary approach is used, it is clear that an adult who disciplines a child as soon as possible after an infraction is more successful in preventing recurrent disobedient behavior. A child disciplined some time after an infraction occurs is generally less able to associate the punishment with the disobedience. Of course, the age of the child should be considered. A five-year-old needs to be disciplined more rapidly than an adolescent for the child to make the connection between the inappropriate act and the chosen discipline, whatever the form.

The most effective means of discipline has proven to be inductive in nature. That is, parents who explain the negative effects of unwanted behavior immediately after the behavior occurs are thought to have a better chance at success in disciplining children than parents who either assert their power through physical means or who withhold and turn away from the disobedient child. Again, however, the age of the child should be considered. A three-year-old does not need and will not benefit from a long discussion of why it was wrong to slam the door or hit a sibling. In contrast, an adolescent may benefit from such a discussion.

See also ABUSERS; CHILD ABUSE.

dismissal   See DISPOSITION.

disposition   In addition to questions of fact surrounding alleged child abuse or neglect, civil courts must decide what actions should be taken on behalf of the child. This type of decision, known as a disposition, is equivalent to sentencing in a criminal case.

Dispositional choices available to judges are different in different jurisdictions. Most dispositions related to child abuse or neglect fall into one of the following categories: dismissal, adjournment in contemplation of dismissal, suspended judgment, issuing an order of protection, removal of the child from the caretaker or termination of parental rights.

Dismissal   When evidence is not sufficient to prove child abuse or the child is no longer in danger a judge may terminate or dismiss the case. No further action may be taken following dismissal.

Adjournment in contemplation of dismissal   Parties to a case may agree to a specific court order (e.g., a family treatment program) before the court makes a decision concerning the facts. Compliance with the agreement is monitored for a specified period of time after which the court may decide that the child is no longer in danger and dismiss the case. If, after a hearing, the court determines that all parties have not complied with the agreement it may then proceed to a DISPOSITIONAL HEARING without completing a full fact-finding hearing.

Suspended judgment   In some areas a court may issue specific orders to the parties and delay its decision for a specified period of time. During this time (usually six months to a year) the court monitors compliance. At the end of the time period, the court may decide to dismiss the case, extend the monitoring period or, in the case of noncompliance, issue an order based on the evidence presented at the original adjudicatory hearing.

An order of suspended judgment is issued after all evidence has been heard. Adjournment in contemplation of dismissal may take place before fact-finding.

Order of protection   The order of protection allows a child to remain at home under the supervision of a designated agency. Conditions that must be met by the caretakers are carefully spelled out in the order. Failure to comply with provisions of the order may result in caretakers being held in contempt of court. The order of protection may be used in conjunction with other dispositions.

Removal of the child   When less drastic measures fail, the abused child may be removed from home and placed in the custody of a public or private agency. Placement orders usually specify time limits and the conditions necessary for the child to return home. In the United States, the ADOPTION ASSISTANCE AND CHILD WELFARE REFORM ACT requires regular review of out-of-home placements.

Termination of parental rights   In extreme cases where it appears that parents will never be able to care adequately for the child, the court may permanently sever the parents' rights to serve as legal guardians of the child. Many states require that separate hearings be held when termination of parental rights is at issue.

See also DISPOSITIONAL HEARING.

dispositional hearing   The dispositional hearing is held to determine what actions should be taken on behalf of the child. In most areas the dispositional hearing is a separate proceeding that follows the ADJUDICATORY HEARING or fact-finding hearing.

Information taken into consideration at the hearing may include medical and mental health evaluations, social assessments and similar materials as well as specific recommendations of the probation officer or child protection worker.

See also ASSESSMENT; DISPOSITION; COURT.

doctrine of sovereign immunity   A professional child protection worker in the United States often works for a state or for a state-sponsored agency. As a MANDATED REPORTER of suspected child abuse or neglect, a professional so employed cannot always expect legal immunity from lawsuits stemming from such reports or cases. Although the agency (or the state itself) may be free of legal liability under the doctrine of sovereign immunity, the individual employee is not. In more than a few situations, however, all professionals who work for the state or state agency receive unqualified immunity. Some individual state provisions for modification in the immunity laws exist as well.

See also APPENDIX I.

Doe, Baby Jane   See BABY DOE.

dolls, anatomically correct   See NATURAL DOLLS.

domestic relations   See COURT.

drug dependence, maternal   See MATERNAL DRUG DEPENDENCE; PARENTAL SUBSTANCE ABUSE.

due process   Due process refers to the fundamental fairness of the law and the procedures by which it is administered. There are two types of due process. *Substantive due process* requires that a law be reasonable, not arbitrary or capricious. *Procedural due process,* more often an issue in child abuse cases, deals with the right of each person to a fair trial. Fairness is often defined in terms of three basic rights: privacy, proper notice of the hearing and an impartial hearing.

Investigations of suspected abuse or neglect often give rise to concerns that the alleged abuser's right to privacy has been violated. The line between a reasonable investigation and invasion of personal privacy is often unclear. Some actions that would normally be construed as privacy violations re permissible if they are clearly in the interest of the child's welfare. For example, it may be necessary for a protective service worker to enter a private home without permission in order to prevent further harm to a child. In general, invasions of privacy are permissible only if an overriding public interest is at stake.

Parties to a child abuse hearing are entitled to timely notice of the hearing. The notice should inform them of the charges, names of the parties involved, where and when the hearing is to be held.

Several rights are subsumed under the general right to a fair hearing. These include the right to be represented by counsel, to confront and cross-examine witnesses, the right to a jury trial and family integrity. Actual application of these rights may vary depending upon the type of proceeding (i.e., civil or criminal), the court in which the case is tried (criminal, juvenile, etc.) and the specific charges made. Criminal proceedings usually adhere closely to due process procedures; juvenile courts are often less strict in adherence.

In keeping with the right to counsel, most states specifically provide for the appointment of a GUARDIAN AD LITEM to represent the interests of the child. The guardian ad litem must act independently of attorneys for both the prosecution and defense.

The right to confront one's accusers and to cross-examine witnesses is often problematic in child abuse trials, particularly when the victim is very young. Normal court procedures may be intimidating to the child; testimony and cross-examination can subject the child to additional trauma. Many courts now allow videotaped or closed-circuit television testimony. Others allow testimony IN CAMERA. Whatever methods are used, provisions for cross-examination must be made.

Some states do not permit trial by jury in juvenile court proceedings. In others a judge may, at the request of one or both parties, make a jury trial available.

United States law requires that reasonable attempts be made by the state to maintain family integrity by offering rehabilitative services. Before PARENTS' RIGHTS can be terminated, the state must prove that attempts have been made to keep a child at home or that the child is in immediate danger.

See also ADVOCACY; CHILDREN'S RIGHTS; IN RE GAULT; TERMINATION OF PARENTAL RIGHTS.

due process, procedural   See DUE PROCESS.

due process, substantive   See DUE PROCESS.

dwarfism   Prolonged abuse or neglect can inhibit the body's secretion of the growth-producing hormone somatotropin, which causes significant physical, emotional and intellectual retardation. This syndrome is known by several names, including: psychosocial dwarfism, abuse dwarfism, deprivation dwarfism, reversible hyposomatotropism, reversible growth failure, and post-traumatic hypopituitarism.

Diagnosis is based on the observation of a significant slowdown in physical growth after infancy. Skeletal growth is severely retarded, and height is below the third percentile as compared to children of the same chronological age.

Endocrinological tests demonstrate a lack of somatotropin (growth hormone) production before the child is removed from the unhealthy environment. The factor that distinguishes these symptoms from other organically induced growth failure is the rapid reversal seen when children are hospitalized. Significant increases in pituitary secretion have been observed as rapidly as two weeks following removal of the child from the abusive situation. Other symptoms may take much longer to improve. SUBDURAL HEMATOMA, often a result of shaking or battering, has also been identified as a cause of hypopituitarism.

Psychosocial dwarfism is in some ways similar to the FAILURE-TO-THRIVE syndrome seen in infants. The major distinction between the two is the age of the child at onset. A generally, but not universally, accepted demarcation point is age three. Growth failure occurring prior to that point is known as failure to thrive, afterward as psychosocial dwarfism.

In addition to a background of especially cruel or neglectful treatment at home, children suffering from psychosocial dwarfism may present a history of unusual behavioral symptoms. They may exhibit an exaggerated desire for food or drink, sometimes eating from trash cans or drinking from toilet bowls. Bouts of excessive eating may be followed by self-starvation or vomiting. These children often lack age-appropriate control of urination and bowel movements and may throw aggressive tantrums or appear socially withdrawn.

Sleep appears to play an important part in producing the growth failure seen in psychosocial dwarfs. Unusual patterns of sleep and wakefulness are frequently observed. Research has shown a direct correspondence between the normalization of sleep patterns and the growth spurt experienced by children when they are removed from the abusive situation.

Retarded motor and intellectual development is frequently present in the psychosocial dwarf. Like skeletal growth, these symptoms usually show remarkable improvement when the child is moved to a healthy living environment. Improvements in IQ scores up to as much as 55 points have been recorded. When deprivation continues into adolescence, a delay in the onset of puberty is usually observed. The exact cause, or causes, of somatotropin deficiency in the psychosocial dwarfism syndrome is not clear. As mentioned earlier, sleep patterns seem to be related to production of the growth hormone, however there is no consistent explanation for the sleeping difficulties. Significant increase in somatotropin production is usually observed when the child is removed from the home in which the initial symptoms occurred. The relative rarity of psychosocial dwarfism coupled with the difficulty of collecting accurate information about the child's treatment prior to intervention has left many questions about this syndrome unanswered.

Money, John. *The Kaspar Hauser Syndrome of "Psychosocial Dwarfism": Deficient Statural, Intellectual, and Social Growth Induced by Child Abuse.* Buffalo, N.Y.: Prometheus Books, 1992.

E

Early and Periodic Screening, Diagnosis and Treatment (EPSDT) The Early and Periodic Screening, Diagnosis and Treatment (EPSDT) program was enacted in 1967 by the Congress of the United States as part of the MEDICAID program. The required services were defined specifically in the Omnibus Budget Reconciliation Act of 1989. EPSDT now requires periodic screening, vision, dental and hearing services. Medicaid is jointly funded by the states and the federal government to provide medical care to low-income families and individuals.

EPSDT was specifically designed to detect potentially disabling physical or mental conditions in poor children. Screening begins in infancy and may continue up to age 21. In addition to screening, the program provides treatment of any medical problems and transportation to and from the medical facility.

All states are required to provide this service to Medicaid-eligible children. Welfare departments are responsible for administration of EPSDT in most areas.

Regular monitoring can help identify cases of maltreatment that might otherwise have gone undetected. Screening programs such as EPSDT can also help reduce the incidence of SITUATIONAL ABUSE AND NEGLECT.

See also POVERTY.

ecchymosis See BRUISES.

edema Bumps or BRUISES can result in edema, a swelling of body tissue caused by an excessive collecting of fluid in the body tissue. Such swelling is a possible indicator of battering but may also be the result of various diseases, malnutrition or allergies.

education, community See COMMUNITY EDUCATION.

education, parent See PARENT EDUCATION.

educational neglect The National Center on Child Abuse and Neglect offers the following definition of educational neglect:

> Failure to provide for a child's cognitive development. This may include failure to conform to state legal requirements regarding school attendance.

Little information is available on the incidence of this problem. Most child protection agencies do not keep separate statistics on this form of neglect. Because educational neglect is not considered life threatening, it may receive less attention from child abuse experts than other forms of abuse and neglect.

In recent years, several proposals have been made that would penalize parents of children who are chronically truant from school. Proposed penalties range from fines and imprisonment to reductions in welfare assistance. These proposals illustrate a growing tendency to deal with the problem of school attendance outside of the child protection system.

emergencies Abused or neglected children may need immediate intervention to protect them from further severe maltreatment or to ensure proper treatment of injuries. All areas of the United States are covered by HOTLINES that provide around-the-clock telephone screening of potential child abuse emergencies. These phone services are usually operated by, or have a direct link with, local child protection agencies and law enforcement authorities.

Assessment of danger to the child is the first and perhaps the most important step in the screening and investigatory process (see INVESTIGATION).

If the child is determined to be in immediate physical or emotional danger several alternatives are available. PARENT AIDES or HOMEMAKER SERVICES may be called to assist the family and ensure proper treatment of the child. The abusing adult may be voluntarily or involuntarily removed from home. When abuse is discovered in a hospital emergency room, the child may be placed on HOSPITAL HOLD for his or her protection.

Removing a child from home is usually the least preferable of emergency interventions. Emergency removal may place additional strain on a child who has already suffered severe emotional trauma. Children often find it difficult to adjust to abrupt changes brought on by out-of-home placement. Emergency placement further disrupts families and may reduce parents' willingness to cooperate with subsequent efforts to protect the child. When emergency removal of a child is necessary, trauma to the child and family may be reduced by placing the child with a friend or relative. Placement in an emergency shelter or foster home is considered only if no suitable alternatives are available.

Most developed countries make legal provisions for placing children in protective custody. In the United States, children may be removed from parents' custody by court order or, in an emergency, by state authority. Many states allow police to take a child into protective custody without prior court approval. When children are removed without a court order, a HEARING must be held to review the decision. Court supervision of protective custody focuses on rights of the child, parents and the state.

emergency custody   Virtually all states have legal provisions for an authorized person to remove a child from a dangerous or abusive situation. This immediate removal into emergency custody can occur either with or without a court order, although states have varying requirements governing this action; some states require that a court order be obtained before emergency custody without parental consent is effected. In addition, each state has different definitions of who is authorized to take emergency custody action.

Despite the clear necessity of emergency custody in some cases, most experts currently agree that, in general, every effort should be made to avoid unnecessary removal of a child from the home. The entire concept of interfering with what has been termed the "sanctity of the home and family" is one that has received increasing judicial scrutiny in recent years.

emergency room   Most severely abused children and many with less serious physical injuries are brought to hospital emergency rooms for treatment. Specialized training both in detection of child abuse and in crisis intervention is considered essential for emergency room personnel.

Emergency room physicians and nurses must often work without benefit of adequate social or medical histories of the child who receives treatment. In urban areas, emergency room personnel must be alert to HOSPITAL HOPPING, a practice employed by some chronic abusers.

Metropolitan hospitals may see 50% to 65% of reported cases of abuse as opposed to the 2% to 5% treated by private physicians. Figures such as these have led some observers to speculate that private physicians tend to underreport abuse.

According to a 1997 report on violence-related injuries treated in hospital emergency departments published by the Bureau of Justice Statistics, about 26% of the violence-related injuries were experienced by children aged 18 and under. Of these, 5.3% were children under age 12 and 6.1% were children ages 12–14.

Although data were not generally broken down into categories of younger children, researchers did note that preschool children were at great risk for injuries. Of children under age 12 who were examined or treated for sexual abuse, approximately half were age four or younger. Of children treated for physical abuse, about half were age five or younger.

The perpetrator of the injury varied according to the age of the individual and is reflected in the chart below. As can be seen from the chart, children age 12 and under who are treated in emergency departments of hospitals are most at risk for abuse from relatives (56.3%), followed by acquaintances (34.1%). In contrast, those who are age 12–19 are most at risk from acquaintances (58.2%), followed by strangers (29.9%). (Adults age 20 and over are also most at risk from acquaintances [43.9%] and strangers [35.2%].)

RELATIONSHIP TO THE PATIENT OF THE PERSON WHO INFLICTED THE INJURY

Age of ED Patient	Total	Relative	Acquaintance	Stranger
Child under age 12	100%	56.3%	34.1%	9.7%
Age 12–19	100%	11.9%	58.2%	29.9%
Adult 20+	100%	20.9%	43.9%	35.2%

Source: Michael R. Rand, "Violence-Related Injuries Treated in Hospital Emergency Departments," Bureau of Justice Statistics Special Report, 1997, page 6.

---

emotional abuse   See PSYCHOLOGICAL/EMOTIONAL MALTREATMENT.

emotional neglect   The National Center on Child Abuse and Neglect defines emotional neglect as failure· to provide the psychological nurturance necessary for a child's psychological growth and development."

Numerous studies have documented the crucial importance of a warm, safe and loving relationship with an adult for the healthy physical and emotional development of children. Early studies of HOSPITALISM in infants separated from their mothers at birth documented physical and cognitive impairment. These deficits appeared to result from a lack of physical contact and emotional interaction. Institutionalized infants in the studies received adequate food, shelter and medical care yet appeared undernourished, listless and withdrawn. In many cases the condition of these infants continued to worsen and eventually resulted in their death. Their FAIL-URE TO THRIVE was attributed to impersonal care received in the hospital. Overburdened nurses had little time to hold or interact with the infants. The sterile hospital environment offered little sensory stimulation. Conversely, infants in another ward who received a good deal of loving attention in a sensory-rich environment appeared happier and followed normal developmental patterns. Similar characteristics have been observed in children who receive insufficient parental attention at home.

Tactile stimulation (touching) appears to be especially important for both cognitive and emotional development of infants and children. Infants whose parents are physically undemonstrative may reach out indiscriminately to strangers at a time when others their age normally exhibit a fear of strangers.

Emotionally neglected children often show signs of psychopathology in later life. As children they may appear depressed and withdrawn or may engage in frantic ACTING OUT in the hopes of attracting some type of attention from caretakers. Norman Polansky, a professor of social work at the University of Georgia, has described a phenomenon that he calls the APATHY-FUTILITY SYNDROME, in which neglected children develop a form of emotional numbness and immaturity that may later result in their becoming neglectful parents.

Despite the potentially devastating effects of emotional neglect, many states do not specifically identify it as a condition to be reported to child protection agencies. Legal definitions of emotional neglect, when they exist, are often so vague as to be useless in a court of law. Further, while the results of emotional neglect can be observed, it is often difficult to prove that parental neglect, rather than other factors, was the cause.

encopresis   Repeated involuntary defecation (soiling) occurring in children over the age of four years is termed *encopresis*. Boys are over three times more likely than girls to suffer from this condition. Encopresis is usually accompanied by chronic constipation. Physical causes of encopresis include neurogenic megacolon, a nerve deficiency that inhibits peristalsis in the bowel, and anatomic megacolon, the obstruction of the bowel by a tumor or lesion. When no physiological cause is found encopresis is sometimes interpreted as the child's attempt to express hostility or resolve conflict. Many encopretic children live in families where open conflict is avoided at all costs.

Some psychotherapists have observed similarities between a parent's somatic concerns and those of the child. For example, the encopretic child may have a parent who suffers from irritable bowel syndrome or from chronic constipation.

Fecal soiling may be seen as both a precipitant and a consequence of abuse. Caretakers find an encopretic child extremely frustrating and enraged parents may resort to harsh punishment in an effort to stop the behavior. Harsh treatment can actually prolong the problem and is almost never helpful.

In a child who has been toilet trained for over one year encopresis sometimes is seen as indicative of internal conflicts that the child cannot address directly. These conflicts may be related to abuse.

A careful assessment, beginning with a thorough medical examination, is recommended as the first step in treating encopresis.

enuresis Repeated involuntary discharge of urine in a child over three years of age. Enuresis is derived from the Greek word meaning "I make water." Approximately 10% of children between the ages of six and 10 in the United States are enuretic.

A number of myths have grown up around the problem of enuresis. Many caregivers believe that bed-wetting is done out of spite, although psychotherapists strongly oppose this interpretation. Most believe enuresis is related to anxiety, usually due to situational stress.

Another myth is that enuretic children are emotionally disturbed. Though the incidence of emotional problems is slightly higher among this group, many of these problems vanish as the enuresis is controlled.

Many cruel and inhumane remedies have been tried in an effort to cure enuresis. Seventh-century parents forced bed wetters to drink a pint of their own urine. Other "cures" included beating, tying a string around the penis, placing the child's buttocks on a hot stove, making the child wear wet garments, shaming or ridiculing the child. All of these methods are ineffective and abusive. There is no evidence that punishment is an effective treatment for enuresis.

Physicians and psychologists generally attribute nonphysiologically based enuresis to situational stress. Punishment usually exacerbates the problem in these cases.

As with ENCOPRESIS, treatment of enuresis should begin with a thorough medical examination.

EPSDT See EARLY AND PERIODIC SCREENING, DIAGNOSIS AND TREATMENT.

evidence Statements by various parties, written documents, material objects and the opinions of experts may all serve as evidence in an investigation of suspected child abuse or neglect. Not all such evidence is allowed in court hearings. Courts have rules that govern the kinds of evidence that may be considered. Types of evidence allowed may differ according to the type of hearing. Preliminary or pretrial hearings are held for the purpose of issuing temporary orders. Evidence allowed at a preliminary hearing may not meet the rules of evidence applicable to a later court proceeding.

Adjudicatory or "fact-finding" hearings usually require that evidence conform to the legal rules of evidence and have a direct bearing on the issue before the court. In general four kinds of evidence are allowed.

Direct evidence is based on the witness's own observations and perceptions and does not depend on proof of any other facts. A neighbor's account of having watched the accused beating the child is direct evidence.

Real, demonstrative or autoptic evidence is concrete physical evidence. A child's injuries, X-rays showing broken bones, instruments used to harm a child and photographs are examples of real evidence.

Circumstantial evidence includes observations that allow the court to reach a specific conclusion, for example, testimony that a parent was shouting, threatening and visibly enraged at a child shortly before the alleged abuse occurred.

Expert or opinion evidence is usually given by someone who has special skills or expertise beyond that of the court. Opinions of expert witnesses are admissible only if they are related to an expert's area of expertise. Physicians are often called upon to give expert testimony concerning the nature and extent of a child's physical injuries.

Evidence that is not based on a witness's direct observations or experience is called "hearsay" and is generally not admissible in a fact-finding hearing. (See TESTIMONY for special cases where hearsay evidence may be allowed.)

In most court proceedings certain conversations such as those between a physician and patient or between psychotherapist and client are considered "privileged" and therefore may be excluded from testimony. Many states have laws specifically abrogating these privileges where child abuse or neglect is involved. Such communications can serve as important evidence in court.

See also PSYCHOLOGICAL/EMOTIONAL MALTREATMENT.

evidence, autoptic   See EVIDENCE.

evidence, circumstantial   See EVIDENCE.

evidence, clear and convincing   EVIDENTIARY STANDARDS.

evidence, demonstrative   See EVIDENCE.

evidence, direct   See EVIDENCE.

evidence, expert   See EVIDENCE.

evidence, opinion   See EVIDENCE.

evidence, real   See EVIDENCE.

evidentiary standards   Different types of court cases require different levels or standards of proof.

The three most common standards are: a fair preponderance of the evidence; clear and convincing evidence; and proof beyond a reasonable doubt.

Jurisdictions differ in the particular evidentiary standard applied to specific types of cases. If a standard is not specified by law, the preponderance of evidence standard is usually applied.

Preponderance of evidence is the least restrictive, or easiest, standard. To meet this standard a party must simply give a greater amount of credible evidence than that provided by the opposing party. Evidence presented may leave some degree of doubt in the minds of the judge or jury. When all evidence presented in court is considered a jury must decide if one side has presented more credible evidence in support of its case than has its opponent. The preponderance of evidence standard is used most often in civil court proceedings.

Clear and convincing evidence requires more confidence on the part of the decision maker than a simple preponderance of evidence. This standard is usually applied to removal of a child from home due to child abuse or neglect. By requiring a somewhat higher standard of proof courts seek to strike a balance between parents' interests in maintaining their children at home and the child's need for protection.

Beyond a reasonable doubt, the highest standard, is applied in criminal court proceedings. Evidence must support a party's contentions to a moral certainty. There must be no "reasonable" doubt in jurors' minds. The word reasonable implies a comparison of the jurors' standards for absolute certainty to those of the average person. This standard is particularly challenging to prosecutors of child sexual abuse cases who often must rely on circumstantial evidence and/or testimony from very young children to prove a case.

Proof beyond a reasonable doubt is also required for TERMINATION OF PARENTAL RIGHTS.

excited utterance   Courts usually do not accept hearsay testimony (observations concerning statements made by someone other than the witness) as evidence. An exception to this rule may be made when a person under great stress (usually the victim of a crime) makes a statement. In such instances a person who heard the statement may be allowed to testify concerning the victim's original exclamation.

The excited-utterance exception to the hearsay rule is frequently applied in trials involving child abuse. Because the credibility of a young child's testimony is often questioned, corroborating testimony from an adult is considered important evidence. Some states require that testimony of a young child be supported by testimony from an adult. A child's statements made shortly after an incident of alleged abuse and in the presence of a child protection worker, teacher or other adult are allowed under the ancient rule of *res gestae*. This rule may be interpreted literally as "things done." It extends to things said, gestures made and thoughts expressed that are so closely related to the occurrence of an event as to be considered a part of the event.

Excited utterances are justified by the theory that a victim's statements immediately following a crime are likely to be truthful because the victim is under stress and unable to construct a false account of events. The victim's mental state (i.e., excitement and the length of time that elapses between the event in question and the victim's statement) are of crucial importance.

Acceptance of excited utterance testimony from children is controversial. Courts are sometimes criticized for allowing this type of testimony when several hours, even days, have passed between the incident and the excited utterance. Another problem associated with reliance on excited utterance testimony is that children often delay reporting abuse out of fear or shame. Very young children may fail to understand an event and therefore do not become upset immediately following abuse. In such cases the child's statements would fail to meet the criterion of being under stress.

See also TESTIMONY.

exhibitionism   Exposure of the sex organs as a means of sexual gratification. Some experts also refer to flaunting of past abuse as exhibitionism.

Sexual Exhibitionism

One-third of all reported sex offenses involve exhibitionism. Research indicates that only 17% of all exhibitionistic episodes are referred to the police.

Victims of exhibitionism include both children and adults but are almost always female. Girls at or near the age of puberty are the most frequent victims. The majority of victims show no long-term effects though a small proportion may be significantly traumatized.

Perpetrators of sexual exhibitionism are most likely to be young adult males with interpersonal difficulties but without serious psychopathology. Exhibitionists usually do *not* progress to more serious sex crimes.

Almost three-fourths of all exhibitionism takes place outdoors. Most incidents occur in streets, alleys and parking lots. Only 5% take place in public parks or school playgrounds. About 14% of exhibitionist incidents occur at home.

Many states have statutes that impose harsher penalties against offenders when the victim is a child.

Children who have been subjected to repeated sexual abuse sometimes engage in seductive or exhibitionistic behavior toward adults. Incest victims may behave seductively as a means of getting love or attention when their emotional needs cannot be met in more conventional ways. These children come to view themselves as dehumanized sexual objects in much the same way that they have been treated by their abusers. Such behavior has contributed to the damaging myths that children enjoy sexual relations with adults and that children are the seducers.

Other Forms of Exhibitionism

A second and rather rare form of exhibitionism has been observed in abused children following their removal from the abusive situation. Displaying an eagerness to describe their abuse to others these children have developed an identity centered around their history of abuse. Self-labeling is used as justification for current negative behavior or as a means of gaining special consideration from others. For example, a child may blame all failures to comply with the wishes of teachers or foster parents on his or her status as an abused child, e.g., "I can't do it because I was abused by my parents." This form of exhibitionism should not be confused with a normal healthy desire to understand past abuse by talking about it with others.

exhibitionism, sexual   See EXHIBITIONISM.

ex parte *Crouse*   In Pennsylvania in 1838, a court ruling upheld the right of the state to determine whether a young girl, Mary Ann Crouse, should remain in the Philadelphia House of Refuge, outside the custody of her parents. Crouse had been remanded to the House of Refuge at her mother's request, although without her father's knowledge or approval. In an attempt to obtain custody of his daughter, the father demanded Mary Ann's release on the grounds of the Sixth Amendment, which provides for due process of law. The institution countered that the young girl was ineligible for such protection since she was a minor and the Pennsylvania Supreme Court subsequently ruled against the father. Mary Ann Crouse was the first juvenile in the United States whose custody was determined by a court that successfully invoked the doctrine of PARENS PATRIAE as a way of removing her from parental jurisdiction.

expert evidence   See EVIDENCE.

expert witness   In any court situation, a witness is called upon to testify according to firsthand knowledge of an event or series of events. Some witnesses may have special education, experience or skills that are valuable in a child abuse or neglect case. These witnesses contribute either to the defense or to the prosecution or are important in terms of general edification of the court. This type of witness may be asked to comment upon details of the case and to give an opinion based on the specialized training or background he or she has in a specific area. In this situation, the witness is called upon to do more than simply state facts as seen or heard. Some expert witnesses in child abuse or neglect cases are physicians, psychiatrists, psychologists and social workers.

Expert Witnesses in Child Abuse Cases: What Can and Should Be Said in Court (American Psychological Association, 1998) is a book that describes the many problems and pitfalls surrounding therapists who act as expert witnesses. For example, a thera-pist who has been counseling a child may see him or herself as the child's advocate and thus objectivity may be problematic.

Another problem may be that the therapist is unfamiliar with the current research on the subject. Richard Lawlor, an author in *Expert Witnesses in Child Abuse Cases* is particularly condemning of psychologists acting as expert witnesses and said,

A significant portion of what passes for expert testimony in child sexual abuse cases is poorly grounded in the psychological research literature, reflects a lack of the knowledge of this constantly expanding literature, and often demonstrates a significant role confusion on the part of many experts who testify in court. Even psychologists, who presumably have both a research and clinical underpinning to their testimony, seem to be prey to the same difficulties as most other expert witnesses in these cases. Of even more concern is the fact that much of the investigation done in cases of child sexual abuse appears to be done by the least trained professionals and paraprofessionals, without adequate knowledge, skills, experience, training, and sometimes even motivation to apply the knowledge and skills that they have been taught.

Lawlor also said some techniques used to determine whether child sexual abuse had occurred could actually result in an iatrogenic effect—meaning that a child who was not abused could begin to believe in imagined abuse and could also exhibit clinical symptoms of distress that were not present in the recent past. Lawlor stated that children who may have been abused but who do not display emotional distress should not be referred to a therapist for investigative purposes.

Another concern has been with the techniques of investigative experts; for example, with using anatomically correct dolls, children's drawings and so forth. Lawlor and others contend that these techniques have not been scientifically validated as indicative of child abuse. In fact, in one of the few controlled studies of the drawings of children who were known to be sexually abused, only 10% (five of 52) drew genitalia in their pictures of people. This 10% was more than the 2% of non-abused children who drew genitalia but it was not statistically significant enough to draw conclusions of evidence of abuse.

In some cases, individuals have been convicted of child abuse primarily on the basis of an expert witness. For example, in a 1986 New Jersey case, Margaret Kelly Michaels was convicted of 155 counts of child sexual abuse on children who had attended the Wee Care Nursery School. The chief prosecution witness was a psychologist who testified that the children exhibited "child sexual abuse syndrome" based on her interviews with them and their behavior. This conviction was reversed in 1993 by the New Jersey Superior Court Appellate Division, which found that the expert testimony was inadequate and stated, "Unquestionably, this erroneously admitted evidence was capable of producing an unjust result and thus requires the reversal of defendant's convictions."

This does not mean that expert witnesses are never useful nor does it mean they are always wrong. Experts report that expert witnesses can be very helpful in explaining facts about child abuse that the jury may not understand; for example, that not all child abuse victims will sob on the stand and in fact, some may behave very stoically. Depending on the state and the jurisdiction, they may also be able to talk about common behaviors of children who have been sexually abused.

Some therapists who have served as witnesses have been accused of overzealously leading children toward the finding that the therapist wants—for or against child abuse. One problem is that the therapist may have uncovered real child abuse, but if a videotape appears to be leading to a judge or jury, they may be unable to find that child abuse occurred.

The main criteria for a good expert witness are knowledge of the topic, an ability to be objective and neutral during the interview(s) with the child and also the capability of reporting any factual data about the child which has been learned and which indicates abuse, particularly data that can be corroborated.

See also SEXUAL ABUSE; WITNESS.

Ceci, Stephen J., and Helene Hembrooke, eds. *Expert Witnesses in Child Abuse Cases: What Can and Should Be Said in Court.* Washington, D.C.: American Psychological Association, 1998.

exposure This procedure is a form of INFANTICIDE in which a newborn is abandoned to die from such indirect causes as hypothermia or starvation. Some ancient cultures positively sanctioned or encouraged exposure of weak, premature or deformed infants. Believing that such children would pass their deformities along to their offspring, Aristotle recommended that rearing of disabled or deformed children be forbidden by law.

Roman law allowed exposure of infants born in cases where marital infidelity was suspected, a practice that continued until outlawed by the emperor Valentinian III in A.D. 434. Exposure was practiced by many other cultures as well. In 19th-century CHINA, female infants were routinely cast into a river or left to die.

In some countries, children are still routinely abandoned. Some abandoned children are adopted.

expungement Judges may order the destruction or expungement of court records. In many states records of juvenile court proceedings are expunged after a predetermined number of years. Some jurisdictions allow either party to a child abuse case to apply for expungement. When requesting expungement a convicted defendant must satisfy the court that he or she has been rehabilitated, i.e., no longer engages in the conduct that led to conviction.

Expungement of unverified reports of abuse has been a hotly debated issue among proponents and critics of child abuse reporting laws. Those in favor of expungement argue that an individual's reputation can be severely harmed by such information, even though an investigation has determined the report to be unfounded. Some child advocates believe it is important to maintain such information for use in future investigations. State policies differ regarding expungement of unverified reports.

eye injuries Vision problems and eye injuries are important and usually easily recognizable indicators of abuse. Close examination of the eyes by a trained physician using an ophthalmoscope can sometimes reveal evidence of trauma and internal injuries that would otherwise have gone unnoticed.

Abuse-related eye injuries can be caused by a number of different kinds of trauma. Sharp objects can lacerate eyelids, cornea and sclera. Subsequent scarring from these cuts can permanently impair vision. Harsh chemicals introduced into the eye can cause burns and scarring. A direct blow from a fist or other blunt object can cause retinal damage as well as external damage to the cornea. Force transferred through the vitreous (jellylike substance inside the eye) to all parts of the eye applies sudden and extreme pressure to delicate internal structures and may damage the optic nerve. Collection of blood and damaged tissue inside the eye following trauma can also impair vision.

Blows to the front of the head may injure the visual cortex, causing blindness or other visual problems. Damage to the optic nerve can occur when head trauma causes cranial bones to splinter or when swelling applies pressure. Gouging can separate the optic nerve from the eye, resulting in permanent vision loss.

A sudden blow to the chest may produce a rapid increase in pressure within the blood vessels, causing retinal hemorrhaging. This condition, known as PURTSCHER RETINOPATHY, is common among young children who have been battered. Though retinal hemorrhages are often found in abused children they can also occur as a result of other childhood activities, such as participation in contact sports or gymnastics.

An ophthalmoscopic examination is an important part of a thorough medical assessment of PHYSICAL ABUSE.

failure to bond   See ATTACHMENT DISORDER.

failure to grow   See GROWTH FAILURE.

failure-to-thrive syndrome   A marked retardation or cessation of growth during the first three years of the life of a child. The most frequently used technical criterion for diagnosing failure to thrive (FTT) is when the child's weight falls below the third percentile on a standard growth chart. Another criterion is if the child's growth rate plummets, as with a child who is in the 90th percentile but then drops to the 50th percentile. At this level of delayed growth, the child has a serious and potentially life-threatening condition.

Some children adopted from overseas orphanages may show growth delays when they are first adopted. Said Miller and Adamec in *The Encyclopedia of Adoption,* "Growth delays are most commonly due to orphanage living, either because of inadequate amounts of food, improper feeding techniques, or lack of nurturing physical contact and affection. It may be surprising, but children need love and affection in order to grow adequately."

Organic and Nonorganic FTT Cases of FTT are divided into two major categories: organic and nonorganic FTT. Organic FTT may be the result of genetic predispositions or of chronic illnesses or diseases that affect the intake, absorption or utilization of food. In children adopted from other countries, parasitic infections may cause growth delays, as may diseases such as tuberculosis. Once diagnosed and treated, most children rapidly improve, given continued loving care and attention and medical treatment.

Nonorganic FTT is caused by a lack of adequate nurturing and maternal rejection syndrome, which may be present in biological families or in children adopted from orphanages.

This lack of nurturing and rejection may have many causes, including

- The parent's lack of knowledge about childrearing
- Inadequate technical advice or support for mothers who breast-feed their babies
- Nutritional deficiencies caused by extended breast-feeding as the sole source of nourishment
- Rigidity in feeding practices
- Maternal depression and anxiety over the ability to care for the infant
- Maternal feeling that the child is in some way damaged or retarded
- The child's colicky and nervous behavior, which damages the parent-child bond
- The failure of the mother and child to bond

According to Dr. Miller in her article for *Pediatric Annals,* "Growth delays result from a variety of causes, including insufficient food, improper feeding techniques such as bottle propping, lack of nurturing physical contact, depression leading to poor appetite or poor absorption and use of calories, or almost any concurrent medical problem."

Some researchers attribute nonorganic FTT in the child solely to insufficient nutritional intake, while others believe it may also be due to a neuroendocrine disturbance that occurs when an infant or child is deprived of emotional nurturance.

The mothers of nonthriving infants with nonorganic FTT are frequently undernourished themselves, and they may live a life of social isolation with little or no help from their friends, family or neighbors. In addition, fathers of these nonthriving children are often absent from the home.

Symptoms and Diagnostic Path

Children suffering from FTT usually appear emaciated, weak, irritable, listless or apathetic. At the same time, infants may display a kind of hypervigilance—looking to anyone who approaches them for nurturance—and be devoid of the customary wariness of strangers exhibited by other children of their age.

Infants suffering from the sensory deprivation that is associated with nonorganic FTT often maintain a posture in which the arms are held out, flexed at the elbow with the hands up and legs drawn in. This position of apparent surrender is held for long periods of time.

Some children with FTT may not appear to be malnourished at first glance, but upon careful examination, they may have poor muscular development, dull or pale skin, sparse, dry hair or similar evidence of poor nourishment. Young victims of FTT often show a remarkable growth spurt upon hospitalization, with rapid gains in both weight and head circumference. Their behavioral manifestations are slower to improve and may linger for some time after the child has regained an adequate rate of physical growth.

Authors Andrew P. Sirotnak, Joyce K. Moore and Jean C. Smith discussed FTT in their chapter on neglect in *Understanding the Medical Diagnosis of Child Maltreatment: A Guide for Nonmedical Professionals*. According to these authors, organic failure to thrive should be considered by physicians as a possible cause of FTT, because problems in organs, including the lungs, the kidneys, the intestines and stomach, the liver, the thyroid, the adrenal glands and the heart can all lead to a FTT.

The authors said that a physical examination of the child and a medical history are crucial: "The minimum studies include a complete blood count; serum electrolytes (an analysis of sodium, potassium, bicarbonate, blood urea nitrogen, and creatinine in the blood); a urinalysis; a stool examination for blood and fat; a thyroid test; a test for cystic fibrosis; and an X-ray of the chest. If any of these preliminary studies suggest an abnormality, they should be followed up with other tests to clarify the reason for the abnormality."

Treatment Options and Outlook

The doctor who diagnoses FTT must decide whether to hospitalize the child. Hospitalization may be needed for weeks or longer, and it may improve (sometimes temporarily) the conditions of malnutrition, dehydration and possible PHYSICAL ABUSE in the home. Sirotnak, Moore and Smith say that the malnutrition of FTT can be resolved with a high-calorie and high-protein diet and frequent feedings, as well as monitoring of the child's height, weight and head circumference.

Unfortunately, the rapid improvement that the child may experience during hospitalization is often reversed when the child is returned home, in the case of nonorganic FTT. Unless significant changes are made in the quality of care that is provided at home, the child may continue to suffer from a retarded physical, psychological and intellectual development.

According to Sirotnik and his colleagues, "The consequences of FTT can be severe. The child, deprived of an adequate intake of calories, will break down fat and muscle to maintain growth of the brain. A child who is failing to thrive usually becomes abnormal with respect to low weight first. Subsequently, the child will slow in height growth. Small head size and delayed growth of the brain are seen as manifestations of severe and prolonged FTT."

The caregiver of a child with FTT should also be evaluated. She may be causing or contributing to the child's FTT because of a problem with SUBSTANCE ABUSE, psychiatric illness or postpartum depression. She may also be experiencing insufficient financial resources and inadequate emotional support from the baby's father and/or her own family.

Risk Factors and Preventive Measures

FTT is diagnosed after the child is exhibiting symptoms and signs. The intervention of child protective services may be necessary, and medical intervention from physicians is crucial. The mother may also need assistance from social services staff in learning how to feed and interact with her child. If the child is in danger, either from neglect or physical abuse, then the child may need to be removed from the family by protective services staff.

If the child is placed with a foster family, where he or she subsequently gains weight and height in the new home, then the problem was likely to have been nonorganic FTT. Some children do well with a new foster family, and then they are returned to the mother, where they lapse back into FTT.

In the past, children with FTT have gone from their mothers to a foster family and back, in almost a revolving door fashion. The child improves with the foster family and is returned to the mother, where the child's progress halts and growth and height become abnormal again. Then the child returns to foster care and improves and so is returned to the mother, where the child's growth and weight deteriorate again, and on and on.

However, with the passage of the Adoption and Safe Families Act in 1997, parental rights can be terminated within about two years (and sometimes sooner). This is especially true in the case of a child with FTT, if the child cannot improve or deteriorates with the biological family but does well with a foster family.

If the child also does poorly with the foster family, then he or she should be evaluated or reevaluated for organic FTT.

See also ATTACHMENT DISORDERS.

Adamec, Christine, and Miller, Laurie C., M.D. *The Encyclopedia of Adoption*. 3rd ed. New York: Facts On File, 2006.

Miller, Laurie C., M.D. "Initial Assessment of Growth Development, and the Effects of Institutionalization in Internationally Adopted Children." *Pediatric Annals* 29, no. 4 (April 2000): 224–232.

Sirotnak, Andrew P., Joyce K. Moore, and Jean C. Smith. "Neglect." In *Understanding the Medical Diagnosis of Child Maltreatment: A Guide for Nonmedical Professionals*. New York: Oxford University Press, 2006.

fallen fontanel (*caida de mollera*) Traditional medicine in many Latin American countries, as well as among Mexican-Americans, holds that fallen fontanel (the soft cranial bones) in infants can result in listlessness, diarrhea and vomiting. There is no evidence, however, that these symptoms are attributable to displacement of the cranial bones.

The traditional cure for this condition is to turn the baby upside down, place the top of the head in water and shake the infant to return the fontanel to its proper position. Though this practice can produce RETINAL HEMORRHAGE, or even SUBDURAL HEMATOMA if applied too forcefully, it is not considered abusive since it is a widely held, culturally based belief.

family court See COURT.

family preservation The concept that it is extremely important to help abusive or neglectful families whose children are in foster care, despite the nature of their problems, so that they may continue to parent their children or so that they may be able to parent them again later after resolution of their problems. This concept was embodied in the ADOPTION ASSISTANCE AND CHILD WELFARE ACT OF 1980, and it was very closely followed by state social services agencies until the late 20th century, when the ADOPTION AND SAFE FAMILIES ACT (ASFA) was passed.

Although it was still considered important to reunite children with their families when possible under ASFA, the federal government instructed state agencies to consider the needs of the children first. In some cases, children had remained in the foster care system for years prior to the passage of ASFA, sometimes entering foster care as babies or small children and later "aging out" of the system at age 18. Adoption was a low priority or not even considered for most children in foster care.

Some experts criticized the concept of family preservation and said that not only did it force children to stay in foster care for very long periods but it also caused them to be returned to and then re-abused by parents who could not or would not resolve the problems that led to the abuse, such as substance abuse or mental illness. Others said family preservation was a workable idea but that the available funds were insufficient to accomplish the therapeutic aims of family preservation. Generally, both sides agreed that children were remaining in the foster-care system for too long.

See also FOSTER CARE.

family violence Physical or sexual attacks on a spouse, live-in partner or sibling by another member of the family unit. Also known as domestic violence. Family violence often leads to or is accompanied by child maltreatment, particularly physical abuse.

Though wives may attack husbands or boyfriends, many of these attacks are made in self-defense. Because their average size and strength is usually significantly greater, men are more likely to inflict serious injury on both women and children.

Violence between siblings may be the most frequent form of family violence. Unfortunately, little information is available on either its incidence or effects. In addition, SIBLING ABUSE is thought to represent a significant proportion of child abuse; however, it is also the type of family violence that is the least likely to be reported to authorities.

Effects of Family Violence on Children

Even if children themselves are not abused, it is traumatic for them to witness the abuse of their parent or other family members. Children may be very conflicted, wishing to defend the family member but being afraid to do so, since the abuser is nearly always much bigger and stronger than the child and is often a parent or parental authority figure. However, when the child does *not* defend the abused person, he or she may feel guilty and conflicted. According to Gail Hornor in her article in the *Journal of Pediatric Care* in 2005, "The child is torn between a desire to help or rescue the victim and the need to keep a family secret. School-aged children may begin to feel responsible for the violence."

School-aged children in homes where violent behavior is occurring may have trouble with their schoolwork and may also exhibit somatic complaints, such as headaches and stomachaches, that are related to the incidents of family violence.

Family violence may be very difficult for adolescents. Said Hornor, "Adolescents in domestically violent homes express rage, shame, and betrayal. These feelings may be manifested by rebellious behaviors such as truancy, dropping out of school, drug/alcohol use, and running away. Adolescents also may exhibit loss of impulse control." She also added that the witnessing of family violence in childhood increases the risk for the child being in a violent personal relationship in adulthood.

Hornor said that primary-care providers should screen families for family violence, and by doing so,

they may play a key role in helping to end family violence, as well as in breaking the cycle of continued violence when children grow into adulthood. She added, "The psychological trauma of the child witnessing domestic violence can be reduced by decreasing the child's exposure to the violence and linking the child and family to mental health resources, thus helping the child and family to heal."

Factors Related to Family Violence

Richard J. Gelles, an expert in child abuse and family violence, has identified four factors that are directly related to family violence. The first is the intergenerational nature of abuse, which means that an abused child is more likely to become an abusive adult than an adult who was not abused in childhood. However, not all abused children grow up to become abusive adults. (See ABUSERS; ADULTS ABUSED AS CHILDREN.)

Next, POVERTY is also related to violence in families. Though the majority of families with incomes below poverty guidelines are not violent, it is also true that the rates of child abuse and spouse abuse in poor families are higher than in families with substantially higher incomes.

A third characteristic of violent as well as neglectful families is social isolation. These families are observed to have infrequent contacts with friends and relatives, participate in few community activities and move often.

A final factor, social stress, may combine some of the three previous factors with other stressful circumstances. Unemployment, low levels of education, high-stress jobs, marital conflict, poor living conditions and many other factors can increase the level of family stress and may lead to family violence.

Physical Violence and Child Abuse

In a study published in *Violence and Victims* in 2004 by Li-Ching Lee, Jonathan B. Kotch and Christine E. Cox, the researchers studied 219 mother-child pairs in which the children were newborns. Of these child-caregiver pairs, 42 families (19.2%) had at least one child maltreatment report within two years following the initial interviews.

The researchers found that physical violence in the families was a predictive factor for child abuse. The researchers also discovered that the family's receipt of Aid to Families with Dependent Children (AFDC)—now known as Temporary Aid to Needy Families (TANF)—was highly associated with family violence and child maltreatment.

Said the researchers, "Agencies that intervene in families to prevent domestic violence would do well to routinely investigate the possibility of child maltreatment. Such efforts could contribute to the development of improved strategies for ameliorating the pernicious effect of domestic violence and maltreatment on children through prevention and early intervention."

See also BULLYING; CHILD ABUSE; PHYSICAL ABUSE; SEXUAL ABUSE.

Hornor, Gail. "Domestic Violence and Children." *Journal of Pediatric Health Care* 19, no. 4 (2005): 206–212.

Lee, Li-Ching, Jonathan B. Kotch, and Christine E. Cox. "Child Maltreatment in Families Experiencing Domestic Violence." *Violence and Victims* 19, no. 5 (October 2004): 573–591.

fatalities, child abuse   Deaths primarily caused by parents and sometimes by others. According to the U.S. Department of Health and Human Services, there were 1,490 fatalities in 2004 that resulted from child maltreatment in the United States.

Many children die from neglect, while others die from physical abuse or a combination of forms of maltreatment. For example, acute neglect may result in a fatal drowning because the parent or other caregiver has left an infant or small child in a bathtub alone for several minutes or longer. A parent may leave a baby or small child in a locked car in the summertime, causing hyperthermia and death. In some cases, children may accidentally cause their own deaths, sustaining fatal injuries when they discover a firearm that has not been locked up properly. A curious child may accidentally kill himself or herself or another child by discovering and then firing a loaded gun.

Some children die as a result of severe shaking, also known as SHAKEN INFANT SYNDROME, although death is not always the consequence of shaking an infant or child. (In some cases, the child continues to live but often suffers severe brain damage from the shaking.)

Malnutrition and starvation cause the deaths of some children, and these are forms of neglect. In 2004, most child fatalities in the United States that resulted from maltreatment were caused by neglect (36%), followed by a combination of different forms of maltreatment (30%) and physical abuse (28%).

Some children are chronically maltreated, and although an acute incident may result in the child's death, such as a battering that had led to brain trauma, it is also true that further investigation may reveal that months or years of severe physical abuse had previously occurred, based on multiple untreated fractures that show up in X-rays of the child after death.

Babies and Small Children Are at Greatest Risk

Babies and small children under the age of four years are the most at risk for experiencing fatalities from child abuse and/or neglect. An estimated 45% of all child maltreatment fatalities occurred to infants younger than one year in 2004, according to the Administration on Children, Youth and Families in their annual report.

According to the National Clearinghouse on Child Abuse and Neglect, infants and small children are most likely to die from chronic abuse over time (battered child syndrome) or by the impulsive acts of others, such as by choking, drowning or suffocating. Babies are also more likely to die from starvation or dehydration than older children. Small children who are unsupervised are also at risk of death from ingestion of toxic substances or other accidents, such as drowning.

Perpetrators

Perpetrators of child fatalities caused by child maltreatment vary in their characteristics, but researchers have found some patterns. Often the person causing the death is a high school dropout at the poverty level who is depressed and in the age group of the mid-20s. However, well-educated and older individuals with no evidence of depression may also commit acts of abuse and/or neglect.

Most perpetrators (about 83%) are one or both parents of the child. Mothers alone represented about a third (31%) of the perpetrators of child fatalities from maltreatment in 2004. Other children in the family should not automatically be ruled out as perpetrators. Although it is not common, sometimes children cause the death of other children.

Indications of Underreporting of Fatalities

In a study reported in the *Journal of the American Medical Association* in 1999, researchers found a serious underestimation of child homicides that were caused by child abuse, in part because of methods of coding child deaths and in part because of the lack of child fatality teams to evaluate the cause of a child's homicide. Other reasons for underreporting were inaccurate death certificates, lack of information on the perpetrator and differing case definitions.

The researchers studied all child homicides in North Carolina from 1985 to 1996. They found that about 85% of all child homicides resulted from child abuse, although almost 60% of the homicides were not defined as caused by child abuse. Based on their findings, the researchers stated, "For the United States, we estimated that 6,494 more children were killed by fatal child abuse from 1985 through 1996 than reflected by vital records coding."

The researchers also looked at the perpetrators of the incidents and said, "Although the public may believe that biological parents are less likely to kill their own offspring, we found they accounted for 63% of the perpetrators of fatal child abuse. The findings from this study indicate that caregiving males, biological parents, and caregivers of children younger than 1 year are the most common perpetrators of fatal abuse and, therefore, need to be especially targeted in prevention efforts."

Differences between Child Abuse Fatalities and Other Homicides

According to Bill Walsh in his Office of Juvenile Justice Delinquency prevention publication on investigating child fatalities, fatalities that stem from child abuse have several unique features that differ from most homicides. These key differences in child fatalities include the following:

- Delayed deaths are common
- Few or no witnesses are common
- Nontraditional weapons are often used

- Trace evidence is less useful
- Circumstantial evidence is important
- Internal injuries may not be obvious
- Motives differ from those in most homicides
- Coordination with non-law-enforcement agencies (such as protective services staff) is necessary

Delayed deaths Delayed deaths are common in child fatalities, especially in the cases of abusive head trauma and internal injuries that were sustained to the child's chest and/or abdomen. After suffering from the injury, the child may live for hours or days or longer. Said Walsh,

> This delayed death scenario can also occur when a child is severely scalded from an immersion burn, suffers an infection or other medical complications arising from the injuries, and then dies weeks or months after the incident occurred. Or a child may suffer severe brain trauma and lapse into a coma for months, only to die eventually from pneumonia or some other medical complication. Although the abuse was not the immediate cause of death in these situations, the manner of death would still most likely be ruled a homicide because the original abuse was the basis for the medical complication that resulted in death.

When a delayed death occurs, there is often more than one crime scene to be investigated, such as the child's home, the vehicle that transported the child to the physician or hospital and the hospital or other place where the child died. It should also be noted that an unreasonable delay in seeking medical attention for a child is a possible indicator of abuse.

Few or no witnesses observe the abuse Another difference between the circumstances of child fatalities sustained from abuse and those of other homicides is that often there are few or no direct witnesses to the child abuse, which often occurs in the child's home. In contrast, many homicides occur outside the home.

Sometimes another individual who lives with the abuser has witnessed the abuse or neglect but will not reveal what is known to investigators, whether from fear or a desire to protect the abuser, or from both motives. Said Walsh, "To obtain cooperation, it is often possible to charge a reluctant witness with failure to report suspect child abuse or failure to protect a child. In some cases, these individuals may actually have been involved in the fatal maltreatment and can be charged as accomplices in the child's death."

When there are witnesses with some information about the abuse that led to the child's fatality, they may include the following types of individuals:

- Parents and stepparents
- Parents' boyfriends or girlfriends (live-in or otherwise)
- Siblings and other children
- Other family members
- Caregivers, such as babysitters and child-care employees
- Teachers (day-care, preschool, school, church)
- Neighbors (current or past)
- Emergency room physicians and nurses
- Medical providers who have seen the child in the past, including school nurses. (Medical records may also provide important information.)
- Protective services workers (Abuse or neglect may have been reported in the past; note that past reports may have been filed under the mother's last name, which may differ from the child's last name.)
- Law enforcement personnel (who may have been in contact with the family for past incidents or allegations)
- First responders (individuals first on the crime scene)

Witnesses should be interviewed as early as possible, and they should also be interviewed separately from each other. It is also important to differentiate between what a witness personally observed from what someone else may have told a witness. For example, if a witness says that a child fell off a couch, he or she should be asked if they observed the fall when it occurred. Sometimes they may be repeating what others have told them, and in some cases, the person who said that he or she observed the child falling off the couch was the perpetrator who caused the child's death in another manner.

Witnesses who appear calm may seem "guilty" to some people, but it is important to note that people react differently to the death of a child; some individuals remain calm while others are hysterical. Hysteria does not negate the possibility of guilt nor does calmness indicate that guilt is likely. The demeanor of direct witnesses should be considered, but it is not conclusive proof of a crime.

Investigators should not wait until the autopsy of the child is released to start interviewing witnesses, because precious time and information can be lost by doing so, and the perpetrator could then have time to destroy valuable evidence of the crime.

Nontraditional weapons are often used In contrast with most homicides, which are committed with a gun, knife or a blunt object, children who die from child abuse are usually injured by the perpetrator's hands or by scalding water or common household items used by the perpetrator. One exception occurs when the perpetrator uses a weapon of abuse such as an electrical extension cord, rope or another weapon that leaves distinctive marks on the child.

Trace evidence is less helpful In most homicides, trace evidence such as fingerprints or DNA is often used to identify the perpetrator; however, in the case of child fatalities, fingerprints and DNA of the parents and others known to the child are both prominently available within the house, and, consequently, their presence does not automatically link those who live in the home with the death of the child. Several exceptions include when the child was sexually assaulted or when the perpetrator bit the child, in which cases DNA evidence is significant.

Circumstantial evidence is important Many child abuse fatalities depend on circumstantial evidence. Prosecutors may use circumstantial evidence to prove that the suspected abuser was the only person who was present when the crime was committed and that the injury was not an accidental one. Circumstantial evidence is often less useful among homicide cases not involving child abuse fatalities.

Internal injuries often are not evident With many homicides, the cause of death may be readily apparent, as with individuals who are killed by a gunshot wound or by a stabbing. Conversely, however, in the case of a child fatality, fatal injuries may involve harm to the brain and internal organs, and these are injuries that can only be detected through radiological procedures such as X-rays, a computed tomography (CT) scan and/or a magnetic resonance imaging (MRI) scan. Investigators should not assume that they know what happened to a dead child based on external evidence, especially when it appears that a child may have died of SUDDEN INFANT DEATH SYNDROME. A further examination and an autopsy are needed to rule out death by maltreatment.

Motivations are different   With child fatalities, the common motivations are usually *not* greed or revenge, and they do *not* generally occur in concert with a robbery, sexual assault or another crime, as is the case with other homicides. Because the majority of child maltreatment fatalities occur as the result of abuse or neglect by a parent, the motive is often anger because the perpetrator is annoyed by the child's behavior, such as crying, bed-wetting or feeding problems with the child. Sometimes the parent or other caregiver has unrealistic expectations of the child, such as expecting a newborn to sleep through the night or assuming that a one-year-old child can be toilet trained. When these expectations are not met, the parent or other caregiver may blame the child and become angry and frustrated to the point of causing harm and the child's death.

Some caregivers have intense feelings of anger or even hatred toward a child, which eventually lead to explosive and sudden violence and to the subsequent death of the child. In some cases, the perpetrator is rageful because of a mental illness, although this is not common.

Coordination with protective services is necessary   In most homicides, it is not necessary to work closely with non-law-enforcement agencies. However, when a child dies from possible or likely child abuse or neglect, law enforcement personnel must work closely with child protective services workers in the state or county social service office. In at least 10% of the cases, and as many as a third of the cases, the child was previously known to protective services workers because of past alleged and/or

substantiated abuse or neglect. The child may have been in foster care and later returned to the parent or other caregiver.

The key role of protective services staff in the case of a child fatality is to determine whether abuse or neglect occurred and, if so, to protect any other children in the household. The key role of law enforcement is to determine whether a crime was committed and, if so, who committed the crime.

In most cases, law enforcement officials should lead the investigation, because they are trained in obtaining search warrants, interviewing witnesses, collecting and evaluating evidence and filing criminal charges. In about half the states, multidisciplinary teams investigate child maltreatment. Most officials agree that one thorough investigation is better than two separate investigations.

See also ABUSERS; IMPULSE CONTROL; INFANTICIDE; PARENTAL SUBSTANCE ABUSE.

Administration on Children, Youth and Families. *Child Maltreatment 2004*, Children's Bureau, U.S. Department of Health and Human Services, Washington, D.C., 2005.

Herman-Giddens, Marcia F., et al. "Underascertainment of Child Abuse Mortality in the United States." *Journal of the American Medical Association* 282, no. 5 (August 4, 1999): 463–467.

Knight, Laura D., M.D., and Kim A. Collins, M.D. "A 25-Year Retrospective Review of Deaths Due to Pediatric Neglect." *American Journal of Forensic Medicine and Pathology* 26, no. 3 (September 2005): 221–228.

Walsh, Bill. *Investigating Child Fatalities*. Office of Juvenile Justice and Delinquency Prevention, Office of Justice Programs, August 2005.

Federal Republic of Germany   See GERMANY.

fellatio   This term refers to oral contact with the male genitals. Fellatio is a form of sexual abuse when a child is forced or encouraged to perform, submit to or observe the activity. Children are sometimes forced to engage in fellatio with another child for the sexual stimulation of a pedophile. In such cases, the adult is responsible for the behavior even though he or she is not physically engaged in the act itself.

See also SEXUAL ABUSE.

felony Crimes punishable by death or by imprisonment for longer than one year are called felonies. In common law, murder, mayhem, arson, rape, robbery, burglary, larceny, escape from prison and rescue of a convicted felon are considered felonies.

Criminal acts of abuse or neglect may be classed as either a felony or a MISDEMEANOR, depending on the severity of the act. Jurisdictions may vary in the specific acts they consider felonies; however, a felony is always a more serious crime than a misdemeanor.

female genital mutilation Although illegal in the U.S. and in many other countries, female genital mutilation (FGM) is still practiced today in some parts of the world. The term refers to purposeful unnecessary surgical procedures performed on female infants, girls and women, usually as a cultural ritual.

The practice is most commonly found in parts of Africa as well as in some areas in Asia and the Middle East. However, it is known that some immigrants to the United States and other countries may practice FGM. Most pediatricians do not believe that such procedures are an acceptable form of "cultural diversity," seeing them instead as child abuse, and nearly all Western pediatricians condemn such procedures.

FGM may be seen as a means to protect a female's virtue or to make her more marriageable. As many as 4 to 5 million such procedures occur each year, often with no anesthesia and by nonmedical personnel using razor blades, broken glass or other sharp objects.

According to a 1998 issue of *Pediatrics,* all forms of FGM are condemned by the American Academy of Pediatrics, which actively discourages physicians from participating in any way in such a procedure. The authors described several key forms of FGM: Type I FGM, or CLITORIDECTOMY; Type II, or excising of all of the clitoris as well as some or all of the

labia minora (similar to infibulation); and Type III, which is the most radical and includes excision of the clitoris and all or part of the labia minora, followed by cuts that are made in the labia majora.

The authors wrote, "The labial raw surfaces are stitched together to cover the urethra and vaginal introitus, leaving a small posterior opening for urinary and menstrual flow. In Type III FGM, the patient will have a firm band of tissue replacing the labia and obliteration of the urethra and vaginal openings.

Another type of FGM includes a variety of practices, such as cutting or stretching the clitoris and labia, cauterizing the clitoris and introducing corrosive substances into the vagina.

The physical effects of various forms of FGM, particularly Type III, are very severe. Females who have just undergone such a procedure may experience severe bleeding, pain, infection, tetanus and other complications. Adult women may later experience painful intercourse, recurrent urinary tract infections, pelvic infections and other complications. An episiotomy is required for a vaginal childbirth.

The psychological effects have not been studied but individuals who have experienced FGM report feeling great terror and anxiety.

Frader, Joel E., et al. "Female Genital Mutilation." *Pediatrics* 102 (July 1998): 153–157.

fetal alcohol syndrome (FAS) A serious condition that is caused by mothers who abuse (or even use) alcohol during pregnancy. FAS is the most serious form of a range of alcohol-caused disorders known as alcohol-related neurodevelopmental disorder (ARND); for example, fetal alcohol effect (FAE) is defined by many experts as a less severe form of FAS. There is considerable variation among children with FAS, and the damage experienced by the child ranges from mild to severe.

According to the Centers for Disease Control and Prevention (CDC), from 1,000 to 6,000 newborns are born with FAS each year in the United States. Children with FAS usually require more attention than other children, and thus, they may be at greater risk for abuse by their frustrated and/or inattentive alcohol-abusing mothers. As a result, these children may be removed from the home for abuse or neglect and subsequently placed in FOSTER CARE. If the parental rights of the mother are terminated, the child may be free for adoption; however, adoptive parents should be fully aware of the challenges that a child with FAS may bring, as well as the possible need for continued care during adulthood.

The condition known as FAS was identified in 1968 by French researcher P. Lemoine, who first described the signs of FAS in 127 children born to alcoholic mothers. However, this research was essentially ignored. In 1973, Kenneth Jones and David Smith at the University of Washington in Seattle also identified this problem among children of alcoholic mothers. They labeled the condition "fetal alcohol syndrome" in their article in *Lancet.* Researchers who followed Jones and Smith have continued to study FAS, and it is expected that much more research will be performed on this condition.

According to the Centers for Disease Control and Prevention, about 10% of pregnant women in the United States drink during their pregnancies, and of these women, about 2% are binge drinkers (those who drink five or more drinks on one occasion), and 2% are heavy drinkers (those who drink seven or more drinks per week or engage in binge drinking). Binge drinking as well as heavy drinking—or even only 0.5 drinks per day—may cause FAS. As a result, doctors urge all pregnant women to avoid alcohol entirely, since there is no known safe amount of alcohol.

Some racial and ethnic patterns have been found among children with FAS. For example, according to Dr. Sokol and colleagues in their article in a 2003 issue of the *Journal of the American Medical Association,* American Indian/Alaska Native children have a 16 times greater risk of having FAS than white children. In addition, black children have a five times greater risk of being born with FAS than white children.

In some states, the presence of FAS signs in a newborn child is regarded as child abuse, and the child may be removed from the home; however, as mentioned, in many cases, it is difficult or impossible to identify FAS in a newborn, even among physicians experienced in diagnosing FAS.

Symptoms and Diagnostic Path

Most children with FAS are not diagnosed until they are older than age six, thus missing an opportunity to engage in an early intervention program that could have provided educational and developmental assistance to the child.

The child with FAS has experienced brain damage as a result of his or her mother's drinking, and other severe birth defects develop as well. Often children with fetal alcohol syndrome are born prematurely and are underweight, with small heads. These children are likely to remain unusually small and thin throughout their life span. They may also experience seizures and a host of other medical problems that they will not outgrow.

Only a physician experienced in diagnosing FAS in an infant or young child should diagnose a child of this age, because diagnosis can be very difficult; however, there are some identifiable facial features, including

- Folds in the eyelids
- A short nose
- A thin upper lip
- A small chin
- An overall "flattened" appearance

Children with FAS may have central nervous system dysfunctions that lead to impulsivity, memory problems and learning disabilities. In addition, they may suffer from other medical and developmental problems, including

- Heart defects or heart murmurs
- Poor physical coordination
- Cleft lip or palate
- Kidney deformities
- Speech delays
- Frequent infections
- Sleep disorders

Treatment Options and Outlook

FAS cannot be cured, but the individual medical problems of the child with FAS should be treated;

for example, children with FAS who have speech delays may improve with speech therapy. Children with heart problems should be treated by a cardiologist, and those with kidney problems should be treated by urologists or nephrologists. As for developmental delays, the child will need additional assistance in school.

Risk Factors and Preventive Measures

The best way to avoid fetal alcohol syndrome in a child is for pregnant women to stop drinking alcohol altogether during their pregnancy. If a woman does not know that she is pregnant in early pregnancy, she should stop drinking immediately when she discovers that she is or even may be pregnant.

Adamec, Christine, and Laurie C. Miller, M.D. *The Encyclopedia of Adoption.* 3rd ed. New York: Facts On File, 2006.

Jones, Kenneth, and David Smith. "Recognition of the Fetal Alcohol Syndrome in Early Infancy." *Lancet* 3, no. 2 (November 1973): 999–1,001.

Sokol, Robert J., M.D., Virginia Delaney-Black, M.D., and Beth Nordstrom. "Fetal Alcohol Spectrum Disorder." *Journal of the American Medical Association* 290, no. 22 (December 10, 2003): 2,996–2,999.

Weinburg, Naimah Z. "The Adverse Effects That Parental Alcohol Use May Have on Children Are Numerous, Pervasive, Costly and Often Enduring." *Journal of the American Academy of Child & Adolescent Psychiatry* 36, no. 9 (September 1997): 177–187.

filicide Murder of a child by the parent is termed *filicide*. Statistics from 1985 show that 3% of all homicides reported in the United States during that year were filicides. This figure may underestimate true incidence, however, because many child abuse-related deaths are reported as accidents. Over twice as many children are killed by their parents than parents killed by their children.

fixated offender This type of male sexual offender presents a pattern, beginning in adolescence, of being sexually attracted to children. Though he may occasionally engage in sexual activity with adults, such an offender rarely initiates the activity. The fixated offender actively seeks the company of children and fantasizes about sexual contact with them.

PEDOPHILIA is deeply ingrained in the psyche of the fixated offender. Unlike regression, fixation is not the result of a frustrated desire for sex with an adult or similar situational cause, and the offender rarely shows any remorse for his sexual attacks on children. Often compared to an addiction, this pattern of abusive behavior is particularly resistant to treatment.

Though the terms fixated and regressed have been widely used to differentiate perpetrators of child sexual abuse, it has been suggested recently that the motivation of the offender can be better understood as a continuum ranging from the appropriate display of affection to brutal rape. David Finkelhor, a noted researcher of child sexual abuse, has suggested that the two major factors that differentiate pedophiles are: (1) the exclusivity of their attraction to children, and (2) the strength of that attraction. This idea is known as a CONTINUUM MODEL OF CHILD ABUSE.

fondling In the context of child SEXUAL ABUSE, fondling refers to touching of the genitals, breasts or buttocks. Fondling may be a prelude to more extensive sexual activity or an end in itself. Adults are most frequently the fondlers; however, some sexual abuse involves encouraging or coercing children to fondle adults.

As is the case with other forms of sexual abuse, men are more likely to be reported for fondling. While men are the most frequent sexual aggressors, some writers speculate that women's role of primary caretaker of children permits inappropriate fondling to go unnoticed. Reports of nurses and child care workers who routinely use fondling as a way of quieting upset infants appear with reasonable frequency but are often difficult to document.

fontanel, fallen See FALLEN FONTANEL.

forensic medicine In cases of suspected child abuse or neglect specialized medical knowledge is often necessary to answer questions of law. A physician may be asked to examine a child and to testify in court whether, in his or her professional opinion, the child has been abused. When a child dies under suspicious circumstances a medical examiner, usually a pathologist, is called upon to conduct an autopsy to determine the probable cause of death. Both of these physicians are practicing forensic medicine.

Forensic medicine requires special training in gathering medical evidence and providing expert court testimony. With respect to child abuse, forensic specialists must have thorough knowledge of various methods of abuse and must be able to distinguish between accidental injuries and those likely to be intentionally inflicted. In such cases the physician is often asked to determine the validity of a caretaker's explanation of the injury. Through careful examination and application of specialized knowledge the physician is often able to find evidence to support or refute the caretaker's claim.

The ability to date injuries is particularly important in determining who was responsible for the child at the time of injury and also in establishing evidence of a pattern of abuse. Physicians frequently rely on microscopic examination of damaged tissue and use of X-rays to determine the approximate date of the abuse. By applying knowledge of the normal healing process, the examiner is able to determine the amount of time that has elapsed since the injury. Multiple injuries or fractures for example, in various stages of healing, are usually indicative of abuse over an extended period of time. Such evidence belies explanations of a "freak accident" or a single episode of abuse.

When neglect is a suspected cause of death, the forensic examiner's task is somewhat different. In addition to looking for evidence of abuse and neglect, the physician must also rule out other medical explanations for the death. Some chronic diseases can inhibit the normal absorption of nutrients, causing a child to die of starvation despite being fed a healthy diet. In some cases, such as SUDDEN INFANT DEATH SYNDROME, no satisfactory explanation of death can be determined.

Evidence presented by the forensic medical examiner is usually presented in combination with other evidence concerning the child's psychosocial history, the parent's history, the current family situation, reports from teachers, neighbors etc.

See also RADIOLOGY, PEDIATRIC.

foster care The state-managed system in which children who are abused and/or neglected are placed, usually under the protests of their parents or other caregivers, because of acts of abuse or neglect. The parents or caregivers may have problems with alcohol abuse, drug abuse, incarceration, mental illness and so forth. In a small number of cases, parents willingly place their non-abused children into foster care because they are unable to care for them.

Many foster children are considered to have "special needs," which means they are developmentally delayed, have a learning disability or experience another problem, such as a psychiatric diagnosis, attention-deficit/hyperactivity disorder or depression. All foster children must have a case plan for their future, which is developed by state workers in the foster-care system. These plans are subject to an independent administrative review at least once every six months.

Each state sets its own laws that define abuse and neglect, as well as the laws under which it is determined whether abuse or neglect has occurred. (See APPENDIX V.)

In 2003, about 15% of children in the United States who were abused or neglected were placed in foster care, according to *Child Maltreatment 2003.* There were about 523,000 children in foster care in 2003, the most recent figures available as of this writing.

Often children who are believed or known to be abused or neglected are placed in foster care as an emergency precaution because PROTECTIVE SERVICES workers are convinced that the problems of the parents or other caretakers cannot be resolved quickly enough for the children to be safe in their home. In some cases, the child is placed with other relatives, while in other cases, the child is placed in a group home or with nonrelatives who are licensed foster parents.

In a court hearing that is held later, a judge will decide if the child should remain in foster care or should be returned to the parents or other caretakers. Many children are placed in KINSHIP CARE, which means that they are placed with a relative of their parents, such as a grandmother or an aunt, in lieu of nonrelative foster care. If more than one child is removed from the family, caseworkers usually attempt to place them together, but this is not always possible.

In many states, the relative receives a monthly payment to help pay for the child's care. (Nonrelative foster parents also receive monthly payments.) In addition, children in foster care are eligible for Medicaid coverage.

When children are placed in foster care, the parents or other caretakers from whom the children were taken are given goals to achieve and time frames during which these goals must be met, such as attending anger-management classes and/or parenting classes within a given period of time. If the parents are drug and/or alcohol abusers, they may be ordered to enter a rehabilitation facility so that they can work to overcome their drug or alcohol problem. Other goals may be set for the parents, depending on the individual case, such as getting a job. If these goals are achieved within about one to two years, depending on state law, the children may be returned to their parents. If the goals are not met, the parental rights may be terminated involuntarily.

While the children are in foster care, their parents or other caretakers usually may visit them at specified times, generally under the supervision of a protective services worker. Whether children will visit an incarcerated or institutionalized relative depends on state law and state social services policy, as well as on practical considerations, such as whether a caseworker has time to transport the child to the facility and back.

Substance Abuse among Parents Is a Major Factor in Foster-Care Entry

It is estimated that as many as one-third to two-thirds of all the substantiated cases of child abuse involve substance abuse. It should also be noted that abused children of substance abusers are at risk for re-abuse: in one study of 95 abusive parents who were also substance abusers, described in *Children & Youth Services Review,* the abusers were 13 times more likely to maltreat their children again than were non–substance abusers.

According to David Howe, author of *Child Abuse and Neglect: Attachment, Development and Intervention,* most substance abusers are individuals who are impulsive, have feelings of inadequacy, are self-centered, and are also depressed. In addition, these individuals often have a low frustration tolerance. These are all traits in the parents or other caregivers that may cause them to be at risk for abusing their children.

Data on Children in Foster Care

As of September 2003 (the latest information as of this writing), according to the Adoption and Foster Care Analysis and Reporting System (AFCARS), the average age of the children in foster care was 10.2 years, and the average length of time that children had been in care was 31 months.

Most of the foster children that were in care in September 2003 lived with nonrelative foster families (46%), followed by relative foster homes (23%). The remaining children were placed in an institution (10%), a group home (9%), or a pre-adoptive home (5%). Some were on a trial home visit with their parents (4%). Two percent were runaways, and 1% were in supervised independent living.

The children in foster care were about equally split between boys (53%) and girls (48%). Note that these figures are rounded off and thus do not equal 100%. In considering the race and ethnicity of the foster children, most were white (39%), followed by African-American (35%) and Hispanic (17%).

The social worker case goal for most of the children (48%) was to be reunited with their families, followed by the goal of adoption (20%). Of the children who exited foster care in September 2003, most were reunified with their parents or primary caretakers (55%), followed by those who were adopted (18%) and those children who moved to live with other relatives (11%). Eight percent were emancipated, 4% were placed with guardians, 2% transferred to another agency and 2% ran away.

Of the foster children who were adopted, 62% were adopted by their foster parents, followed by those who were adopted by relatives (23%). Only 15% of the children were adopted by nonrelatives.

Types of Foster Homes

Depending on the circumstances, children who are placed in foster care may be placed with licensed foster parents, with relatives or in a group home or another facility.

Background on Foster Care

Foster-care placement was actually intended to provide short-term substitute care until a child could return home; however, because of interpretations and misinterpretations of the ADOPTION ASSISTANCE AND CHILD WELFARE REFORM ACT OF 1980, many children remained in foster care for most of their lives, leaving foster care only by virtue of attaining the age of 18. This situation changed with the passage of the ADOPTION AND SAFE FAMILIES ACT (ASFA) in 1997.

Prior to ASFA, in many cases, children who entered the foster system were eventually "reunited" with their families, and many of them were also re-abused, entering the foster-care system again, in a seemingly revolving door fashion.

Alarmed at the large numbers of children in foster care, Congress passed the Adoption and Safe Families Act in 1997. This act enabled states to involuntarily terminate parental rights if parents were unable or unwilling to resolve their severe family problems. It also enabled the TERMINATION OF PARENTAL RIGHTS if the parents had murdered another child in the family, and the act also provided for the termination of parental rights in other circumstances as well, such as infant abandonment. ASFA did not preclude efforts to continue to provide assistance to families; however, it did put time limits on families.

Health Problems of Foster Children

Studies have indicated that foster children have many medical problems. This problem is compounded by the fact that it may be difficult or impossible for foster parents to obtain the child's past medical records, although foster parents should always ask social workers for this information.

According to an article by Moira Szilagyi, medical director of Foster Care Pediatrics in Rochester, New York, about 80% of foster children have one or more chronic medical problems. Chief among them are respiratory problems, with about 18% experiencing asthma. Blood disorders such as anemia are found in about 20% of foster children.

Other common problems cited by Szilagyi included hearing impairments, visual impairments, neurological disorders from mild to serious, sexually transmitted diseases and other infectious ailments. In many cases, children have not received their recommended childhood immunizations.

Foster children may also have developmental delays, language disorders, learning disabilities and behavioral problems. In addition, the children may experience emotional problems such as oppositional defiant disorder, attention-deficit/hyperactivity disorder or anxiety disorders. However, experts say that despite the severe problems that many foster children have experienced in the past, as well as the existing emotional disorders they often struggle with, they often do not receive appropriate psychiatric or psychological services.

Long-Term Impacts of Foster Care

Studies have revealed that children who remain in foster care for years often experience many problems as adults. For example, according to the 1996 book *Assessing the Long-Term Effects of Foster Care*, only half of all foster children graduate from high school, compared to 78% in the general population. As many as 40% will receive welfare benefits as adults or will be incarcerated. In addition, adults who were former foster children have a homeless rate that is at least four times that of the general population.

Despite its problems, foster care is an important resource for abused children. The majority of foster families offer competent, warm and loving care. Under good conditions, foster families receive adequate support from caseworkers and in turn provide a stable environment for the child. To be effective, foster care must be part of a comprehensive system of treatment involving the child, biological family and foster family.

Adoption of Foster Children

Since the passage of the Adoption and Safe Families Act in 1997, many more children who cannot return to their families from foster care are adopted. Most of the adoptive parents are also the children's foster parents, with the adoption providing the children with a continuity of care. Others are adopted by relatives and a small percentage are adopted by nonrelatives. Most of the new adoptive parents of the children (about 88%) are given an adoption subsidy to help them pay for the children's care, and the children are also continued on Medicaid.

There is also a generous tax credit of about $10,000 per child when children with special needs from the U.S. foster-care system are adopted, even if no money was expended by the adoptive parents in the course of the adoption. As a result, parents who adopt two siblings with special needs from foster care are entitled to a tax credit of over $20,000. In contrast, families who adopt children not in foster care must have expended adoption fees in order to obtain an adoption credit, and the credit is tied to income limitations, the amount of the fees and other factors. (See the most recent edition of IRS Publication 968 for current information.)

Data on children adopted from foster care In fiscal year 2003, about 50,000 foster children were adopted. Half were boys, and half were girls. Many children had been in foster care for years: the average time in foster care was seven years. However, after parental rights were terminated, the children were adopted in an average of 16.3 months.

Most of the adopted children were white (42%), followed by African-American (33%) and Hispanic (16%).

Most of the children were adopted by married couples (67%), followed by single females (28%). In 3% of the cases, the children were adopted by single males, and in 2% of the cases, they were adopted by an unmarried couple.

In 2003, many children were waiting to be adopted: 119,000. A slightly higher percentage of children available to be adopted, also known as "waiting children" (53%) were boys, compared to the 47% female foster children available for adoption. About 62% of the children waiting to be adopted were from under one year to five years old.

Children abused by foster parents Sometimes children who are placed in foster care are neglected or abused by their foster parents. This is very traumatic because some have already faced abuse or neglect at the hands of their parents or other long-term caretakers, compelling them into the foster-care system. In most cases, children are frightened and do not wish to enter foster care. Few children voluntarily leave their own homes, even when the environment is very abusive and harsh.

Foster parents are usually screened, but sometimes the screening is a cursory one. When maltreatment occurs by foster parents, their foster children are more likely to be neglected than abused; according to *Child Maltreatment 2003,* of foster parents who abused their foster children, 50% were neglectful, followed by 19.6% who committed multiple maltreatments and 16.9% who physically abused their foster children. (See the table.)

TABLE
PHYSICAL ABUSE, NEGLECT AND SEXUAL ABUSE OF CHILD VICTIMS OF MALTREATMENT, 2003,
BY PERCENTAGE AMONG DIFFERENT CATEGORIES OF CHILD ABUSERS

	Parent	Other relative	Foster parent	Residential facility staff	Child day-care provider	Unmarried partner of parent	Friend or neighbor
Physical abuse only	11.0	10.4	16.9	19.0	12.9	16.6	3.4
Neglect only	62.0	37.5	50.0	46.3	48.4	37.9	9.7
Sexual abuse only	2.7	29.9	6.3	11.5	23.0	11.5	75.9
Psychological maltreatment only, other only, or unknown only	9.1	5.8	7.3	8.4	2.5	14.4	2.7
Multiple maltreatments	15.2	16.4	19.6	14.7	13.1	19.6	8.3
Total percent	100.0	100.0	100.0	100.0	100.0	100.0	100.0

Source: Adapted from Administration on Children, Youth and Families, *Child Maltreatment 2003.* Children's Bureau, U.S. Department of Health and Human Services, Washington, D.C., 2005, page 68.

If abuse or neglect is discovered by protective services workers, the child is usually removed to another home or facility for foster children.

See also ABUSERS; ADOPTING ABUSED CHILDREN; ADULTS ABUSED AS CHILDREN; CHILD ABUSE; FAMILY VIOLENCE; NEGLECT; PARENTAL SUBSTANCE ABUSE; PHYSICAL ABUSE; PSYCHOLOGICAL/EMOTIONAL MALTREATMENT; SEXUAL ABUSE; SUBSTANCE ABUSE.

Adamec, Christine, and Laurie C. Miller, M.D. *The Encyclopedia of Adoption.* 3rd ed. New York: Facts On File, 2006.

Administration on Children, Youth and Families. *Child Maltreatment 2003.* Children's Bureau, U.S. Department of Health and Human Services, Washington, D.C., 2005.

Fuller, Tamara L., and Susan J. Wells. "Predicting Maltreatment Recurrence among CPS Cases with Alcohol and Other Drug Involvement." *Children and Youth Services Review* 25, no. 7 (2003): 553–569.

Howe, David. *Child Abuse and Neglect: Attachment, Development and Intervention.* New York: Palgrave Macmillan, 2005.

Internal Revenue Service. "Tax Benefits for Adoption," Publication 968, U.S. Department of Treasury, 2005.

McDonald, Thomas P., et al. *Assessing the Long-Term Effects of Foster Care: A Research Synthesis.* Washington, D.C.: CWLA Press, 1996.

Szilagyi, Moira. "The Pediatrician and the Child in Foster Care." *Pediatrics in Review* 19, no. 2 (February 1998): 39–50.

Takayama, John I., M.D., et al. "Relationship between Reason for Placement and Medical Findings among Children in Foster Care." *Pediatrics* 101, no. 2 (February 1998): 201–207.

founded report Reports of suspected child abuse or neglect are considered founded if verified by an investigation. The process of verifying reports is called SUBSTANTIATION.

Statistics from several states indicate a wide variation in the percentage of reports that are founded. Differences in rates of substantiation may reflect legal definitions of abuse and neglect or variations in protective service agencies policies.

foundling hospital The first known foundling hospital for unwanted children was established in A.D. 787 by Datheus, Archpriest of Milan. During the late 19th century, a large foundling hospital in St. Petersburg, Russia, handled an average of 25,000 babies annually.

Although they were established to care for large numbers of unwanted babies who were being killed or abandoned by their parents, the foundling hospitals themselves often provided inadequate care or engaged in exploitation. About one in every four babies placed in early foundling hospitals died there. Early studies of the FAILURE-TO-THRIVE SYNDROME by Rene A. Spitz, John Bowlby and others were conducted in foundling hospitals. These studies concluded that even when infants were provided with excellent physical and medical care they often became listless, failed to grow at the normal rate and sometimes died—apparently as a result of inadequate emotional nurturance.

New methods of birth control, legalized abortion, the availability of public financial support for the poor and an expanded interest in adoption have combined to reduce the need for foundling hospitals in most Western nations since World War II.

fractures Breaks in bones. The ability of physicians to identify and date fractures was greatly enhanced by advances in the use and interpretation of X-rays. By employing X-ray technology, pediatric radiologists are able to tell approximately when a fracture occurred and often what type of force caused the fracture. By comparing this information with the caretaker's explanation of an injury the physician can often identify cases of suspected abuse.

While certain types of fractures are indicative of abuse, a diagnosis of abuse requires information about the child's environment, how the injury occurred, the child's caretakers and medical history. Some childhood diseases can render the bones brittle and thus more susceptible to injury. Conditions such as OSTEOGENESIS IMPERFECTA and congenital insensitivity to pain must be ruled out in the process of diagnosing child abuse. It is not uncommon for infants, particularly breech deliveries, to sustain fractures during childbirth. As a general rule, fractures incidental to childbirth will be visible on X-rays by the 11th day of life. Bone trauma appearing after this time is assumed to have occurred following birth.

In evaluating the possibility of child battering, consideration of the child's age is important. While it is quite possible for a child to sustain certain types of fractures while learning to walk, the presence of a transverse (crosswise) or spiral fracture in a child who is not yet able to walk may arouse suspicion.

Bone fractures related to child abuse are caused by a direct blow, twisting (usually of a limb), shaking or squeezing. The particular kind of force used may produce a characteristic type of fracture. A direct blow often produces a transverse or spiral fracture to the shaft of a long bone. Blows to the head often produce internal injuries in addition to fractures of the cranium, mandible and maxillary bones. Swelling due to increased pressure inside the cranium can cause the sutures of the skull to separate.

Twisting forces may produce spiral fractures in the long bone shaft. This type of fracture, like those resulting from direct blows, occurs frequently from accidental causes. A spiral fracture of the tibia (one of two bones in the forearm) is somewhat more likely to be the result of abuse than similar fractures of other bones.

Fractures at the epiphyseal-metaphyseal junction are also produced by twisting and are more frequently related to abuse. The epiphysis, the cartilaginous end of a child's long bones, can be detached from the relatively stronger metaphysis by twisting or vigorous jiggling of a child's limbs. This type of injury is difficult to identify in the early stages of healing. In some cases a fragment of bone or cartilage may be visible on an X-ray, in others the only visible sign is swelling of tissues around the joint. Epiphyseal-metaphyseal injuries to the hip and shoulder sometimes cause the joint space to fill with blood. Widening of the hip or shoulder joint space usually indicates this type of injury. As healing progresses formation of CALLUS becomes visible in X-rays, allowing easier identification of the injury.

Violent shaking of a child can cause spinal damage as well as epiphyseal-metaphyseal fractures. Spinal fractures usually follow hyperflexion (exaggerated twisting or bending) of the vertebral column. Typical injuries are compression, notching and/or dislocation of the vertebrae.

Squeezing injuries usually involve rib fractures. According to Dr. Sills et al., "Rib fractures are seen in 5–26% of abused children with 90% of abuse-related fractures occurring in children under 2 years

FRACTURES ASSOCIATED WITH BATTERING

Transverse	
—Long Bones	Often accidental in children who are old enough to walk, rarely accidental in nonambulatory children; may result from a direct blow
Spiral	
—Long Bones	Can be caused by twisting or a direct blow; often accidental in older children
Fractures of the Cranium	Young children and infants are especially susceptible to these injuries; may result in macrocephaly, separation of the cranial sutures, CNS damage
Vertebral Fractures	
—Compression, Notching	Often caused by shaking; may also be associated with CNS injury, subdural hematoma, internal organ damage
Epiphyseal Metaphyseal Injury	
—Long Bones	Caused by twisting forces; most frequently associated with battering; may not be immediately detectable on X-rays
Rib Fractures	May result from squeezing of the chest; sometimes associated with shaking injuries; frequently concomitant with internal organ injury
Humerus Fractures	May result from twisting or rotating the child's arm, commonly results from abuse when child is three years or younger.

of age." Fractures resulting from squeezing are usually bilateral, caused by an adult grasping both sides of the chest and applying pressure. They may also be caused by twisting or shaking the child. When rib fractures are detected internal injuries may also be present.

Determining When Fractures Are Present

Dating of fractures is especially important in detecting child abuse. By comparing physical evidence of the fracture's age with the caretaker's explanation of the accident the physician can detect discrepancies that might lead to a suspicion of battering. Presence of multiple fractures in various stages of healing is a hallmark of the BATTERED CHILD SYNDROME.

Determination of the age of a particular fracture usually depends on observation of soft tissue changes, observation of a visible fracture line, formation of CALLUS around the fracture and ossification of the periosteum (membrane covering the bone, which is usually damaged by trauma and the resulting bleeding). Immediate soft tissue manifestations of a fracture are EDEMA and swelling. Four to five days after the injury the first stages of new bone growth begin. Actual calcification is not visible on X-rays until 10 to 14 days following the injury.

While a fracture line may be immediately visible following the injury some fractures are difficult to detect and are identifiable only after calcification begins to occur. Bone resorption along the line of the fracture during the first few days following the injury usually makes the fracture easier to detect. Most long bone fracture lines remain visible on X-rays for four to eight weeks.

Detection of child battering involves the use of information obtained from several sources. When bone fractures are detected information from visual and X-ray examination can help determine the type of force that caused the injury and the approximate date of its occurrence. A SKELETAL SURVEY can also detect the presence of other fractures that may not have been reported. Medical information is then compared to accounts of the injury provided by the caretaker, other witnesses and the child (if old enough). Use of clinical data increases the accuracy with which a diagnosis of child battering can be made. Increased accuracy of diagnosis can help prevent further abuse as well as false accusations of caretakers.

Sills, Robert M., et al. "Bones Breaks, and the Battered Child: Is It Intentional or Is It Abuse?" *Pediatric Emergency Medicine Reports Archives,* January 1998.

France   According to the *Country Reports on Human Rights Practices, 2004: France,* from the Bureau of Democracy, Human Rights, and Labor, which was released by the United States State Department on February 28, 2005, data from 2003 shows that there are some child maltreatment issues in France.

Child abuse is strictly forbidden in France; however, it is estimated that there were 18,000 cases of child abuse in 2003, which included 5,200 cases of SEXUAL ABUSE.

Forced marriages among children and adolescents are also a problem in France, and according to the High Council on Integration, about 70,000 girls in France ranging in age from 10 to 18 years old were threatened with a forced marriage. Most of the girls emigrated from North Africa, sub-Saharan Africa and Turkey. The threatened girls may seek refuge in a shelter, and their parents, who are usually the perpetrators, may be prosecuted. It should be noted that there is a difference between an arranged marriage and a forced marriage; in the circumstances of a forced marriage, the girl is compelled to marry someone, while in an arranged marriage, she willingly agrees to marry the individual her parents have chosen.

Forced Begging

Compelling children to beg is illegal in France, and individuals who are found to have engaged in a criminal network that forces children to beg may be imprisoned for three to 10 years and be fined up to $6.1 million (4.5 million euros). In 2003, the French police arrested 67 adults in a Roma encampment and charged them with sexually enslaving children. The children had been kidnapped from Romania, brought into France, raped and then sent into Paris to prostitute themselves and steal. The children were forced to earn $272 per day (200 euros) or they were severely punished.

Child prostitution   CHILD PROSTITUTION is illegal in France, and the penalty for soliciting a child prostitute is up to 10 years' imprisonment. Despite the severe penalties related to child prostitution, it is estimated that 3,000 to 8,000 children were trafficked into France in 2003 and forced into prostitution or begging. SEXUAL TRAFFICKING in girls and adolescents continues to be a problem and is punishable in France by imprisonment of up to seven years and a fine of $204,360 (150,000 euros).

Bureau of Democracy, Human Rights, and Labor. *Country Reports on Human Rights Practices, 2004: France.* United

States State Department, released on February 28, 2005. Available online. URL: http://www.state.gov/g/drl/rls/hrrpt/2004/41681.htm. Downloaded September 1, 2005.

frustration-aggression theory One explanation of physically abusive behavior focuses on the link between biological factors, characteristics of the particular situation and learned response patterns. Seymour Feshbach, a leading proponent of the frustration-aggression approach, focuses primarily on situational factors and learned responses in his explanation of abuse. Aggressive biological impulses are mentioned only as innate impulses to strike out when provoked.

Situational factors that contribute to abusive behavior are broken down into three subgroups: intent, responsibility and perceived justification. Immature or inexperienced parents often have unrealistic expectations of children. A parent may believe an infant intentionally soils a clean diaper or purposely refuses to go to sleep at the appointed time. The parent believes the child is responsible for these actions in the same way an older child or adult would be accountable. Finally, instead of seeing the situation as a normal part of child-rearing the abusive parent feels treated unfairly by the child. These three perceptions combine to intensify the parent's frustration.

Feshbach credits social learning for increasing the likelihood of an aggressive response. Abusive parents learn, through various means, aggressive ways of dealing with frustration. While frustration does not automatically trigger aggression, parents who have learned aggressive responses are more likely to be abusive.

Following the frustration-aggression approach, treatment of the abusing parent would focus on changing unrealistic perceptions and expectations of the child's behavior and on learning new ways of responding to frustration. Many treatment programs incorporate these elements.

gastrointestinal injuries   The stomach and intestines are frequently damaged by forceful blows to the child's abdomen. Hollow organs, particularly the stomach and colon, are most susceptible to injury when they are filled with gas or partially digested food. Rapid compression of these viscera resulting from a blow to the abdomen can rupture organ walls. Such damage to the stomach causes its contents to spill into the peritoneal cavity. Hydrochloric acid from the stomach is highly irritating to other body tissues and can cause a child to go into shock. If the peritoneal cavity is not cleansed, spillage of stomach contents may cause abscesses to develop. Surgical repair of stomach and intestinal ruptures is necessary to prevent further contamination of the peritoneal cavity.

Rapid acceleration when a child is thrown or pushed is likely to tear connective tissue attaching the small intestine to the abdominal wall. Such injuries may cause hemorrhaging of damaged blood vessels.

HEMATOMA (buildup of blood) of the duodenum may result from a blunt blow to the abdomen. This type of injury occurs when the duodenum, with a rich blood supply, is crushed against the vertebral column. The resulting buildup of blood in the walls of the bowel obstructs normal flow of material through the gastrointestinal tract. Indicators of duodenal hematoma include vomiting of greenish material and complaints of tenderness in the upper abdomen. Laboratory tests and X-rays are required to confirm the diagnosis.

This type of injury can usually be treated without surgery. With proper medical treatment the hematoma usually dissipates in 10 to 14 days.

See also ABDOMINAL INJURIES.

gatekeepers   Professionals, agencies and institutions in frequent contact with children are the "gatekeepers" of child protection services. Gatekeepers are often mandated by state or federal law to report cases of suspected child abuse or neglect. Doctors, teachers, child-care workers, social workers, counselors, psychologists, dentists and others are often the first to identify and report abuse. Unfortunately, many individuals in these positions lack adequate training in detection and reporting of suspected abuse and neglect. Widespread efforts are underway in many areas to provide training to those who work with children on a regular basis.

Gault   See IN RE GAULT.

genital mutilation   See CASTRATION; CLITORIDECTOMY; FEMALE GENITAL MUTILATION; INFIBULATION.

Germany   The *Country Report on Human Rights Practices, 2004* released by the United States State Department in 2005, discussed the child abuse problem in Germany in 2003. No statistics were available on physical abuse, although some individual cases of abuse received considerable media attention.

With regard to fatalities, 95 children were the victims of homicide or murder in 2003, and there were also some statistics on sexual abuse. According to the report, there were 15,430 cases of recorded sexual abuse in Germany in 2003. Even when sexual abuse is perpetrated by German citizens in another country, the abuse is illegal and punishable in Germany despite whether the abuse is legal in the other country.

According to the report, the Criminal Code in Germany has laws against child pornography and sexual abuse. For example, the sentence for possession of child pornography is one year in prison, while the sentence for distributing child pornography is five years in prison.

The number of cases of possessing or distributing child pornography increased from 2,002 in 2002 to 2,868 in 2003; however, according to the police, the increased number of cases resulted from greater awareness and reporting rather than an actual increase in sexual abuse.

An area of Germany that borders on the Czech Republic is considered a "haven for pedophilia," and the two countries have worked together to resolve this problem; however, it continues to persist.

Trafficking in girls and women is a problem in Germany, and organized crime rings routinely force girls and women into prostitution, particularly using threats of deportation, physical violence and other tactics. Most of the trafficked women range from age 16 to 25, but some are younger.

Bureau of Democracy, Human Rights, and Labor. *Country Reports on Human Rights Practices, 2004: Germany.* United States State Department, released on February 28, 2005. Available online. URL: http://www.state.gov/g/drl/rls/hrrpt/2004/41683.htm. Downloaded September 1, 2005.

gonorrhea   The most common venereal disease. Gonorrhea is caused by a bacterium commonly known as gonococcus. It infects the mucous membranes causing them to become inflamed. A discharge of pus is also common to cases of gonorrhea.

Gonococcus bacteria are spread through direct contact, predominantly during sexual intercourse. In addition, infants may contract gonorrhea at birth when passing through the vagina of an infected mother. If so infected and left untreated, infants can be blinded by the disease. As a part of a complete physical examination for child SEXUAL ABUSE, cultures are obtained from the genitals, rectum and throat of victim children—regardless of reported method of sexual contact. These cultures are then examined for gonococcus bacteria, which, if present, may indicate sexual abuse.

See also SEXUALLY TRANSMITTED DISEASE.

Greece   The Bureau of Democracy, Human Rights, and Labor's *Country Reports on Human Rights Practices,* *2004* discussed problems with child abuse. Child maltreatment does occur in Greece, and there are penalties that are enforced for abuse violations of Greek laws. There are no national statistics on the incidence of child abuse; however, there are welfare laws that provide help for abused and neglected children. Children's rights groups have alleged that the government residential centers are inadequate. The number of children in residential centers is reportedly declining, while the numbers of children placed in foster care are said to be increasing; however, statistical information is not available.

Trafficked Children

The trafficking of children for use in the sex trade or forced labor is a problem in Greece, and the country is both a destination site and a transit area to other countries for human trafficking in general. The areas from which most people were trafficked in 2003 were Albania, Belarus, Bulgaria, Moldova, Romania and Russia.

Most of the children who were trafficked to Greece for the purposes of begging, stealing and forced labor were from Albania. It was also reported that some Albanian Roma parents sold or "rented" their children. It was estimated by Albanian police that in 2003, more than 1,000 children were trafficked into Greece and forced to beg.

Trafficking is a criminal offense in Greece. The penalties for the trafficking of adults are up to 10 years' imprisonment, and the penalties are even harsher for the trafficking of children. For example, in 2003, two child traffickers received prison sentences of 13 and 14 years, and they were fined more than $94,000 each.

Trafficked minors are often jailed as criminals by the police in Greece. Children younger than age 12 are placed in Greek government orphanages, but older children are arrested and/or detained and deported as illegal immigrants. Often they are deported in groups of children.

Some children are kidnapped from their native countries and brought to Greece, where they are sold to individuals who operate prostitution businesses. Others voluntarily enter the country trying to find a job, but they are then forced into prostitution by people who threaten to get them deported if they refuse to prostitute themselves. In some cases, traffickers confine trafficked children and women against their will in hotels, clubs or apartments.

CHILD PORNOGRAPHY is also a problem in Greece. In 2003, Greek police broke up a massive child pornography ring on the INTERNET, which had customers in 20 countries.

Bureau of Democracy, Human Rights, and Labor. *Country Reports on Human Rights Practices, 2004: Greece.* United States State Department, released on February 28, 2005. Available online. URL: http://www.state.gov/g/drl/rls/hrrpt/2004/41684.htm. Downloaded September 1, 2005.

growth failure   Failure to meet age-appropriate milestones for physical development is primarily caused by inadequate nutrition. A number of organic problems, such as malabsorption of vital nutrients, genetically linked characteristics, disease or infection can interfere with a child or infant's maturation. In some cases, inadequate nutrition is linked to nonorganic factors, such as lack of knowledge by parents, rigid feeding practices or parental neglect and rejection.

Between birth and age three, significant growth failure is most often referred to as FAILURE-TO-THRIVE SYNDROME. After age three, growth retardation is known as DWARFISM.

Though Rene A. Spitz, John Bowlby and other researchers hypothesized that growth failure could result directly from a lack of emotional nurturance, it is now believed that this phenomenon is primarily related to poor nutrition. However, emotional factors frequently contribute to inadequate nutrition. Clinical evidence shows that when children suffering from psychosocial dwarfism are removed from the abusive situation, they experience a rapid growth spurt. This is also true of infants suffering from nonorganic failure to thrive syndrome.

growth failure, reversible   See DWARFISM.

guardian   An adult other than the biological parent may be appointed by a court of law to serve as a child's guardian. A guardian has virtually the same legal powers and responsibilities as a parent; however, guardianship is subject to change or termination by the court. In some cases, the guardian may not have actual CUSTODY of the child.

See also GUARDIAN AD LITEM.

guardian ad litem   In a child protection case involving suspected abuse or neglect, a child is granted an adult advocate, usually but not always an attorney. This individual represents the child for the duration of the litigation, with primary responsibility to ensure that procedural aspects of the case are legally correct. A guardian ad litem is appointed by the court when circumstances dictate that the best interests of the child would be served by so doing.

State laws differ concerning the right to counsel in juvenile proceedings. However, some state courts have found that in cases of child abuse or neglect, the right to counsel is required by the United States Constitution, which calls for due process and equal protection. The guardian ad litem—literally, guardian at law—is charged with protecting only legal rights. This differs from a guardian of the person, whose responsibility is to safeguard the physical and emotional well-being of a child in abuse or neglect proceedings.

guilt and shame   Common negative emotions felt by children who have been abused (especially when they have been sexually abused) that often continue or emerge in adults who were abused as children. Feelings of guilt and shame are the reason why many children fail to report their victimization to others, such as their parents, teachers or law enforcement authorities.

Guilt is a feeling of self-reproach in which an individual takes at least partial responsibility for involvement in (or observation of) an activity that he or she knows or senses was wrong, whether the abuse was sexual or physical.

Shame is a negative emotional response that is directly linked to guilt. That is, the person feels guilt (responsibility) and then shame (sadness and distress stemming from guilt). Shame is often linked to a fear that others will discover what one has done, and that they will be angry or condemning.

Thus guilt is more of an internal blaming process, while shame is more often tied to what others will think about one's behavior. Sometimes the words *guilt* and *shame* are used interchangeably.

Both guilt and shame can play a positive role in some cases, because they may prevent people from committing harmful acts that they contemplate, or, if such acts are committed, they may prevent any recurrences of such behavior. However, when it is an abused child who feels guilt and shame, usually out of proportion to the circumstances, then such emotions can cause serious problems.

In some cases, media exposure provides a great deal of information about the victim to the public. For example, some newspapers have a policy to specifically name crime victims of any age. In addition, if the child's name has already appeared in the media, if and when a similar crime is committed, such as a newly missing child, then the previously victimized child's name may also be mentioned, even though that child had no connection with the new crime. Surprisingly, some newspapers may not name victims, but instead they may name close family members and even include the address of the child in a story or release other information that would make it easy to identify the child.

Abusers Use Guilt and Shame to Their Own Ends

Most people who abuse children or adolescents are very aware of feelings of guilt and shame, and they readily manipulate these emotions. For example, the abuser often tells the abused child or adolescent that the abuse was his or her fault and that no one will believe otherwise. In the case of physical abuse, the child may be told that he or she "deserved it," or even that the child is a bad person and must have the badness beaten out of him or her.

If the abuse was sexual, it may be described by the abuser as normal, or the abuser may tell the child that it was the child's own fault and that he or she was a willing participant. If the child was a willing participant, it is usually from fear or the feeling that he or she must comply with the demands of the abuser. After several incidents of abuse, a pattern has been established that can be very difficult for the child to break.

The abuser will not tell the child that the behavior is, in fact, abnormal and that, even if it were

consensual, children do not have the legal right to consent to sex with anyone, including relatives.

If the abuse does come to the attention of others, the abuser will often actively deny it, stating that the child is lying, imagining the abuse or seeking to punish the parent because of normal parental limits, such as setting a curfew, refusing to buy the child an extravagant item and so forth. It is true that children occasionally do lie about abuse, often because of the manipulation by others. In the past, overly zealous therapists found abuse where it did not exist. However, any allegation should be investigated.

Other types of emotional manipulation often occur in addition to the purposeful use of guilt and shame in the course of abuse, such as the use of fear. The abuser may tell the child that if he or she refuses to participate in an act that the child does not wish to perform (often a sexual act), then the abuser will kill or harm the child or will kill or harm people close to the child, such as parents. He may also manipulate the child's shame subsequent to the abuse and tell the child that parents and others will be disgusted by the child's behavior and will not want him or her anymore because *they* will feel shame and disgust about the child's actions and will blame the child. This approach is often used effectively with runaway adolescents.

Because of their guilt and shame, children may accept such irrational statements, and the cycle of abuse will likely continue until the child shares the information with someone. However, often the abuser tells the child not to tell anyone, or the abuser will know that the secret has been revealed. Since children and sometimes adolescents as well are prone to magical thinking, the child may attribute special powers to the abuser, and the abuse will therefore continue.

It is important for parents, teachers and others to tell children and adolescents that if anyone insists upon touching them in a private place (using language geared to the child's age), this is a form of emotional manipulation. It is wrong and the adult's fault, and the abuse should be reported to a trusted person who is an adult. In addition, children should be forewarned that although parents and others will be very upset to learn of the abuse that has occurred (or has been threatened), they will not be angry with the child but will instead wish to help the child.

The problem is further complicated, however, because often the abuser *is* the parent, trusted relative, neighbor or friend, and it is very hard for children to report to others about their own parents' abusive behavior as well as trusted others. In addition, children may not realize that the abuse is abnormal, since it has occurred for so long. Thus it is helpful if teachers, doctors and other professionals who suspect abuse has occurred or is occurring tell children that it is wrong and illegal for children to have sex with their parents or other relatives, and it is not the child's fault if sexual abuse occurs. Teachers may wish to discuss child abuse in the classroom and explain the tactics that abusers use to keep children silent about the abuse.

In most cases, doctors, teachers and other professionals are MANDATED REPORTERS of child abuse, and thus they are compelled by law to report suspected child abuse. However, sometimes they fear reporting the abuse because they are not sure if their suspicions are accurate.

Shame and the Internet

Sometimes abusers shame or manipulate the abused child by threatening to post pornographic pictures of the child on the Internet. Children and adolescents may experience extreme dread that their family, neighbors and peers will see the photographs on the Internet and then shun or mock them. In some cases, children's photographs have been posted on a pornographic Web site, which can be mortifying to the child upon discovery.

Abusers also use the Internet to attempt to convince children that adult-child sex is normal, often by showing the child photographs of adults and children engaging in sexual acts on the Internet.

See also ABUSERS; ADULTS ABUSED AS CHILDREN; CHILD MOLESTER; CHILD PORNOGRAPHY; CHILD PROSTITUTION; DENIAL; INCEST; INTERNET AND CHILD SEX ABUSE; PEDIATRICIANS; PEDOPHILIA; SEX OFFENDERS, CONVICTED; SEXUAL ABUSE; SEXUAL TRAFFICKING; STATUTORY RAPE.

Hague Convention on the Civil Aspects of International Child Abduction   In order to address issues of concern relative to the return of abducted children and international visiting rights, on October 6, 1980, delegates and representatives of 36 nations convened in the 14th session of the Hague Conference on Private International Law. Their intent was to submit to their governments a comprehensive statement concerning the protection of children in matters relating to custody. On October 24, the assembly adopted the Hague Convention, which was subsequently signed by the United States on December 23, 1981.

The stated desire of the convention was to "protect children internationally from the harmful effects of their wrongful removal or retention." Among other things, the convention establishes a central authority in each country to help individuals who seek return of children abducted from or retained outside the nation in which they are legal residents. In 1986, the United States Senate gave "advice and consent" to the Hague Convention, and in 1987, legislation was introduced to implement policies and procedures outlined in the international document.

According to the U.S. Department of State, the following countries (as well as the United States) are parties to the Hague Convention of 1980 on the Civil Aspects of International Child Abduction as of 2005:

Country	Effective Date
Argentina	June 1, 1991
Australia	July 1, 1988
Austria	October 1, 1988
Bahamas	January 1, 1994
Belgium	May 1, 1999
Belize	November 1, 1989

Country	Effective Date
Bosnia and Herzogovina	December 1, 1991
Bulgaria	January 1, 2005
Burkina Faso	November 1, 1992
Canada	July 1, 1988
Chile	July 1, 1994
China:	
Hong Kong Special Administrative Region	September 1, 1997
Macau	March 1, 1999
Colombia	June 1, 1996
Croatia	December 1, 1991
Czech Republic	March 1, 1998
Cyprus	March 1, 1995
Denmark	July 1, 1991
Ecuador	April 1, 1992
Finland	August 1, 1994
France	July 1, 1988
Germany	December 1, 1990
Greece	June 1, 1993
Honduras	June 1, 1994
Hungary	July 1, 1988
Iceland	December 1, 1996
Ireland	October 1, 1991
Israel	December 1, 1991
Italy	May 1, 1995
Luxembourg	July 1, 1988
Former Yugoslav Republic of Macedonia	December 1, 1991
Malta	February 1, 2003
Mauritius	October 1, 1993
Mexico	October 1, 1991
Monaco	June 1, 1993
Netherlands	September 1, 1990
New Zealand	October 1, 1991
Norway	April 1, 1989
Panama	June 1, 1994
Poland	November 1, 1992
Portugal	July 1, 1988
Romania	June 1, 1993

Country	Effective Date
St. Kitts and Nevis	June 1, 1995
Slovak Republic	February 1, 2001
Slovenia	April 1, 1995
South Africa	November 1, 1997
Spain	July 1, 1988
Sweden	June 1, 1989
Switzerland	July 1, 1988
Turkey	August 1, 2000
United Kingdom	July 1, 1988
Bermuda	March 1, 1999
Cayman Islands	August 1, 1998
Falkland Islands	June 1, 1998
Isle of Man	September 1, 1991
Montserrat	March 1, 1999
Uruguay	September 1, 2004
Venezuela	January 1, 1997
Zimbabwe	August 1, 1995

For further information, contact

United States Central Authority
U.S. Department of State
The Office of Children's Issues
2401 E Street NW, Room L127
Washington, DC 20037
202-736-7000
Fax: 202-663-2674
http://travel.state.gov/family/abduction/hague_
    issues/hague_issues_1487.html

hair pulling   Hair pulling may result in traumatic ALOPECIA (hair loss) and SUBGALEAL HEMATOMA.

Head Start   A nationwide, comprehensive educational program for disadvantaged preschool children that is funded by the United States government, Head Start provides a range of educational enrichment services to young children. Recent studies have shown it to be an effective tool in countering the effects of poverty on children's educational readiness.

As a matter of federal policy, all Head Start staff are MANDATED REPORTERS of child abuse and neglect.

health visitor   In Britain, National Health Service provisions include education and prevention programs and general promotion of good health through the services of a health visitor. Most generally, a health visitor's primary concern is with preschool children and their families. In this capacity, the health visitor may be involved in surveillance of child health and welfare, making regular and routine exams of children. British law requires that newborns be seen by a health visitor at least once during the first 12 months of life; high-risk cases are visited more often.

See also PARENT AIDES.

hearing   Any proceeding where evidence is considered for the purposes of determining an issue of fact is known as a hearing. Usually a hearing takes the form of a formal trial; however, administrative hearings may take place outside of the court process.

Judicial hearings may be held for the purpose of issuing temporary orders (preliminary hearing), fact-finding (adjudicatory hearing) and to determine what action should be taken (dispositional hearing). Emergency removal of a child from home and changes in custody also require hearings. In emergencies a hearing must take place within a specified period of time following removal of the child.

See also ADJUDICATORY HEARING; CUSTODY; DISPOSITIONAL HEARING; EMERGENCY CUSTODY.

hearing, adjudicatory   See ADJUDICATORY HEARING.

hearing, dispositional   See DISPOSITIONAL HEARING.

hebephilia   Sexual desire and responses directed exclusively toward pubescent children by an adult are termed *hebephilia*. Hebephiles are often mislabeled as pedophiles, adults who are sexually attracted to prepubescent children (see PEDOPHILIA). The hebephile usually shows little interest in young children and will engage in sexual activity with adults or children only when adolescents are unavailable.

See also ADOLESCENT ABUSE; CHILD MOLESTER; SEXUAL ABUSE.

helpline   Telephone counseling services are often called helplines. Usually staffed by trained volunteers, helplines offer information, referral and paraprofessional counseling. Unlike HOTLINES, which are frequently connected to protective service agencies, helplines usually do not directly report suspected abuse or neglect. Calls to these services are often anonymous. If abuse or neglect is suspected the callers are encouraged to seek help on their own.

Helplines can serve an important early intervention function. By helping families cope with stress and relieving the social isolation many parents feel, these services can prevent abuse and neglect.

hematemesis   The vomiting of blood, usually as a result of abdominal trauma. Hematemesis can be indicative of internal battering injuries when no external signs are observable.

hematoma, jejunal   See JEJUNAL HEMATOMA.

hematoma, subdural   See SUBDURAL HEMATOMA.

hematoma, subgaleal   See SUBGALEAL HEMATOMA.

hematuria   Trauma to the kidneys or bladder can frequently be detected by the presence of hematuria—blood in the urine. Hematuria may be a sign of serious internal injury. It may also indicate an infection in the bladder or kidneys. Children who present this symptom should be examined by a knowledgeable physician for other evidence of abuse when battering is suspected.

hemoptysis   Spitting or coughing of blood, usually caused by damage to the lungs. Hemoptysis is sometimes observed in battered children.

hemorrhage, intradermal   See INTRADERMAL HEMORRHAGE.

hemorrhage, retinal   See RETINAL HEMORRHAGE.

herpes, genital   Genital herpes is a contagious viral disease, and once contracted, it occurs in the genitals or anal area. There are two forms of herpes simplex virus: HSV-1 and HSV-2.

HSV-1 usually causes cold sores on the lips or nose, and it is not considered a sexually transmitted disease (STD); however, it is possible for HSV-1 to be transmitted to the genitals through oral sex. In most cases, however, genital herpes is caused by HSV-2, and it is transmitted through vaginal, oral or anal sexual contact. According to Willis and Levy in their 2002 article on CHILD PROSTITUTION in the *Lancet*, the risk for contracting herpes is significant during unprotected sex. Said the authors, "Without use of condoms, the risk of transmission of STDs is high; during one act of unprotected sex with an infected partner, an adolescent girl has a 30% risk of acquiring genital herpes simplex virus and a 50% risk of acquiring gonorrhoea."

Herpes is an inflammatory disease that causes clusters of small vesicles to form on the skin at the infection site. If the disease is found in a child or adolescent, this may indicate that SEXUAL ABUSE has occurred. However, sometimes adolescents contract STDs from other adolescents. Regardless, children or adolescents with genital herpes should be screened by a physician for evidence of sexual abuse.

According to the Centers for Disease Control and Prevention (CDC), genital herpes is more common among women (one in four) than men (one in five). It is estimated by the CDC that as many as 45 million people in the United States ages 12 and older are infected with HSV-2.

The presence of genital herpes can increase the risk for infection with the HUMAN IMMUNODEFICIENCY VIRUS (HIV), because herpes lowers the body's resistance to pathogens. As a result, if a person with genital herpes has unprotected sexual contact with a person infected with HIV, he or she has a greater risk of contracting HIV than does a person without herpes.

Symptoms and Diagnostic Path
Genital herpes is characterized by blisters or sores on the penis or vagina. These blisters break and

then heal over several weeks. The disease alternates between periods of inflammation and remission. During periods of remission when there are no skin lesions, herpes is considered less transmissible.

The infection may present within two to 10 days of exposure to an infected partner. The symptoms of the first outbreak may extend for two to three weeks, after which the virus becomes dormant until the next outbreak.

The herpes virus is usually transmitted to others when an individual has herpes sores present; however, it can also be transmitted when no sores are visible.

Some or all of the following symptoms may be present with an initial outbreak of genital herpes (some individuals have no symptoms or do not notice the sores characteristic of herpes because they may be very small and not bother the individual):

- Small, reddish sores on or near the genitals or anus that become watery blisters that break
- Fever
- Swollen glands in the groin
- Flu-like symptoms
- Painful urination
- Vaginal discharge
- Itching or burning in the genitals or anal area
- Headache

If a physician suspects that a patient may have genital herpes, there are several blood tests that can detect the virus; however, the results will not be known for another one to two weeks.

Treatment Options and Outlook

Genital herpes is incurable, and outbreaks may occur up to five times a year; however, some patients have fewer or greater numbers of outbreaks. For many people, unless they have a compromised immune system, the outbreaks will become milder with the passage of years. In fact, in many people, the symptoms are so mild that they are unaware that they are infected. Unfortunately, they may then unknowingly infect their sexual partners.

Medications are available to control the symptoms of herpes and prevent future outbreaks, including Zovirax (acyclovir), Famvir (famciclovir) and Valtrex (valacyclovir).

Risk Factors and Preventive Measures

Children and adolescents who have been sexually abused are at risk for infection with genital herpes.

The only way to prevent contracting genital herpes is to refrain from having unprotected (or any type of) sex or to have sex with a long-term partner who has tested negative for herpes.

Once genital herpes has been diagnosed, the following recommendations are given by the National Institute of Allergy and Infectious Diseases, in order to avoid transmitting the infection:

- Keep the infected area clean.
- Do not touch the sores.
- Wash hands if the sores are touched.
- Avoid all sexual contact from the first symptoms of an outbreak until the herpes sores are healed.

See also GONORRHEA; SEXUAL ABUSE; SEXUALLY TRANSMITTED DISEASE; SYPHILIS.

Willis, Brian M., and Levy, Barry S. "Child Prostitution: Global Health Burden, Research Needs, and Interventions." *Lancet* 359 (April 20, 2002): 1,417–1,422.

homelessness   Lack of adequate, stable shelter is a significant problem for children in industrialized as well as developing countries, In the United States families comprise over 25% of the homeless population. Most of these families are headed by a young single mother with two to three young children. The typical child in a homeless family is subject to a great deal of poverty, stress and disruption.

Homeless children suffer from poverty, abuse and neglect in addition to instability and lack of adequate housing. In some developing countries homeless children, abandoned by their families, must live on their own, supporting themselves by whatever means are available. Because of its connection to POVERTY, homelessness may be seen as a form of societal or SOCIAL ABUSE. Responsibility for such abuse is often seen as resting with the society, which denies children the basic requirements for healthy development.

See also INDIA.

Bassuk, Ellen, and Leonore Rubin. "Homeless Children: A Neglected Population." *American Journal of Orthopsychiatry* 57, no. 2 (April 1987): 279–286.

homemaker services—home health-aide services

The origin of homemaker–home health-aide programs in the United States can be traced at least as far back as the 1920s. There are also some reports detailing groups in the late 19th century that provided in-home care to children and families. These were often affiliated with a religious organization, e.g., the Little Sisters of the Poor, a Roman Catholic order, or the Jewish Welfare Society in Philadelphia. In general, these early services were available to new mothers who needed help with infants or to mothers too ill to convalesce and care for their families simultaneously.

Not until the 1960s was there any large-scale federal funding for regular in-home care to children and families. In 1965, Title XVIII of the Social Security Act included benefits for homemakers–home health aides under Medicare.

The range of services that homemaker–home health aides provide includes help for families in which situational neglect has been identified. This neglect is often the result of an overburdened caretaker. Respite care is another role assumed by the homemaker–home health aide. In families where a child is disabled, terminally ill, retarded or mentally disturbed, such respite care can alleviate parental stress. The homemaker–home health aide can both teach and assist, in order to alleviate the parental stress and the neglect to children. Also, in cases of suspected or known abuse, homemaker–home health aides play multiple roles. These may include observation and reporting, as well as the above-mentioned assistance and education. In cases of suspected child abuse and neglect, the homemaker–home health aide may be asked to provide TESTIMONY in court.

Many professionals recognize the value of homemaker–home health aide services as an alternative to less costly forms of care. Foster care or other out-of-home care for children is also less desirable, since it is disruptive to family life. Homemaker–home health aides can play an important part in diminishing potential disruption in family settings, particularly those in which real or suspected abuse and neglect may already have caused disruption.

Guidelines and accreditation for training and employing homemaker–home health aides are advocated by the National Home-Caring Council, an organization that had its inception in the early 1960s. In 1986, the National Home Caring Council merged with the National Association for Home Care and Hospice. They are located at 228 7th Street SE, Washington, DC 20003.

hospital hold

In many areas hospitals are granted broad powers to hold children in custody for up to 24 hours when, in the opinion of the administrator, a child's safety is in danger or the parents may leave before a protective service worker can make a home visit. A hospital hold is used as an interim measure to protect abused children who are brought to hospital EMERGENCY ROOMS for treatment. The procedure allows child protection agencies sufficient time to act on cases when a child is in immediate danger.

hospital hopping

Abusive parents and caretakers often go to great lengths to avoid detection. Chronic child abusers sometimes engage in an evasive practice called hospital hopping. While fearing detection, the abuser will avoid using the same hospital or doctor twice when seeking medical care for the abused child. Medical personnel have greater difficulty recognizing a pattern of abuse when they are unfamiliar with the child's medical and social history.

See also MUNCHAUSEN SYNDROME BY PROXY.

hospitalism

High mortality rates among infants in European and American hospitals became a cause for concern during the early part of the 20th century. The FAILURE-TO-THRIVE SYNDROME observed in institutionalized infants, known then as hospitalism, was initially attributed to poor nutrition and infection. Later, physicians began to suspect that lack of social and sensory stimulation might be related to this plight of institutionalized infants.

A well-known study conducted by Rene Spitz during the 1940s compared four groups of infants—three raised by their mothers in different settings and a fourth group raised in a FOUNDLING HOSPITAL. Infants who were cared for by their mothers all received similar types of attention. The foundling hospital provided a much different kind of care. Infants in this setting spent their days in cribs located in separate cubicles. Human contact was limited to brief visits from custodial and medical staff. After the first year of life infants reared by their mothers were within normal developmental limits. Foundling infants were retarded in their physical development, withdrawn, apathetic, less active and scored poorly on infant intelligence tests (these characteristics are sometimes referred to as MARASMUS).

Later studies of maternal deprivation showed that infants raised at home by severely neglectful mothers exhibited characteristics similar to those of the foundling infants. Subsequent research showed that retardation of physical growth was more likely related to inadequate feeding habits rather than lack of physical and emotional stimulation. Intellectual, developmental and emotional impairment associated with the deprived infants appeared to be more closely related to the lack of social and sensory stimulation.

Spitz, Rene A. "Hospitalism." *The Psychoanalytic Study of the Child* 1 (1945): 53.
———. "Hospitalism: A Follow-up Report." *The Psychoanalytic Study of the Child* 2 (1946): 113.

hotlines Hotlines play an important role in child protection. These telephone services provide around-the-clock information and referral for victims and reporters of suspected child abuse or neglect.

Telephone crisis services were originally designed to facilitate a quick response to emergencies that required a child to be removed immediately from an abusive situation. Many hotlines now provide non-emergency information and referrals as well.

Hotlines are an important part of a comprehensive child protection system. Most government-sponsored child protection programs around the world maintain some form of 24-hour availability, usually in the form of a telephone hotline. Hotlines are usually staffed by professional child protection workers or trained volunteers backed up by an on-call professional. Workers are trained to screen reports and to respond appropriately to emergency situations. By necessity, hotline workers are called upon to provide counseling to callers in crisis. However, unlike HELPLINES, which are intended to provide telephone counseling, the role of the hotline worker is to match the caller to the appropriate service. This requires workers to be skilled in assessing calls quickly and knowledgeable concerning the range of resources available.

In the United States, most state-affiliated child protection agencies operate hotlines with 24-hour availability.

human immunodeficiency virus A serious infection that is transmitted by a person who is infected with the virus to another individual, either by blood or through sexual fluids. HIV may progress to acquired immunodeficiency syndrome (AIDS). Children who have experienced SEXUAL ABUSE are at risk for contracting HIV, despite their age. Some children contracted HIV while in utero; however, the medical treatment of pregnant women with HIV can reduce the risk of the development of HIV in their infants. In fact, HIV appears on the decline in the United States among infants and young children, probably due to treatment of pregnant women with drugs that suppress the virus.

Worldwide, an estimated 700,000 children are newly infected with HIV each year, primarily due to contraction of the virus during their mothers' pregnancy or in childbirth. About 90% of these children live in sub-Saharan Africa.

Many children die when the disease progresses to AIDS. In the United States, more than 5,000 children have died of AIDS through 2003.

Exposure to drugs in utero is common among children in foster care. According to Susan Vig, Susan Chinitz and Lisa Shulman, M.D., in their 2005 article on young children in foster care in *Infants & Young Children*, about 80% of children in foster care were exposed prenatally to maternal drugs. Said the authors, "Maternal drug use places a child at increased risk for congenital HIV infection. This maternal population most likely did not seek timely prenatal care and therefore was not offered the now-available treatments for HIV positive mothers to significantly diminish transmission of the virus to their fetus."

They noted that foster children also have an increased risk for other congenital infections, such as hepatitis, SYPHILIS and HERPES.

Children adopted from other countries may test positive for HIV; usually, they were infected in utero by their mothers.

HIV Is on the Decline among Children

The number of infants who were diagnosed with HIV/AIDS in 33 states, Guam and the Virgin Islands has significantly declined since 2001, according to the Centers for Disease Control and Prevention (CDC), declining from 306 in 2001 to 145 in 2004.

In considering children younger than age 13 who were newly diagnosed with HIV/AIDS over the same period, the numbers declined to about half, from 360 in 2001 to 174 in 2004. In considering children younger than age 13 in the reporting states, there were 2,634 children with HIV in 2004. In contrast, almost a hundred times more adolescents and adults were HIV-positive in the reporting areas (209,641) in 2004. (See table.)

Symptoms and Diagnostic Path

Many children have no symptoms when they are in the early stages of the virus; however, they may test positive for HIV. When symptoms occur, they may be as follows:

• Frequent infections and infections that are not normally seen in most children
• Developmental delays
• FAILURE TO THRIVE

HIV is usually diagnosed with the enzyme-linked immunosorbent assay (ELISA). Other tests may also be used to test for HIV, such as DNA polymerase chain reaction (PCR) tests.

Treatment Options and Outlook

There is no cure for HIV as of this writing, but children can be treated with antiviral medications, such as lamivudine (3TC), nevirapine (NVP) and zidovudine (ZDV). Some physicians combine several different antiviral drugs to treat HIV, creating a "cocktail" of drugs.

Risk Factors and Preventive Measures

The following groups of children have a greater risk of contracting HIV:

• African-American children
• Children whose parents are sex workers (prostitutes)
• Children whose parents are intravenous drug users
• Sexually abused children
• Children in foster care

In most cases, children cannot help being infected with HIV if their mothers have the virus and the mothers transmit it to them during pregnancy or childbirth. Some mothers may not know that they harbor HIV because they have received no prenatal care and no HIV testing. Women who know that they are HIV-positive or have AIDS should inform their obstetricians so that they can receive medication and reduce the risk of transmitting the infection to their babies.

Adolescents who are sexually active and all children who are sexually abused have an increased risk for contracting HIV, especially if they engage in CHILD PROSTITUTION or if they are compelled into SEXUAL TRAFFICKING.

Adolescents who willingly engage in sex can reduce the risk of contracting HIV by using condoms; however, adults who force children or adolescents into sex often do not use condoms. Programs that actively seek to protect children against sexual abuse could help to decrease the spread of HIV and AIDS.

See also FOSTER CARE; SEXUAL ABUSE; SUBSTANCE ABUSE.

Centers for Disease Control and Prevention (CDC). "Cases of HIV/AIDS, by Area of Residence, Diagnosed in 2004—33 Sites with Confidential Name-Based HIV Infection Reporting." *HIV/AIDS Surveillance Report* 16. Atlanta,

ESTIMATED NUMBERS OF PERSONS LIVING WITH HIV INFECTION
(NOT AIDS) AT THE END OF 2004, BY AREA OF RESIDENCE AND AGE CATEGORY, UNITED STATES,
AS REPORTED BY 33 STATES

Area of residence	Adults or adolescents	Children younger than age 13	Total
Alabama	5,232	26	5,258
Alaska	241	1	242
Arizona	5,288	45	5,342
Arkansas	2,154	9	2,163
Colorado	5,650	14	5,664
Florida	33,331	268	33,599
Idaho	333	1	334
Indiana	3,651	24	3,675
Iowa	506	3	509
Kansas	1,099	7	1,106
Louisiana	7,518	103	7,621
Michigan	5,945	62	6,007
Minnesota	3,038	21	3,059
Mississippi	4,041	34	4,075
Missouri	4,701	34	4,735
Nebraska	605	6	611
Nevada	3,076	13	3,089
New Jersey	14,933	263	15,196
New Mexico	872	0	872
New York	38,083	1,046	39,129
North Carolina	10,886	71	10,957
North Dakota	81	0	81
Ohio	7,829	55	7,884
Oklahoma	2,251	16	2,267
South Carolina	6,491	55	6,546
South Dakota	170	2	172
Tennessee	6,414	68	6,482
Texas	22,460	307	22,767
Utah	744	9	753
Virginia	9,105	49	9,154
West Virginia	630	5	635
Wisconsin	2,206	17	2,223
Wyoming	78	1	79
Subtotal	209,641	2,634	
Total			212,275

Source: Adapted from Centers for Disease Control and Prevention (CDC), "Cases of HIV/AIDS, by Area of Residence, Diagnosed in 2004—33 States with Confidential Name-Based HIV Infection Reporting." *HIV/AIDS Surveillance Report* 16. Atlanta, Ga.: Department of Health and Human Services, Public Health Services, 2005, page 22. Available online. URL: http://www.cdc.gov/hiv/STATS/2004SurveillanceReport.pdf. Downloaded on December 22, 2005.

Ga.: Department of Health and Human Services, Public Health Services, 2005. Available online. URL: http://www.cdc.gov/hiv/STATS/2004SurveillanceReport.pdf. Downloaded on December 22, 2005.

Vig, Susan, Susan Chinitz, and Lisa Shulman, M.D. "Young Children in Foster Care: Multiple Vulnerabilities and Complex Service Needs." *Infants & Young Children* 19, no. 2 (2005): 147–160.

hydrocephaly   Enlargement of the head caused by a buildup of cerebrospinal fluid. Increased pressure within the cranial cavity can result in permanent central nervous system injury and death.

Hydrocephaly can develop as a result of disease or trauma. Child abuse should be considered as a possible cause in cases where explanation of the head trauma seems implausible and where no evidence of disease is present.

hypervigilance   Severely abused children may become hypervigilant as a result of the random nature of past abuse. These children are watchful and withdrawn, constantly on guard, lacking an ability to trust others yet seeking emotional nurturance. Lengthy treatment and much patience on the part of the therapist and caretaker are usually required to overcome this manifestation of abuse.

A form of hypervigilance is also observed in infants suffering from FAILURE-TO-THRIVE SYNDROME. These infants sometimes lack the wariness of older children, seeking affection indiscriminately from anyone who approaches.

See also WITHDRAWAL.

hyphema   Hemorrhage in the front portion of the eye is known as hyphema. Observable as a "blood-shot" eye, hyphema may be the result of a blow directly to the eye or other head trauma.

hypopituitarism, post-traumatic   See DWARFISM.

hyposomatotropism, reversible   See DWARFISM.

hypovitaminosis   See AVITAMINOSIS.

identification with the aggressor Psychoanalytic theory explains aggressive behavior of abused children as an ego defense mechanism. In an attempt to cope with feelings of powerlessness the abused child often adopts a violent mode of relating to others. Rage that cannot be expressed toward the abuser for fear of retaliation is redirected at other, less powerful individuals. Identification with the aggressor may explain the high degree of SIBLING ABUSE in families where one or both parents are abusive.

Though adopting an aggressive self identity may give the child a temporary sense of control over a situation that is largely beyond control, it ultimately causes the child to feel even worse. In becoming the aggressor the child may also internalize negative feelings toward the abuser. When others condemn the child for violent acts the child, remembering anger at the abuser, feels that he or she is also hopelessly bad. The child becomes trapped in a cycle in which feelings of low self-worth lead to acts of aggression that, in turn, bring confirmation of the child's badness from others.

See also GUILT AND SHAME.

identification with the victim Passive, dependent behavior of abused children may result from identification with a parent who is also the victim of abuse. Though this form of ego defense appears to be less common than IDENTIFICATION WITH THE AGGRESSOR it can be observed in many children who are withdrawn and who appear to be perpetual victims.

Psychoanalytic theorists believe identification with the victim is likely to occur when the child forms a strong early attachment to a passive-dependent parent. Identity as a victim offers a clearly defined, though maladaptive, role. Unlike the child who identifies with the aggressor, the child who copes with abuse in this way may be less burdened by feelings of guilt. Both types of ego defense are likely to lead to deep, long-lasting feelings of low self-esteem.

immunity, legal Most jurisdictions that have laws specifically requiring individuals to report suspected abuse and neglect also protect reporters from legal liability for such reports. MANDATED REPORTERS are typically granted immunity from criminal and civil charges arising from a report made in good faith. In many areas all reports are presumed to be in good faith unless it can be proven that the reporter knowingly filed a false report. Immunity from criminal and civil prosecution removes a significant legal barrier to reporting suspected abuse and neglect.

Critics of immunity for reporters argue that it leads to overreporting and abuse of reporting laws. In particular, opponents argue that the difficulty of proving a report was filed in bad faith encourages divorced parents to use false reports as a tactic in custody disputes. Some states have attempted to address this problem by increasing penalties for false reports.

Besharov, Douglas J. "Child Welfare Liability: The Need for Immunity Legislation." *Children Today,* September–October 1986.

impetigo A highly contagious skin disease occurring primarily in young children and infants, impetigo produces rapidly spreading red blisters. Severe cases of impetigo are often indicators of neglect and unsanitary living conditions.

impulse control Poor impulse control may be both a precipitant and a result of abuse. Parental immaturity, reflected in an inability to separate emotions from actions, is often blamed for abuse. Impulse control is lacking when the parent's frustrations and emotional needs are translated directly into action. In psychoanalytic terms, impulsive behavior reflects a weak superego (internal control mechanism).

When parents become frustrated or angry they may lash out at the first convenient target—usually the child. Though they may later regret their actions, abusive parents often lack sufficient control to avoid impulsive maltreatment of their children. Pedophiles and repeat sexual offenders are also cited as having poor control, in their case, over sexual impulses. Development of internal controls is an important goal in treatment of abusers. Until sufficient internal controls are developed, protection of the child may depend on external controls exercised by another adult or a child protection agency.

Learning to control aggressive impulses is a normal task in child development. Children of abusive parents usually lack adequate role models for controlling or sublimating anger. Though a child may develop a kind of pseudo-impulse control founded on fear of punishment, this mechanism quickly breaks down under stress. The resulting behavior often takes the form of unpredictable temper tantrums. Failure to master aggressive impulses leads the child to feelings of hopelessness and negative self-worth. If the abused child does not later develop adequate internal controls, he or she may grow up to be an abusive parent.

See also ABUSERS.

in camera In some cases of suspected child abuse or neglect, a legal hearing is held in the judge's chambers. This closed hearing is described by *in camera*, the Latin term meaning, literally, in secret.

incest A sexual act between an adult and child who are related to each other. In the case of adoptive parents with no biological relationship to the child, most people consider sexual acts between an adoptive parent and an adopted child to be incest because of the parental relationship; however, state law varies on this point.

Mother-son incest accounts for a much smaller proportion of incest than father-daughter incest, while cases of reported mother-daughter incest are the least frequently documented. Incest involving siblings as both perpetrators and victims is less likely to be reported than incidents involving parent-child exploitation. This may reflect an attitude that such occurrences are less serious or a parental preference for handling such matters within the family.

Incest has a long-lasting and profound effect on children, increasing the risk for SUBSTANCE ABUSE in the victim as well as depression, anxiety and even SUICIDE. (See ADULTS ABUSED AS CHILDREN.) It also increases the risk for the victim of childhood abuse becoming a child abuser in adulthood.

Younger-Victim Incest Offenders v. Older-Victim Incest Offenders

Most of the research on incest offenders includes offenders of children of all ages; however, in one unique study, reported in the *Journal of the American Academy of Psychiatry and Law* in 2005, the researchers compared data on incest offenders of two groups, including one group who had been convicted of sexually abusing relatives from infancy to age five and another group who had abused relatives who were 12–16 years old. (Researchers did not study sex offenders who had abused children who were six to 11 years old.)

Said the researchers, "Sexual abuse of an infant or toddler not only represents the same breach of society's values and laws that a similar crime against an adolescent does, but it also contravenes any semblance of adaptive sexual behavior, biologically or otherwise. With this difference in mind, it is reasonable to predict that a person who offends against a very young child would differ, on one or many levels, from a person whose sexual assault victims appear to be limited to adolescents." The researchers found that this assumption was a valid one.

In this study, girls were the most common victims. Said the researchers, "In fact, in the entire database from which the two groups in this study were sampled, only 19 of 342 offenders did not have a female victim."

There were 48 men who were sex offenders of infants and young children in one group and 71 men whose youngest victims were 12–16 years old in the other group. About 40% of the men said that they had been sexually or physically abused children.

The researchers found significant differences between the men in the two groups, with the sexual abusers of infants and small children having a greater rate of psychopathology than the sexual abusers of adolescents. For example, of the men who sexually abused young victims, 85% had a history of drug dependency, compared to the rate of drug dependency among men who had sexually abused adolescent victims (9%). Half the men who victimized young victims had a history of alcohol dependency, compared to 27% of the men who had victimized adolescents.

There was almost a four times higher rate of a history of criminal behavior (33%) among men who had abused infants and young children, compared to the rate for the men who had abused adolescents (9%). The abusers of young children also had a higher rate of a family history of violence (62%) compared to the rate for the adolescent abusers (43%).

Those who sexually abused infants and young children had a higher rate of abusing males (26%) than the abusers of adolescents (10%). In addition, they had a higher rate of making threats of violence or causing injury (38%) than the victimizers of adolescents (9%). The sex offenders of young children also had a higher rate (49%) of having more than two victims than the offenders of adolescents (18%), although most offenders of multiple victims had no more than two victims.

The abusers of young victims were more likely to have abused their nephews, nieces and grandchildren than the offenders of older children, who were more likely to abuse sons or daughters. For example, 47% of the abusers of young children had abused nephews, nieces and/or grandchildren, compared to 16% of the abusers of adolescents. In contrast, 29% of the abusers of infants or young children had abused their sons or daughters, compared to 41% of the abusers of adolescents.

Interestingly, both groups had high rates of being married: 79% of the abusers of infants and young children and 91% of the abusers of adolescent family members.

Sibling Offenders

When the offender is a sibling, in the majority of cases, it is a male and often a brother who instigates or forces the incest. According to John V. Caffaro and Allison Conn-Caffaro, authors of *Sibling Abuse Trauma: Assessment and Intervention Strategies for Children, Families, and Adults* (Haworth Maltreatment and Trauma Press, 1998), the following are characteristics of sibling incest:

• Forced sexual contact on a child by an older brother or sister

• Attempts at intercourse, oral/genital contact or other compulsive sexual activity

• May extend over long periods

• May include unwanted sexual references in conversation, indecent exposure, forcing a sibling to observe sex, forcing a sibling to view pornography or taking pornographic pictures of a sibling

• Behavior is not limited to age-appropriate developmental curiosity. It may not appear to be forced but nonetheless is based on manipulation, fear, threats and/or coercion or may occur while the victim is unconscious.

• Sexual contact occurs when both participants are engaging in the behavior as an attempt to cope with unmet needs for affection.

Other characteristics found among families of sibling incest were a lack of parental warmth, a lack of supervision and a confusion of normal boundaries between individuals. In many cases, the children have observed their parents openly having sex with each other.

It is also true that occasionally females are the perpetrators in incest cases. This problem has been studied very little by clinicians but is known to exist. When a boy is sexually pursued by his sister, evidence indicates that he is much less likely to reveal the incest than is a sister who is abused by a brother.

Brother-brother incest also occurs, particularly when there is little supervision and in large families. Older brothers may rape or allow others to rape the child. Sister-sister incest is known to happen but is considered very rare. Indications are that in such cases, the sisters have been sexually abused by their father or older brothers before the onset of the sister-sister incest.

Treatment of Sibling Incest Is Important

In an article in a 1998 issue of *Child Welfare,* Janet DiGiorgio-Miller described how the family and offender should be treated by therapists. She pointed out the necessity of involving child protective services workers. If the parents refuse to contact protective services, then the therapist must contact them. She also pointed out the necessity of ensuring that the offender never be left alone with the victim. This may mean that the offending sibling must go live with a relative or other family member during treatment. Trial visits may be arranged at a later date.

It is also important to make sure that the offender considers factors that led to the abuse (such as low self-esteem, excessive preoccupation with sex and other factors) and that he (or she) acknowledge the negative effect his (or her) actions had on the sibling.

Incest through History

The phenomenon of incest has a long and complex history. The story of Oedipus, who unknowingly married his own mother, is often cited as an example of early attitudes toward incest. When finally faced with the knowledge that he had married his mother, Oedipus gouged out his eyes. His mother committed suicide. Both acts illustrate the extreme shame and disgrace felt as a result of a strong cultural prohibition against incestual relations.

Biblical references to incest range from sympathetic, in the case of Lot—who engaged in sexual relations with his daughters after the death of his wife—to a strong injunction against incest in the book of Leviticus. Among ancient Egyptian royalty, marriage between brothers and sisters was expected as a way of maintaining the purity of blood lines. Generally, however, sexual relations between close relatives have been looked upon with disgust and have been subject to strong negative sanctions throughout history.

Victim Is Often Not Believed

A serious problem faced by victims of incest, particularly adolescent girls, is that often when they *do* tell someone in authority about the incest, they are not believed. This may be partly because it is hard for many people to believe that a family member would sexually abuse another family member. But other factors come into play as well.

For example, when the incest has occurred for years before it is reported, the victim may not exhibit much emotion during the telling; rather, she may exhibit a very "flat," unemotional appearance. Many individuals, including those with knowledge of abuse, expect to see crying and distress, and when such behavior is not apparent, they may assume that the individual is lying about the abuse. Leslie Feiner explained this problem in her 1997 article for the *Journal of Criminal Law and Criminology.*

> The incest dynamic itself can also affect the credibility of the traumatized teenage storyteller, because such victims do not tend to testify in ways that jurors would typically expect. Just as victims of long-term abuse tend to become more passive over time with their abusers, so too can they withdraw from others; they are plagued by low self-esteem, and their communication and social skills are often weak. Jurors who expect an incest survivor to relate a narrative in an expressive, direct and tearful way are likely to be disappointed. On the contrary, it is entirely likely to see such a witness testify flatly, without emotion, tears or even eye contact.

Feiner further stated,

> Teenage girls are particularly vulnerable to negative judgments regarding their credibility. In simulated sexual abuse trials where only the age of the victim was manipulated, researchers found that jurors tended to find girls over twelve years of age to be significantly less credible than adolescent girls under the age of twelve. As researchers polled their jurors, they found that as victims entered adolescence, jurors perceived them as partly responsible for the abuse they were subjected to, and that

belief correlated with a decrease in their perceived credibility. . . .

In this respect the skepticism people demonstrate toward teenage sexual abuse victims is similar to the skepticism that greets adult victims of acquaintance rape. However, even if adult women face serious obstacles in pressing claims of rape, teenage incest victims face even more.

See also ABUSERS; ADULTS ABUSED AS CHILDREN; SEXUAL ABUSE; SIBLING ABUSE.

Caffaro, John V., and Allison Conn-Caffaro. *Sibling Abuse Trauma: Assessment and Intervention Strategies for Children, Families, and Adults.* New York: The Haworth Maltreatment and Trauma Press, 1998.

DiGiorgio-Miller, Janet. "Sibling Incest: Treatment of the Family and the Offender." *Child Welfare* 77, no. 3 (May 1998): 335–338.

Feiner, Leslie. "The Whole Trust: Restoring Reality to Children's Narrative in Long-Term Incest Cases." *Journal of Criminal Law and Criminology* 87, no. 4 (Summer 1997): 1,385–1,429.

Firestone, Philip, et al. "A Comparison of Incest Offenders Based on Victim Age." *Journal of the American Academy of Psychiatry and Law* 33, no. 2 (November 2, 2005): 223–232.

Indecency with Children Act 1960   Provisions of this act of Parliament specifically dictate the criminal nature of sexual behavior toward children. The acts states that, "Any person who commits an act of gross indecency with or towards a child under the age of 14, or who incites a child under that age to such an act with him or another, shall be liable on conviction."

indenture   In previous centuries, those in Europe and colonists in America devised a way to handle neglected children. This was to place them in the care of a family who provided food and shelter in exchange for a legal promise that the children would act as servants until a certain age or, in the case of girls, until marriage. Many children placed in indenture were either orphans or from poor families who could not afford to provide food and shelter.

The indenture system was originally formalized in the 17th century to permit adults without money a means of immigrating to the North American colonies. These individuals would enter an agreement, similar in some ways to an apprenticeship, in which they contracted with an employer for a specific period. This system soon accommodated children, many but not all of whom were orphans, who had no other means of support.

Indentured servants were under the absolute control of a master or mistress, who was bound by law to provide for the indentured servant's basic needs. In 17th-century North America, the usual term of labor for an indentured servant was about five years, after which the servant received his or her freedom. Terms of indenture and conditions under which servants were bound varied widely from colony to colony. In some areas, indentured servants were treated quite harshly, in others they received fair and reasonable treatment.

In 19th- and early 20th-century Canada, nearly 100,000 poor children under the age of 14 were sent from Britain to serve terms of indenture on farms and as household servants. This trend reflected concerns of philanthropic reformers who wanted to save children from working in mines and factories under conditions considered unsafe and unhealthy. Eventually, other reformers agitated for changes in these programs, which essentially deprived school-age children of their education and placed many of them in situations devoid of comfort, where they performed menial and arduous agricultural or domestic tasks. By 1925, indenture arrangements effectively ended when British policies were changed to prohibit emigration of children under age 14 not accompanied by parents.

India   According to the *Country Reports on Human Rights Practices, 2004* on India, released by the United States State Department in 2005 on behavior that occurred in 2004, the country has serious problems with child maltreatment. For example, honor killings are a problem in India. These are murders perpetrated by one or more family members who believe that a female adolescent or adult has shamed the family; for example, by being raped or by having sex outside of marriage. In some parts of India, up to 10% of all murders are honor killings.

CHILD PROSTITUTION is common in India, although it is illegal. Some experts say that as many as 500,000 children are involved in prostitution in India, which is approximately equivalent to half of all child prostitution worldwide.

The SEXUAL TRAFFICKING of children and adolescents from other countries occurs in India. The Immoral Trafficking Prevention Act (ITPA) in India prohibits human trafficking, but trafficking goes on nonetheless. In some cases, it is aided and abetted by law enforcement officials who ignore the trafficking or even actively participate in it.

The ITPA has tough penalties for offenders, especially for the trafficking of children, and a conviction for an offense against a child under age 16 can result in imprisonment from seven years to a life sentence. Despite these penalties, it has been estimated that as many as 50,000 women and children are trafficked into India each year for the purpose of sexual exploitation. As many as 10,000 children are trafficked from the neighboring countries of Nepal and Bangladesh each year. Girls who are seven years old and older are trafficked from the economically depressed parts of these countries to major prostitution centers in New Delhi, Calcutta and Mumbai.

In some cases, family members in India sell their young daughters into prostitution. Some parents believe that they are giving their children to strangers who will then employ them or marry them.

Boys four years old and older are trafficked into the Persian Gulf to serve as camel jockeys there or in the Middle East. Camel racing is an extremely popular sport in some countries, such as Qatar, where it is considered a national pastime, and some races have the prestige of the Kentucky Derby in the United States. However, often the weight limit for a camel jockey is 60 pounds or less, precluding the use of adolescent males. As a result, male children are purchased or kidnapped from India, Pakistan and Bangladesh so that they can work as camel jockeys. Because

of extreme pressure from human rights groups, countries such as Qatar have sought an alternative solution to enslaving children, such as creating a robotic camel jockey, as described in the *Wall Street Journal.*

The aborting of females on a large scale is an ongoing problem in India, where male children are valued much more highly. The law in India bans the use of amniocentesis or ultrasound to determine the sex of the fetus; however, experts report that this law is frequently violated by family planning centers, and the government does not intervene in the law prohibiting termination of a pregnancy because of a sex preference. When female children are born, many mothers give health care and nutrition preference to their male children.

Marital issues are related to the maltreatment of children and adolescents in India; half of all women in India marry before they are age 15, although the legal age of marriage is 18 years, according to the Health Ministry. Thousands of child marriages occur each year.

In addition, dowries, which are payments from a bride's family to the groom's family, are prohibited by the Dowry Prohibition Act of 1961, but they continue to be offered and accepted. In some cases, dowry disputes have led to harassment and even violence, sometimes causing the death of the bride. There were 6,285 dowry deaths in 2003, down from 6,822 such deaths in 2002. Some women have committed SUICIDE because of pressure over their dowries.

Bureau of Democracy, Human Rights, and Labor. *Country Reports on Human Rights Practices, 2004: India.* United States State Department, released on February 28, 2005. Available online. URL: http://www.state.gov/g/drl/rls/hrrpt/2004/41740.htm. Downloaded on September 1, 2005.
El-Rashidi, Yasmine. "Ride 'Em, Robot: Qatar Offers Solutions to a Jockey Shortage." *Wall Street Journal* CCXLVI, 68 (October 3, 2005): A2, A12.

indictment   Criminal prosecution for child abuse begins with a written accusation known as an indictment. The document is prepared by a public prosecuting attorney and submitted, under oath, to a grand jury for review. Members of the grand jury must determine whether the accusations, if proven true, would be sufficient to convict the accused of a crime. An indictment approved by a grand jury is known as a true bill.

Indictments serve as formal notices to parties accused of crimes. Charges must be spelled out clearly enough to allow the defendant to prepare an adequate defense.

See also PETITION.

infanticide   Infanticide is the purposeful murder of infants. In most cases, the infant is killed by a parent, usually the mother. Perpetrators of infant maltreatment have been identified throughout history and in virtually every society. Infanticide may take the form of violent trauma, such as strangulation or battering, or the child may be left to die of starvation or hypothermia (this form of abandonment is also known as exposure). In some cases, babies have been sacrificed as part of a religious ritual.

Of all the children who die from abuse and/or neglect in the United States, infants represent the largest percentage of fatalities: about 44% of all child maltreatment fatalities in the United States in 2003 occurred to babies younger than one year, according to the Administration on Children, Youth and Families in their annual report. Infants who die from neglect are more likely than children in other age groups to die from starvation or dehydration.

Worldwide, infants and young children have the greatest risk of suffering from fatal abuse, according to the *World Report on Violence and Health,* published by the World Health Organization in 2002. The risk for death from abuse is greater than double among infants and young children compared to the risk of death among children who are five to 14 years old.

Historical Background of Infanticide

History is replete with accounts of infanticide. Biblical accounts of the mass murder of infants include the pharaoh's order that all male children be drowned and King Herod's attempt to slaughter all Jewish males under the age of two. Ancient Roman law permitted the destruction of unwanted infants.

Aristotle advocated infanticide as a way of dealing with disabled or deformed infants.

Some societies did not consider an infant to be a person until the child was ritually confirmed. In ancient Rome, a newborn was placed on the floor in front of the mother's husband. If he picked the child up, it was considered his offspring; if not, the child was often killed. The Romans viewed this as a way of protecting the purity of their race. Vikings presented the male infant with a spear. If the infant grasped the spear, he was allowed to live. Viking brothers were also obligated to kill their sister's infant if she died during childbirth.

Medieval English society protected the child's right to live only after it had consumed earthly nourishment. Many early Christians did not consider a child fully human until the infant was baptized, and children who died before baptism occurred were not allowed to be buried in sanctified ground. Excluded from church cemeteries, these children were given the same burial afforded a domestic animal.

In the Middle Ages, a common method of infanticide was overlaying, in which the mother lay on top of the infant until it smothered to death. However, overlaying was considered a sin by the priests of the time.

Until the 19th century, the Indian practice of casting female infants into the Ganges River was widespread. Polynesians expected mothers of lower social status to destroy all newborns immediately following birth, but babies born to upper-class mothers were protected from slaughter. A particularly brutal form of infanticide is said to have been practiced in rural Ireland in the 20th century. So-called changeling babies, or infants born with congenital anomalies or who were simply unattractive (and thought to be bewitched), were roasted alive over an open fire.

Though prevalent, infanticide was by no means always condoned. In 18th-century Prussia, infant murderers were punished by sacking. Sewn into a cloth sack and weighted with heavy rocks and/or with a snake, a dog and a cock, perpetrators were thrown into a river to drown. Sacking was forbidden by Frederick the Great, who thought decapitation was a more appropriate punishment. Other punishments for those who committed infanticide included being burned at the stake or being impaled.

In 1871, the infant death toll at baby farms, where infants were given into the care of others, usually by unwed mothers, had reached such proportions that the British House of Commons appointed a special committee to investigate the problem. As a result of the inquiry, the Infant Life Protection Act was passed. For the first time, minimum standards for child care were established in Britain.

In some civilizations, infants were placed in building foundations or in dikes to ensure the structure's strength. Brazilian tribes have been reported, as recently as 1977, as casting children from a high ledge into the ocean. The stated purpose of this ritual slaying was to ensure a bountiful harvest.

Infanticide has also long been practiced as a means of population control. Australian aboriginal mothers have been reported to kill a child when there was insufficient food or water to sustain the family. This phenomenon is not limited to historical or primitive cultures. Infanticides committed by unwed mothers have been documented in Japan, the United States and other industrialized countries.

Current Worldwide Problems with Infanticide

According to the International Society for Prevention of Child Abuse and Neglect, in considering regions that identify female infanticide as a form of maltreatment, 100% of individuals in the Americas (North and South) as well as Oceania (Australia and New Zealand) regard infanticide in this manner. Ninety-five percent of Europeans also share this view. Other regions, however, have a significantly different view. For example, 67% of those surveyed in Asia view female infanticide as child abuse or neglect, as do 82% of those surveyed in Africa. In general, 90% of developed countries regard female infanticide as a problem, as do 79% of developing (poor) countries.

Research Studies

In a study reported in a 2003 issue of the *Journal of the American Medical Association*, of 34 newborns know to have been discarded or killed by a parent older than 16 years in North Carolina, the researchers estimated that at least two children per 100,000 newborns were either killed or left to die, in most cases, by their mothers (29 out of 34 cases).

Said the researchers, "The risk of homicide on the first day of life (neonatacide) is 10 times greater than the rate during any other time of life." The researchers found that there were more male victims (59%) than female victims. Half the mothers were age 20 and younger. About 21% of the mothers who committed infanticide were married women. About 24% of the mothers had received prenatal care. The most common causes of death among the infants were either asphyxiation/strangulation (41%) or drowning (27%).

Based on a study published in 1998 in the *New England Journal of Medicine*, about 50% of infanticides occur by the time the baby is four months old, and two-thirds have occurred by the sixth month of the infant's life. The researchers investigated 2,776 homicides among children in the first year of life over the period 1983–91. One-third of the babies were killed as a result of battering or another form of maltreatment, such as suffocation or strangulation, drowning, the use of firearms, criminal neglect, arson and cuts and stabbing.

The researchers identified some key risk factors associated with infant homicides. These include the following:

- A second or subsequent infant born to a mother less than 19 years of age
- Maternal age of less than 17 years
- No prenatal care received by the mother

Postpartum Psychosis

Some experts believe that maternal infanticide often occurs as a result of mental illness. According to Margaret Spinelli, in a 2004 article in the *American Journal of Psychiatry*, there are five different categories of maternal infanticide.

The first category includes infant homicides committed by young women who do not want to have the baby and who have kept the pregnancy secret from those around them. The baby is born with the mother receiving no assistance. The mothers may report experiencing a temporary psychotic dissociation, saying that it was as if they were watching themselves delivering the child, while experiencing no pain. The baby is either murdered or dies without receiving resuscitation.

The second category includes women who perform the murder with an abusive male partner. The third category is that of infants who die from neglect because the mother is preoccupied with other tasks. The fourth category is that of mothers who are attempting to DISCIPLINE their babies, and the child dies as a result. The fifth and last category is that of purposeful homicide. This may occur (although it need not) as a result of the mother's mental illness, such as postpartum depression, postpartum psychosis or schizophrenia.

The most commonly cited case of postpartum psychosis is that of Andrea Yates, who drowned her five children, ages seven, five, three, two and six months, in 2001 in a bathtub at her home in Houston, Texas. Yates was subsequently sentenced to life imprisonment for the homicides, but her conviction was overturned in 2005. After a second trial in July 2006, Yates was found not guilty by reason of insanity and committed to a state mental hospital.

Noted Spinelli, "Mrs. Yates had a history of psychiatric illness and a first reported psychotic episode after Noah's birth in 1994. At that time she told no one because she feared Satan would hear and harm her children. Two suicide attempts after her fourth pregnancy were driven by attempts to resist satanic voices commanding her to kill her infant."

Spinelli said that there are lessons and risk factors to be learned from the Yates case. Some of these which should be considered are

- A history of psychiatric illness in the mother
- The mother's childbearing history (Yates was either pregnant or breastfeeding from 1994 to 2001)
- A family history of psychiatric illness
- Past psychiatric interventions (Yates was hospitalized in a psychiatric facility in 1999. A social worker filed a report with PROTECTIVE SERVICES, but no investigation occurred.)
- Inadequate education about mental illness (Mr. Yates stated that he believed Mrs. Yates would spring back from her mental illness.)
- Inadequate education about mental illness among medical professionals (Many health-care professionals do not realize that postpartum psychosis

is a medical emergency; psychiatrists, nurses, social workers and other professionals missed the signs among Mrs. Yates.)
- Poor psychiatric management of postpartum psychosis (Mrs. Yates's psychiatrist discontinued her antipsychotic medication two weeks before the tragedy, for unknown reasons.)

See also ABUSERS; CORPORAL PUNISHMENT; DISCIPLINE; FATALITIES, CHILD ABUSE; SHAKEN INFANT SYNDROME; SUDDEN INFANT DEATH SYNDROME.

Administration on Children, Youth and Families. *Child Maltreatment 2003*. Children's Bureau, U.S. Department of Health and Human Services, Washington, D.C., 2005.

Herman-Giddens, Marcia E. "Newborns Killed or Left to Die by a Parent." *Journal of the American Medical Association* 289, no. 11 (March 19, 2003): 1,425–1,429.

International Society for Prevention of Child Abuse and Neglect. *World Perspectives on Child Abuse*. 6th ed. Carol Stream, Ill.: International Society for Prevention of Child Abuse and Neglect, 2004.

Krug, E. G., et al, eds. *World Report on Violence and Health*. Geneva, Switzerland: World Health Organization, 2002.

Overpeck, Mary D., et al. "Risk Factors for Infant Homicide in the United States." *New England Journal of Medicine* 339, no. 17 (1998): 1,211–1,216.

Radbill, S. "A History of Child Abuse and Infanticide?" In Ray Heifer and C. Henry Kempe, eds. *The Battered Child*. Chicago: University of Chicago Press, 1980, pp. 3–20.

Spinelli, Margaret G., M.D. "Maternal Infanticide Associated with Mental Illness: Prevention and the Promise of Saved Lives." *American Journal of Psychiatry* 161, no. 9 (September 2004): 1,548–1,557.

infantile addiction   See ADDICTION, INFANTILE.

infantile cortical hyperostosis   A condition, also known as Caffey's disease, in which new bone forms beneath the periosteum of infants. A healed lesion of infantile cortical hyperostosis is similar in appearance to a fracture suffered during battering. In 95% of cases of this condition, the mandible (jawbone) is affected—a bone unlikely to be fractured as a result of battering.

Infant Life Protection Act, 1872 (Britain) The 19th-century practice of "baby farming" gave rise to the Infant Life Protection Act. Mothers unable or unwilling to care for their children often entrusted their care to women who ran BABY FARMS. These infants were frequently subjected to cruel treatment and were even sold by women who ran these farms. In two cases of such maltreatment, involving Margaret Waters and Sarah Ellis, such a public outcry was raised that Parliament passed the act.

Although by itself a somewhat ineffective statute, it received a great deal of publicity and set the precedent for a series of reforms affecting the care and well-being of infants. Among them were registration of homes in which infants were cared for, compulsory registration of births and deaths and more stringent regulations governing burial of stillborn infants.

infibulation This brutal ritual is practiced on young females in many cultures but is particularly prevalent on the African continent. It involves the complete removal of the clitoris and labia. The sides of the vulva are then sewn together leaving only a small opening for discharge of fluids. At marriage, infibulated females have their vaginas reopened to permit intercourse and childbirth. The main function of this procedure is to ensure that the female will be a virgin at the time of marriage.

Some have linked CLITORIDECTOMY and infibulation to the widely practiced custom of male circumcision; however, both infibulation and clitoridectomy are more extensive and more dangerous. Removal of the clitoris effectively eliminates the female's capacity for sexual stimulation. Many young girls die or suffer painful, chronic problems as a result of these operations. Though the practice is defended by some as an important cultural, religious or social ritual, it is widely condemned around the world. Elimination of sexual mutilation has been the topic of several international health conferences.

See also FEMALE GENITAL MUTILATION; INITIATION RITES.

Ingraham v. Wright An important United States Supreme Court decision in 1977 held that CORPORAL PUNISHMENT in schools was not inherently cruel or abusive. This ruling was based on common-law precedents establishing disciplinary corporal punishment in public schools. The case, *Ingraham v. Wright,* was one that received a great deal of public attention, as it was argued and decided on the basis of the Eighth Amendment, which provides for protection against cruel and unusual punishment.

The plaintiff in the case, James Ingraham—a 14-year-old junior high school student—received hospital treatment for bruises received after being "struck repeatedly by a wooden instrument." The school principal responsible for Ingraham's corporal punishment was absolved of legal responsibility by the court ruling. The court held that "the administration of corporal punishment in public schools, whether or not excessively administered, does not come within the scope of Eighth Amendment protection."

Many child abuse and neglect experts denounced this finding as one that further validates violence against children—and legalizes child abuse—in one of the nation's most influential social institutions, its public schools.

initiation rites Virtually all cultures have rituals to mark the transition to adulthood. These events are sometimes referred to as puberty rites or rites of passage. Though initiation rites are often harmless ceremonies, rituals practiced by some primitive societies have been widely denounced as forms of institutionalized child abuse.

In New Guinea for example, boys are subjected to a series of increasingly painful rites before they can be officially recognized as adults. Bloodletting plays an important role both as a cleansing ritual and as a symbol of the male's ability to withstand pain. Passage to manhood may also include ritual scarification of the back, face or chest, sleep deprivation, burning, forced vomiting and verbal harassment. Some New Guinea tribes, the Sambia and the Keraki for example, force boys to serve as sexual partners for older initiates. These practices are attributed to a cultural belief that ingestion of semen is necessary for boys to acquire strength. By contrast, initiation of girls into womanhood appears much less abusive. The traditional ritual of defloration, once practiced by tribal elders, appears to have ended in New Guinea.

Conversely, some African tribal groups engage in brutal mutilation of females. CLITORIDECTOMY and INFIBULATION are still practiced as initiation rites among remote tribes like the Gusii. Both males and females are expected to endure mutilation and other extremely painful acts unflinchingly.

Though Western child abuse experts classify many initiation rites as abusive, these practices may be seen as normal, even essential, in the societies where they are practiced. Practices such as clitoridectomy and infibulation, and sexual exploitation, are almost universally condemned. However, experts are less likely to agree that practices such as scarification and psychological humiliation constitute abuse. Some even speculate that these institutionalized forms of abuse are responsible for a lower incidence of idiosyncratic (deviating from cultural norms) abuse in non-Western societies.

injuries, abdominal   See ABDOMINAL INJURIES.

injuries, cord   See CORD INJURIES.

injuries, eye   See EYE INJURIES.

injuries, gastrointestinal   See GASTROINTESTINAL INJURIES.

injuries, mental   See MENTAL INJURY; PSYCHOLOGICAL/EMOTIONAL MALTREATMENT.

injuries, mouth   See MOUTH INJURIES.

in loco parentis   Literally, in place of the parents—this term is applied when either the state or a court-appointed individual acts on behalf of a child in cases of suspected abuse or neglect.

innoculation   Since the development of modern vaccines, the innoculation of children against life-threatening and debilitating disease has become standard practice. Innoculation against disease has significantly reduced child mortality and increased the average life span. Many pediatricians now recommend that children be innoculated by 18 months to two years of age. Some consider failure to innoculate by age two to be MEDICAL NEGLECT.

This form of prevention has proven so effective that a majority of states and countries have laws requiring that all children be vaccinated against certain diseases. Legally required innoculation has not, however, been without controversy. Some parents dispute such requirements on the basis of religious beliefs. Others believe such vaccinations are dangerous or an infringement on their right to do what they think is best for their children.

In the United States, laws requiring innoculation vary from state to state. Most states tie innoculation to school attendance. Children are denied entry into the school system until they can produce evidence that they have received the required vaccinations. Parents who refuse to allow their children to be innoculated may be charged with medical and/or EDUCATIONAL NEGLECT. In some cases physicians, educators or child welfare workers can petition the court to order the parents to have their child innoculated.

Though widely practiced, mandatory innoculation continues to be a controversial subject in many areas.

in re Gault   Due to the lack of a clearly defined body of legal rights for children, the United States Supreme Court in 1967 established basic principles governing those rights. In re *Gault*, the legal case that prompted the court's decision, concerned itself with the rights of juveniles charged with delinquency. Specifically, the case involved a 15-year-old Arizona boy, Gerald Francis Gault, who was accused of making an obscene telephone call to a neighbor. After an informal hearing in juvenile court, he was committed to a state institution for juvenile delinquents until age 21. Had he been an adult he would have received DUE PROCESS protections and a maximum incarceration of two months. The Supreme

Court overturned the juvenile court's decision and found that juveniles—who could possibly be jailed if found guilty—had the right to notice, counsel, confrontation and cross-examination. They were protected as well against self-incrimination.

Establishing this precedent in the Gault case meant that the traditional PARENS PATRIAE view taken by juvenile court was no longer viable. Gault provided judicial guarantees that children's rights would be protected in the same way that adults' rights were preserved under the Constitution. This ruling bears directly on child abuse and neglect cases, since legal rights of children in such court proceedings can be considered independent of those of their parents.

institutional abuse and neglect Sometimes social policies and institutions designed to help children do more harm than good. As the number of children enrolled in day care, treatment facilities, correctional institutions and foster care increases so does concern with institutional maltreatment.

Some child advocates argue that any institutionalization of children is abusive. Placement of children with adults in jails, correctional facilities or treatment centers puts children at significant risk of abuse and is prohibited in many areas.

Children placed in treatment and correctional facilities must be given a label. Designation as retarded, delinquent, emotionally disturbed or mentally ill can enable a child to receive special services that may benefit him or her. Such a label also places a child at significant risk of subsequent maltreatment. Some advocates say that institutional labeling is itself a form of abuse. Others point to the deprivation of freedom and denial of legal protection that often goes with institutional care.

Abuse within institutions may take several forms. Residents of full-time, 24-hour residential institutions may suffer physical neglect associated with poor nutrition, lack of exercise and idleness due to a lack of programmed activities. Medical abuse and neglect may also occur when health problems go untreated or when medication is dispensed without adequate monitoring or controls.

Many institutions, due to their age or lack of adequate funding, do not meet minimal standards

for safety. Children living in these institutions may suffer burns from unprotected radiators, lacerations or fractures from poorly designed or defective buildings and furnishings and numerous other environmentally induced injuries.

Children in institutional settings may suffer physical abuse at the hands of staff, other residents or outsiders. Some children suffering developmental disabilities or mental illness must be protected from self-inflicted injuries.

In recent years, a number of child sexual abuse cases in residential facilities and day care centers have received media attention. Historical accounts indicate that sexual exploitation of children in institutions has long been a problem. Recent publicity has caused institutions and lawmakers to consider new ways of protecting children from sexual abuse outside the family.

Problems associated with institutional abuse stem from many different sources. Treatment and correctional facilities are often inadequately funded. Lack of funds may lead to neglect of physical facilities and inadequate supervision of children. Poor recruitment procedures for child care workers and foster families also share blame for the increased risk of maltreatment. Finally, many institutions have simply failed to realize or acknowledge real or potential abuse.

Residential facilities have a responsibility to protect children from abuse. Most governmental, licensing and accreditation authorities require specific procedures for investigation of alleged maltreatment of children. Institutions are typically required to involve a neutral third party, in most cases a child protection or licensing agency, in the investigation of all such complaints. Recent civil suits have forced child care facilities to screen applicants for employment more carefully and to develop more thorough procedures for ensuring the safety of children.

interdisciplinary team See MULTIDISCIPLINARY TEAM.

intergenerational cycle of abuse Numerous studies have documented the increased risk that abused children will become abusive parents when they reach adulthood.

Abused children are not condemned to become abusive parents. However, under stress the parent with a history of abuse appears to be more likely to lash out at a child than to find other ways of expressing frustration and anger.

Many parents who were abused as children find ways of breaking the cycle of abuse. Parents who do not repeat the abuse they received as children appear to have more extensive social supports (friends, family etc.), have fewer negative feelings about pregnancy, give birth to healthier babies and are better able to express anger over their past abuse. These parents are also more likely to have suffered abuse from only one parent and have frequently reported a satisfactory relationship with the non-abusive parent.

Many mental health professionals agree that early intervention with abused children is an effective way to break the cycle of abuse. In the absence of such intervention it is still possible for parents with a history of abuse to avoid maltreating their children by developing a network of friends and family to call on in time of crisis, by developing appropriate ways of expressing anger and frustration and by learning new child-rearing techniques.

Self-help organizations seek to help parents break the cycle of abuse by providing social support on a 24-hour basis.

See also ABUSERS; ADULTS ABUSED AS CHILDREN.

Internet and child sex abuse   The Internet is the medium through which people using computers can interact with others, obtain information on virtually any subject, and buy and sell items. The Internet is also used to convey information about sex offenders; for example, the National Sex Offender Public Registry (http://www.nsopr.gov) provides a searchable database of sex offenders in all states in the United States. The information is provided by the states to the Department of Justice for this purpose. Individuals can search the database to discover if sex offenders live in their communities.

Sometimes the Internet is used to purvey CHILD PORNOGRAPHY. It has also become a medium by which pedophiles and others interested in child SEXUAL ABUSE may identify and contact children

and adolescents, with the ultimate goal of inducing them to create sexual materials and of possibly meeting in person to engage in sexual activity.

In some cases, police officers posing as minors have engaged pedophiles in online relationships that proceed to sex talk, and they have subsequently made arrangements to meet these prospective abusers in a public place. Sometimes, expecting to meet the "child," the pedophile actually flies to the appointed place from a remote site, only to be met and arrested by a police officer. According to a 2005 article in *Sexual Abuse: A Journal of Research and Treatment,* police officers posing as juveniles represent about 25% of all Internet sex crimes arrests. In addition, many such prosecutions have led to convictions, with a low risk of cases that are dropped or dismissed.

Child Pornography and the Internet

Until the Internet became widely popular, child pornography was thought to be largely disappearing, primarily because of the active crackdown of postal authorities and police. However, individuals using their computers to gain access to children and child pornography online are usually invisible to law enforcement authorities, and the child pornography business can be highly profitable. Often the children are induced into creating sexual images of themselves, which they provide to the abusers. As a result, child pornography has become a serious global problem.

A major problem with controlling child pornography on the Internet is that some adults have protested that they have the right to view pornographic materials (although in the United States, they do not have the right to view child pornography). Such individuals have alleged that any constraints or active policing of Web traffic would infringe upon their rights of free speech.

This premise was upheld when the Communications Decency Act, signed in 1996 by U.S. president Bill Clinton, was found unconstitutional by the U.S. Supreme Court in 1997 because it was deemed to be an intrusion on the rights of adults to view pornography depicting adults. (Child pornography is still illegal in the United States, and laws against child pornography are enforced.)

Federal law also bans adults from producing or selling child pornography created or transported by mail, computer or any other means (18 U.S.C.A. § 2252 [West Supp. 1999]).

Another complication to controlling access by and to children who may connect with pedophiles is that the Internet has an extensive global reach. Thus, if one country creates strict rules restricting access to child pornography and increases governmental control over who may use the Internet, users may transfer their access to other countries that allow them more (or total) freedom.

The Process of Enticing Child Victims

There are different ways in which ABUSERS arrange to abuse children, such as with pornography, sex talk and prostitution. However, often the initial process follows a common path. For example, some abusers seek out children and adolescents on the Internet, particularly lonely or bored children and adolescents. Abusers tell children they are beautiful, smart and wonderful people, usually initiating the contact in a nonsexual manner. They may tell the child that they understand him or her and care deeply, unlike the parents. (Many adolescents are convinced that their parents do not care about them and do not understand them.)

Abusers often make the first encounter in a public chatroom, and then urge the child to move to a private chatroom where what is said will not be monitored. Once the conversation is no longer public, the pedophile may communicate with the child online in private chatrooms, instant messages or text messages via cell phones. Some pedophiles have arranged to send a child a cell phone so that there is no record of the calls available.

Grooming of Child Victims by Abusers

Abusers gradually "groom" the child by a careful choice of words and progressively lead into the subject of sex, moving into increasingly explicit sex talk. They continue to use very positive language to maintain the dialogue. Eventually, they may convince the child to send them sexually explicit photographs or videos.

In one case, an abuser sent a male adolescent a Web camera and offered to pay the child $50 if he posed with his shirt off for a few minutes. This seemed like an easy and nonthreatening way to make money to the child, so he complied. The abuse later escalated to nudity and to sex acts in front of the Web camera.

Abusers may use photographs of the child for personal erotic arousal or they may sell or trade the photographs. The child's sexually explicit photographs may eventually appear on Web sites, much to the mortification and horror of the child. Even the fear that such images may appear on the Internet is a devastating thought to most children.

Eventually, an abuser may seek an in-person meeting with the child, warning the child not to tell others about the meeting, particularly their parents. Abusers may also solicit the child to run away to another city where the abuser is located, and where the abuser may have direct control over the child. When in-person meetings occur, the abuser may encourage the child to use alcohol or illegal drugs that the abuser supplies, to further increase the control of the abuser over the child and the ease with which the child may be induced into committing sexual acts.

In some cases, an abuser will lead a child into prostitution, after which the child's self-esteem has usually plummeted while dependence on the abuser remains high. The abuser may blackmail the child into prostitution by telling him or her that the photographs will be shown to parents or others if the child fails to comply with whatever demands the abuser imposes.

Once initiated into drug abuse and/or child prostitution, the abuser will often tell the child that the behavior must continue or parents or others will be notified of this behavior. In addition, the abuser may tell the child that the parents would not want the child back, since he or she has engaged in behavior that would shock or horrify parents or other caretakers. Because the child is ashamed and embarrassed about his or her behavior, such statements are believed.

Secretiveness Is Crucial to the Abuser

Said John Carr in his report on child abuse and child pornography over the Internet, "Secretiveness is generally essential to the abuser's strategy. In the course of their initial discussions with a child, a paedophile will often take care to establish the exact location of the computer in the home. He will be anxious to discover how easily their conversations could be overlooked or overheard. He will also often be keen to ensure that the child does not keep any record of their conversations on the computer, as sooner or later he will seek to sexualize the contact and conversations as part of the grooming process."

Carr said that organized crime has become involved with online child abuse and child pornography. These criminals are usually not pedophiles themselves, but those willing to commit child sex crimes in order to make a profit. Some sites run by criminals accept credit card payments for images of child pornography. Criminals engaged in the sexual trafficking of children may also use such sites to exhibit the victimized children.

Victimized Children and Their Victimizers

Often those who are enticed by online abusers are teenage girls. According to a national survey reported in a 2004 issue of the *Journal of Adolescent Health*, based on local, state and federal law-enforcement investigations of 129 sexual offenses that began with Internet encounters, most victims were girls ages 13–15 (75%) who met the offenders in Internet chatrooms. Female victims may believe themselves to be in love with the offender.

Most of the offenders (76%) were more than 25 years old. In the cases of male victims, nearly all offenders were male. Most victims did meet with the offenders and had sex with them.

According to the National Juvenile Online Victimization Study, two-thirds of the online sex offenders studied owned child pornography, and 83% of them had owned images of children six to 12 years old. In addition, 80% of the offenders had images depicting the sexual penetration of minors.

The researchers analyzed the characteristics of 2,577 offenders, and they found that nearly all (99%) were males and most (92%) were non-Hispanic whites. The majority (86%) were 26 years old or older. Most of the offenders (97%) acted alone. Nearly half (45%) had committed a sex crime against a child, and 11% were known to be violent.

See also PEDOPHILIA; SEXUAL TRAFFICKING.

Carr, John. *Child Abuse, Child Pornography and the Internet.* London: NCH. Available online. URL: http://www. net. make-it-safe.net/eng/pdf/Child_pornography_Internet_Carr2004.pdf. Downloaded October 15, 2005.

Mitchell, Kimberly J., Janis Wolak, and David Finkelhor. "The Exposure of Youth to Unwanted Sexual Material on the Internet: A National Survey of Risk, Impact, and Prevention." *Youth & Society* 34, no. 3 (March 2003): 330–358.

———. "Internet-Initiated Sex Crimes Against Minors: Implications for Prevention Based on Findings from a National Study." *Journal of Adolescent Health* 35 (2004): 424e11–424e20.

———. "Police Posing as Juveniles Online to Catch Sex Offenders: Is It Working?" *Sexual Abuse: A Journal of Research and Treatment* 17, no. 3 (July 2005): 241–267.

Office of Juvenile Justice and Delinquency Prevention. *Child Pornography Possessors Arrested in Internet-Related Crimes: Findings from the National Juvenile Online Victimization Study.* Washington, D.C.: U.S. Department of Justice. Available online. URL: http://www.missingkids.com/en_US/publications/nC144.pdf. Downloaded October 15, 2005.

intervention, voluntary   See VOLUNTARY INTERVENTION.

intradermal hemorrhage   Bleeding within the skin.

See also BRUISES.

intraocular bleeding   Bleeding inside the eye can be caused by a blow directly to the eye or head. In the case of PURTSCHER RETINOPATHY, sudden compression of a child's chest due to hitting, shaking or squeezing can cause a hemorrhage of the retina. The most common cause of intraocular bleeding is head trauma. Retinal hemorrhage is frequently a symptom of child battering, although it may be caused by accidental injury or participation in sports such as football and gymnastics. Studies of battered children have shown that the presence of bleeding inside the eye—especially the retina—is an indicator that a SUBDURAL HEMATOMA may also be present. Small clots that appear in the retina as a result of trauma generally last approximately two weeks. Other forms of intraocular bleeding may indicate serious damage to the eye, possibly resulting in blindness.

investigation Once a report of suspected child abuse or neglect has been made, an investigation is necessary to determine: (1) if the report is accurate and (2) if the child is in danger. Investigations of suspected abuse and neglect are typically conducted by child protection workers; however, in some areas law enforcement officers are responsible for investigation of such reports.

The first responsibility of the investigator is to assess the level of danger to the child and, if necessary, take immediate steps to ensure the child's safety. Situations such as those listed below suggest a child is in immediate danger:

- The maltreatment in the home, present or potential, is such that a child could suffer permanent damage to body or mind if left there.
- Although a child is in immediate need of medical or psychiatric care, the parents refuse to obtain it.
- A child's physical and/or emotional damage is such that the child needs an extremely supportive environment in which to recuperate.
- A child's sex, age, physical or mental condition renders the child incapable of self-protection—or for some reason constitutes a characteristic the parents find completely intolerable.
- Evidence suggests that the parents are torturing the child or systematically resorting to physical force, which bears no relation to reasonable discipline.
- The physical environment of the home poses an immediate threat to the child.
- Evidence suggests that parental anger and discomfort with the investigation will be directed toward the child in the form of severe retaliation against him or her.
- Evidence suggests that the parent or parents are so out of touch with reality that they cannot provide for the child's basic needs.
- Evidence suggests that a parent's physical condition poses a threat to the child.

- The family has a history of hiding the child from outsiders.
- The family has a history of prior incidents or allegations of abuse or neglect.
- The parents are completely unwilling to cooperate in the investigation or to maintain contact with any social agency and may flee the jurisdiction.
- The parent or parents abandon the child.

The investigation centers on allegations specified in the report of suspected abuse. While evidence of other maltreatment may be collected in the course of an investigation it is important to determine the accuracy of each allegation contained in the original report.

A typical investigation begins with a check of available records to see if the child or family has been the subject of other investigations. The child protection worker may then interview the child, family, the alleged abuser (if not a family member) and others who may have special knowledge of the child or family.

Interviewing the Child

It is usually best that a child be interviewed alone to minimize embarrassment or intimidation; however, in some cases a parent or other trusted adult may facilitate questioning. Though parental permission is not required to interview a child concerning suspected abuse or neglect, a parent should be notified that the child will be interviewed. When sexual abuse is suspected it is recommended that the interviewer and child be of the same gender.

Children are frequently reluctant to discuss alleged abuse with a stranger. Interviewers should make every attempt to put the child at ease. A child may need to be reassured that he or she has done nothing wrong and will not be punished. Criticism of the parent(s) may cause the child to become defensive and uncooperative with the interviewer. As much as possible, children should be allowed to tell their own story in their own words, without leading questions, prompts or undue pressure. Some child protection workers have found anatomically correct dolls useful in interviewing young children who are thought to have been sexually abused.

Reliving abuse through an interview can be traumatic for a child. Often child protection workers, law enforcement officers, lawyers and judges can combine questioning into one interview, thereby reducing trauma to the child. In some cases videotaped interviews may be used as evidence in court.

Direct observation of any injuries is an essential part of an interview. If it is necessary for the child to remove his or her clothing, care should be taken to explain the reasons for disrobing in a nonthreatening, careful manner. In some cases it may be necessary to have the child examined by a physician to determine the existence and extent of injury.

Care must be given to explain to the child both the purpose of the interview and what to expect next. The child's questions should be answered truthfully and in language appropriate to his or her age.

Interviewing Adults

Adults should be informed of the reason for the interview and their legal rights with regard to the investigation. When possible, family members should be interviewed both separately and as a group. Separate interviews allow the child protection worker to compare accounts of an incident and may encourage the interviewee to share information more freely. Observing the family together often supplies important data on family interaction patterns.

Parents accused of abuse and neglect are often hostile and uncooperative. Interviewers who convey a neutral attitude toward the alleged abuse and who avoid direct confrontation are often successful in securing a reasonable level of cooperation. Keeping the focus on the child's welfare and asking open-ended questions are also useful strategies for soliciting necessary information. The child protection worker must be supportive of parents without appearing to condone inappropriate behavior.

Other Methods of Obtaining Information

Direct observation of a child's environment can supply useful information. Cleanliness of the home, presence of nutritious food, cooking and sanitary facilities, adequate sleeping arrangements, lighting, heat and water are all important.

Behavior of the child and family members should also be observed. An angry outburst or emotional coldness toward a child may belie a parent's description of a close relationship with the child.

Secondary information may be obtained from medical, school and police records. These kinds of data can help verify information obtained from interviews and observation.

A medical or mental health evaluation of a child may help identify or confirm evidence of abuse or neglect.

Observable physical evidence of injury should be documented with carefully taken photographs. Photographs should be identified accurately (name of subject, time, location, age etc.) and should include distinguishing features that allow identification of the child as well as a clear view of the injury itself. Color film is preferred to black and white. Infrared film may increase visibility of injuries where dark skin coloring inhibits clear observation of trauma. Production of photographs that are acceptable as evidence in court requires the careful attention of a skilled photographer.

Outcome of the Investigation

After all relevant information has been collected the investigator must make a decision concerning the accuracy of the alleged abuse or neglect and the need for further intervention.

The investigator may conclude that abuse or neglect exists, does not exist or that further information is necessary to make a determination. When abuse or neglect is substantiated interventions vary depending on the level of risk to the child, the child's needs and the family's willingness to cooperate. If the family refuses to cooperate, a court order may be necessary to ensure treatment. In some cases the investigator may conclude that abuse or neglect does not exist but that services should be offered to the family.

isolation See SOCIAL ISOLATION.

Italy There are some problems with child abuse in Italy, according to a report released by the United States State Department in 2005 on problems in 2003. The Telfono Azzuro, a nonprofit organization dedicated to preventing child abuse and neglect, received about 350,000 calls on child abuse. There were also estimates of from 1,800 to 2,300 children who worked in CHILD PROSTITUTION. Of these children, 1,500 to 2,300 of them were trafficked into Italy and forced into prostitution. (See SEXUAL TRAFFICKING.) There were also an estimated 29,000 Web sites in Italy devoted to CHILD PORNOGRAPHY and related crimes. The police shut down 36 pornographic Web sites in 2003 and arrested nine people for child pornography crimes.

Trafficking of humans is illegal in Italy, and those who violate the law face from eight to 20 years in prison. If the trafficked individuals are minors, the sentence is increased by about one-third to one-half. In the report, it was estimated that about 200 of the trafficked individuals were minors. In one case, a Romanian father sold his 10-year-old daughter for sex and was arrested. A Bulgarian man was arrested for bringing pregnant Bulgarian women into Italy. The women gave birth in Italy, and the babies were sold to Italian families for about $13,500 (10,000 euros) each.

Most of the trafficking for the purposes of sexual exploitation occurred with women and children from China, eastern Europe, Nigeria, North Africa and South America. Children were also trafficked into the country for sweatshop labor, especially with Chinese immigrant children.

Bureau of Democracy, Human Rights, and Labor. *Country Reports on Human Rights Practices, 2004: Italy.* United States State Department, released on February 28, 2005. Available online. URL: http://www.state.gov/g/drl/rls/hrrpt/2004/41688.htm. Downloaded October 19, 2005.

J

Japan Based on a United States State Department report on human rights practices for 2004, released in 2005, in general, the rights of children in Japan are protected by the government. If children are abused, local child-welfare officials may remove children from the home and also may prevent parents from meeting or communicating with their children. In addition, doctors, teachers and welfare officials are MANDATED REPORTERS of suspected child abuse. According to the Ministry of Health, Labor, and Welfare, 108 children died from child abuse over the period 2000–03. There were also about 24,000 reports of child abuse in 2003, up 2% from 2002.

BULLYING in school was a problem in Japan in 2003, and the Education, Culture, Sports, Science and Technology Ministry reported that there were about 35,000 acts of violence in 2003 in elementary, junior high and high schools, and overall acts of bullying rose by 5.2%.

CHILD PROSTITUTION, particularly among teenagers, and CHILD PORNOGRAPHY, were both problems in 2003. Ready availability of the Internet as well as the ability to access Web sites using cellular phones enabled strangers to contact children and make dates with them. In 2003, the government passed a law making it a crime for anyone to use the Internet for child prostitution or child pornography.

The SEXUAL TRAFFICKING of adolescents continued to be a problem in Japan. In some cases, underage girls and women were trafficked from other countries, such as Thailand, the Philippines and eastern Europe, and they were sexually exploited or forced into labor. Illegal immigrants from China were trafficked into Japan by organized crime groups, where they were held in debt and either sexually exploited or forced to perform indentured service in restaurants and factories.

In one case, a brothel owner and a sex club boss were charged with human trafficking after they compelled two Japanese girls to work for them as prostitutes in order to repay club debts.

Bureau of Democracy, Human Rights, and Labor. *Country Reports on Human Rights Practices, 2004: Japan.* United States State Department, released on February 28, 2005. Available online. URL: http://www.state.gov/g/drl/rls/hrrpt/2004/41644.htm. Downloaded September 1, 2005.

jejunal hematoma The collection of blood in the jejunum or middle part of the small intestine. Usually the result of a blow to the abdominal area.

See also ABDOMINAL INJURIES and GASTROINTESTINAL INJURIES.

Johnson and Wife v. State of Tennessee In the 1830s, a Mr. and Mrs. Johnson were convicted of excessively punishing their daughter. This case was one of the earliest recorded occasions where parents in the United States were tried for child maltreatment. The conviction was later overturned because an overzealous judge issued an improper charge to the jury.

juvenile court See COURT.

juvenile court movement The origins of the juvenile court in the United States date to the early 19th century. At that time, children over age 14 were treated as adults by the court systems, arrested, brought to trial, sentenced and punished according to criminal laws framed with adult offenders in mind. Even children between the ages of seven and 14 years were not always guaranteed immunity from criminal prosecution. It was the state's prerogative to hold a child legally accountable in criminal court if it preferred to do so, and judicial mechanisms for this purpose existed prior to establishment of a juvenile court.

Juvenile court system supporters worked to make judicial law more responsive to the needs of children. In recognition of these needs, by 1875 New York state prohibited placement of children with adults in almshouses for more than 60 days. Proponents of separate and special judicial treatment for children urged use of psychology, social work and medical science when sentencing, treating and rehabilitating youth. As a result, the first juvenile court in the United States was established in 1899 in Chicago, Illinois.

By the early 1900s, the juvenile court movement had been successful in permanently estab-

lishing this separate arena where the child's unique needs were taken into account. Wanting to guard the child against societal dangers, the juvenile court movement emphasized rehabilitation rather than retribution. Establishment of a juvenile court system was also to keep children separate from adult offenders. Much earlier, New York City had founded the House of Refuge in 1825, a correctional facility that segregated children from older, more hardened criminals. The juvenile court movement supported this and also sought more informal court procedures, as compared to the legalistic formality of a criminal court. The juvenile court movement desired also that the court consider each child's needs separately. More specifically, the juvenile court movement recognized that children must be protected if they are unable to seek and find their own protection. The juvenile court, therefore, was charged with acting as a substitute parent.

key masters See UNDERGROUND NETWORKS.

kidnapping Any unlawful seizure of a person and detention against that person's will is generally described as kidnapping. In modern times and in most nations of the world, kidnapping is a crime punished by death or lengthy imprisonment. In the United States, federal laws governing kidnapping were amended following the 1932 abduction and subsequent murder of aviator Charles A. Lindbergh's infant son. The Lindbergh baby kidnapping was the most famous among numerous early 20th-century abductions, many of which involved wealthy or well-known families and a large number of which had extortion as a key factor. The notoriety surrounding the Lindbergh case led directly to federal legislation that imposed the death penalty for anyone convicted of transporting a kidnap victim across state lines. When a noncustodial parent resorts to this type of action in order to secure unlawful custody of a child or children, it is termed CHILD STEALING.

Historically, abducting female children or young women for the purpose of selling them into prostitution was considered in many cultures a form of kidnapping.

See also MANN ACT; PARENTAL KIDNAPPING PREVENTION ACT OF 1980; SEXUAL TRAFFICKING.

kinky hair syndrome See MENKES' KINKY HAIR SYNDROME.

kinship care When children are abused and neglected and removed from their primary caretakers, sometimes they are placed with extended-family members: this is referred to as *kinship care.*

In some states, caregiver relatives may receive the same foster care payment as would an unrelated foster parent. The advantage of kinship care is that it provides continuity for the child, who may be able to stay with people he or she already knows and who care about him or her. There is an advantage to society itself because it is difficult to recruit sufficient numbers of nonrelative foster parents.

The disadvantages are that kinship care providers are usually women living alone, such as grandmothers or aunts, who have few financial resources. Often they are less closely monitored than are nonrelative foster parents and thus the potential for abuse may be greater, either by the visiting biological relative who abused the child in the first place or by the kin caregiver herself, in a case of intergenerational abuse. In addition, kinship care providers are less likely to obtain medical treatment for foster children, including immunizations, well-child visits and appointments when the child is ill. Thus the child may be at risk for medical neglect.

laboratory tests   Several routine tests are used by doctors to aid in the diagnosis of child abuse. Included are:

Partial thromboplastin time and *prothrombin time* tests measure blood-clotting factors. Knowledge of clotting time helps distinguish between bruising and bleeding associated with hemophilia and trauma-induced injuries.

Urinalysis helps detect sugar, protein, blood or other substances in the urine. Blood in the urine may be evidence of internal injury that may not be immediately apparent to the casual observer.

A complete *blood count* yields information about the level of red and white blood cells. This test may give evidence of poor nutrition or infection.

The *Rumpel-Leede* or *tourniquet* test is used to measure the plasticity of capillaries. Fragile capillaries may cause a child to bruise more easily than other children. Abusive parents frequently claim "the child bruises easily." This test helps verify claims of bruisability.

Landeros v. Flood   This 1976 ruling by the California Supreme Court established the liability of physicians and hospitals when they negligently fail to diagnose and report child abuse.

Gita Landeros, the plaintiff, was severely and repeatedly beaten by her mother and her mother's common-law husband. When brought to the San Jose Hospital for treatment the infant showed clear evidence of suffering from BATTERED CHILD SYNDROME, including a fractured tibia and fibula (apparently from severe twisting) and multiple bruises and abrasions. The physician, A. J. Flood, failed to perform a full SKELETAL SURVEY and therefore did not discover a skull fracture. In failing to properly diagnose the child's condition the physi-

cian also did not report the case to the proper law enforcement and child protection authorities.

The child was returned to the mother and her partner who continued to abuse her until she was brought to another hospital for treatment of blows to her eyes and back, puncture wounds, bites on her face and burns on a hand. At the second hospital a physician properly diagnosed the child's condition and reported the case to local authorities who took her into protective custody.

The court reversed a dismissal by a lower court and held the physician and the hospital responsible for failing to diagnose and report child abuse. This ruling opened the door for future malpractice suits against physicians and medical institutions who fail to report suspected child abuse.

least detrimental alternative   See BEST INTERESTS OF THE CHILD.

legal immunity   See IMMUNITY, LEGAL.

legal rights of persons identified in reports   In the United States persons criminally accused of child abuse have a right to be represented by a lawyer. In juvenile or family court proceedings, the right to counsel varies from state to state. Approximately one-half of all states grant the right to counsel in civil as well as criminal proceedings.

Some critics of present child abuse laws argue that persons accused of child abuse should be entitled to counsel in all proceedings. Civil proceedings can establish the basis for removal of a child from the home and for further criminal charges. Even when a civil proceeding does not result in criminal charges or removal of the child, some believe that the investigation itself and subsequent supervision by a child protection agency is likely to infringe on the parent's legal rights.

lesion   A term frequently used to describe injuries resulting from abuse, lesion can refer to an injury of any type to any part of the body.

liability of reporters   The fear of being sued could prevent some people from reporting suspected abuse or neglect to child protection authorities. This is especially true when abuse is suspected but cannot be proven without further investigation. In an effort to remove this barrier to reporting, all MANDATED REPORTERS in the United States are granted immunity from civil and criminal prosecution when reports are made in good faith. Further, in at least 40 states voluntary (nonmandatory) reporters are exempt.

Communications between doctor and patient, psychologist or social worker and client, and clergy and parishioner often receive special legal protection under the law. Although some jurisdictions require these professionals to report confessions of dangerous crimes, most states classify information passed between these parties as privileged communication. However, reports of suspected abuse or neglect are not afforded this protection. In fact, these professionals are usually classified as mandated reporters and are therefore required to report all cases of suspected maltreatment, A majority of states in the United States impose criminal and/or civil penalties on mandated reporters for failure to report such cases. In at least one case (*LANDEROS V. FLOOD*) a physician has been found legally liable for failing to report suspected abuse.

lice   Head lice are not uncommon in children. These small parasitic insects attach themselves to the scalp and survive by sucking blood through the skin. Children frequently acquire them from casual contact while playing or at school.

Treatment of an infested child involves repeated application of medicated shampoo and careful inspection of the hair for the insects or their eggs. This process requires persistence and usually takes place at home under a physician's instructions. If untreated, lice can cause significant discomfort to the child and may result in infection. Neglected children are sometimes found to have severe infestations of head or body lice that have gone untreated for a lengthy period of time.

Pubic lice are found in the groin area and sometimes produce bluish spots on the skin that disappear when the lice are treated. The presence of pubic lice on a child who has not reached sexual maturity is a strong indicator of possible SEXUAL ABUSE. When pubic lice are discovered on a child of any age, a careful examination should be conducted to determine how the insects were transmitted and whether there is other evidence of sexual abuse.

local authorities   In the United States, the child protection agency designated by the mandated state agency to serve a particular area is known as the local authority. A local authority may be a branch of the state agency, a private agency under government contract or a county department of social services. The term may also be applied to a community council for child abuse and neglect.

Local authorities have primary responsibility for child protection in Britain. Specifically, local authorities include councils of nonmetropolitan counties and metropolitan districts, the London boroughs and the common council of the City of London. Local social service authorities are under the general supervision of the secretary of state for social services or the secretary of state for Wales. Policy making for management of child abuse cases is the responsibility of an Area Review Committee appointed by the local authority. In addition to child protection, local authorities have responsibility for child care, delinquency prevention, foster care, legal advocacy for children and adoption.

See also PROTECTIVE SERVICES.

loss of childhood   See PARENTIFIED CHILD.

low birth weight Premature birth, inadequate prenatal care or SUBSTANCE ABUSE by the mother during pregnancy can cause infants to be significantly below normal weight at birth. Low birth weight may require an extended hospital stay until infants are healthy enough to be cared for at home. Premature infants often spend the first days, weeks or even months of their lives in an incubator.

Many experts believe treatment for low birth weight and other medical problems can interfere with the natural mother-infant bonding process, placing the child at increased risk of abuse (bonding failure). Many hospitals are now taking steps to increase contact between mothers and infants who require intensive medical attention.

malabsorption syndrome Any of a number of specific conditions, often inherited, that interfere with the absorption of nutrients in the intestines. Malabsorption can be caused by a number of childhood diseases, many of them fatal. It is a frequent cause of organically based FAILURE-TO-THRIVE SYNDROME.

malpractice Failure to diagnose and report child abuse or neglect may leave physicians and other professionals open to malpractice suits. In *LANDEROS V. FLOOD*, the California Supreme Court held a physician and hospital liable for failure to diagnose abuse in an infant who showed clear signs of BATTERED CHILD SYNDROME.

mandated reporters People who, by virtue of their professional or occupational status, are specifically required by state or federal law to report all cases of suspected child abuse or neglect to the mandated central agency in the state. Legal penalties are imposed for failure to report, and some mandated reporters have been sued successfully for failing to report cases.

The occupational and professional categories whose practitioners are mandated reporters vary slightly according to different state laws but usually include health-care worker, mental health professional, social worker, counselor, education staff, law enforcement officer and child-care worker. In some states, other professions are required to report suspected abuse, such as firefighter, veterinarian (children who abuse animals may be child abuse victims, or the abuser may have harmed the animal), funeral director and commercial film processor. Some states require all persons to report suspected child maltreatment, regardless of their profession.

Penalties for failure to report vary from state to state. There are also gray areas that concern experts; for example, if abuse *may* have occurred, but the reporter is unsure. Generally, if abuse is likely, it must be reported and then others will determine if the abuse actually occurred.

The mandate to report child abuse overrules husband-wife privilege as well as physician-patient privilege. Only attorney-client privilege or clergy-penitent privilege is upheld in most states. However, some states specifically exclude privileges for clergy, and some states recognize no privilege. For details about mandatory reporters by state, see the table on the following pages.

Mann Act In response to concern over what was termed *white slavery*, in 1910 the U.S. Congress passed the Mann Act. This legislation made inter-state transportation of females for prostitution or enticement for immoral purposes a federal offense. If found guilty under the terms of the Mann Act an individual can be fined up to $5,000, receive five years in prison, or both. In some circumstances, cases involving SEXUAL ABUSE of children can incur judicial action under the terms of the Mann Act.

See also CHILD SLAVERY; STATUTORY RAPE.

marasmus, nutritional A lack of sufficient protein in the diet causes a condition known as nutritional marasmus. Characterized by emaciation, an apparently enlarged head, wide, staring eyes, shrunken buttocks and loose skin folds, it is the product of prolonged and severe dietary inadequacy. Nutritional marasmus may occur when breast-feeding is reduced or ended and not replaced by an adequate

MANDATORY REPORTERS OF CHILD ABUSE AND NEGLECT IN THE UNITED STATES

State	Professionals who must report	Others	Standard	Privileged communications
Alabama	• Health-care professionals • Mental health professionals • Social work professionals • Education/child-care professionals • Law enforcement professionals	Any other person called upon to give aid or assistance to any child	Known or suspected (abuse or neglect)	Attorney/client
Alaska	• Health-care professionals • Mental health professionals • Social work professionals • Education/child-care professionals • Law enforcement professionals	• Paid employees of domestic violence and sexual assault programs and drug and alcohol treatment facilities • Members of a child fatality review team or multidisciplinary child protection team • Commercial or private film or photograph processors	Have reasonable cause to suspect	Not granted in statutes reviewed
Arizona	• Health-care professionals • Mental health professionals • Social work professionals • Education/child-care professionals • Law enforcement professionals	• Parents • Anyone responsible for care or treatment of children • Clergy/Christian Science practitioners • Domestic violence victim advocates	Have reasonable ground to believe	• Clergy/penitent • Attorney/client
Arkansas	• Health-care professionals • Mental health professionals • Social work professionals • Education/child-care professionals • Law enforcement professionals	• Prosecutors • Judges • Department of Human Services employees • Domestic violence shelter employees and volunteers • Foster parents • Court-appointed special advocates • Clergy/Christian Science practitioners	• Has reasonable cause to suspect • Have observed conditions which would reasonably result	• Clergy/penitent • Attorney/client
California	• Health-care professionals • Mental health professionals • Social work professionals • Education/child-care professionals • Law enforcement professionals	• Firefighters • Animal control officers • Commercial film and photographic print processors • Clergy • Court-appointed special advocates	• Have knowledge or observation of • Know or reasonably suspect	Clergy/penitent
Colorado	• Health-care professionals • Mental health professionals • Social work professionals • Education/child-care professionals • Law enforcement professionals	• Christian Science practitioners • Veterinarians • Firefighters • Victim advocates • Commercial film and photographic print processors • Clergy	• Have reasonable cause to know or suspect • Have observed conditions that would reasonably result in such abuse	Clergy/penitent

(continues)

MANDATORY REPORTERS OF CHILD ABUSE AND NEGLECT IN THE UNITED STATES

State	Professionals who must report	Others	Standard	Privileged communications
Connecticut:	• Health-care professionals • Mental health professionals • Social work professionals • Education/child-care professionals • Law enforcement professionals	• Substance abuse counselors • Sexual assault counselors • Battered women counselors • Clergy • Child advocates	Have reasonable cause to suspect or believe	Not addressed in statutes reviewed
Delaware	• Health-care professionals • Mental health professionals • Social work professionals • Education/child-care professionals • All persons	Not addressed in statutes reviewed	Know or in good faith suspect	• Attorney/client • Clergy/penitent
District of Columbia	• Health-care professionals • Mental health professionals • Social work professionals • Education/child-care professionals • Law enforcement professionals	Not addressed in statutes reviewed	Know or have reasonable cause to suspect	Not granted in statutes reviewed
Florida	• Health-care professionals • Mental health professionals • Social work professionals • Education/child-care professionals • Law enforcement professionals • All persons	• Judges • Religious healers	Know or have reasonable cause to suspect	Attorney/client
Georgia	• Health-care professionals • Mental health professionals • Social work professionals • Education/child-care professionals • Law enforcement professionals	Persons who produce visual or printed matter	Have reasonable cause to believe	Not granted in statutes reviewed
Hawaii	• Health-care professionals • Mental health professionals • Social work professionals • Education/child-care professionals • Law enforcement professionals	Employees of recreational or sports activities	Have reason to believe	Not granted in statutes reviewed
Idaho	• Health-care professionals • Mental health professionals • Social work professionals • Education/child-care professionals • Law enforcement professionals • All persons	Not addressed in statutes reviewed	• Have reason to believe • Have observed conditions that would reasonably result in such abuse	• Clergy/penitent • Attorney/client
Illinois	• Health-care professionals • Mental health professionals • Social work professionals • Education/child-care professionals • Law enforcement professionals	• Homemakers • Substance abuse treatment personnel • Christian Science practitioners • Funeral home directors • Commercial film and photographic print processors • Clergy	Have reason to believe	Clergy/penitent

MANDATORY REPORTERS OF CHILD ABUSE AND NEGLECT IN THE UNITED STATES

State	Professionals who must report	Others	Standard	Privileged communications
Indiana	• Health-care professionals • Mental health professionals • Social work professionals • Education/child-care professionals • Law enforcement professionals • All persons	Staff member of any public or private institution, school, facility or agency	Have reason to believe	Not granted in statutes reviewed
Iowa	• Health-care professionals • Mental health professionals • Social work professionals • Education/child-care professionals • Law enforcement professionals	• Commercial film and photographic print processors • Employees of substance abuse programs • Coaches	Reasonably believe	Not granted in statutes reviewed
Kansas	• Health-care professionals • Mental health professionals • Social work professionals • Education/child-care professionals • Law enforcement professionals	• Firefighters • Juvenile intake and assessment workers	Have reason to suspect	Not addressed in statutes reviewed
Kentucky	• Health-care professionals • Mental health professionals • Social work professionals • Education/child-care professionals • Law enforcement professionals • All persons	Not addressed in statutes reviewed	Know or have reasonable cause to believe	• Attorney/client • Clergy/penitent
Louisiana	• Health-care professionals • Mental health professionals • Social work professionals • Education/child-care professionals • Law enforcement professionals	• Commercial film or photographic print processors • Mediators	Have cause to believe	Clergy, Christian Science practitioner/penitent
Maine	• Health-care professionals • Mental health professionals • Social work professionals • Education/child-care professionals • Law enforcement professionals	• Guardians ad litem and court-appointed special advocates • Fire inspectors • Commercial film processors • Homemakers • Humane agents • Clergy	Know or have reasonable cause to believe	Clergy/penitent
Maryland	• Health-care professionals • Mental health professionals • Social work professionals • Education/child-care professionals • Law enforcement professionals • All persons	Not addressed in statutes reviewed	Have reason to believe	• Attorney/client • Clergy/penitent

(continues)

MANDATORY REPORTERS OF CHILD ABUSE AND NEGLECT IN THE UNITED STATES

State	Professionals who must report	Others	Standard	Privileged communications
Massachusetts	• Health-care professionals • Mental health professionals • Social work professionals • Education/child-care professionals • Law enforcement professionals	• Drug and alcoholism counselors • Probation and parole officers • Clerk/magistrates of district courts • Firefighters • Clergy/Christian Science practitioners	Have reasonable cause to believe	Clergy/penitent
Michigan	• Health-care professionals • Mental health professionals • Social work professionals • Education/child-care professionals • Law enforcement professionals	Clergy	Have reasonable cause to believe	• Attorney/client • Clergy/penitent
Minnesota	• Health-care professionals • Mental health professionals • Social work professionals • Education/child-care professionals • Law enforcement professionals	Not addressed in statutes reviewed	Know or have reason to believe	Clergy/penitent
Mississippi	• Health-care professionals • Mental health professionals • Social work professionals • Education/child-care professionals • Law enforcement professionals • All persons	• Attorneys • Ministers	Have reasonable cause to suspect	Not addressed in statutes reviewed
Missouri	• Health-care professionals • Mental health professionals • Social work professionals • Education/child-care professionals • Law enforcement professionals	• Persons with responsibility for care of children • Christian Science practitioners • Probation/parole officers • Commercial film processors • Internet service providers • Clergy	• Have reasonable cause to suspect • Have observed conditions that would reasonably result in such abuse	• Attorney/client • Clergy/penitent
Montana	• Health-care professionals • Mental health professionals • Social work professionals • Education/child-care professionals • Law enforcement professionals	• Guardians ad litem • Clergy • Religious healers • Christian Science practitioners	Know or have reasonable cause to suspect	Clergy/penitent
Nebraska	• Health-care professionals • Social work professionals • Education/child-care professionals • All persons	Not addressed in statutes reviewed	• Have reasonable cause to believe • Have observed conditions that would reasonably result in such abuse	Not addressed in statutes reviewed

MANDATORY REPORTERS OF CHILD ABUSE AND NEGLECT IN THE UNITED STATES

State	Professionals who must report	Others	Standard	Privileged communications
Nevada	• Health-care professionals • Mental health professionals • Social work professionals • Education/child-care professionals • Law enforcement professionals	• Religious healers • Alcohol/drug abuse counselors • Clergy/Christian Science practitioners • Probation officers • Attorneys • Youth shelter workers	Know or have reason to believe	• Clergy/penitent • Attorney/client
New Hampshire	• Health-care professionals • Mental health professionals • Social work professionals • Education/child-care professionals • Law enforcement professionals • All persons	• Christian Science practitioners • Clergy	Have reason to suspect	Attorney/client
New Jersey	All persons	Not addressed in statutes reviewed	Have reasonable cause to believe	Not addressed in statutes reviewed
New Mexico	• Health-care professionals • Mental health professionals • Social work professionals • Education/child-care professionals • Law enforcement professionals • All persons	• Judges • Clergy	Know or have reasonable suspicion	Clergy/penitent
New York	• Health-care professionals • Mental health professionals • Social work professionals • Education/child-care professionals • Law enforcement professionals	• Alcoholism/substance abuse counselors • District attorneys • Christian Science practitioners	Have reasonable cause to suspect	Not addressed in statutes reviewed
North Carolina	All persons	Any institution	Have cause to suspect	Attorney/client
North Dakota	• Health-care professionals • Mental health professionals • Social work professionals • Education/child-care professionals • Law enforcement professionals	• Clergy • Religious healers • Addiction counselors	Have knowledge of or reasonable cause to suspect	• Clergy/penitent • Attorney/client
Ohio	• Health-care professionals • Mental health professionals • Social work professionals • Education/child-care professionals • Law enforcement professionals	• Attorneys • Religious healers • Agents of humane societies	Know or suspect	• Attorney/client • Physician/patient
Oklahoma	• Health-care professionals • Education/child-care professionals • All persons	Commercial film and photographic print processors	Have reason to believe	Not granted in statutes reviewed

(continues)

MANDATORY REPORTERS OF CHILD ABUSE AND NEGLECT IN THE UNITED STATES

State	Professionals who must report	Others	Standard	Privileged communications
Oregon	• Health-care professionals • Mental health professionals • Social work professionals • Education/child-care professionals • Law enforcement professionals	• Attorneys • Clergy • Firefighters • Court-appointed special advocates	Have reasonable cause to believe	• Mental health/ patient • Clergy/penitent • Attorney/client
Pennsyl-vania	• Health-care professionals • Mental health professionals • Social work professionals • Education/child-care professionals • Law enforcement professionals	• Funeral directors • Christian Science practitioners • Clergy	Have reasonable cause to suspect	Clergy/penitent
Rhode Island	All persons	Not addressed in statutes reviewed	Have reasonable cause to suspect	Attorney/client
South Carolina	• Health-care professionals • Mental health professionals • Social work professionals • Education/child-care professionals • Law enforcement professionals	• Judges • Funeral home directors and employees • Christian Science practitioners • Film processors • Religious healers • Substance abuse treatment staff • Computer technicians	Have reason to believe	• Attorney/client • Clergy/penitent
South Dakota	• Health-care professionals • Mental health professionals • Social work professionals • Education/child-care professionals • Law enforcement professionals	• Chemical dependency coun-selors • Religious healers • Parole or court services officers • Employees of domestic abuse shelters	Have reasonable cause to suspect	Not granted in statutes reviewed
Tennessee	• Health-care professionals • Mental health professionals • Social work professionals • Education/child-care professionals • Law enforcement professionals • All persons	• Judges • Neighbors • Relatives • Friends • Religious healers	• Knowledge of/reasonably know • Have reason-able cause to suspect	Not granted in statutes reviewed
Texas	• Health-care professionals • Education/child-care professionals • All others	• Juvenile probation or detention officers • Employees or clinics that provide reproductive services	Have cause to believe	
Utah	• Health-care professionals • All persons	Not addressed in statutes reviewed	• Have reason to believe • Have observed conditions which would reasonably result	Clergy/penitent

MANDATORY REPORTERS OF CHILD ABUSE AND NEGLECT IN THE UNITED STATES

State	Professionals who must report	Others	Standard	Privileged communications
Vermont	• Health-care professionals • Mental health professionals • Social work professionals • Education/child-care professionals • Law enforcement professionals	• Camp administrators and counselors • Probation officers • Clergy	Have reasonable cause to believe	Clergy/penitent
Virginia	• Health-care professionals • Mental health professionals • Social work professionals • Education/child-care professionals • Law enforcement professionals	• Mediators • Christian Science practitioners • Probation officers • Court-appointed special advocates	Have reason to suspect	Not granted in statutes reviewed
Washington	• Health-care professionals • Mental health professionals • Social work professionals • Education/child-care professionals • Law enforcement professionals	• Any adult with whom a child resides • Responsible living skills program staff	Have reasonable cause to believe	Not granted in statutes reviewed
West Virginia	• Health-care professionals • Mental health professionals • Social work professionals • Education/child-care professionals • Law enforcement professionals	• Clergy • Religious healers • Judges, family law masters or magistrates • Christian Science practitioners	• Reasonable cause to suspect • When believed • Have observed	Attorney/client
Wisconsin	• Health-care professionals • Mental health professionals • Social work professionals • Education/child-care professionals • Law enforcement professionals	• Alcohol or drug abuse counselors • Mediators • Financial and employment planners • Court-appointed special advocates	• Have reasonable cause to suspect • Have reason to believe	Not addressed in statutes reviewed
Wyoming	All persons	Not addressed in statutes reviewed	• Know or have reasonable cause to believe or suspect • Have observed conditions that would reasonably result in such abuse	• Attorney/client • Physician/patient • Clergy/penitent

Source: National Clearinghouse on Child Abuse and Neglect Information. *Mandatory Reporters of Child Abuse and Neglect.* Washington, D.C.: U.S. Department of Health and Human Services, 2003.

source of nutrition. Repeated severe infection can also cause symptoms similar to those of marasmus.

masked deprivation   See EMOTIONAL NEGLECT.

masturbation   Masturbation refers to the manipulation of one's own or another's genitals for sexual gratification. Exhibitionists may seek to obtain sexual gratification by masturbating in the presence of a child. Other CHILD MOLESTERS may force or encourage children to masturbate in their presence or may participate in the masturbation. Nurses, babysitters and parents have been reported, on occasion, to masturbate infants and young children as a way of quieting them.

Though self-masturbation by children is not considered a damaging behavior, frequent or open masturbation may be an indicator that the child is a victim of sexual abuse. This is especially true in the case of young children.

Masturbation also plays an important role in the practice of PEDOPHILIA. Pedophiles are strongly aroused by children and often maintain large collections of CHILD PORNOGRAPHY as a fantasy aid to masturbation.

maternal drug dependence   Use of drugs, including alcohol, during pregnancy can cause severe and lasting damage to the fetus. Facial malformation, growth retardation and damage to the central nervous system are all present in children suffering from FETAL ALCOHOL SYNDROME. Infants born to mothers addicted to opiates may also become addicted, and they experience painful withdrawal symptoms at birth.

Many states now require that pregnant women who are drug or alcohol dependent be reported to a mandated agency for investigation of child abuse or neglect. Instances in which an infant is removed from the mother's care at birth are, however, rare.

See also ADDICTION, INFANTILE; PARENTAL SUBSTANCE ABUSE; SUBSTANCE ABUSE.

maternal rejection syndrome   See FAILURE-TO-THRIVE SYNDROME.

matricide   This term refers to the murder of one's mother. Matricide is relatively rare. Statistics show that most matricides are committed by sons. Though little is known about the motivation of children who kill their mothers, information from case studies suggests a strong link between matricide and child abuse. Most such murders occur during or shortly after an episode of child abuse.

Psychiatric profiles of mothers murdered by a son show a pattern of overly restrictive and harsh treatment of the son. Close examination of these profiles often indicates a strong sadistic component of the relationship. Also, mothers in these studies often behaved seductively toward the son yet quickly followed such behavior with brutal treatment. Despite the strong erotic component of these relationships INCEST was rarely consummated. Further, in most of these cases fathers were typically absent or extremely passive.

See also PARRICIDE, REACTIVE; PATRICIDE.

media coverage of child abuse   It has long been true in the United States that there is widespread public response to media coverage of child abuse and neglect. Newspapers and magazines in the 19th century and, more recently, radio and television coverage of child maltreatment issues have been useful and effective means of publicizing needs in this area.

As early as the 1870s, when the now-famous MARY ELLEN WILSON case was written about in the *New York Times,* reporters and editors recognized the public's interest in child abuse. Some observers have drawn a correlation between the increase in media coverage of abuse and neglect and the response via private organizations and public agencies that seek to protect children and prevent child maltreatment. Whether or not there is a cause-and-effect relationship and despite some critics' charges that sensational reporting often does little more than titillate its audience, it is clear that, beginning in the late 19th century, the media in all its forms has promoted greater public awareness of child abuse and neglect.

Following C. Henry Kempe's report, "The Battered-Child Syndrome," in the July 7, 1962, issue of the

Journal of the American Medical Association, many professional journals, popular magazines and newspapers increased their coverage of a wide range of child maltreatment issues. Numerous articles detailed the problem, focusing particularly on the psychopathology of abusing parents and varieties of physical abuse cases but also reported on other facets such as sexual abuse and corporal punishment.

According to one source, over the last three decades there have been over 1,700 articles published in professional journals alone, pieces that focus on child abuse and attendant issues. Likewise, newspaper coverage of the topic has grown enormously. In the 30-year period between 1950 and 1980, the *New York Times Index* lists 652 articles on child abuse. And popular magazine coverage of abuse and neglect increased as well. For the 10 years following publication of Kempe's article in the AMA journal, 28 articles about child abuse were printed in magazines read by the general public, a figure contrasting sharply with the previous decade during which only three stories on abuse were published.

It is apparent to many experts that, in the 1970s and 1980s, changes in public policy regarding child abuse and neglect were precipitated to some degree by greater coverage of the subject. In this respect, the 20th century is similar to the previous century, when public and private agencies were established in apparent response to news coverage of child protection issues. In this sense, the media has positively influenced the heightened public awareness of and interest in child abuse and neglect.

Gerbner, George, Catherine J. Ross, and Edward Zigler, eds. *Child Abuse: An Agenda for Action.* New York: Oxford University Press, 1980.

Medicaid   Title XIX of the Social Security Act—known as Medicaid—was signed into law by President Lyndon B. Johnson on July 30, 1965. Medicaid is jointly funded by the federal government and the states. It provides a range of medical services to low-income individuals who meet state criteria for that category. Of particular relevance to child abuse is the inclusion of families who participate in the Temporary Aid to Needy Families Program (TANF).

Children in those eligible families receive a number of medical services under Medicaid. Among those services are early and periodic screening, diagnosis and treatment (EPSDT). EPSDT provides medical screening to children on a regular basis, beginning in infancy. Medicaid and TANF are credited with making a strong contribution toward eliminating or reducing SITUATIONAL ABUSE AND NEGLECT associated with POVERTY and poor health care.

See also SOCIAL SECURITY ACT.

medical evaluation   A thorough medical evaluation is important in the identification of abuse or neglect as well as the treatment of injuries resulting from maltreatment. The physician conducting the evaluation should be trained in recognition of medical conditions associated with abuse. Serious injury may be overlooked due to a lack of visual evidence or because the examiner fails to recognize subtle signs of trauma.

Thorough assessment requires the involvement of several different disciplines, including psychiatry, pediatrics, social work and nursing. In many cases a specialist in pediatric neurology, radiology, ophthalmology, dentistry or other area is necessary to evaluate the existence and the extent of injury fully. When abuse or neglect is suspected as the cause of death, an AUTOPSY by a pathologist trained in FORENSIC MEDICINE is appropriate.

In many cases evidence of trauma is easily recognizable. Since one purpose of the medical evaluation is to gather evidence for the existence of nonaccidental injury, the physician must be skilled in determining the possible causes of a particular injury as well as the approximate time it was inflicted. While it is not often possible to say with absolute assurance precisely how a child was injured, it is often possible to rule out certain causes. Suspicion of abuse is often aroused when a caretaker's account of how a child was injured does not coincide with medical evidence.

More often a physician is called upon by parents to treat a sick or injured child when no suggestion of maltreatment is made. A physician must constantly be aware of suspicious explanations or behavior by caretakers as well as physical evidence of abuse.

A complete medical evaluation may involve a SKELETAL SURVEY to detect any FRACTURES and evidence of other internal injury. When SEXUAL ABUSE is a possibility, a thorough examination of the genitalia, mouth and anus, with appropriate tests for sexually transmitted disease and, in adolescents, pregnancy, is conducted. Other tests may reveal inadequate nutrition or other evidence of NEGLECT.

Frequently, more than one form of maltreatment is observed in a child. Presence of PHYSICAL ABUSE will alert the medical specialist to look for other evidence of maltreatment such as neglect or PSYCHOLOGICAL/EMOTIONAL MALTREATMENT.

The medical specialist must be skilled in differentiating abuse-related trauma from disease-related symptoms that mimic abuse. Various diseases, congenital conditions and even birthmarks can be confused with indicators of abuse or neglect. Certain folk medicine remedies (see CAO GIO) also produce lesions that are frequently interpreted as evidence of abuse by examining physicians.

Despite the difficulty of confronting a parent with the information that the child could not have injured him or herself, the physician's first responsibility is to protect the child. This involves notifying the proper child protection authorities and, in some cases, arranging for the child to be hospitalized for treatment observation and/or protection. Honest and sensitive discussion of the problem with caretakers immediately following diagnosis may improve the likelihood that they will cooperate in efforts to prevent further maltreatment. The primary purpose of the medical evaluation is to identify evidence of abuse or neglect, not specifically to identify the abuser. Evidence obtained by the physician should be presented to the proper law enforcement or child protection authorities charged with the INVESTIGATION of child abuse.

medical model   Since World War II, the medical model has greatly influenced public perceptions of child abuse and neglect. By presenting abuse as a form of psychopathological illness, the medical model held out hope that it, like other sicknesses, could be isolated and cured. Dominance of the medical approach to child abuse may stem in part from developments in pediatric radiology (see RADIOL-OGY, PEDIATRIC) that allowed physicians to diagnose unusual patterns of bone trauma that appeared to be the result of battering.

Popularization of the term BATTERED CHILD SYNDROME by C. Henry Kempe and his associates further strengthened the perception of child abuse as illness. Subsequent attention by the popular media created the perception of all abused children as victims of sadistic PHYSICAL ABUSE. This vision of child abuse played an important role in mobilizing political action on behalf of abused children. Within five years of publication of an article entitled "The Battered Child Syndrome" in the *Journal of the American Medical Association,* each of the 50 states had adopted a law that required reporting of suspected child abuse and neglect. The medical image of child abuse continues to heavily influence approaches to treatment and prevention.

In spite of its usefulness in generating public action the medical model is frequently criticized for ignoring societal causes of abuse and neglect. Focusing attention on individual pathology while useful and appropriate in many situations, may not be sufficient to eliminate underlying causes of child maltreatment. Some critics of the medical model argue that it amounts to BLAMING THE VICTIM and call for a more balanced approach to the problem.

See also DEFECT MODEL OF CHILD ABUSE; PSYCHOPATHOLOGY.

medical neglect   Failure of parents or other custodial caregivers to provide for or permit necessary medical treatment. This failure may be based on religious beliefs, fear, ignorance, misunderstanding of the care that is needed or a lack of concern. It may also be based on the abuser's fear of arrest and incarceration should physicians observe the extent of the injuries the child has suffered and the likely PHYSICAL ABUSE that occurred.

In 2003, 39 states reported on cases of medical neglect, according to *Child Maltreatment 2003,* a report from the Administration on Children, Youth and Families. Of the entire child population in the United States in 2003, less than 1% (0.3%) of all children were reported as experiencing medical neglect. In contrast, 7.5% of all maltreated children suffered from another form of NEGLECT.

Some examples of medical neglect were discussed by Andrew P. Sirotnak, Joyce K. Moore and Jean C. Smith in the book *Child Victimization.* For example,

A young asthmatic boy is repeatedly brought to the emergency room only when his condition is so severe that he immediately goes into intensive care. The parents of a girl with congenital cataracts refuse to consent to eye surgery, which would prevent her eventual blindness. When a child with a treatable serious chronic disease or handicap has frequent hospitalizations of significant deterioration because the parents ignore medical recommendations, court-enforced supervision or even foster placement may be required.

Other examples of medical neglect are seriously inadequate preventive care, such as the failure to obtain treatment for a recognized visual impairment, or allowing a child to suffer painful tooth decay without seeking dental treatment. (However, if the parents are on Medicaid, which may not provide children with dental or vision care, and/or they are poor, this factor is taken into consideration.)

A significant percentage of seriously abused children do not receive medical attention, usually before they are brought to the attention of child protective services. For example, as noted by Sirotnak, Moore and Smith in a study of children who had been abused, among children ages 11–14 who reported being abused and suffering serious burns, 60% said they were *not* taken to see a nurse or a doctor. Of children who said that they were bitten by another person or an animal, 52% were *not* taken to see a nurse or doctor.

Medical Neglect Is a Subject of Continuing Controversy

The issue of medical neglect has been the subject of much heated debate and many legal battles. In cases of serious acute illness and life-threatening or disabling chronic disease, the state social services department may sometimes decide that is necessary to obtain a court order to allow treatment.

When ongoing treatment is required, court supervision or foster placement may be necessary to ensure proper medical care. A distinction is usually (but not always) made between those situations in which medical intervention has a reasonable possibility of succeeding and those cases of children with fatal diseases, such as cancer, in which medical procedures are mostly palliative.

See also ABUSERS; FAMILY VIOLENCE; SEXUAL ABUSE.

Administration on Children, Youth and Families. *Child Maltreatment 2003.* Children's Bureau, U.S. Department of Health and Human Services, Washington, D.C., 2005.

Sirotnak, Andrew P., Joyce K. Moore, and Jean C. Smith. "Neglect." In *Understanding the Medical Diagnosis of Child Maltreatment: A Guide for Nonmedical Professionals.* New York: Oxford University Press, 2006.

medicine, forensic   See FORENSIC MEDICINE.

Megan's Law   This term was first used to describe a law requiring community notification of released sex offenders, which was passed in 1994 in New Jersey (New Jersey State Sex Offender Registration Act) subsequent to the abduction and murder of a child, Megan Kanka. Megan was killed by a twice-convicted sex offender who had completed his prison term and had moved in with two other sex offenders to a house across the street from the Kanka's house. He asked Megan to come over and see his puppy. She was subsequently kidnapped, raped and murdered.

In 1996, the federal government passed its own version of Megan's Law as an amendment to the Violent Crime Control and Law Enforcement Act of 1996. This law ordered all states to establish a form of community notification of child sex offenders. This information must be released to the public when necessary for public safety. (Each state's interpretation of the federal law varies.) Opponents of the law believed it was tantamount to double jeopardy for the offender, that it gave neighborhood residents a false sense of security and that it simply did not work—even with this law, repeat sex offenders have been released and victimized more children. They also point out that most abuse (80% or more) is perpetrated by individuals known to the child, such as family members, and that "stranger danger" is not the main problem. Supporters of Megan's Law, however, counter that Megan Kanka knew her abuser, as he was a neighbor, but the family did not know he had been convicted of sex offenses in the past.

Another act, the WETTERLING ACT, requires released child sex offenders to register their addresses with the state and to report any changes of address.

See also CIVIL COMMITMENT LAWS; RAPE.

"National Conference on Sex Offender Registries: Proceedings of a BJS/SEARCH Conference." Bureau of Justice Statistics, April 1998, NCJ-168965.

Menkes' kinky hair syndrome This rare inherited disease inhibits the absorption of copper into the system, resulting in brittle bones and possibly death. Due to the multiple fractures present in infants suffering from this disease, it is often confused with the BATTERED CHILD SYNDROME. The name derives from characteristic changes in the hair of those with this disease. Hair is stubby, coarse and ivory in color.

mental cruelty Often used as grounds for divorce, mental cruelty may also form the basis for intervention in a family by child protection agencies. As a legal term, mental cruelty refers to a pattern of behavior by an individual that threatens the mental and physical health of another. Courts differ in the type and severity of actions they consider to be mental cruelty. In recent years, the definition has generally expanded to include behavior that was not previously considered abusive. A child who is the target of mental cruelty by a parent or caretaker is a victim of PSYCHOLOGICAL/EMOTIONAL MALTREATMENT.

mental injury A term used in some child abuse laws, mental injury refers to intellectual or psychological damage. Determination of the existence and extent of mental injury is usually based on a comparison of a child's performance and behavior with that of other children of the same age and cultural background.

Legal definitions of mental injury usually depend upon evaluation by a qualified psychiatrist, psychologist or pediatrician. Further, the impairment must be attributable to an act or acts of omission or commission by an adult responsible for the child. Pennsylvania law (Act 124, 1975) defines mental injury as "a psychological condition . . . which: (1) renders the child chronically and severely anxious, agitated, depressed, socially withdrawn, psychotic, or in reasonable fear that his/her life and/or safety is threatened; (2) makes it extremely likely that the child will become chronically and severely anxious, agitated, depressed, socially withdrawn, psychotic, or be in reasonable fear that his/her life is threatened; or (3) seriously interferes with the child's ability to accomplish age-appropriate developmental milestones, or school, peer, and community tasks."

Mental injury may result from PSYCHOLOGICAL/EMOTIONAL MALTREATMENT well as PHYSICAL ABUSE, SEXUAL ABUSE and NEGLECT.

mental retardation Ironically, mental retardation is seen as both a cause and a result of child abuse.

Mental retardation can result from child battering, nutritional and medical neglect, drug or alcohol use during pregnancy and other forms of maltreatment. SUBDURAL HEMATOMA due to battering is perhaps the major cause of traumatically induced mental retardation among children. Battered infants are especially susceptible to brain damage because the infant cranium is soft and does not afford the same protection provided by the fully developed adult bone structure.

Mentally retarded or developmentally delayed children are often singled out as targets for abuse by their caretakers. Parents may feel angry, frustrated and/or guilty as a result of having a retarded child. These feelings are sometimes directed toward the child in the form of abusive behavior. The child is also more likely to be the recipient of abuse connected with family stress, alcohol and drug abuse and mental illness on the part of the parent or primary caretaker. Mentally retarded children and adults are more vulnerable to physical and sexual assaults from outside as well.

Because many children suffering from mental retardation are cared for in institutions or community-based programs, they are often the victims of INSTITUTIONAL ABUSE AND NEGLECT. For centuries, these children and adults were subjected to imprisonment, beating, sexual misuse and starvation and were sometimes put to death. Even now, vast differences exist in the quality of care provided for mentally retarded individuals in different communities and countries around the world.

microcephaly A condition in which the cranial capacity is abnormally small, microcephaly may develop following a blow to the head. Damage caused by microcephaly is usually irreversible.

Minnesota Multiphasic Personality Inventory Psychometric tests are sometimes used to detect emotional disturbance in children who have been abused. Most such tests can be administered and interpreted only by trained psychologists. The Minnesota Multiphasic Personality Inventory (MMPI) is one of the most popular tests used in the assessment of older children.

The MMPI consists of over 500 items that must be answered true, false or "cannot say." Originally developed as a means of classifying patients in mental hospitals, the test is divided into 10 basic scales that measure characteristics such as hypochondria, depression, hysteria, paranoia, hypomania and schizophrenia.

minor See CHILD.

Miranda warnings In cases of alleged child abuse and neglect, as in other alleged crimes, an accused person is protected against self-incrimination by the so-called Miranda warnings, based on the 1966 U.S. Supreme Court decision in *Miranda v. Arizona.* In that ruling, the court held that statements made by an individual who has been taken into custody cannot be used by the prosecution *against that individual* unless procedural safeguards

against self-incrimination have been exercised. Briefly stated, the Miranda warnings cover the following points:

1. An individual has the right to remain silent.
2. Anything said by an individual can and will be used against that individual in a court of law.
3. An individual has the right to talk with a lawyer and to have the lawyer present during questioning.
4. If an individual cannot afford to hire a lawyer, one will be appointed to represent that individual prior to any questioning, if the individual so desires.

misdemeanor In criminal court proceedings offenses are distinguished according to how serious they are perceived to be. FELONIES are considered most serious and are punishable by more severe penalties. Misdemeanors are treated less severely, traditionally receiving prison sentences no longer than one year. In some cases, misdemeanors and felonies are tried in different courts, with alleged felons receiving greater procedural safeguards.

See also COURT, DUE PROCESS.

molestation See CHILD MOLESTER.

Mongolian spots Birthmarks are sometimes mistaken for bruises on young children and infants, arousing the suspicion of child abuse. Mongolian spots appear on some children at birth. These are grayish blue in color and last from two to three years. These spots can appear on any part of the body, but are most commonly found on the back and buttocks. Though Mongolian spots are found on children of all races, they appear more frequently on dark-skinned infants.

mouth injuries Injuries to the mouth and surrounding area are relatively common in children. Determination of whether trauma is due to accident or abuse often depends on the plausibility of the caretaker's explanation of the accident and on the age of the child. While some types of oral injuries are common in children learning to walk, such injuries are less likely to be accidental in pretoddlers or children who have been walking for some time.

Mouth injuries include tearing of the frenum (the small, V-shaped muscle joining the lip to the gum at the front of the mouth); cuts, abrasions and contusions of the lips; loosening, intrusion (forcing back into the gum), avulsion (total removal) and fractures of the teeth; and laceration of the tongue or gums. Fracture of the mandible (lower jaw), and less frequently the maxillary bone (upper bone structure), may also result from a forceful blow to the mouth area.

Prompt attention to oral injuries by a physician or dentist is important. Avulsed teeth have a 90% chance of being saved if replaced in the socket within 15 minutes of removal. The success rate of reimplantation drops 15% after one hour. Tooth fractures should also receive prompt attention from a dentist to avoid loss of the tooth.

Neglect of proper oral hygiene can cause unnecessary pain and discomfort as well as permanent damage to a child's mouth. Though it is often difficult to determine whether neglect of dental needs is intentional, poor oral hygiene is often indicative of more general MEDICAL NEGLECT.

Dentists can be especially helpful in early identification of possible abuse or neglect involving oral damage and hygiene. Many areas require that dentists report suspected child maltreatment to local child protection or law enforcement authorities.

multidisciplinary team   Identification and treatment of child abuse and neglect often requires a variety of different skills and perspectives. Multidisciplinary teams have been found to be an effective way of helping professionals work together in diagnosing and treating child abuse. Such teams are used widely in many different countries. In the United States some states specifically require the use of multidisciplinary teams.

Composition of teams may vary but most teams include representatives from the fields of social service and medicine. Members of the mental health, nursing, education, legal and law enforcement professions are frequently included. Inclusion of a representative of the agency legally charged with investigation of reported abuse is recommended as a means of improving coordination of services and reducing conflict.

In addition to identification and treatment planning, multidisciplinary teams may also provide consultation, community education and prevention services. Many teams are based in hospitals. Other models include interagency programs and teams directly connected to a government agency.

Though some teams experience relatively high levels of disagreement between members and occasional disputes over turf, most experts agree that the advantages of the multidisciplinary approach outweigh the disadvantages. Use of multidisciplinary teams has been credited with improving the quality and coordination of treatment, lessening the need for out-of-home placement, strengthening families, reducing the chance of reinjury and lowering the overall cost of treatment.

multiple maltreatment   Child abuse is rarely confined to a single incident or mode of abuse. Investigation of suspected abuse often reveals forms of maltreatment other than that reported. Physically abused children are also often neglected. Victims of sexual abuse may also be subjected to psychological or physical abuse.

The combination of several forms of maltreatment often presents special problems for the treatment of abused and neglected children. Failure to identify all forms of maltreatment may lead to inappropriate intervention. Unrecognized or untreated abuse may have lasting effects. Careful ASSESSMENT of each child's situation is essential to ensure proper treatment and protection.

Munchausen Syndrome by Proxy (MSBP)   A form of child abuse that refers to recurrent severe illnesses, usually among children, that are actually induced by another person, most frequently the biological mother. Once a therapeutic separation occurs from the abusive person, the child usually recovers, often quite dramatically. Munchausen Syndrome by Proxy (MSBP) is the common name for this disorder, but the formal term used by psychiatrists is *Factitious Illness by Proxy.*

The person who is causing the illness may inject the child with bacteria or even feces or other contaminated material or may harm the child by injecting unneeded drugs and dangerous drugs (such as insulin in a child who is not diabetic) or other substances that cause illness. Sometimes the child's own blood is used to cause apparently bloody stools in a diaper or the parent may inject contaminated blood into the child's bloodstream. There are many different ways in which caregivers may cause severe harm, and even death, to children.

The syndrome received its name in an odd way. Baron K. F. H. von Munchausen was an 18th-century German mercenary with a penchant for telling tall tales. Accounts of his adventures were further embellished in a pamphlet entitled "Baron Munchausen's Narrative of His Marvellous Travels and Campaigns in Russia." In the early 1950s, Richard Asher, an English physician, used the term *Munchausen Syndrome* to describe a psychiatric disorder characterized by dramatic and untruthful medical histories and feigned symptoms.

The first paper on Munchausen Syndrome by Proxy was described in a paper by British pediatrician Roy S. Meadow, who had a patient with frequent and puzzling illnesses and whose urine was apparently infected by one type of bacteria in the morning and yet another in the evening. However, some urinalyses would be normal. The mystery was solved when it was discovered that the bacteria were present only when the mother helped to collect the urine specimen. She was purposely contaminating the child's urine with bacteria.

It is unknown how many children suffer from Munchausen Syndrome by Proxy, but it is believed to be rare. When it occurs, an infant or toddler is the usual victim, but it can be present in older children as well. This problem is often very difficult to detect. The perpetrator may present false medical histories, inflict physical symptoms on the child, alter laboratory specimens and directly induce disorders in the child. As a result of these fabrications, the child may be subjected to frequent unnecessary hospitalizations, painful tests, potentially harmful treatment, and even death.

In one case, an eight-year-old with severe hypoglycemia received a partial pancreatomy (partial removal of the pancreas) to resolve the problem. It was later discovered, however, that the parent had administered drugs prior to the child's surgery to induce hypoglycemia, and after the surgery, the child's symptoms occurred again because the parent administered insulin. The mother was a nurse who had falsified prescriptions for sulfonamides and insulin. In another case, a small child received a pancreatomy because of symptoms induced by a parent. It was believed that his mother, a person with Type 2 diabetes, had injected insulin into the child to induce the symptoms.

A Florida child was hospitalized more than 200 times and had suffered 40 operations before her mother's abuse was discovered. Other children have suffered equally harrowing experiences. In an article in a 1997 issue of *Pediatrics,* a discussion of MSBP is followed by a distressing account of an adult who had as a child experienced repeated and purposeful abuse at the hands of her mother, whose usual modus operandi was to break or injure bones with a hammer.

In an article about a child ultimately diagnosed with MSBP, published in a 2005 issue of *AACN Clinical Issues* by Lieder et al., the researchers reported on a two-year-old child from South America who had been evaluated repeatedly in South American hospitals and was ultimately sent to the United States with his mother for further evaluation, with fees financed by corporations to which the mother, a nursing assistant, had appealed. In the first 17 months of his life, the child had experienced numerous invasive tests and had received many antibiotics for infections. Yet no cause for his illness was identified.

Upon the second admission to the hospital with a 104-degree fever, the staff began to suspect MSBP because of the numerous types of bacteria in his blood that were commonly found in the intestinal tract. The hospital alerted child protective services, who led the mother out of the room. As she left, the nurse noticed that the mother had a vial of blood in her purse. It was confiscated and was later identified as the child's blood. The mother offered no explanation for why she had the vial of blood.

After the child was separated from the mother, he quickly recovered and his body temperature dropped to normal and remained there. He began eating normally. Said the authors,

> The mother of the South American child reported here exemplifies the characteristics of the MSBP perpetrator as described in the literature. She was knowledgeable of medical terminology. She was cooperative and friendly with the staff and loyal and attentive to her child, staying with him most of the time throughout hospitalization. Her behavior, consistent with that of a concerned parent, made the diagnosis of MSBP remote in the early phases of his evaluation. However, with the recurrence of polymicrobial bacteremia [many different types of bacteria in the blood] from unlikely pathogenic organisms, suspicions emerged from the nursing and medical providers for contamination of blood samples.

The child was placed in temporary foster care in the United States. Because he was a South American citizen, he was ultimately sent to foster care in his native country.

Symptoms and Diagnostic Path

According to the *Diagnostic and Statistical Manual of Disorders (DSM-IV)*, the four criteria are that an illness in another person is either caused or faked, the motivation of the perpetrator is to obtain sympathy from others, the motivation is not a desire for economic gain, and the behavior cannot be explained by another psychiatric diagnosis.

The underlying reason for the abuse appears to be the attention that the perpetrator receives. The perpetrator may have been a victim of abuse in childhood, although this is not always the case. Lieder et al. advised that "a detailed and objective medical history of the child and family is imperative from the immediate caregivers and any other neutral sources, including medical records from all previous institutions. Attention to unusual illnesses, deaths in siblings or parents, and the condition of the child when not in the care of the suspected perpetrator is noted."

In addition, the authors also recommended that "Any samples, specimens, potentially contaminated lines or materials should be retained for future analysis, with care taken to establish a chain of evidence for law enforcement purposes (including proper sealing, labeling, and storing of specimens to prevent tampering)." They also noted that caregiving nurses are mandated reporters of suspected child abuse, and they may not delegate this responsibility to others.

In some cases, videotapes can be used if nursing staff or doctors are suspicious that the parents or other caregivers may be inducing illness in the child. In one study of 41 patients whose rooms were monitored over the period 1993–97, reported in *Pediatrics* in 2000, a diagnosis of MSBP was made in 23 cases. In four patients, the parents' innocence was actually established by the videotapes.

It can be difficult to diagnose MSBP because the mother usually appears to be a loving and caring person, and experts say that if and when MSBP is suspected, hospital staff can become very polarized between accusers and defenders. The underlying reason for the abuse is the attention the mother receives. Often she may be a person with medical training or even a nursing degree.

A very thorough description of this disorder is provided in a 1999 issue of *Critical Care Nursing Quarterly*. The authors reported that children under five are at greatest risk. They provided clinical profiles of both the victim and the perpetrator. According to the authors, the typical child victim profile is as follows:

1. Persistent or recurrent illness cannot be explained readily by the consulting physician despite a thorough medical workup. The illness presents as an atypical pattern, even to experienced clinicians. Usually, the symptoms are associated with only one system; for example, gastrointestinal problems of vomiting, diarrhea and bloody stool; and neurological problems of seizures, apnea and lethargy. On occasion, a presentation will consist of many different symptoms representing a multisystem disorder.
2. A diagnosis is merely descriptive of the symptoms or a diagnosis of an extremely rare disorder.
3. Symptoms do not respond to the usual treatment regime. Incidents may occur that interfere

with treatment effectiveness, such as intravenous lines coming out, repeated line infections or persistent vomiting of medications.

4. Physical or lab findings are not consistent with the reported history. Lab findings may be unusual or physiologically impossible.
5. Physical findings and reported symptoms conflict with the child's generally healthy appearance.
6. A temporal relationship exists between the child's symptoms and the mother's presence. The reported symptoms fail to occur in the parent's absence and may not have been observed by anyone other than the parent.
7. Pertinent medical history cannot be substantiated. The parent may be unable to provide sufficient information about previous medical care or the records conflict with the parent's report.
8. Presenting complaints include bleeding, seizures, unconsciousness, apnea, diarrhea, vomiting, fever and lethargy. These most commonly reported symptoms should serve as warning signs.

The clinical profile of the abusive perpetrator is as follows, according to the authors:

1. The MBPS parent is reluctant to leave the child while hospitalized. The parent may refuse to leave the child's beside for even a few minutes or to take care of his or her own personal needs. He or she often will attend to the child-victim to the exclusion of his or her other children to a degree that it is detrimental to them.
2. The parent develops close personal relationships with hospital staff. The parent may spend the little time when he or she does leave his or her child's side socializing with the health-care staff and parents of other ill children. Nurses and physicians may find themselves becoming emotionally involved with the parent, blurring practitioner/patient boundaries.
3. The parent's educational or employment background is in the medical field or he or she aspires to be a health-care provider. Often the parent is medically knowledgeable and well versed in medical terminology and procedures.
4. The parent displays an unusual calm when facing problems related to the child's health. Although the parent expresses concern for the child, when an emergency occurs, he or she remains unaffected. The parent actually may be highly supportive and encouraging of the medical/nursing practitioner, even when the practitioner expresses confusion about the child's problems. A minority of MBPS parents goes to the opposite extreme and becomes angry, degrading the staff and demanding additional procedures that are not medically indicated.
5. The medical problems of the parent are similar to those of the child. A substantial number of MBPS parents exhibit some or all of the features of Munchausen Syndrome.
6. Information fabrication may not be confined to the child's symptoms or history but may include aspects of the parent's family, education, previous employment, illness and other historical data.
7. In some cases, prominent religious beliefs, superstitions or cultural beliefs are integral parts of the parent's presentation and personality.

Treatment Options and Outlook

The child suffering from MSBP will not recover unless and until the abuse is detected and stopped. The child may have experienced many invasive procedures prior to that point and, as mentioned earlier, may even had serious surgeries. However, after the MSBP is detected, usually with the collaboration of child protective service workers and the hospital staff, the child's medical condition will remit. The child will need to be placed in foster care, and if any visits are allowed between the child and the mother, they must be monitored extremely closely by social workers and/or foster parents, because the abusive behavior is likely to occur again without such monitoring.

Risk Factors and Preventive Measures

Few parents induce MSBP, and there are few known risk factors other than child abuse in the parent's past history. However, of those that are known, the parents are usually female and, as mentioned, they often have medical knowledge. If MSBP is suspected, the best course of action is to isolate the child from the parent to see if the child's health improves. This action is likely to be vigorously contested by the parent, who will try to enlist the staff to help him or her see the child. In some cases, the hospital staff has been bitterly divided by this issue, between those who think that the parent may be guilty and others who think it is unimaginable that such abuse could have occurred at the hands of a parent or other caregiver who they perceive as very loving, devoted and caring.

Bryk, Mary, and Patricia T. Siegel. "My Mother Caused My Illness: The Story of a Survivor of Munchausen by Proxy Syndrome." *Pediatrics* 100, no. 1 (July 1997): 1–7.

Hall, David E., et al. "Evaluation of Covert Video Surveillance in the Diagnosis of Munchausen Syndrome by Proxy: Lessons from 41 Cases." *Pediatrics* 105, no. 6 (2000): 1,305–1,312.

Lieder, Holly S., et al. "Munchausen Syndrome by Proxy: A Case Report." *AACN Clinical Issues* 18, no. 2 (2005): 178–184.

Pasqualone, Georgia A., and Susan M. Fitzgerald. "Munchausen by Proxy Syndrome. The Forensic Challenge." *Critical Care Nursing Quarterly* 22 (May 1999): 52–64.

mutilation, genital See CASTRATION; CLITORIDECTOMY; FEMALE GENITAL MUTILATION; INFIBULATION.

mysopedic (misopedic) offender This type of pedophile (see PEDOPHILIA) is the most sadistic of all sexual offenders. Mysopeds are sometimes referred to as "child haters" and are responsible for most brutal rapes and murders of children. Though quite uncommon, mysopeds have often been the focus of a great deal of media attention. Some of the more widely publicized cases involve mentally disordered men with long histories of molesting children, who commit a number of rape/murders before being apprehended.

One well-known case involved an Illinois man, John Wayne Gacy, who worked as a clown entertaining children in hospitals and at home. When finally arrested for a sexual offense, he confessed to sexually assaulting and strangling 32 teenage boys and young men.

national register The idea of a nationwide repository of child abuse reports has often been advanced as a way to monitor trends, conduct research and track offenders who move from place to place to avoid apprehension. It has not been possible to establish such a register in the United States because differences in state laws, definitions of abuse and rules regarding confidentiality have made this information difficult to collect and compare. Similar impediments to a national register of child abuse reports exist in Canada and in Great Britain, which consist of separate territories, provinces and/or countries.

natural dolls These are also known as "anatomically correct" dolls. A young victim of SEXUAL ABUSE may not have developed verbal skills to communicate accurately her/his experience or may simply find it very difficult or threatening to tell anyone about the episode. Hence, gathering information from the child is a difficult and sensitive task and dolls are sometimes used.

In past years, some therapists felt that such dolls were a useful tool in the diagnosis and treatment of young victims of sexual abuse because they believed that children found it less difficult to act out the abuse using the dolls or to point to the doll's sexual organs when discussing the abuse. Many therapists still use the dolls, although they have come under criticism. For example, in their chapter on the validity of child sexual abuse allegations in the book, *Expert Witnesses in Child Abuse Cases: What Can and Should Be Said in Court* (American Psychological Association, 1998), Celia B. Fisher and Katherine A. Whiting question the validity of findings from the use of such dolls. The authors write that the "rapid, widespread use of the dolls evokes popu-

lar concern over the appropriateness of presenting explicitly sexual material to children, professional concern over their potentially coercive and suggestive nature, and judicial concern regarding their ability as assessment tools for the validation of child sexual abuse. . . ."

They add that although sexually abused children are more explicit in their play with the dolls, sex play has also been found with children who had not been sexually abused. There is also some concern that the use of the dolls could be regarded as a form of entrapment. The authors said that research has revealed that asking non-abused children detailed questions about sexual behavior increases the incidences of such behavior in doll play. But they said that leading questions are common in sexual abuse cases. In other words, if the interviewer asks many questions related to genitalia, the questions themselves can increase the child's attention to the doll's oversized genitalia. This behavior then "proves" to the interviewer that the child was abused, but in fact the child's interest and behavior was piqued by the questioning of the interviewer. The authors said "psychologists using these dolls as a diagnostic instrument risk operating in an ethically indefensible manner."

neglect A serious failure, usually on the part of the parent or other custodial caregiver, to meet the minimal standards of a child's nutritional, clothing, shelter, medical, educational and safety needs. As a result of this failure, harm occurs or is highly likely to occur to the child. Neglect also encompasses the failure to act on the child's behalf, such as allowing or encouraging a child to use alcohol or drugs. A parent is not able to prevent a child from using drugs or alcohol when away from home (although all parents should actively discourage this use), but a parent should refrain from giving substances to a child or encouraging a child to consume alcohol and/or drugs at home.

The category of neglect may also include the failure to protect the child sexually, such as allowing the child to prostitute himself or herself or to have sex with adults, with the parent's knowledge and tacit permission.

Child abuse experts Murray A. Straus and Glenda Kaugman Kantor devised their own definition of caregiver neglect in a 2005 issue of *Child Abuse & Neglect*. According to these experts, "Neglectful behavior is behavior by a caregiver that constitutes a failure to act in ways that are presumed by the culture of a society to be necessary to meet the developmental needs of a child and which are the responsibility of the caregiver to provide."

Neglect is the most frequently occurring form of child maltreatment in the United States. In addition, nearly two-thirds (61%) of all children removed from their homes in 2003 suffered from neglect. According to *Child Maltreatment 2003*, children who were neglected were 31% more likely than children who were physically abused to suffer from a reexperience of neglect

State Laws on Neglect Vary

Each state has its own definition of what constitutes neglectful behavior toward children, and some are more specific than others. (See APPENDIX VI.)

In some states, parents are regarded as neglectful when they are incarcerated or otherwise institutionalized, and thus, they cannot provide any care to the child. Parental substance abuse may be considered neglect, and in some states, the finding of drugs in a newborn baby or a physician observing a newborn child with apparent FETAL ALCOHOL SYNDROME are both grounds for the TERMINATION OF PARENTAL RIGHTS. Violent behavior in the presence of a child, even when the child is not harmed or threatened, may be considered neglectful. (If the parent attacks the child beyond the use of accepted CORPORAL PUNISHMENT, this is PHYSICAL ABUSE.)

Some states consider the manufacturing of a drug in the presence of a child to be neglectful, particularly when the drugs are highly volatile and dangerous illegal drugs such as methamphetamines.

Neglectful Behavior: Acts of Omission

In contrast to other forms of child maltreatment, such as SEXUAL ABUSE or physical abuse, the category of neglect encompasses acts of omission, such as the failure to provide food, shelter and clothing or the failure to supervise the child based on the child's age (such as failing to watch a two-year old, who then wanders into the street outside her home) as well as the failure to meet the child's developmental needs.

Omissions can be as serious—or even more serious—than maltreatment commissions with regard to child care. In the most serious cases, such failures may lead to the child's death. In 2003, about 36% of all child maltreatment fatalities were caused by neglect, followed by about 29% of the deaths caused by multiple maltreatment types and 28.4% caused by physical abuse.

Types of Neglect

The most common type of neglectful behavior toward a child is the failure to provide food, clothing and/or shelter. If parents are homeless, they should seek help from others. Such a failure can be fatal to a newborn or young child as they cannot ask others for help. There are other common types of neglect, such as medical neglect, safety neglect, abandonment and educational neglect.

Medical neglect Some parents may refuse to obtain appropriate medical care for their children when the children are ill, which could be deemed MEDICAL NEGLECT. (However, religious exemptions are sometimes made if the religion prohibits medical intervention and if state law allows for such an exemption.) Children in the United States and other Western countries usually need not die of malnutrition, rickets and other diseases that can be easily treated by physicians—but if no one intervenes on behalf of children suffering from these diseases, they can and do suffer from such ailments and may die.

Neglect in infants and small children can cause poor growth, as seen with FAILURE TO THRIVE. This may be caused by a failure to provide proper nutrition as well as the psychological neglect of the child. See PSYCHOLOGICAL/EMOTIONAL MALTREATMENT.

Safety neglect Parents and other caregivers may also be neglectful when they fail to provide a safe environment, especially for small children.

As authors Andrew P. Sirotnak, Joyce K. Moore and Jean C. Smith said in their chapter on neglect in *Understanding the Medical Diagnosis of Child Maltreatment: A Guide for Nonmedical Professionals,* "This might involve leaving poisons, open heaters, knives, or guns with the child's reach. Repeated dog bites by the family dog also represent a dangerous home environment."

The authors said that one indicator of safety neglect can be observed by the physician: "Watch how they [the parents] handle the child and react to his injury. If a baby who has fallen off the sofa is brought to the medical provider and then left unattended on the examining table, one should be concerned about the parents' ability or desire to protect that child."

Safety neglect is a significant cause of death among young children. Children under the age of three have not developed a safety consciousness, and they are especially susceptible to accidents. While all children are likely to suffer preventable accidents on occasion, repeated serious accidents indicate that a child's caretaker is unable or unwilling to take the necessary steps to protect the child.

Considering abandonment ABANDONMENT is a form of neglect, and it may be criminal, depending on state laws and the circumstances of the case. Often children as young as two or three years (or younger) are left in charge of their younger siblings with no food, no instructions and no idea where their parents are.

Abandonment can be fatal, as when the child is left alone with no food and starves, or a child who is severely harmed by an accident when left alone is unable to seek help from others.

Educational neglect Educational neglect is the failure to ensure that a child attends school in accordance with state law. If the parent does not encourage or even discourages a child from going to school without a valid reason, this act is neglectful and harmful to the child, potentially preventing the child from learning important skills, such as how to read and how to make calculations.

Victimized children Boys or girls may be neglected; however, most maltreated children (including all forms of abuse) are young children. Small children are also the most likely to die of neglect.

See FATALITIES, CHILD ABUSE.

TABLE I
VICTIMS OF NEGLECT ONLY BY RACE, 2003

Race	All victims	Numbers	Percentage
African-American	159,361	81,651	51.2
American Indian or Alaska Native	7,469	5,061	67.8
Asian	3,933	1,873	47.6
Pacific Islander	1,390	329	23.7
White	334,965	161,703	48.3
Multiple Race	10,133	5,669	55.9
Hispanic	78,207	39,740	50.8
Unknown or Missing	34,224	18,236	53.3
Total	629,682	314,262	

Source: Adapted from Administration on Children, Youth and Families, *Child Maltreatment 2003.* Children's Bureau, U.S. Department of Health and Human Services, Washington, D.C., 2005, page 48.

In considering all categories of abuse and neglect, the victimization rate (per 1,000 children) was highest among children ages 0–3 years, or a rate of 16.4 children per 1,000. The rate steadily declined with age; for example, the rate for children ages four to seven years was 13.8 per thousand. The rate for children ages eight to 11 years was 11.7 per 1,000, and the rate of victimized children ages 12–15 years was 10.7 per 1,000. Children ages 16–17 years had the lowest rate of 5.9 per 1,000 children in this age group.

In considering the race and ethnicity of neglected children, the highest percentage of children who experienced neglect only (and not other forms of child maltreatment) in 2003 were American Indian or Alaska Native (67.8%), followed by children of multiple races (55.9%). See Table I for information on the race and ethnicity of children who experienced neglect only in 2003.

Categories of neglectful perpetrators Neglect was the largest maltreatment category among perpetrators, according to *Child Maltreatment 2003,* and more than half of all perpetrators (57%) had neglected children. Parents were the largest category of neglectful perpetrators (62%); however, parents and custodial caregivers were not the only individuals who may be neglectful of children.

In considering different categories of perpetrators, as can be seen from Table II, various types

TABLE II
PHYSICAL ABUSE, NEGLECT AND SEXUAL ABUSE OF CHILD VICTIMS OF MALTREATMENT, 2003
BY PERCENTAGE AMONG DIFFERENT CATEGORIES OF CHILD ABUSERS

	Parent	Other relative	Foster parent	Residential facility staff	Child day-care provider	Unmarried partner or parent	Friends or neighbors
Physical abuse only	11.0	10.4	16.9	19.0	12.9	16.6	3.4
Neglect only	62.0	37.5	50.0	46.3	48.4	37.9	9.7
Sexual abuse only	2.7	29.9	6.3	11.5	23.0	11.5	75.9
Psychological maltreatment only, other only, or unknown only	9.1	5.8	7.3	8.4	2.5	14.4	2.7
Multiple maltreatments	15.2	16.4	19.6	14.7	13.1	19.6	8.3
Total percent	100.0	100.0	100.0	100.0	100.0	100.0	100.0

Source: Adapted from Administration on Children, Youth and Families, *Child Maltreatment 2003*. Children's Bureau, U.S. Department of Health and Human Services, Washington, D.C., 2005, page 68.

of people may maltreat children (parents, other relatives, foster parents and so on). However, despite the disparity of maltreatment perpetrators, in almost every category, neglect is the most frequently occurring category of child maltreatment.

For example, among maltreating other relatives, 37.5% were neglectful. Among maltreating foster parents, 50% were neglectful. Among maltreating child day-care providers, 48.4% were neglectful. Among unmarried partners of the parent, 37.0% were neglectful. The same pattern of the dominance of neglect among all forms of maltreatment was found among most other categories, with the one exception of the category of friends and neighbors. Of people in this category who harmed children, they were most likely to be sex abusers (75.9%) rather than be guilty of other forms of maltreatment.

Neglect may cause long-lasting harm Some longitudinal research indicates that neglected children may suffer more lasting emotional damage than physically abused children. In addition, studies have revealed that neglected children, along with children who have been abandoned or are in failed placements, suffer from more health problems and worse health overall than children who were sexually or physically abused.

Neglect may also affect a child's cognitive development. Said Patricia Yashima in her chapter in *Child Victimization*, "Among school-age children, neglect is associated with decreases in children's cognitive functioning, as measured by IQ scores,

standard academic achievement tests, language ability, and school performance."

Purposeful v. nonpurposeful neglect Neglect may be willful, as when a parent refuses to send a child to school, refuses to take a very sick child to the doctor or refuses to buy the child winter clothes in a cold environment, despite having sufficient funds to do so. Neglect may also be unintended, as in the case of a caretaker who is suffering from a severe mental illness or a developmental delay and who is incapable of providing adequate care to a child.

Parents may lack education or knowledge about child care, as with younger teenage parents and, as a result, may neglect their children. Parents may also live in poverty and/or may have substance abuse problems. However, whether the neglect was intentional or not, the end result is the same: the child suffers from neglect. PROTECTIVE SERVICES workers who discover neglect will seek to help the parents rectify the problems that led to the neglect of their children.

In some cases, and especially if the parent or other caregiver acknowledges the problem, children who have been placed in foster care can return home. In other cases, the problems at home cannot be resolved, and children must be placed with other relatives or foster parents. If the parental problem cannot be resolved within about one to two years, the parent's parental rights may be involuntarily terminated, and the child may be then permanently placed with relatives or placed for adoption with relatives, foster parents or nonrelatives.

Mentally ill caregivers Various forms of mental illness or emotional disturbances can play a role in parental neglect. Actively psychotic parents are usually unable to care for children, and they may become neglectful or abusive.

Parents who are developmentally delayed may be very well intentioned but may be unable to provide for the needs of their children; however, they may be able to manage parenting with the assistance of others.

Norman Polansky, author of several studies on child neglect, described a condition known as APATHY-FUTILITY SYNDROME, similar to psychological depression, which may be observed in severely and chronically neglectful mothers. This syndrome is characterized by emotional numbness, limited intellectual ability and other factors that are often related to the mother's own deprivation during childhood.

Neglect caused by lack of knowledge Parents who neglect a child's needs because they lack an adequate knowledge of parenting often respond to teaching when it is given sensitively, although sometimes they refuse to comply with appropriate guidance for child care and safety. Ignorance of proper child care can often be corrected by arranging for instruction from a visiting nurse or PARENT AIDE.

In some cases, however, it is necessary to terminate the parents' parental rights, so that the child can have a chance at a normal life with another family member, foster parent or adoptive parent.

Living in poverty POVERTY may affect parents' ability to provide the physical necessities for their children. By itself, poverty does not provide a sufficient reason for labeling parents as neglectful. Studies show that the majority of children living in poor families are not neglected. Often conditions that are unhealthy for children can be corrected by the provision of adequate support for food, clothing and housing. The failure by a society to provide an adequate minimum level of support for all children is sometimes called SOCIAL ABUSE.

Substance abuse SUBSTANCE ABUSE is another major cause of child neglect, because addicts are often more centered on obtaining their next "fix"

TABLE III
REPORTERS OF CHILD NEGLECT BY
REPORT SOURCE, 2003

Report source	Number	Percent
PROFESSIONALS		
Educational personnel	45,487	10.8
Legal, law enforcement, criminal justice personnel	108,363	25.7
Social services personnel	56,282	13.4
Medical personnel	32,430	7.7
Mental health personnel	8,063	1.9
Child day-care providers	2,832	0.7
Foster-care providers	1,825	0.4
Total professionals	255,282	60.6
NONPROFESSIONALS		
Anonymous reporters	35,012	8.3
Other reporters	34,161	8.1
Other relatives	35,382	8.4
Parents	19,283	4.6
Friends or neighbors	22,321	5.3
Unknown reporters	17,769	4.2
Alleged victims	1,435	0.3
Alleged perpetrators	688	0.2
Total nonprofessionals	166,051	39.4
Total	421,333	
Total percent		100.0

Source: Adapted from Administration on Children, Youth and Families, *Child Maltreatment 2003*. Children's Bureau, U.S. Department of Health and Human Services, Washington, D.C., 2005, page 37.

than on feeding or clothing their children. Experts say that as many as 75 percent of children in foster care have been removed from their families because of problems with substance abuse, primarily alcohol and/or cocaine as well as other illegal drugs.

Reporters of neglect Most individuals who report neglectful behavior toward children to the authorities are individuals who are professionals (60.6%), and in 2003, individuals in the legal, law enforcement or criminal justice fields represented 25.7% of all reporters of maltreatment. As seen in Table III, among individuals who were nonprofessionals, the largest percentage of reporters of neglect were other relatives (8.4% of the total), anonymous reporters (8.3%) and other reporters (8.1%)

Signs of neglect in children According to the National Clearinghouse on Child Abuse and Neglect Information, there are signs that may signal the child is neglected, such as when the child

- Is frequently absent from school
- Begs or steals food or money
- Lacks needed medical or dental care, immunizations or glasses
- Is consistently dirty and has severe body odor
- Lacks sufficient clothing for the weather
- Abuses alcohol or other drugs
- States that there is no one at home to provide care

Adult caregivers who are neglectful may exhibit particular behaviors as well. Child neglect may be a problem when the parent or other adult caregivers

- Appears indifferent to the child
- Seems apathetic or depressed
- Behaves irrationally or in a bizarre manner
- Is abusing alcohol or other drugs

Investigation of child neglect Any INVESTIGATION of suspected neglect should take into account each child's unique situation. A thorough evaluation includes a medical examination; a review of medical records for evidence of immunization status, a discovery of the number of a child's accidental injuries and the frequency of medical checkups; a report from day care or school officials concerning attendance, academic performance, behavior and diet; and a family assessment that is conducted by a trained social worker, including home visits to assess the child's environment.

See also ABUSERS; ADULTS ABUSED AS CHILDREN; FOSTER CARE; INFANTICIDE.

Administration on Children, Youth and Families. *Child Maltreatment 2003.* Children's Bureau, U.S. Department of Health and Human Services, Washington, D.C., 2005.

Hashima, Patricia Y. "Prevention of Child Neglect—Toward a Community-Level Approach." In *Child Victimization.* Kingston, N.J.: Civic Research Institute, 2005, pp. 17-1–17-14.

National Clearinghouse on Child Abuse and Neglect Information. "Recognizing Child Abuse and Neglect: Signs and Symptoms," September 2003. Available online. URL: http://nccanch.acf.hhs.gov/pubs/factsheets/signs.pdf. Downloaded December 15, 2005.

Sirotnak, Andrew P., Joyce K. Moore, and Jean C. Smith. *Understanding the Medical Diagnosis of Child Maltreatment: A Guide for Nonmedical Professionals.* New York: Oxford University Press, 2006, pp. 169–170.

Straus, Murray A., and Glenda Kufman Kantor. "Definition and Measurement of Neglectful Behavior: Some Principles and Guidelines." *Child Abuse & Neglect* 29 (2005): 19–29.

neglect, community See COMMUNITY NEGLECT.

neglect, emotional See EMOTIONAL NEGLECT.

neglect, institutional See INSTITUTIONAL ABUSE AND NEGLECT.

neglect, medical See MEDICAL NEGLECT.

neglect, neurological manifestations See NEUROLOGIC MANIFESTATIONS OF ABUSE AND NEGLECT.

neglect, prediction of See PREDICTION OF ABUSE AND NEGLECT.

neglect, situational See SITUATIONAL ABUSE AND NEGLECT.

neglectful parents See ABUSERS.

neonaticide The killing of an infant immediately following birth is known as neonaticide. In some cultures neonaticide has been considered an acceptable form of limiting family size or eliminating malformed infants. Historically, some societies drew a sharp distinction between neonaticide and INFANTICIDE. These groups often developed rituals by which a child was accepted or rejected by the mother's husband. Until ritually accepted, an infant was not considered human and could therefore be murdered or abandoned with impunity.

Today neonaticide is relatively rare; however, reports of murdered or abandoned newborns are still heard from time to time in most countries.

neurologic manifestations of abuse and neglect

Over half of all abused or neglected children show signs of impaired cognitive, language, learning, motor or psychological development. Physical abuse of children is a significant cause of mental retardation and cerebral palsy. Studies have shown that even in the absence of retardation, abused children tend to score lower than non-abused children on intelligence tests.

Neurologic impairment may be caused by obvious damage to the central nervous system, such as microcephaly or spinal cord injury; however, neurologic injury is often the result of more subtle trauma. Nerve damage caused by shaking may not be readily apparent to an examining physician but may be reflected later in developmental delays.

Neglect also plays an important role in the production of neurological and developmental impairment. Poor nutrition and lack of social and sensory stimulation is associated with retarded intellectual, motor and emotional development. These forms of neglect are typical in battered children but are also found when no evidence of physical abuse is apparent. Infants who do not receive adequate TACTILE STIMULATION may exhibit signs of motor and intellectual impairment and later may have difficulty forming emotional attachments. Failure to provide adequate medical treatment for illness or injury may also cause neurological damage.

Because of the high rate of neurological problems associated with abuse and neglect, all child victims should be screened for neurodevelopmental deficits. A careful neurologic examination includes assessment of cranial nerve and cerebellar functioning, reflexes and local damage, as well as evaluation of gross and fine motor skills, sensory-motor abilities, activity level and attention span.

Developmental screening can involve compiling a careful history of the child's development from a caretaker, observation by a medical practitioner trained in the identification of neurologic impairment, use of developmental checklists, and formal developmental screening tests. Using screening tests, such as the Denver Developmental Screening Test (DDST), is the preferred method of assessment.

Neurologic impairment can be both the cause and the result of abuse. Developmentally delayed children require additional time and patience from parents. Frustrated parents especially those with unrealistically high expectations for their child's behavior, are more likely to abuse their children. Abuse increases the likelihood of neurological impairment which, in turn, increases the probability of abuse.

nutritional deficiency   See MARASMUS, NUTRITIONAL; RICKETS; SCURVY.

nutritional marasmus   See MARASMUS, NUTRITIONAL.

offender, fixated See FIXATED OFFENDER.

opinion evidence See EVIDENCE.

opu hule **(turned stomach)** Originating among Native Hawaiian islanders, this culturally based belief stipulates that tossing or jiggling a young child up and down will result in *opu hule,* or a "turned stomach." This term means that the stomach has been twisted or displaced. Children who suffer from symptoms of indigestion, fussiness or general discomfort are often thought to be suffering from *opu hule.* Tossing or bouncing a child is considered to be a form of child abuse and is frowned upon in the Native Hawaiian culture.

order of protection In the United States, the legal basis for court intervention in the family of an abused or neglected child is an order of protection. The order is typically issued by a juvenile court and places the child under the supervision of an authority, usually the designated child protection agency. Typically, children are allowed to remain at home while under an order of protection, provided the family meets specific conditions spelled out in the order. Failure to comply with these terms may result in the parents being held in contempt of court, fined and/or imprisoned. Violation of such orders is also likely to prompt the court to take custody of the child.

The National Center on Child Abuse and Neglect lists the following conditions that are usually included in an order of protection:

- Refrain from any conduct that is detrimental to the child.

- Refrain from any conduct that would make the home an improper place for the child.
- Give adequate attention to the care of the home.
- Comply with visitation terms if the child has been removed from the home.
- Comply with the treatment plan.

ossification Formation of new bone, known as ossification, is visible on X-rays and can be an important clue in the detection of child battering. A trained physician can determine if there is a history of multiple fractures by examining a series of X-rays for evidence of ossification, which indicates the healing of old fractures, as well as searching the X-rays for more recent trauma.

See also FRACTURES.

osteogenesis imperfecta Osteogenesis imperfecta is an inherited condition that causes bones to be very brittle and easily fractured. It is sometimes mistaken for BATTERED CHILD SYNDROME.

overlaying Overlaying refers to the suffocation of an infant by an adult lying on top of the baby. Prior to the 20th century many infants were thought to have died as a result of overlaying (also known as stifling). Deaths that are now attributed to SUDDEN INFANT DEATH SYNDROME were frequently thought to be the result of the mother intentionally or accidentally overlaying the infant during the night. Overlaying was considered a negligent act by a mother and was punished in the Roman Catholic and Anglican churches. Fear of accidental suffocation led to the custom of mothers and infants sleeping in separate beds, an uncommon practice in earlier times.

A special device was developed in 17th-century Europe to prevent accidental overlaying. This device, called an *arcuccio*, consisted of a metal and wood arch. The infant, protected underneath the *arcuccio*, could sleep in the same bed with the mother without the possibility of accidental suffocation. Some countries made failure to use the *arcuccio* a punishable offense. References to the use of the *arcuccio* can be found as late as 1890.

paddling One of many forms of CORPORAL PUNISH-MENT, paddling is a variation of CANING in which school officials (teachers or administrators) some-times strike students with the flat side of a wooden paddle to promote discipline. Although the practice is a time-honored one, it has numerous detractors and several international children's rights organiza-tions work to prohibit paddling and other forms of corporal punishment.

In the United States, the practice of paddling was challenged in a case brought before the United States Supreme Court by three junior high school students in Dade City Florida. The case, INGRAHAM V. WRIGHT, exposed the potential and real injuries accruing from the practice of paddling. Ultimately, the Supreme Court found that public schools had the constitu-tional right to exercise paddling or any other form of "reasonable" corporal punishment. To date, there are only nine states in the United States in which paddling or any other means of corporal punishment is prohibited. In many other countries of the world, corporal punishment in any form is illegal.

pancreatitis This term refers to damage to the pancreatic ducts, usually caused by abdominal trauma. Laceration of the pancreas causes the enzymes amylase and lipase to be released into the peritoneal cavity causing a large buildup of fluid and inflammation of the peritoneum (the mem-brane enclosing the abdominal cavity).

Occasionally pancreatitis is contained within a smaller area, causing an abscess or a fibrous cap-sule called a pseudocyst to develop. These develop-ments result in the appearance of a painful lump in the upper abdomen two to three weeks after the injury. Surgical intervention is required to correct such lesions.

Pancreatitis is rare in childhood. When it is present, child abuse is strongly suspected. A radio-graphic study of long bones to detect other evi-dence of battering can be helpful in confirming this suspicion.

parens patriae This legal doctrine provides the foundation for a court's entry into the realm of the family. When parents are determined to be unable or unfit to provide adequate and proper care for a child, the court can step in to safeguard the BEST INTERESTS OF THE CHILD. Parens patriae literally means "guardian of the community" and rests on the principle that the state is the ultimate and absolute protector of all citizens, especially children.

This doctrine was first established in the United States in 1838 in the case of Mary Ann Crouse. At that time, the court ruled that a child's parents, "when unequal to the task of education or unwor-thy of it, be supplanted by the parens patriae." The ruling was widely upheld in the courts throughout the 1800s. By the early 20th century, it had become the legal basis on which the juvenile court was established. Its acceptance as a fundamental pre-rogative of a court means that in cases of suspected child abuse or neglect, the court is the best judge of a child's home environment and that environ-ment's effect on a child's welfare.

In 1968, passage of the UNIFORM CHILD CUSTODY JURISDICTION ACT limited use of parents patriae in cases of CHILD STEALING. The exception occurs in cases where a child requires emergency protec-tion. Under the UCCJA, an emergency condition can result in the court's instituting immediate mea-sures to protect the child. In custody dispute cases that involved child stealing, the doctrine of parens patriae was found to contribute directly to multiple child custody adjudications.

See also EX PARTE *CROUSE*.

parent aides   Many child abuse treatment programs provide special assistance to families in the form of paraprofessionals who serve as role models to parents. These parent aides may be paid or may volunteer their time. Aides perform many different services, such as modeling appropriate parenting techniques, helping to identify problems, teaching specific skills, serving as advocates and giving emotional support and nurturance. Most of all, parent aides serve as friends of the family.

Parent aides are sometimes described as surrogate parents. They provide emotional support for both parents and children. Some experts believe it is necessary for parents to go through a REPARENTING process in which they experience the warmth, acceptance and positive learning they did not receive from their parents. Parent aides are usually older adults or couples who, in addition to having been parents themselves, have had special training in working with abusive or neglectful parents.

This type of family support works best in combination with a comprehensive treatment program. Parent aides are often members of a MULTIDISCIPLINARY TEAM. Some hospitals in the United States use parent aides to perform a role similar to that of the HEALTH VISITOR in Britain. Aides are assigned to parents within a few days of the child's birth and continue assisting the parents as long as necessary, usually six to 18 months.

parental substance abuse   Some children are abused or neglected as a result of the drug and/or alcohol abuse of their parents or other caregivers. According to the National Survey on Child Drug Use and Health, about 5 million parents in the United States who abused alcohol had at least one child younger than age 18 living in the household in 2002. Alcohol abuse alone is associated with violence toward children and is estimated to be a factor in about 30% of all child abuse cases, according to the National Institute on Alcohol Abuse and Alcoholism (NIAAA). An estimated one-third to two-thirds of all child maltreatment cases involve some form of substance abuse. As a result, children of substance-abusing parents are more likely to enter the foster-care system, and they are also more likely to stay in the system longer than children whose parents do not abuse alcohol and/or drugs.

Some drugs make it difficult or impossible for parents to manage an appropriate caregiving role, either because the drugs are heavily sedating (such as with marijuana, barbiturates and many narcotic painkillers) or are very stimulating (such as methamphetamine and cocaine).

For example, methamphetamine, which is an increasingly popular drug of abuse in the United States, stimulates the central nervous system and can induce many psychological effects, such as anger, panic and irritability, as well as psychotic features, such as paranoia and hallucinations. As a result, users may become violently aggressive to those around them. The drug can also cause heart failure, stroke, seizures and other severe health problems.

It is also true that methamphetamine laboratories, where the drug is clandestinely manufactured, are very dangerous because of the highly flammable materials that are needed to produce the drug. Clearly, a child is not safe in such an environment, and some states have passed laws making it illegal for a child to be in an environment where methamphetamine and/or other illegal drugs are produced.

States that consider it abuse or neglect to manufacture a controlled substance in the presence of a child or on the premises occupied by a child include Colorado, Indiana, Iowa, Montana, South Dakota, Tennessee and Virginia. States that consider it abuse or neglect if the chemicals or equipment used to manufacture controlled substances are used or stored where children are present include Arizona and New Mexico.

According to a report on methamphetamine abuse from the National Association of Counties, reported in 2005, the results of 500 counties in 45 states revealed that, "In an alarming number of meth arrests, there is a child living in the home. These children many times suffer from neglect and abuse." According to the research, 71% of the responding counties in California and 70% in Colorado reported an increase in children being placed out of their home because of methamphetamine abuse. In addition, when asked if the particular nature of the parent who was a methamphetamine user increased the difficulty of reuniting the children with their parents, the majority (59%) of the respondents said that it did.

Cocaine is another drug of abuse that stimulates the central nervous system. Cocaine is associated with depression, anxiety, panic attacks, violent rage and paranoid behavior. It is also associated with an increased risk for domestic violence. Cocaine use may increase the risk for suicidal behavior among users. It can also induce a psychotic break with symptoms that are difficult to distinguish from the symptoms found in a person with schizophrenia, such as hallucinations and paranoid behavior. In some cases, the individual will suffer a psychotic break from which he or she will not recover.

Clearly, such symptoms and behaviors are not conducive to even marginally effective parenting, and consequently, children who are living with a person dependent on cocaine are at risk for abuse and/or neglect.

State Laws

In 12 states and the District of Columbia, if there is evidence of drugs, alcohol or other controlled substances that are identified in newborn infants, this exposure is included under the state definition of child abuse or neglect. These states include Florida, Illinois, Indiana, Iowa, Massachusetts, Minnesota, North Dakota, South Carolina, South Dakota, Texas, Virginia and Wisconsin. In addition, 12 states have specific reporting procedures for infants who were born exposed to drugs or alcohol, including Arizona, California, Illinois, Iowa, Kentucky, Maryland, Massachusetts, Michigan, Minnesota, Missouri, Oklahoma and Utah.

Predicting the Recurrence of Child Abuse in Cases Involving Substance Abuse

Two researchers sought to identify the key factors that predicted maltreatment recurrence, reporting their findings in *Children and Youth Services Review* in 2003.

The researchers collected data from 95 investigations in Illinois that involved alcohol or other drugs as part of the maltreatment allegation. Most

subjects were African-American (60%), and the other subjects were about evenly split between Caucasians and Latinos. Most families (68%) were headed by a single parent. The most common form of maltreatment was neglect (38%), followed by exposing an infant to a substance (37%). Physical abuse (7%) and sexual abuse (2%) were much less frequently found.

The researchers found that there were several significant factors that were related to the recurrence of abuse or neglect; for example, among families in which protective service workers initially found the presence of parental substance use, these parents were 13 times more likely to maltreat their children again. Twenty-six percent of the parents with an alcohol or drug problem had another maltreatment report filed on them within 60 days of the first report.

Another highly predictive factor for repeated child abuse was whether criminal activity was present. If the protective worker noted a "high risk" for criminal activity in the initial report, the children in these cases were found to be 770 times more likely to be abused and/or neglected again than among the cases that were noted by the worker as having no risk for criminal activity. Since many illegal drug users engage in criminal activity to obtain illicit substances, this is yet another factor that increases the risk of child abuse to children of parents who abuse illegal drugs.

The Psychiatric Impact of Parental Substance Abuse

In addition to the greater risk of child abuse and neglect among children living with substance-abusing parents, some studies have shown that such children also have a significantly greater risk for the development of psychiatric disorders. In their study on psychiatric disorders among children living with drug-abusing, alcohol-abusing and non–substance abusing fathers, reported in a 2004 issue of the *Journal of the American Academy of Child & Adolescent Psychiatry*, researchers Michelle L. Kelley and William Fals-Stewart found that children with substance-abusing fathers had a significantly higher risk for psychiatric disorders.

The researchers studied 120 two-parent couples with biological children, including 40 families that included fathers who met the American Psychiatric Association's criteria for having a cocaine or opiate use disorder; 40 fathers who met the criteria for alcohol dependence (alcoholism) but who did not have a drug abuse or drug dependence problem; and 40 fathers who had neither an alcohol nor a drug dependency. Twenty-five of the 40 fathers in the drug-abusing group (62.5%) had criminal or legal problems, compared to 22 of the fathers in the alcoholism group (55%) and two (5%) of the fathers in the non–substance abusing group.

The researchers also found that more than half the children (53%) of the drug-using fathers had a psychiatric diagnosis, compared to 25% of the alcoholic fathers and 10% of the non–substance abusing fathers. In considering depression alone, 38% of the children of the drug-using fathers were depressed, compared to 13 percent of the children of alcoholic fathers and 3% of the children whose fathers were not substance-dependent.

It should be pointed out that another possibly significant factor may be the presence of a psychiatric disorder among the alcohol- or drug-dependent parents. It may be possible that substance-abusing parents are themselves more likely to have psychiatric disorders than those who are not substance abusers, which may then indicate the presence of a genetic link that may be passed on to their offspring. Experts who study social problems and consider either genetic predispositions or environmental factors in causing psychiatric disorders continually study this issue and debate it among themselves. However, whatever the cause, substance-abusing parents are more likely to have children with emotional disorders, and this issue should be further studied.

See also FAMILY VIOLENCE; PROTECTIVE SERVICES.

Fuller, Tamara L., and Susan J. Wells. "Predicting Maltreatment Recurrence among CPS Cases with Alcohol and Other Drug Involvement." *Children and Youth Services Review* 25, no. 7 (2003): 553–569.

Gwinnell, Esther, M.D., and Christine Adamec. *The Encyclopedia of Addictions and Addictive Behaviors.* New York: Facts On File, 2005.

Kelley, Michelle L., and William Fals-Stewart. "Psychiatric Disorders of Children Living with Drug-Abusing, Alcohol-Abusing, and Non-Substance-Abusing Fathers."

Journal of the American Academy of Child & Adolescent Psychiatry 43, no. 5 (May 2004): 621–628.

Kyle, Angelo D., and Bill Hansell. *The Meth Epidemic in America: Two Surveys of U.S. Counties: The Criminal Effect of Meth on Communities, The Impact of Meth on Children.* Executive Summary, National Association of Counties, July 5, 2005.

Office of Applied Studies. "Alcohol Dependence or Abuse among Parents with Children Living in the Home." *NSDUH Report,* Substance Abuse and Mental Health Services Administration, February 12, 2004.

Parental Kidnapping Prevention Act of 1980   In order to address more effectively issues related to child stealing in custody disputes, this federal law requires that each state honor other states' custody determinations.

parent education   Special programs designed to teach parenting skills are used to treat and prevent child abuse and neglect. Specific parenting skills taught in these programs vary. Many courses for young or neglectful parents focus on basic skills such as proper hygiene and feeding. Abusive parents often expect children to perform beyond their developmental capabilities. Learning about normal developmental patterns helps create more realistic expectations and may help reduce frustration. Programs for parents of older children often focus on improving communication skills. Parent Effectiveness Training, developed by Thomas Gordon, Ph.D., is an example of such a program.

During the past decade, many public schools have begun to offer family life education classes as part of the regular school curriculum. These programs are designed to help adolescents make informed choices about marriage and child rearing.

Many child protection experts believe parent education programs are ineffective for unmotivated parents. Further, some abusive parents have sufficient knowledge but need assistance of other kinds. However, when used as part of a comprehensive treatment and prevention effort, parent education is an important resource for many families.

Gordon, Thomas. *Parent Effectiveness Training: The Proven Program for Raising Responsible Children.* New York: Three Rivers Press, 2000.

parenthood, psychological   See PSYCHOLOGICAL PARENTHOOD.

parentified child   Children inappropriately placed in the role of parent are said to be parentified. A parentified child may be expected to behave as an adult or be given primary responsibility for care of younger siblings. In some cases children are expected to take care of a parent's emotional or physical needs. Forcing children into adult roles too soon may lead to impaired emotional development sometimes referred to as the loss of childhood.

See also PSEUDOMATURITY; ROLE REVERSAL

parent-infant traumatic syndrome (PITS)   The combination of subdural hematomas and specific types of bone lesions was labeled the parent-infant traumatic syndrome by radiologist John Caffey in 1946. By using improved X-ray techniques, Caffey and his associates were able to detect a pattern of trauma that they believed to be of suspicious origin.

Specifically, the PITS, also called the battered baby syndrome, involves multiple fractures and other lesions of bone and cartilage in various states of healing. Bone damage typically occurs at joints and often appears to be the result of twisting or vigorous shaking. The combination of bone lesions and head trauma suggests a specific type of injury that is unlikely to be accidental.

The ability to detect unusual patterns of bone injury was an important advance in the recognition and treatment of physical child abuse. Physicians who suspected nonaccidental injury could examine full skeletal X-rays for additional evidence of abuse. Radiologic evidence is still an important tool in the diagnosis of battered children and is often presented in court as physical evidence of abuse.

See also BATTERED CHILD SYNDROME; RADIOLOGY; PEDIATRIC.

parents' rights   Legal rights of parents often come into conflict with those of children and the state during the course of INVESTIGATION or treatment of child abuse or neglect. Parents have the right to custody and supervision of children and to make decisions on behalf of a child under the legally established age of majority.

In the United States, the balance between the rights of parents and those of the state has been defined in several court cases. *PRINCE V. MASSACHUSETTS* limited a parent's discretion in requiring or allowing a child to work. *Wisconsin v. Yoder* confirmed the right of Amish parents to educate children at home rather than send them to secondary school. Other decisions have allowed parents to withhold permission for nonessential medical treatment for religious reasons, established parents' right to use reasonable physical force in disciplining children and have denied parents the right to prevent school officials from using CORPORAL PUNISHMENT on their child.

Parents' rights are frequently at issue when a government agency seeks to remove a child from parental custody. Most states require an agency to provide clear and convincing evidence that a child is at risk before parental custody can be terminated. Concern over the legal rights of parents has led many child protection agencies to seek alternatives to removal of children from parental custody.

In the United States a group of parents and professionals calling themselves Victims of Child Abuse Laws (VOCAL) has formed to promote parents' rights and to combat what they believe are overzealous attempts to protect children.

While some countries do not operate according to a concept of individual rights, most have laws pertaining to a parent's role. In SWEDEN, for example, parents are not allowed to use physical force in disciplining their children.

See also TERMINATION OF PARENTAL RIGHTS.

parents' rights, termination of   See TERMINATION OF PARENTAL RIGHTS.

parricide, reactive   A rare and extreme reaction to child abuse is murder of the abusive parent by the victim. Parricide accounts for approximately 1% of all murders.

Most children maintain a strong, albeit conflicted, attachment to the parent even in the face of repeated abuse. Profiles of children who murder an abusive parent or parents generally show that these children have no significant history of violent behavior. In most cases, there is a long history of abuse. Murders usually occur shortly after, or during, an abusive episode. Handguns or rifles are the most frequent murder weapons in such cases.

Little is known about the reasons for reactive parricide. Theorists disagree as to the motivation of children who kill their parents. Some attribute the phenomenon to a preference for violent behavior learned from the parents themselves. Others believe these murders to be the desperate reaction of extreme rage committed by a child who feels powerless.

passive abuser Child abuse can include other perpetrators, in addition to the person who actually beats or otherwise abuses the victim. It also includes the parent or caretaker who stands by and fails to take action to protect the child from abuse. Termed a *passive abuser*, this person is also responsible for the abuse and may face legal charges.

patria potestas According to the terms of this early Roman law, a father had full and absolute power over his children. Historically, this legal power originally included INFANTICIDE, but that was gradually eliminated from the law.

patricide The murder of one's father is termed *patricide*. In 1985, 209 fathers in the United States were murdered by one of their children. Patricide accounted for about three-fourths of 1% of all homicides. Case studies suggest a strong connection between child abuse and patricide.

Fathers who are murdered by a son tend to be cruel, dominant, critical and competitive with them. Mothers are often passive, sometimes dependent, sometimes overprotective of the son. Fathers frequently display jealousy of the son's attachment to the mother. In many cases, the father is physically abusive to the mother in the presence of the son. The son, unable to gain the father's approval, becomes the mother's protector. Patricide usually occurs during or shortly following an episode in which the father abused a family member. Murder of a parent by a daughter is rare.

pederasty Anal intercourse between an adult male and a boy (usually between the ages of 12 and 16 years) is known as pederasty. Men who engage in this practice are known as pederasts. Though others may label the pederast as homosexual this may be a misnomer. Many pederasts also have sexual relations with women and are often repelled by the thought of intercourse with other adult males. Likewise it is improper to assume that homosexuals are pederasts. Most homosexuals are not pederasts and strongly disavow the practice.

The term *pederasty* is derived from the Greek roots *ped*, meaning boy, and *erastes*, meaning lover. Originally, the word had much the same meaning as pedophile, and the two words are sometimes used interchangeably.

See also PEDOPHILIA.

pediatricians Medical doctors who specialize in the diagnosis and treatment of children and adolescents. Because pediatricians have numerous medical encounters with children, they are also likely to see possible instances of abuse and/or neglect, and state laws require them to report suspected abuse. (See MANDATED REPORTERS.) A pediatrician can be a child's lifeline away from abuse and neglect. However, in one study, reported by Gunn and her colleagues, more than a quarter of the physicians surveyed (28%) said that they had suspected child abuse in some cases but had failed to report it to the authorities.

In this study, 195 pediatricians completed a survey regarding the reporting of suspected abuse to the authorities. The researchers found that male physicians were significantly less likely to report suspected abuse than female doctors. In addition, physicians who had been threatened with a lawsuit for reporting suspected cases of child abuse in the past were less likely to report abuse (48% of this group failed to report suspected abuse), even though these physicians (all from one unidentified southeastern state) had been granted absolute immunity from prosecution. Another key factor that the researchers found was that the physicians who had been previously deposed or who had testified in court in a maltreatment case were less likely to report later suspected cases of abuse.

Said the researchers, "The most commonly expressed reasons for not reporting included concerns about consequences of reporting for the provider, the child, or for the family." They further stated that, "Throughout the qualitative portion of the survey, fear was a recurrent theme: fear of lawsuit, fear of physical harm from families, and fear of the apparent impact of reporting on children and families." In addition, the comments from the pediatricians revealed that they were unclear on the level of certainty of abuse that was needed before they should make a report to protective services officials. The researchers recommended further education and training of pediatricians with regard to child abuse laws and the reporting process.

See also ASSESSMENT; CENTRAL REPORTING AGENCY.

Gunn, Veronica L., M.D., Gerald B. Hickson, M.D., and William O. Cooper, M.D. "Factors Affecting Pediatricians' Reporting of Suspected Child Maltreatment." *Ambulatory Pediatrics* 5, no. 2 (March–April 2005): 96–101.

pedophilia   Pedophilia refers to a psychiatric disorder causing a sexual preference for and attraction to children. Specifically, the pedophile is an adult who is sexually attracted to children who have not yet reached the age of puberty. However, the term *pedophile* is often used to refer to any adult who is sexually attracted to males or females below the legal age of consent. (See STATUTORY RAPE.) Most pedophiles are not violent toward children, instead leading and enticing children to willingly perform sexual acts, although some are violent to the point of rape and murder.

Experts believe that most pedophiles are males. Some female adults (and male adults) are sexually attracted to boys or girls, but these children are usually at or beyond the age of puberty. Sometimes, however, females sexually abuse children

in concert with males, or they will knowingly allow males to abuse their own children or other children. (See SEXUAL ABUSE.) This is more likely to occur if the women are abusing drugs and/or alcohol.

Pedophiles may believe that their behavior is normal and that it helps teach children how to become loving and affectionate. Such individuals avoid such words as *pedophilia,* preferring to use such terms as *adult-child sex.* They believe that others who do not understand their behavior are unreasonably rigid. Some organizations of pedophiles claim large memberships and actively support the practice of pedophilia.

Pedophiles may fail to consider the short- or long-term consequences of their actions; for example, in one case, a pedophile was told by a child whom he had met on the Internet that her mother was a police officer (which was a true statement), yet he molested the girl anyway.

Much Is Unknown about Pedophiles

In her article on the roots of pedophilia, published in the *Journal of the American Medical Association* in 2005, Lynne Lamberg pointed out that much is yet unknown about pedophiles. Most studies of pedophiles are performed on people in jail or prison, and it is also true that many acts of sexual abuse are never reported.

Lamberg stated that in one study of pedophiles at Beth Israel Hospital, some individuals reported just one sexual act with a child, while others said they had committed thousands of such acts. About 60% of the subjects said they were themselves sexually abused as children. In addition, the study revealed that pedophiles have a greater likelihood than others of justifying their actions with cognitive distortions. Pedophiles may convince themselves that they have done nothing wrong.

Pedophiles may go to great lengths to gain the child's confidence before attempting a sexual act. However, in some cases a pedophile's desires are confined to fantasy only, and they are not manifested in any sexual acts with children. According to Cynthia Crosson-Tower in her book, *Understanding Child Abuse and Neglect,* fantasy is very important to the pedophile. Said Crosson-Tower, "He may fantasize sexual and emotional involvement with children and often act out his fantasies. Interestingly, the perpetrator projects his feelings of powerlessness and often perceives that it is the child who initiates the relationship."

Parents May Not Realize a Person Is a Pedophile

The pedophile is often a person who is known to the child's parent(s) and is one who seeks to gain their trust as well as the child's trust. Of course the parents are completely unaware of the pedophile's intentions, in part because he or she hides the motives extremely well and also because pedophilia is beyond the imagining of most parents. The parents may also believe erroneously that they could detect a person who is a pedophile, because they imagine that such an individual would look or act like a bad person. They do not realize that evil intentions can be masked in a normal-looking and normal-acting person.

When their child is molested and sometimes murdered, these parents often blame themselves for failing to know that the person they trusted was a pedophile, and they greatly suffer as a result. However, pedophiles may be very clever, and in most cases, others would not have known that the individual was a pedophile unless he or she was previously convicted and they were aware of the conviction. Yet since the parents trust the individual, it does not occur to them to check out whether the individual has a criminal record—nor would it have occurred to others.

In one case, prior to the passage of laws on the registration of sex offenders, a pedophile thoroughly incorporated himself into a family by befriending the son. The son and the pedophile shared an active interest in sports, and the pedophile took the child to games and advised him on how to play better. When the trust of the child and the family was clearly obtained, the pedophile told the child's elementary school that he was supposed to pick up the child from school. The school allowed the child to leave with this individual, who subsequently raped and murdered the child.

Note that even with legal requirements of sex offenders to register with authorities, some offenders may move to another location or state, where they fail to register as a sex offender. As a result, children in the new community are at risk.

How Pedophiles Meet Children

Pedophiles frequently develop a great deal of skill in meeting children and developing their trust. Formal and informal networks of child molesters are often used to share information on individual children or Internet sites.

Some pedophiles choose a job such as teaching or managing a video arcade that will bring them into contact with children. Others may volunteer to coach a children's team, serve as a scout leader or a babysitter or work in a similar capacity. Some pedophiles prey on children who use the INTERNET.

Child Pornography and Child Prostitution

CHILD PORNOGRAPHY and CHILD PROSTITUTION also play an important role in pedophilia. Pedophiles are the primary purchasers of child pornography. They are also frequently the suppliers of such material, often exchanging or selling material among themselves. In the past, such material was sent through the mail (which is illegal). Although it is also illegal to purvey child pornography on the Internet, it is far more difficult to monitor such activities.

Children are in great demand as prostitutes among pedophiles, who may travel to other countries primarily so that they may molest children.

See SEXUAL TRAFFICKING.

Types of Pedophiles

According to Crosson-Tower, there are several different types of pedophiles. Fixated pedophiles regard themselves as children. Said Crosson-Tower, "As children, these perpetrators' needs were unmet, and having lost faith in adults they now look to children to meet their dependency and nurturing needs. They may find themselves at ease with children and become 'sexually addicted' to them."

Another type of pedophile is the regressed pedophile, who has no sexual interest in children unless adult relationships fail. Said Crosson-Tower, "He is often married, and, in fact, may prefer an adult partner if she validates his need to feel adequate. When relationships with peers are too conflictual, he chooses children. Frequently the onset of his molestation behavior can be traced to a crisis in his life. His relationship with a child becomes an impulsive act that underlies his desperate need to cope."

Tactics of Pedophiles

Pedophiles may entice children with gifts and affection or seek to convince the child of his or her importance to the pedophile. They may also use entrapment, to make the child feel obligated to the pedophile.

Said Fagan et al, in their article on pedophilia in a 2002 issue of the *Journal of the American Medical Association*, in describing information obtained from a study of child sex offenders, "the initial social contact with the child involved some nonsexual enticements such as purchases or flattery. Sexual conversation generally followed. A gradual progression from nonsexual touch to sexual touch happened with the purposeful desensitization of the child to the purpose of the touch."

Most pedophiles do not use physical force but rather rely upon psychological manipulation. When pedophiles do use physical force, it is used so that they may complete a sexual act. However, some pedophiles prefer physical force, and they are primarily those who are angry and who seek power.

Said Crosson-Tower, "The power rapist sees the child as weak, vulnerable, and unable to resist . . . Some rapists who have unsuccessfully tried to take their aggression out on adults may make children their targets."

Treatment of Pedophilia

Pedophilia is difficult to treat and dropouts and non-compliance to treatment are common, according to Cohen and Galynker in their 2002 article for *Journal of Psychiatric Practice*. Treatment involves individual therapy, group therapy and, among males, the use of androgen-suppressing hormones. In extreme cases, male pedophiles may opt for CASTRATION. Therapy may help with the cognitive distortions that pedophiles often use, such as the excuse that the child wanted sex or even that it was the child's fault because he or she had enticed the pedophile.

According to Fagan et al., "On average, 10% to 17% of offenders commit another offense after 4 to 5 years when untreated." As a result, treatment is extremely important. It is not always effective, but ignoring the problem will not prevent it in the future.

Formerly Imprisoned Pedophiles

In the case of pedophiles who are on parole from prison, electronic surveillance and polygraphs (lie detectors) may be helpful in preventing further crimes.

Pedophiles who have been convicted of sexual acts against a child must register as sex offenders, which also involves complying with many rules; for example, they must notify law enforcement officials or other specific authorities of where they are living. If they move, sex offenders must notify the authorities in the new area that they are registered sex offenders. In addition, they may not take a job where there are children, such as driving a school bus or serving food at a school cafeteria. Law enforcement officials often notify the families of children living nearby that there is a registered sex offender among them.

States may also restrict convicted sex offenders on where they may live; for example, they may be restricted from living near schools, parks or other places where children congregate.

In extreme cases, sex offenders may be compelled into a civil commitment, wherein they must live in a prison or other institution because they are considered to be at very high risk of committing more sex offenses if they reside in the community, beyond the controlled environment of an institution. Some sex offenders have challenged this compulsion to be civilly committed after they have already served their prison sentences, but to date, they have lost all court challenges.

See also ADULTS ABUSED AS CHILDREN; CHILD MOLESTER; CIVIL COMMITMENT LAWS; SEX OFFENDERS, CONVICTED.

Cohen, L. J., and I. Galynker. "Clinical Features of Pedophilia, and Implications for Treatment." *Journal of Psychiatric Practice* 8, no. 5 (September 2002): 276–289.

Crosson-Tower, Cynthia. *Understanding Child Abuse and Neglect.* Boston: Allyn & Bacon, 2005.

Fagan, Peter J., et al. "Pedophilia." *Journal of the American Medical Association* 288, no. 19 (November 20, 2002): 2,458–2,465.

Lamberg, Lynne. "Researchers Seek Roots of Pedophilia." *Journal of the American Medical Association* 294, no. 5 (August 3, 2005): 546–547.

People's Republic of China   See CHINA, PEOPLE'S REPUBLIC OF.

periostitis   Inflammation of the periosteum (the fibrous membrane covering bones) is periostitis. Presence of periostitis in a child is evidence of physical trauma. Twisting of a limb or a blow directly to the bone can tear the periosteum away from the bone, causing blood to collect in the newly created cavity. Periostitis is not immediately detectable on an X-ray but begins to appear as new bone forms in the affected area.

See also BATTERED CHILD SYNDROME; RADIOLOGY, PEDIATRIC.

perjury   False testimony under oath, given with the knowledge that it is untrue, constitutes the crime of perjury. In child abuse trials, perjury is most often a concern with the testimony given by adults. Groups representing divorced parents express concern that false accusations of SEXUAL ABUSE are increasingly used as a tactic in bitter custody disputes. Proving sexual abuse of young children often depends on the testimony of adults close to the alleged victim. Even when no corroborating evidence is found, it is often difficult to prove that a witness intended to deceive the court.

Young children may become confused and may be more susceptible to coercion than adult witnesses. However, many experts believe that perjury is rarely an issue when children testify concerning their own abuse. Controversy over the reliability of young children's testimony continues to build as more and more courts allow children to testify.

See also TESTIMONY.

petechiae   Very small bruises, caused by broken capillaries, are called petechiae.

See also BRUISES.

petition   A petition filed in juvenile or family court serves a purpose similar to that of an INDICTMENT in a criminal court. Sometimes referred to as a COMPLAINT, the petition spells out specific conditions that give rise to charges of abuse or neglect as well as the time, date and place where each event was observed. Filing a written petition is the first step in initiating court action. The petition serves as a formal notice of charges to the alleged abuser.

In most jurisdictions, the petitioner is the child protection worker; however, law enforcement officers and physicians may file a petition. A few states allow anyone to file child abuse or neglect petition.

Child protection workers usually do not file a petition until after an initial INVESTIGATION has been conducted and the report is considered to be founded. FOUNDED REPORTS do not necessarily result in a petition. If the child protection worker believes parents will comply voluntarily with recommendations, or that the conditions that precipitated maltreatment no longer exist, it is unlikely that a petition will be filed. Civil court intervention is usually initiated for the purpose of ensuring compliance with recommendations and/or removing a child from home.

Before filing a petition the child protection agency, usually in consultation with an attorney, may attempt to determine whether: (1) there is sufficient admissible evidence to obtain a favorable judgment; (2) whether the complainants, witnesses and victim are available for trial; (3) whether the witnesses are credible; and (4) whether there is physical evidence to support the charges. Child protection workers must also consider the probable effects of a trial on the victim and his or her family.

physical abuse   An act of commission by a parent or other person that may or may not be accidental and that results in physical injury. Injuries caused by physical abuse can result from punching, biting, shaking, throwing, stabbing, choking or kicking a child. Injuries include fractures, BURNS, severe bruises, welts, cuts and/or internal injuries. In the most severe cases, the injuries result in death. Internal traumas such as SUBDURAL HEMATOMA or ABDOMINAL INJURIES, though serious, are not immediately apparent. Physical abuse is often accompanied by

PSYCHOLOGICAL/EMOTIONAL MALTREATMENT, such as extremely negative and/or threatening verbal comments made to the child.

Child abuse reporting laws now require a wide range of professionals to report all forms of suspected abuse. In at least one case, *Landeros v. Flood*, physicians were held liable for civil penalties for failure to report abuse. Still, cases of physical abuse are sometimes overlooked.

Injuries that are incurred by CORPORAL PUNISHMENT (such as spanking) rarely constitute physical abuse under state laws, unless the child's injuries are severe. Corporal punishment is lawful in all states in the United States.

States vary in their definitions of child abuse and also in whether abuse is covered in a separate child-abuse statute. In many states, the degree of harm that is inflicted is a major factor in ascertaining the level of abuse. In addition, in some states, even if a parent does *not* abuse a child, if the child is abused by another person, the law addresses the failure of the parent to protect the child from a known abuser. Sometimes the age of the child is also a factor in determining the category and severity of crime with which the perpetrator is charged.

Demographics of Physical Abuse

In the United States, according to *Child Maltreatment 2003*, published by the Administration on Children, Youth and Families Children's Bureau in 2005, most maltreated children are neglected (61%) rather than physically abused (19%). In considering the entire child population in the United States in 2003, 2.3% suffered from physical abuse, compared to 7.5% who were neglected.

According to *Child Maltreatment 2003*, most reports of suspected physical abuse in 2003 (69.9%) were received from professionals, with the greatest percentage of reports coming from educational personnel (21.8%) or law enforcement/criminal justice professionals (21.5%).

In considering race or ethnicity only, according to *Child Maltreatment 2003*, the greatest percentage of children who were physically abused were Asian (16.6%), followed by African-American children (15.3%) and those whose race was unknown (14.3%). (See Table I.) However, among child fatalities caused by abuse, 43% of the perpetrators were white, followed by 31% who were African-American.

Perpetrators of Physical Abuse

In considering the perpetrators of physical abuse in 2003, 11% of 550,015 of all parental abusers physically abused their children. (Note that only abusive parents are considered among this percentage.) This contrasts with the 62% in this category who neglected their children and 15.2% who committed multiple maltreatments.

In contrast to the parent, the unmarried partner of the parent was more likely to commit physical abuse. Of the 27,888 unmarried partners of the parent, 16.6% committed physical abuse, while 37.9% of those in this category were neglectful.

When considering other types of abusers, residential facility staff are more likely than parents to use physical abuse. Of the 1,225 residential staff who maltreated children, 19.0% physically abused them. (See Table II.) As can also be seen from the table, among the 3,107 foster parents who maltreated children, 16.9% physically abused them. Friends or neighbors committed the least percentage of physical abuse (3.4%). In contrast, of all the 1,571 friends or neighbors who abused children in

TABLE I
VICTIMS OF PHYSICAL ABUSE BY RACE, NUMBERS AND PERCENTAGES, 2003

Race	Number of all abuse victims	Number of physical abuse–only victims	Percentage of physical abuse–only victims
African-American	159,361	24,354	15.3
American Indian or Alaska Native	7,469	728	9.7
Asian	3,933	653	16.6
Pacific Islander	1,390	119	8.6
White	334,965	40,956	12.2
Multiple race	10,133	1,124	11.1
Hispanic	78,207	10,383	13.3
Unknown or missing	34,224	4,898	14.3

Source: Adapted from Administration on Children, Youth and Families, *Child Maltreatment 2003*. Children's Bureau, U.S. Department of Health and Human Services, Washington, D.C., 2005, page 48.

TABLE II
PHYSICAL ABUSE, NEGLECT AND SEXUAL ABUSE OF CHILD VICTIMS OF MALTREATMENT, 2003,
BY PERCENTAGE AMONG DIFFERENT CATEGORIES OF CHILD ABUSERS

	Parent	Other relative	Foster parent	Residential facility staff	Child day-care provider	Unmarried partner of parent	Friend or neighbor
Physical abuse only	11.0	10.4	16.9	19.0	12.9	16.6	3.4
Neglect only	62.0	37.5	50.0	46.3	48.4	37.9	9.7
Sexual abuse only	2.7	29.9	6.3	11.5	23.0	11.5	75.9
Psychological maltreament only, other only, or unknown only	9.1	5.8	7.3	8.4	2.5	14.4	2.7
Multiple maltreatments	15.2	16.4	19.6	14.7	13.1	19.6	8.3
Total percent	100.0	100.0	100.0	100.0	100.0	100.0	100.0

Source: Adapted from Administration on Children, Youth and Families, *Child Maltreatment 2003*. Children's Bureau, U.S. Department of Health and Human Services, Washington, D.C., 2005, page 68.

some manner in 2003, 75.9% sexually abused the children.

Do Social Workers Sometimes Overreact to Abuse Allegations?

Occasionally, child welfare workers err by removing children from families that have not been abusive. This may occur in the wake of community anger over the death of a child who clearly *should* have been removed from the family. In reaction, child protective services workers subsequently decide not to make such an error again and instead operate on the other end of the scale and remove children prematurely.

It is also true that, in past years, some individuals working at child-care centers were unfairly accused of child abuse. The furor of unproven physical and sexual abuse charges against day-care centers in the mid-1980s was later seen as a witch-hunt by many in the legal and medical community.

Sometimes workers err in the eyes of their own court system: in 1999, a Massachusetts minister who was also a father was charged with child abuse for admittedly spanking his son with a strap. The Massachusetts Supreme Judicial Court held that it was his right to discipline his child.

The court added, "Today, we conclude only that, on the totality of the record presented in this case, the effects of the plaintiff's physical discipline on his minor child did not satisfy the department's own regulatory definitions of physical injury and abuse.

However, a method of corporal punishment similar to the plaintiff's could, in different circumstances, rise to a level of severity that would result in the actual infliction of impermissible injuries."

In most cases, however, physical abuse can be identified and documented by trained physicians. Sometimes medical expertise is not even necessary, however. When a parent punishes a toddler by resting her bare buttocks on a hot oven and holding her there until she has permanent burn marks on her buttocks, it is evident to virtually everyone that this is physical abuse. (This is a true case.) When a child is cut or wounded in some other way, it is also clearly physical abuse.

Reasons for Physical Abuse

Experts debate endlessly the reasons why parents abuse their children. Some believe that abusive parents feel caught in a negative spiral of POVERTY and hopelessness. It is believed that parents may become extremely frustrated and angry about their own life and may allow their anger to boil over onto their children. Another reason for some physical abuse stems from ignorance and immaturity; for example, some young parents may have little knowledge about child development. It may seem reasonable to a 14-year-old girl to spank an 18-month-old child harshly for wetting her pants if she does not realize that most children are not toilet trained until they are two or three years old. In addition, the teenage mother may have a lower level of frustration than older mothers.

In some cases, the parent or other abuser was abused during childhood and assumes that physical abuse is acceptable. Even when the abuser knows that abuse is unacceptable, he or she may find themselves acting out old patterns, albeit with different roles. (The adult who was a victim of child abuse may assume the role of the abuser in adulthood.) However, it should be noted that the majority of adults who were abused as children do not become abusers in adulthood.

Sometimes the violence escalates far beyond what the perpetrator had intended. The act of hitting the child seems to make some abusers increasingly violent and angry and may cause them to lose control. Many abusers have said that they "lost it" and that they did not mean to harm the child as severely as they did. However, even unintended or unplanned abuse is an act of abuse.

Substance abuse is another major problem among many parents who physically abuse their children. If the parent is intoxicated on drugs or alcohol, his or her normal inhibitions are gone and negative impulses may take over. This is particularly true with alcohol and drugs such as amphetamine, cocaine and methamphetamine.

Sometimes mental illness can be a causal factor in acts of child abuse. One woman was repeatedly abused as a child by her mother, who thought the child was the "spawn of Satan."

It is also true that, although most people do not like to think about it, there are some parents who exhibit sadistic tendencies and who will expose their children to severe and unspeakable injuries. Some experts have called these parents "untreatable."

Abused Children Sometimes Do Not Receive Needed Medical Treatment

When a child is brought for medical treatment, whether to the child's physician or to an emergency room doctor, the caretaker's account of the injury often can alert the examining physician to the possibility of abuse. An unexplained injury, in which the parent may state that, "I just found him this way," is sometimes an attempt to deny abuse. Explanations that do not seem plausible merit further investigation.

Allegedly self-inflicted injuries of young children may be suspicious in origin. Often children will readily state to an investigator that an adult caused the injury. Experts believe that children rarely lie about such matters.

Most concerned parents bring their children to a physician or hospital immediately after an injury. In contrast, abusive parents often delay seeking medical attention for their child, hoping that the child will not need treatment and/or fearing that they will be punished for child abuse. They may know or suspect that doctors who suspect child abuse are required to report such incidents to child protective services personnel, because they are MANDATED REPORTERS.

In cases of abuse, often the person who brings the child for treatment is not the same person who was with the child at the time of injury. If the abusive parent does bring in the child, the story that he or she relates about the cause of the injury is often not credible to a doctor or sometimes even to nonmedical personnel and should be further investigated.

Findings from a Sample Drawn from the National Survey of Child and Adolescent Well-Being

In a chapter in *Child Victimization* on children investigated by child protective services, drawn from child subjects from the National Survey of Child and Adolescent Well-Being, researchers analyzed the types of injuries children received. The study was comprised of 5,504 children whose families had been investigated for child abuse. About half of the children (51%) were re-abused children from families previously investigated.

Children ages 11 and older were asked about serious injuries that had occurred in the past 12 months, and the injured children were also asked if they were seen by a doctor or nurse subsequent to the injury. Of the 1,155 children who said that they were injured, 11.1% said that they suffered a broken bone, dislocated joint or broken nose. About 80% of these children were seen for this injury by a doctor or nurse.

Of the children who said they were bitten by another person or animal, less than half (48%) received medical attention. Of the children who said they suffered a bad burn, only 40% received medical professional help.

The researchers also compared the percentage of the injuries of their abused subjects to children in the general population. They found that about 9% of the study children ages 11–14 years had suffered broken bones, compared to 4% of children in the general population. About 6% of children of the abused children had suffered burns, compared to less than 1% (0.05%) in the general population.

Said the researchers, "Overall, children age 11 and older who have undergone an investigation for child maltreatment report high levels of violence at the hands of their parents. About one in four of these children are experiencing severe violence at the hands of their caregivers, a much higher rate than the one in ten children found to have experienced this level of violence among children in the general population."

See also ABUSERS; ADULTS ABUSED AS CHILDREN; BATTERED CHILD SYNDROME; BRUISES; BURNS; CORD INJURIES; EYE INJURIES; FATALITIES; FRACTURES; INFANTICIDE; MOUTH INJURIES; MUNCHAUSEN SYNDROME BY PROXY; POISONING; SEXUAL ABUSE; SHAKEN INFANT SYNDROME; SUDDEN INFANT DEATH SYNDROME.

Administration on Children, Youth and Families. *Child Maltreatment 2003.* Children's Bureau, U.S. Department of Health and Human Services, Washington, D.C., 2005.

Gibbons, Claire B., et al. "Safety of Children Involved with Child Welfare Services." In *Child Victimization.* Kingston, N.J.: Civic Research Institute, 2005.

placement of abused children   Removal of maltreated children from their parents may be necessary to ensure proper treatment and to prevent further abuse. Governments base their authority to assume custody of a child on the doctrine of PARENS PATRIAE. Under this doctrine the state assumes a vital interest in ensuring the safety and welfare of children. However, many critics charge that in some cases, the state governments have overstepped this responsibility by removing children unnecessarily.

When a child is in immediate danger, law enforcement officials and, in most states, protective service agencies have authority to take EMERGENCY CUSTODY of the child. Prior approval of a court is not necessary in most areas; however, emergency placement decisions must be reviewed by a judge within 48 to 72 hours after the child is removed.

In Britain, children can be removed from home for up to 28 days under a PLACE OF SAFETY ORDER. The order can be obtained by anyone but must be approved by a magistrate.

Placement decisions are difficult. Child protection authorities must balance possible benefits of removal against the inevitable trauma that will be experienced by both children and parents.

See also ADOPTING ABUSED OR NEGLECTED CHILDREN; FOSTER CARE; KINSHIP CARE.

place of safety order   Under provisions of the Children and Young Persons Act of 1969, anyone in Britain can apply for an order to remove a child from a dangerous place. The emergency order, known as a place of safety order, may be issued by a magistrate at any time. Magistrates can authorize applicants to take custody of the child for a period not to exceed 28 days.

Applicants for such an order do not have to prove abuse or neglect; however, the magistrate must have reasonable cause to believe that: (1) the child's proper development is being avoidably prevented or neglected; (2) his or her health is being avoidably impaired or neglected; or (3) the child is being ill-treated.

A place of safety order may also be used to prevent removal of a child from a safe place. Siblings of the identified child are also covered by the order. Children may be taken without parents' knowledge, but applicants are expected to inform them as soon as possible after removal. Parents have little opportunity to appeal a place of safety order.

Place of safety orders are typically used in emergencies where a child is in immediate danger. Concern has been expressed by some experts that these orders are too easy to obtain, increasing the possibility of unnecessary removal.

poisoning   Abuse-related poisoning of children is relatively rare; however, a significant number of accidental poisonings are a result of parental NEGLECT of normal safety precautions.

Deliberate poisoning of children may be due to a disturbed parent's impulsive act or desire to get revenge. More frequently, intentional poisoning involves a drug overdose, ostensibly for the purpose of quieting an upset child.

The failure of caretakers to exercise adequate safety precautions is more often a cause of child poisoning than deliberate acts. Specifically, improper storage of chemicals and medications significantly increases the likelihood of accidental poisoning. Multiple accidental poisonings occur most often in households characterized by high levels of stress, including illness, recent death of a family member, marital discord and parental drug or alcohol abuse. Children whose caretakers abuse alcohol or drugs are particularly at risk. The easy accessibility of these substances increases the risk of accidental ingestion. Substance abusers also have a diminished capacity to provide adequate care and are frequently neglectful.

Poison centers offer immediate telephone consultation in the event of poisoning. There are over 650 such centers in the United States. Telephone numbers of nearby centers are usually listed under emergency numbers at the front of most telephone directories. In addition to providing lifesaving emergency advice these centers can be especially helpful in identifying victims of repetitive poisoning (approximately one-fourth of all poisonings).

polymorphic perverse offender   Sexual offenders are sometimes classified according to the type of victim and/or sexual acts they prefer. PEDOPHILES, for example, direct their sexual feelings and actions primarily (in many cases exclusively) toward children. Most rapists attack only female victims. However, some sexual offenders appear to be indiscriminate in their choice of victims or sexual acts. They may be described as polymorphic perverse offenders.

This description follows a classification used by Sigmund Freud to describe indiscriminate sexuality. Freud coined the term polymorphous perversity to describe the behavior of individuals who had been seduced as children.

As currently used, the term refers to sex offenders who engage in many different forms of sexual assault (i.e., vaginal rape, sodomy, exhibitionism) and who may attack people of any age. This type of offender accounts for a very small percentage of all child SEXUAL ABUSE.

pornography, child   See CHILD PORNOGRAPHY.

post-traumatic hypopituitarism   See DWARFISM.

poverty   Although child abuse and neglect has been described as a classless phenomenon by numerous writers, researchers and clinicians, the problem of child abuse is most evident among the poor, particularly when there is a problem of substance or drug abuse. While it is true that abuse and neglect can be found in every socioeconomic stratum, statistics show that a disproportionate number of reported cases of abuse and neglect involve low-income families. Studies have shown that poverty status is strongly related to neglect. Poor children are also highly represented among victims of more serious forms of abuse.

It has been argued that low-income families are more likely to be investigated and reported on than middle- and upper-income families. Suggestions have been made that if higher income families were subjected to the same scrutiny, an equal amount of abuse would be found. To date no significant evidence has been presented to support this position. In fact, a comprehensive analysis of possible bias was provided in a 1998 issue of the *American Journal of Orthopsychiatry,* and the researchers found no grounds for such bias. Indeed, they stated their concern that the "myth of classlessness" in child abuse maltreatment could act to prevent poor families and their children from receiving assistance from social service authorities. The authors wrote

> We can no longer afford to cling to untenable positions regarding the equitable distribution of risk to children across class boundaries. We must concentrate our efforts in those areas in which the prob-

lems are most severe, and we must devise tools for working with poor families that address the special concerns, problems, and stresses they face. Ultimately, the close association between poverty and child maltreatment suggests that the most effective way to prevent child abuse will be to reduce the number of families in poverty. If child maltreatment is born largely of the stresses and wants associated with being poor, then primary prevention efforts might best target the underlying political, social, and economic structure that perpetuate poverty.

A Global Look at Poverty and Abuse

Cross-cultural evidence from Western and Eastern societies also supports the assertion that poverty and child abuse are related. Anthropological studies from New Guinea, Africa, Turkey and South America all have documented the increased risks to children raised in poverty.

The mere existence of poverty has been labeled as a form of societal abuse. Poor children who are denied the basic elements necessary for healthy development suffer many of the same consequences as those from whom these elements are intentionally withheld. Social policy researchers David Gil, Leroy Pelton and others have argued that attributing abuse and neglect to individual or family pathology masks true societal causes of the phenomenon. Further, the individual, as opposed to societal, view of child abuse is seen as a means of promoting certain professional and political interests at the expense of a more lasting solution.

High Stress Levels Contribute to Problem

Increased stress is often given as the reason for the association between poverty and abuse. Families with severely restricted incomes are constantly faced with difficult choices and may suffer from inadequate housing, poor health care and malnourishment. Such conditions are seen as neglectful and may contribute to physical, emotional or sexual abuse.

Not All Poor People Are Abusers

Despite its obvious contributions to increased stress and poor living conditions, poverty is by no means synonymous with abuse or neglect as statutorily defined. Only a relatively small proportion of children living in impoverished families are reported to child protection agencies. Parents of such children, through skill, determination and luck, are frequently able to overcome the burdens of poverty. It is clear, however, that poverty places children at significant risk.

Drake, Brett, and Susan Zuravin. "Bias in Child Maltreatment Reporting: Revisiting the Myth of Classlessness." *American Journal of Orthopsychiatry* 68, no. 2 (April 1998): 295–304.

———. *In the Shadow of the Poorhouse* New York: Basic Books, 1986.

Pelton, Leroy H. *The Social Context of Child Abuse and Neglect.* New York: Human Sciences Press, 1981.

———. "Child Abuse and Neglect: The Myth of Classlessness." *American Journal of Orthopsychiatry* 48 (October 1978): 607–617.

prediction of abuse and neglect   Several researchers have attempted to develop screening tests that will predict the likelihood of abuse. Various methods used include pencil and paper questionnaires, standardized interviews and direct observation of parent-child interaction. Presently, all screening is voluntary. High-risk groups such as teenaged parents are most often targeted for screening; however, some hospital programs have attempted to screen all parents of newborns.

Many tests focus on parental characteristics such as emotional deprivation, history of abuse as a child and intelligence. Others examine characteristics of the child. Studies indicate that developmental disabilities, irritability and other traits increase the likelihood that a child will be abused. Several screening devices attempt to measure stress factors, such as POVERTY and SOCIAL ISOLATION. Some researchers attempt to measure the quality of interaction between parent and child. Finally, various attempts have been made to combine these approaches.

To date no completely accurate screening method has been developed. Experts caution that although screening may be useful in targeting prevention efforts, it should not be considered a diagnostic tool. Identification of people as potentially abusive does not mean they are in fact abusing a child. Parents cannot be forced to submit to screening tests nor can potentially abusive parents be required to accept help. Concern over PARENTS' RIGHTS has caused many practitioners to be very cautious in use and interpretation of various screening methods.

preponderance of evidence See EVIDENTIARY STANDARDS.

presentment In some situations, usually an emergency, a grand jury may issue a written accusation of a crime without having received a COMPLAINT from a prosecutor. This document is the equivalent of an INDICTMENT.

prevention Efforts to prevent child abuse and neglect are often classified as either primary or secondary. Primary prevention seeks to protect children from maltreatment before it occurs. This approach may be directed at the general public or at specially targeted high-risk families. Secondary prevention attempts to prevent the recurrence of maltreatment or to keep a potentially abusive situation from getting worse. Subjects of secondary prevention are usually identified through reports of suspected abuse or neglect.

Prevention can take many different forms. Methods frequently used in *primary prevention* include hospital-based neonatal programs that promote mother-infant bonding, home visitors (also called home HEALTH VISITORS or PARENT AIDES), parent education and counseling programs. Most such programs are directed at parents and operate from the premise that by learning more about child rearing they will be less likely to abuse or neglect their children. SEXUAL ABUSE prevention usually directed at children often takes the form of school-based programs that use books, films, plays and puppetry to inform children about the dangers of sexual abuse and ways in which they might protect themselves.

Secondary prevention often involves the entire family in some form of counseling, behavior modification or treatment. Intervention is usually tar-geted to specific family problems, such as a parent's ways of disciplining children or stress management, that are thought to underly the abuse.

Michael Wald and Sophia Cohen, in a review of prevention efforts published in the *Family Law Quarterly,* identified four problems that must be addressed in developing successful prevention programs. First, abuse must be clearly defined. There is much disagreement as to what sorts of situations constitute abuse or neglect. Programs must have a clear definition of the type(s) of behavior they wish to prevent if they are to be successful. Second, some understanding of the causes of abuse and neglect is necessary. Causes are often complex and poorly understood. Third, prevention strategies should be directed where they will do the most good. Most primary prevention efforts are too costly to allow inefficient use. Fourth, there is little accurate information about the effectiveness of various prevention techniques. Prevention of child abuse and neglect is a relatively new field. Adequate evaluation of programs would require large, carefully designed studies.

Treatment after confirmation of child abuse or neglect is sometimes referred to as *tertiary prevention.*

Wald, Michael S., and Sophia Cohen. "Preventing Child Abuse—What Will It Take." *Family Law Quarterly* 20, no. 2 (Summer 1986): 281–302.

prevention, primary See PREVENTION.

prevention, secondary See PREVENTION.

prevention, tertiary See PREVENTION.

Prevention of Cruelty to and Protection of Children Act of 1889 (Britain) As a direct result of actions taken by the National Society for the Prevention of Cruelty to Children (NSPCC), in 1889 the British Parliament enacted a law that established penalties for the ill-treatment and neglect of children. The act was amended in 1894 and again in 1904. In cases where neglect or abuse of a child meant the parent or guardian could benefit financially from a child's life insurance policy, legal penalties were increased.

prima facie   Literally, this means "at first sight." Prima facie evidence is that which is sufficiently strong to prove the allegations in a case of suspected child abuse or neglect. It is considered proof of the suspected charges; however, this evidence is only considered proof in the absence of contradictory or rebutting evidence.

In virtually all states, admissible evidence in a child abuse or neglect case must fall within one of the two following standards of proof. Either clear and convincing evidence must be presented or a preponderance of the evidence must fall in favor of either the plaintiff or the defendant. Prima facie evidence could come under either of these two standards.

See also EVIDENTIARY STANDARDS.

primary prevention   See PREVENTION.

Prince v. Massachusetts   In 1944, a landmark United States Supreme Court case determined that "the custody, care, and nurture of the child resides first in the parents, whose primary function and freedom include preparation for obligations that the state can neither supply nor hinder." However, the court went on to say that, in some cases, the state has an overriding interest in protecting children.

This decision involved a child whose aunt permitted her to sell religious literature on the streetcorner. At legal issue in the case was the charge that parents, guardians or custodians are not free to make martyrs of their children. Sarah Prince, a Jehovah's Witness, was charged with violating Massachusetts's child labor laws by having her nine-year-old niece, of whom she had custody, sell copies of *Watchtower* and *Consolation* on the street. The court affirmed Prince's conviction by a lower court. Its assertion that "the power of the state to control the conduct of children reaches beyond the scope of its authority over adults" affirmed the state's right to intervene against the wishes of parents and children when necessary for a child's protection.

The findings in *Prince v. Massachusetts* provided the basis for subsequent judicial rulings in which the rights of other individuals (i.e., parents) or groups (i.e., schools) take precedence over those of children.

See also RELIGIOUS ASPECTS; *WISCONSIN V. YODER; TINKER V. DES MOINES.*

Mnookin, Robert H. *Child, Family and State: Problems and Materials on Children and the Law.* Boston: Little, Brown, 1978.

prisons, child victimizers in   A 1996 report from the Office of Juvenile Justice and Delinquency Prevention provided a wealth of information about prison inmates who were imprisoned as violent child victimizers. Prisoners had committed such crimes as homicide, kidnapping, rape and sexual assault and other abuses. Researchers surveyed inmates in state prisons who had been convicted of violent crimes and found that 61,000, or about 19% of all state prisoners, had been convicted of a crime against a victim under the age of 18. More than half of the violent crimes were perpetrated against a child under the age of 12. About 70% of the child victimizers in prison were in jail for a rape or sexual assault against a child.

General Characteristics of Imprisoned Child Victimizers

Researchers found that 97% of the offenders were male. Nearly a third had never been arrested before. About 19% of the offenders had been convicted of prior acts such as statutory rape, child abuse or lewd acts with a child. Most did not carry a weapon; only 14% were armed. About a third had committed their crimes against their own child and approximately half had some other relationship with the child such as a friend, relative or acquaintance. Most of the violent victimizations (75%) occurred in either the victim's home or the victimizer's home.

Demographic Characteristics

The majority of the violent child offenders, about 70%, were white. Most, or 78%, had been employed in the month before they were arrested. Their marital status varied: about 37% had never married, 33% were divorced and 23% were married. The others were widowed or separated. The mean age for child victimizers was 33 years.

The educational status of the child victimizers varied. The majority of offenders, about 55%, had less than a high school education; however, about 27% were high school graduates and about 18% were college graduates.

Background as a Child

The majority of the offenders (54%) grew up with both parents and only about 17% had ever spent time in a foster home or institution. Most (69%) said their parents or guardians did not abuse drugs or alcohol. Most (64%) said their immediate family members had never served any jail time.

Most of the offenders (69%) said they had never been physically or sexually abused. Of the ones who reported abuse as a child, most knew their abuser, who was usually a parent or guardian or other relative or acquaintance.

Drug Use

Most of the violent child offenders (57%) said they were not abusing drugs or alcohol at the time of the crime. About 24% were using alcohol and about 5% were using drugs only. About 14% were using both alcohol and drugs. Of those who were drinking at the time of the offense about 79% had been drinking for three or more hours.

Special Sentencing

Judges ordered special sentencing conditions in a greater percentage of cases of child victimizers than of adult victimizers. About 13% of the child victimizers were ordered to participate in a sex offender treatment program or to receive psychological or psychiatric counseling. Only about 2% of those who victimized an adult received such a special sentence.

See also CHILD MOLESTERS; CIVIL COMMITMENT LAWS.

Greenfeld, Laurence A. "Child Victimizers: Violent Offenders and Their Victims." U.S. Department of Justice, Office of Justice Programs, Bureau of Justice Statistics, 1996.

private zone   *Private zone* is a term used in teaching young children how to identify and avoid sexual advances. Breasts, buttocks and genitalia (areas covered by a bathing suit) are all considered to be part of the private zone, which should not be touched by anyone other than the child. Obvious exceptions are made for situations such as examination by a physician or bathing by a parent or appropriate caretaker. In such instances, the quality of the touching is emphasized, and the child is encouraged to use various means to avoid contact that makes them feel uncomfortable. Among other options, children are taught to call for help loudly and to run to a safe place nearby, such as a neighbor's house or a police station, for help. *Private Zone* is also the title of a read-aloud book for children written by Frances S. Dayee (New York: Warner Books, 1984).

privileged communications   In many countries the patient or client may refuse to allow information revealed in a personal conference with his or her physician, pyschotherapist or lawyer to be presented in court. This legal protection is sometimes called the doctor-patient privilege. Child abuse reporting laws often override privileged communications in situations where the reporting of abuse or prosecution of an abuser might be inhibited. Most jurisdictions, however, continue to protect communications between lawyer and client.

See also CONFIDENTIALITY.

probate court   See COURT.

procedural due process   See DUE PROCESS.

proceeding, civil   See CIVIL PROCEEDING.

projection   Psychodynamic explanations of abuse emphasize the abusing parent's reliance on projection as a mechanism for coping with stress. Projection can be described as a process whereby an individual ascribes his or her own feelings to another person. A parent may project feelings of self-hatred onto a child. The child then becomes a scapegoat for the parent's anger and low self-esteem.

Often a particular child becomes unconsciously associated with painful earlier events in the parent's life. The TARGET CHILD may be described as a monster or a demon, suggesting a symbolic association between the child and the parent's own uncontrollable rage. Externalizing feelings of self-hatred is a form of denial that prevents the parent from acknowledging and confronting these feelings. The parent's unconscious need to avoid confronting internal rage may be so strong that when the target child is removed from home another child becomes the object of projection.

Psychodynamic treatment of abusers often centers on helping them acknowledge and understand their own feelings. If treatment is successful the abuser learns to differentiate between his or her own feelings and the child's behavior.

proof, burden   See BURDEN OF PROOF.

proof, standards of   See EVIDENTIARY STANDARDS.

property, children as   See CHILDREN AS PROPERTY.

prosecution, criminal   See CRIMINAL PROSECUTION.

prostitution, child   See CHILD PROSTITUTION.

protection, order of   See ORDER OF PROTECTION.

Protection of Children Against Sexual Exploitation Act of 1977 (P.L. 95-225)   Enacted into law in February of 1978, this was the first piece of federal legislation in the United States to deal directly with CHILD PORNOGRAPHY. Prosecutors found it difficult to obtain convictions due to a provision that limited the law's application to pornographic material produced for commercial purposes. Most child pornographers were able to avoid prosecution by trading material rather than selling it.

In 1984, Congress deleted the commerciality requirement as well as a provision that required the material to be legally obscene. This amendment, known as the Child Protection Act of 1984, greatly increased the number of convictions for production and distribution of child pornography. In the two years following enactment of the Child Protection Act, 164 child pornographers were convicted compared to 64 convictions in the five-plus years preceding the amendment.

protective custody   Physicians, social workers and certain other professionals often have the power to detain a child until a DETENTION request can be filed with the court. In some cases oral permission of a judge must be obtained before a child is held in protective custody.

See also EMERGENCIES; EMERGENCY CUSTODY.

protective services   Refers to the state or county organization that provides assistance to abused and neglected children, and either investigates CHILD MALTREATMENT allegations or works with local law-enforcement personnel to investigate allegations of the abuse and/or neglect of children.

In the United States, every state has a legally designated child protection agency. Each Canadian province provides for child protective services. In Britain, child protection is the responsibility of LOCAL AUTHORITIES.

Child protective services are distinguished from other social services by their involuntary nature. Few abusive parents request intervention from a protective services agency. Typically, clients are resistant and hostile toward protective service workers.

However, they are required to cooperate, or they may risk losing custody of their children and sometimes the termination of their parental rights.

As a result, protective service workers have the legal authority to intervene against parents' wishes in order to determine whether a child is being abused or neglected. If sufficient evidence of abuse or neglect is found, the protective service agency may petition a court for additional powers to act on behalf of the child. When a child is in immediate danger of serious injury, the child protective worker may be granted EMERGENCY CUSTODY powers. Many children are removed from the home under this authority.

Child protective service workers may respond to an allegation of child maltreatment within a few hours to a few days, depending on the severity of the allegation. Once the maltreatment investigation is launched, the workers may talk to the parents of the child as well as other people who know the child, such as child-care providers, teachers and physicians. Depending on the child's age and the severity of the injury, workers may also interview the child alone or in the presence of the parents. If the injury is deemed serious enough, the child will be temporarily (for weeks or months or sometimes for several years or longer) placed with other relatives or in a foster home.

Despite their legal authority, child protective services focus on rehabilitation rather than punishment. Though most parents initially resist help, protective service workers attempt to engage them in a cooperative effort to eliminate conditions that contributed to maltreatment of their children. Often these conditions are difficult to resolve, however, such as SUBSTANCE ABUSE and/or psychiatric problems.

The key tasks of protective service workers can be divided into five categories: investigation of complaints, assessment of the client's needs, case planning, treatment of the parents or other caretakers and case monitoring. Agencies often have separate units that perform investigatory and treatment-related functions. In practice, the investigation phase often comprises a large proportion of protective services. (See the flowchart of the steps followed by child protective services, from the reporting of an incident of abuse or neglect to the final outcome.)

Experts believe that if the punitive arm of protective services were transferred to law enforcement, then families would be more likely to see child welfare workers as family advocates. They also believe this is a more logical choice and point out that a stranger would be arrested for the same kinds of abuse that a parent inflicts upon a child. If that same parent assaulted another child outside the family, then he or she would likely be arrested. In effect, the value of children within the family appears somehow diminished.

Part of the reason for this is that for many years, child welfare officials and social service agencies have believed that their therapeutic intervention could work, if only they had the right mix: enough money, caseworkers, or other resources. Yet clinical studies have revealed that even intensive efforts with groups that perform massive interventions with families, helping them shop, advising them on financial affairs, providing parenting tips, etc., often fail to provide any better results.

Some individuals and organizations believe protective services should be privatized while others believe the function should remain state run and be expanded. Despite the difference in opinion, one point seems clear: few people are satisfied with the protective services system as it stands.

With the passage of the ADOPTION AND SAFE FAMILIES ACT in 1997, protective services workers were still encouraged to preserve families whenever possible, but the law also required states to consider terminating parental rights within a quicker time frame than before, if families could not be reunited. The child would then be adopted or remain in long-term foster care.

For a better understanding of the process whereby a child is reported as abused and enters the system to the final outcome (return to parent, adoption, etc.), see the flowchart.

Guilty Until Proven Innocent

Another problem with protective services units in general is that if a charge is made, it is up to the accused person to prove his or her innocence. Issues of due process and individual rights can be disregarded. In many cases, children who are severely abused are removed from their homes and thus, they are protected. In a few cases, the system is abused by overly zealous therapists and protective services workers. In one noted case in Wenatchee, Washington, a police detective, who was also a foster parent, arrested his foster child's biological parents after she had been with his family for six months. The allegations did not end there, however. The girl and her sister subsequently accused many others in the town of abuse.

Many more children were taken from their families, interviewed, and, after repeated questioning, the children spun elaborate, but similar, tales of

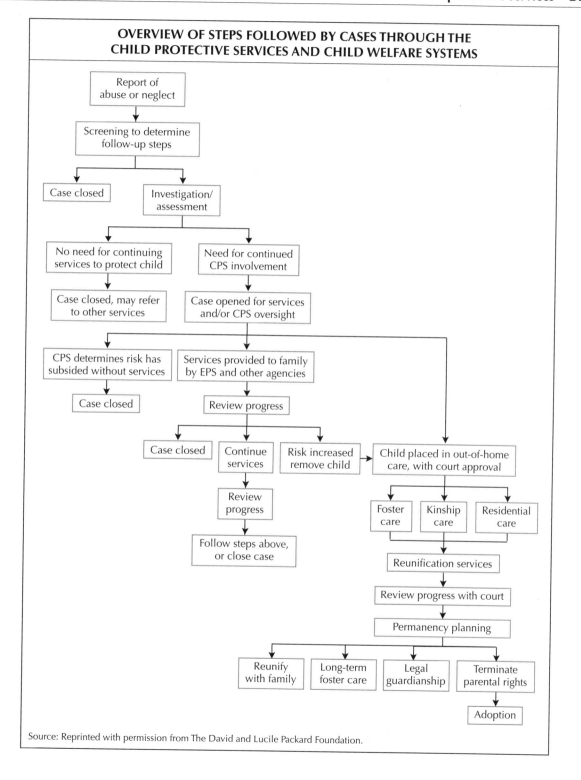

OVERVIEW OF STEPS FOLLOWED BY CASES THROUGH THE CHILD PROTECTIVE SERVICES AND CHILD WELFARE SYSTEMS

Report of abuse or neglect

Screening to determine follow-up steps

Case closed

Investigation/ assessment

No need for continuing services to protect child

Need for continued CPS involvement

Case closed, may refer to other services

Case opened for services and/or CPS oversight

CPS determines risk has subsided without services

Services provided to family by EPS and other agencies

Case closed

Review progress

Case closed

Continue services

Risk increased remove child

Child placed in out-of-home care, with court approval

Review progress

Foster care

Kinship care

Residential care

Follow steps above, or close case

Reunification services

Review progress with court

Permanency planning

Reunify with family

Long-term foster care

Legal guardianship

Terminate parental rights

Adoption

Source: Reprinted with permission from The David and Lucile Packard Foundation.

satanic worship and sexual abuse eventually involving a minister, his wife and their entire Pentecostal church. Those children—sometimes members of the same family—who refused to corroborate the stories were diagnosed with post-traumatic stress disorder and placed in therapy, sometimes in out-of-state institutions. Anytime a member of the community (including the pastor) protested that the charges were fabricated, they found themselves charged in the conspiracy and had their children removed as well.

Said Susan Orr,

Many of the children later recanted. But not before 43 adults—most of whom were desperately poor, unable to read, write, or afford good attorneys—were charged with 30,000 counts of rape involving 60 children. Not understanding what they were doing, some even signed confessions, fearing that unless they cooperated, they would never see their children again. Over a two-year period, ten were convicted while 18 pled to lesser felony charges.

According to Orr, a social worker was fired because she challenged the manner of the investigation. She later filed a civil suit against the Washington Department of Social and Health Services for wrongful termination and was awarded $1.57 million in damages.

Orr, Susan. "Child Protection at the Crossroads: Child Abuse, Child Protection, and Recommendations for Reform." Policy Study No. 262, Reason Public Policy Institute, 1999.
Schene, Patricia A. "Past, Present, and Future Roles of Child Protective Services." In the special issue, "Protecting Children from Abuse and Neglect," *The Future of Children* 8, no. 1 (Spring 1998): 23–38.

pseudomaturity   Neglected children sometimes appear to be much more mature than other children of their age. This pseudomaturity is usually the result of ROLE REVERSAL in which an immature parent looks to the child for care and nurturance. Immature parents may have unrealistic expectations of their children, which place them in the role of caretaker to younger siblings, protector of the parent or even the parent's romantic partner.

Pseudomaturity exacts a high price from children. Forced to forgo their own emotional development in order to care for parents, they typically grow into adults lacking the emotional resources to form healthy, close relationships. They may be extremely dependent on others for emotional support and as parents may follow a pattern similar to that of their own upbringing.

psychological/emotional maltreatment   A type of maltreatment that refers to acts that caused or may have caused conduct, cognitive, affective or other mental disorders. Often the terms *psychological maltreatment* and *emotional abuse* are used interchangeably. Most experts agree that psychological maltreatment involves a pattern of destructive behavior—not a single incident—on the part of an adult. Though virtually all children will be exposed to some form of emotional abuse or neglect at times, those who are *repeatedly* subjected to such treatment may suffer permanent psychological or intellectual damage.

Psychological maltreatment includes emotional neglect, psychological abuse and mental injury. An example of an act of the commission of psychological maltreatment would be a pattern of frequently telling a child that he or she is stupid, evil or hated by the parent.

Acts of omission that may cause psychological maltreatment can be seen with infants who receive basic care and feeding but receive little or no affection or attention and may eventually develop a FAILURE TO THRIVE.

This is a common problem among infants in orphanages but may also occur in infants with families who do not like or are indifferent to the baby. Sometimes severely mentally ill parents psychologically maltreat their children. In one case, a mentally ill woman was raising her toddler son as a cat who ate from bowls on the floor. He was later removed to foster care, and the woman's parental rights were subsequently terminated by the state.

Psychologically maltreated children may also suffer from physical abuse and neglect. When psychological abuse alone occurs, it is often difficult for PROTECTIVE SERVICE workers to identify and document.

Children who are emotionally abused may develop problematic behaviors, such as being destructive (by starting fires), exhibiting anger (abusing animals), abusing alcohol or drugs or even contemplating or committing SUICIDE.

BULLYING one's peers in childhood and adolescence may be considered as a form of psychological maltreatment.

Some experts have provided their own definition of emotional/psychological maltreatment. For example, Steven W. Kairys, M.D., Charles F. Johnson, M.D., and the Committee on Child Abuse and Neglect defined psychological maltreatment in a 2002 issue of *Pediatrics* as "a repeated pattern of damaging interactions between parent(s) and child that becomes typical of the relationship. In some situations, the pattern occurs only when triggered by alcohol or other potentiating factors. Occasionally, a very painful singular incident, such as an unusually contentious divorce, can initiate psychological maltreatment."

Demographics of Victims and Perpetrators of Psychological Maltreatment

In the United States, according to *Child Maltreatment 2003*, a government report released in 2005 by the Children's Bureau of the U.S. Department of Health and Human Services, about 5% of all maltreated victims, or an estimated 38,603 children, were psychologically maltreated in 2003.

The rates of psychological (as well as "other" types of maltreatment that do not fit other categories) maltreatment vary considerably among races and ethnicities. For example, according to *Child Maltreatment 2003*, nearly 42% of Pacific Islander children suffered from this category of abuse, while only 5% of American Indian or Alaska Native children were victims of this type of maltreatment. The rate for African-American children and white children was about 15% each.

Among perpetrators, of all unmarried partners of parents who were abusers, about 14% were perpetrators of psychological abuse (the highest percentage of all perpetrators), followed by parental abusers (about 9%). (See Table I.)

Reporters of Psychological Abuse

Among those who reported psychological maltreatment to authorities, according to *Child Maltreatment 2003*, the largest percentage of reporters were legal, law enforcement and criminal justice personnel (29.9%), followed by educational (13.0%) and social services personnel (12.2%). As can be seen from Table II, most reporters of psychological maltreatment were professionals (65.9%).

State Laws on Psychological Abuse Vary

At least half the states have laws against psychological maltreatment, although this form of abuse is difficult to document and prove. Despite the ambiguity of child protection laws on psychological maltreatment, some children have been removed

TABLE I
PERPETRATORS BY RELATIONSHIP TO VICTIMS AND TYPES OF MALTREATMENT, BY PERCENT 2003

Maltreatment type	Parent	Other relative	Foster parent	Child day-care provider	Unmarried partner of parent	Legal guardian	Friends or neighbors
Psychological maltreatment only, or unknown only	9.1	5.8	7.3	2.5	14.4	5.9	2.7
Physical abuse	11.0	10.4	16.9	12.9	16.6	14.0	3.4
Neglect only	62.0	37.5	50.0	48.4	37.9	55.7	9.7
Sexual abuse only	2.7	29.9	6.3	23.0	11.5	4.2	75.9
Multiple maltreatments	15.2	16.4	19.6	13.1	19.6	20.2	8.3
Total percent	100.0	100.0	100.0	100.0	100.0	100.0	100.0

Source: Adapted from Administration on Children, Youth and Families, *Child Maltreatment 2003*. Children's Bureau, U.S. Department of Health and Human Services, Washington, D.C., 2005, page 68.

TABLE II
DISTRIBUTION OF PSYCHOLOGICAL MALTREATMENT BY REPORT SOURCE, 2003

Report source	Number	Percentage
PROFESSIONALS		
Educational personnel	5,385	13.0
Legal, law enforcement, criminal justice personnel	12,412	29.9
Social services personnel	5,057	12.2
Medical personnel	2,003	4.8
Mental health personnel	2,025	4.9
Child day-care providers	238	0.6
Foster-care providers	232	0.6
Total professionals	27,352	65.9
NONPROFESSIONALS		
Anonymous reporters	2,472	6.0
Other reporters	2,489	6.0
Other relatives	4,099	9.9
Parents	2,427	5.8
Friends or neighbors	1,545	3.7
Unknown reporters	717	1.7
Alleged victims	358	0.9
Alleged perpetrators	53	0.1
Total nonprofessionals	14,180	34.1
Total	41,512	
Total percent		100.0

Source: Adapted from Administration on Children, Youth and Families, *Child Maltreatment 2003*. Children's Bureau, U.S. Department of Health and Human Services, Washington, D.C., 2005, page 37.

from their homes due to the parents' emotional instability or after being allowed to witness acts of cruelty inflicted on another family member.

In Minnesota, emotional maltreatment is defined as the consistent, deliberate infliction of mental harm on a child by a person responsible for the child's care, and which harm has an observable, sustained and adverse effect on the child's physical, mental or emotional development. In Vermont, emotional maltreatment refers to a pattern of malicious behavior that results in impaired psychological growth and development.

Five Categories of Psychological Maltreatment

In an attempt to create a better understanding of the types of behavior that constitute psychologi-

cal maltreatment, Dr. James Garbarino, president of the Erikson Institute for Advanced Study in Child Development, Chicago, Illinois, and his colleagues have identified five categories of psychological abuse/neglect: rejecting, isolating, terrorizing, ignoring and corrupting.

Rejecting refers to an attitude of hostility toward the child or a total indifference to the child's needs. Cross-cultural studies have shown that this type of behavior exists in many different cultures and is frequently associated with high levels of social and economic stress.

Isolating a child from normal social experiences may also constitute abuse. An example of isolation is the parent who consistently denies a child the opportunity to interact with his or her peers.

Terrorizing involves repeated verbal assaults on a child, causing the child to live in constant fear. Threats of abandonment, severe punishment or death fall into this category.

Ignoring a child can inhibit normal emotional and intellectual development. This type of maltreatment may be especially damaging to infants, who need emotional, tactile and intellectual stimulation for healthy development. The failure to provide such stimulation to an infant may lead to FAILURE TO THRIVE.

Finally, corrupting refers to the parent or caregiver who encourages a child to engage in behavior that is destructive, antisocial or damaging. Two obvious examples of corrupting are encouraging a child to engage in CHILD PROSTITUTION or stealing. Both activities place the child at significant risk of harm and deny him or her a normal social experience.

Signs of Emotional Abuse in Children and Parents

According to the National Clearinghouse on Child Abuse and Neglect Information, signs of emotional maltreatment of a child may occur when the child

- Shows extremes in behavior, such as exhibiting overly compliant or demanding behavior, extreme passivity or aggression
- Acts as either an inappropriate adult (parenting other children, for example) or an inappropriate infant (frequently rocking or head-banging, for example)
- Is delayed in physical or emotional development

- Has attempted suicide
- Reports a lack of attachment to the parent

Signs of emotional maltreatment exhibited by the parent or other caretaker may include

- Constantly blaming, belittling or berating the child
- A lack of concern about the child and refusal to consider offers of help for the child's problems
- Overt rejection of the child

See also ADULTS ABUSED AS CHILDREN; CHILD ABUSE; DEPRESSION; FAMILY VIOLENCE; PHYSICAL ABUSE; SEXUAL ABUSE.

Administration on Children, Youth and Families. *Child Maltreatment 2003.* Children's Bureau, U.S. Department of Health and Human Services, Washington, D.C., 2005.

Garbarino, James. "Psychological Maltreatment Is Not an Ancillary Issue." *Brown University Child and Adolescent Behavior Letter* 14, no. 8 (August 1998): 2–4.

Garbarino, James, Edna Guttmann, and Janis Wilson Seeley. *The Psychologically Battered Child.* San Francisco, Calif.: Jossey-Bass, 1986.

Kairys, Steven W., Charles F. Johnson, and Committee on Child Abuse and Neglect. "The Psychological Maltreatment of Children—Technical Report." *Pediatrics,* 2002. Available online. URL: http://www.pediatrics.org/cgi/content/full/109/4/e8. Downloaded December 9, 2005.

National Clearinghouse on Child Abuse and Neglect Information. "Recognizing Child Abuse and Neglect: Signs and Symptoms." September 2003. Available online. URL: https://nccanch.acf.hhs.gov/pubs/factsheets/signs.pdf. Downloaded December 9, 2005.

psychological parenthood Psychological parenthood plays an important role in decisions concerning removal of an abused child from the home. The concept is based upon the idea that a child may establish close psychological bonds with an adult other than a biological parent. An adult becomes a psychological parent through daily interaction and sharing with a child. A parent who is absent, rejecting or inactive is unlikely to fulfill a child's need for a psychological parent.

In their influential book, *Beyond the Best Interests of the Child,* Joseph Goldstein, Anna Freud and Albert Solnit argue that such a close relationship is crucial for healthy development of a child. They advocate restraint in removing children from psychological parents. Since the book's publication, many courts have given greater consideration to the quality of the relationship between a child and his or her primary caretaker.

Separation from a psychological parent is usually painful and upsetting to a child. Child protection workers and courts usually avoid interrupting ties between a child and his or her psychological parent unless separation is absolutely necessary for the protection of the child or a judge requires it.

Goldstein, Joseph, Anna Freud, and Albert Solnit. *The Best Interests of the Child: The Least Detrimental Alternative.* New York: Free Press, 1996.

psychological tests A variety of psychological tests are used to evaluate emotional and adjustment problems in children who have been abused. The four most commonly used tests are the Minnesota Multiphasic Personality Test (MMPI), Rorschach, Thematic Apperception Test (TAT) and Draw a Person Test (DAP).

The MMPI presents a number of statements to the subject, who is asked to respond "true," "false" or "cannot say." In the Rorschach children are asked to interpret a series of inkblots. These interpretations are used as an aid in understanding the child's perceptions of reality and social interaction patterns. The TAT consists of a series of pictures suggesting some type of social interaction. Respondents are required to describe what they think is happening in the picture. Children taking the DAP are directed to draw a picture of themselves, a family member, friend or group of people. Interpretation of the drawings is based on the details included (or excluded), the relationships among the figures and the story the child tells about the drawing. All of these tests may be used in the assessment of a variety of emotional problems and are designed to be administered by persons specifically trained in psychometry.

In addition to these tests, several tests have been designed especially for the assessment of PSYCHOLOGICAL/EMOTIONAL MALTREATMENT or related problems. Many of these tests were originally developed as research instruments. While most focus on maltreatment in the home, some were specifically designed for out-of-home settings.

psychopathological abuse See PSYCHOPATHOLOGY.

psychopathology The importance of mental illness and emotional disturbance as factors contributing to child abuse and neglect is the subject of an ongoing debate among experts. While virtually all scholars and practitioners admit that mental illness may cause parents to neglect or abuse their children, there is widespread disagreement as to the prevalence of psychopathological abuse.

A rather extreme view holds that all child abuse is, by definition, psychopathological. Labeling child abuse as a specific form of illness ignores the complex interplay between intrapsychic factors and external forces that may lead to abuse in some situations but not in others. Further, traditional ways of treating mental illness, such as psychotherapy or drug therapy, are not always effective in changing abusive behavior.

Several psychologists and psychiatrists have attempted to isolate a diagnostic category similar to the medical classification, BATTERED CHILD SYNDROME. Though some have been successful in identifying relationships between various diagnostic categories, for example depression (or schizophrenia) and child abuse, the specific role of psychopathology continues to be elusive. Though it is relatively easy to understand how severe depression may lead to parental neglect, it is more difficult to explain why many parents who suffer from this and other forms of mental illness do not neglect or abuse their children.

Many researchers argue that psychopathology is secondary to cultural and environmental factors as a contributor to child maltreatment. Indeed, a great number of abusers do not appear to suffer from any serious mental disorder as defined by currently accepted diagnostic categories. Some experts have argued that preoccupation with the notion that abuse reflects psychopathology has diverted attention from underlying problems of poverty and family stress. Critics charge that by identifying the individual rather than society as the root of child maltreatment, efforts to combat abuse and neglect have been misdirected. Current approaches to treatment and prevention seem to take a middle ground in this debate, combining psychotherapeutic approaches with education, public awareness programs and support services.

In individual cases, severe mental illness of a caretaker may form the basis for temporary removal of a child from home. Parents who are prone to frequent psychotic breaks or deep depression may be unable to care for their children during these episodes. However, most forms of mental illness are cyclical, and parents are usually quite capable during periods of remission.

psychosocial deprivation See EMOTIONAL NEGLECT.

psychosocial dwarfism See DWARFISM.

puberty rites See INITIATION RITES.

punishment, corporal See CORPORAL PUNISHMENT.

purpura A purplish collection of petechiae less than one centimeter in diameter.
See also BRUISES.

Purtscher retinopathy This term refers to retinal hemorrhaging as a result of sudden compression of a child's chest. Pressure applied to the chest by hitting, grasping or shaking can produce Purtscher retinopathy without the additional intracranial bleeding that normally occurs in conjunction with ocular hemorrhaging.
See also EYE INJURIES.

radiology, pediatric   Documentation and development of the BATTERED CHILD SYNDROME owes a great deal to advances in pediatric radiology. As early as 1906 physicians began to study X-rays of infants. The first X-ray department in a children's hospital was established in 1926. Twenty years later John Caffey, a pediatric radiologist, published an article describing the joint occurrence of SUBDURAL HEMATOMAS and FRACTURES of the long bones in infants. Though he lacked confirming evidence, Caffey suggested that the injuries might have been the result of unreported child abuse. Subsequent findings by Caffey, Frederick Silverman (Stanford University) and others established a strong link between certain types of infant fracture and abuse. This phenomenon of multiple fractures in various stages of healing, accompanied by subdural hematomas, was subsequently called the PARENT-INFANT TRAUMATIC SYNDROME, the battered baby syndrome and the Caffey-Kempe syndrome.

In 1979, several papers were written on the use of the computed tomography (CT) scan in identifying injuries stemming from child abuse. Experts say that CT scans are especially effective in diagnosing abdominal injuries. CT scans can also detect liver, spleen, kidney, pancreatic and adrenal injuries caused by child abuse. Thoracic injuries caused by abuse may also be found using the CT scan.

Other diagnostic radiologic tools for child abuse are ultrasound and magnetic resonance imaging (MRI).

According to the authors of *Diagnostic Imaging and Child Abuse: Technologies, Practices and Guidelines,* some types of fractures are particularly likely to be caused by abuse. "These include metaphyseal 'chip' or 'bucket handle' fractures of the long bones, posterior and lateral rib fractures in infants, fractures of the acromion process and scapula, sternal frac-

tures and spinous process fractures. Fractures moderately specific for child abuse include compression fractures of the vertebrae, multiple fractures, fractures of different ages in the same child, epiphyseal separations, digital fractures, and complex skull fractures."

X-rays may be used as evidence in a courtroom trial and it is up to the judge to determine whether they are admissible or not. Experts say that in general, photographs, X-rays and the results of CT and MRI scans are admissible.

Telemedicine in Child Abuse Diagnosis

Some experts believe that remote assistance from physicians expert in diagnosing child abuse may play a part in assisting physicians in diagnosing children who may have been abused. For example, in Florida, Dr. J. M. Whitworth, professor of pediatrics at the University of Florida, assists physicians in detecting child abuse through a teleconferencing system which allows for microscopic examinations. Qualified physicians at participating sites in Florida conduct and send data to the University of Florida site. Experts hope that the system will be expanded to all counties in Florida.

"Diagnostic Imaging and Child Abuse: Technologies, Practices, and Guidelines." Medical Technology and Practice Patterns Institute, Washington, D.C., 1996.

rape   Though some writers refer to any unwanted sexual contact as rape, the term is most often understood to mean sexual attack involving penile penetration. Laws often distinguish two different types of rape: forcible and statutory. Forcible rape is defined by the combination of penetration, use of force or threat and nonconsent of the victim. Statutory rape involves sexual assault on a child under the age of consent. Since a child is not considered capable of giving informed consent to sexual relations prior to a specific, legally defined age, the use of force and the child's agreement are irrelevant in cases of statutory rape. The actual age at which a child may legally consent to sexual relations varies. In most locations, children may give legal consent at age 14 or 16.

Emergency assessment and treatment of child rape victims focuses on three separate areas: (1) treatment of physical and psychological trauma; (2) collection of evidence for legal prosecution; and (3) prevention of pregnancy and venereal disease. A thorough medical examination is standard procedure for rape victims. It is preferable that the physician be of the same sex as the victim. A trained counselor and/or supportive relative may also help put the child at ease. Virtually all rape victims can benefit from counseling or psychiatric services.

For subsequent legal prosecution, it is important that physical evidence be collected by a trained examiner as soon after the assault as possible. Many hospital emergency rooms have rape kits available for gathering legal evidence. Specimens are collected, labeled and sealed in the kit, usually a manila envelope or box. The sealed container is then given to the investigating police officer.

Specimens are taken from the vagina, mouth and anus and tested for evidence of sperm and/or gonorrhea. Serological tests for syphilis and HIV are also ordered. When the victim is of child-bearing age, a pregnancy test is also performed.

Rape is a criminal act and, as such, should be reported to law enforcement officials immediately. Reports to a child protection agency are necessary if the perpetrator is a family member or person living in the household or when there is reason to believe the child will not receive adequate treatment or protection.

Because of differing legal definitions of rape it is difficult to determine the number of children who are victimized. Reports of child sexual abuse often involve acts other than penetration. Further, some jurisdictions do not include male victims in their statistics. Incestuous rapes often go unreported.

Though some laws make a distinction between penetration and other acts of sexual assault, the psychological effects of such abuse may not be that different. Studies show that factors such as the level of violence involved, the relationship of the perpetrator to the victim and the period of time over which the abuse took place are more significant than the specific type of sexual act.

Statistics on Child Rape

According to data provided by the Bureau of Justice Statistics (BJS) in 1998, a self-report study of 14,000 state prisoners revealed that two-thirds of all sex offenders (for rape or sexual assault crimes) had victimized a child under the age of 18. In the majority of cases, the victims were age 12 and under.

The BJS also reported on a study of rapists and their victims based on FBI data for Alabama, North Dakota and South Carolina. Children under age 12 represented 15% of all rape victims of all ages. (Adults were included in the population of rape victims.) Twenty-nine percent of all rape victims of all ages were ages 12–17. In the cases of the youngest victims, the victim and offender knew each other in 90% of the cases. No racial differences were found; and blacks and whites were equally victimized.

A pattern of when rapes occurred was also revealed. In looking at specific times, a rape was most likely to occur between 8 P.M. on Friday and 8 A.M. on Saturday. As for the method of force, 5% of the rapists used a gun, 7% used a knife and 80% relied on their own physical force.

See also INCEST; SEXUAL ABUSE; STATUTORY RAPE.

"National Conference on Sex Offender Registries: Proceedings of a BJS/SEARCH Conference." Bureau of Justice Statistics, April 1998, NCJ-1 68965.

reactive parricide   See PARRICIDE, REACTIVE.

real evidence   See EVIDENCE.

reasonable doubt   See BEYOND A REASONABLE DOUBT.

receiving home When temporary PLACEMENT OF ABUSED CHILDREN is needed, a receiving home may be used. The home may be a family, a group home or shelter. Receiving homes are intended to provide temporary housing while more permanent plans are being made.

records, sealing of See SEALING OF RECORDS.

regressed offender The regressed offender represents one of two categories commonly used to describe male perpetrators of child SEXUAL ABUSE. Unlike the FIXATED OFFENDER, who has a long-standing preference for children, the regressed offender is primarily attracted to adults as sexual partners. He may continue to have relations with adults after he becomes sexually involved with children.

The psychosexual development of the regressed offender usually gives few indications of later sexual deviance. However, it appears that he may harbor strong doubts about his sexual adequacy. A particularly stressful situation or series of events, such as marital difficulty, a physical ailment or financial strain, may cause these doubts to resurface. As a way of coping with what he experiences as an overwhelming situation, the regressed offender engages in sexual activity with children, hoping to regain control. Sexual assault on children may be temporary or it may become a permanent regression to deviant behavior.

Though they usually express regret for their actions later, regressed offenders are often deeply depressed and may not think or care about the consequences of their behavior during the actual molestation.

religious aspects From time to time, questions arise as to whether certain religious practices constitute child abuse. Religious beliefs concerning punishment, child labor, medicine and sexuality may conflict with social norms of child rearing and, sometimes, with the law. Such conflicts usually pit parents' rights to raise their children according to their own beliefs against the state's duty to protect children.

The question of when to intervene in religiously motivated childrearing practices is often decided on a case-by-case basis. In the United States, where freedom of religion is guaranteed by the First Amendment, the Supreme Court has traditionally been reluctant to interfere with parents' religious practices. WISCONSIN V. YODER established the right of Amish parents to remove their children from school after the eighth grade. In PRINCE V. MASSACHUSETTS, the high court affirmed parents' right to require their children to engage in certain religious practices. Several medical neglect cases have affirmed the right of parents to withhold medical treatment on religious grounds in all but life-threatening circumstances.

Religious practices involving punishment or deprivation of children may constitute abuse. In such cases the actual and potential harm done to the child must be weighed against parents' rights and any possible benefits the child might derive from this type of religious training. Public agencies are most likely to intervene in situations where children are severely abused or neglected. Child protection workers are sometimes placed in the position of having to distinguish legitimate religiously based child-rearing practices from idiosyncratic abuse. Situations in which parents are responding to religious delusions or are not members of any recognized religious group are not considered to constitute grounds for special consideration. For example, Texas penal code in 1999 on this issue stated, "It is an affirmative defense to criminal injury to a child that an act or omission was based on treatment in accordance with the tenets and practices of a religious method of healing with a generally accepted record of efficacy."

Internationally, differing religious and cultural beliefs pose a significant problem for comparing childrearing practices of different nations. Attempts to launch an international campaign against child abuse have been hampered by disagreement over certain practices that have religious significance yet are considered abusive by most standards. Nevertheless, some practices such as genital mutilation have been widely condemned.

removal of child See DISPOSITION.

reparenting   Many parents who abuse or neglect their children did not receive adequate parenting during their own childhood. Reparenting is an attempt to intervene in the intergenerational cycle of abuse by providing parents with the nurturance and structure they missed in their early years. Parents are provided with a surrogate parent such as a PARENT AIDE who can provide the necessary emotional support while serving as a positive parenting role model. Through identification with appropriate role models, the abusive parents are able to become more effective in raising their own children.

reporting   Most countries now require reporting of suspected child abuse and neglect to law enforcement authorities or a child protection agency. In the United States, the CHILD ABUSE PREVENTION AND TREATMENT ACT, a federal law enacted in 1974, encouraged states to strengthen laws specifically requiring reporting of child abuse and neglect.

Reporters of suspected abuse or neglect are usually asked to supply the name and address of the child, the parents' names and addresses, the type and extent of injuries suffered, any evidence of previous abuse and information that may lead to the identification of the perpetrator. In most areas, reports can be filed anonymously. Others require that the reporter identify him/herself to the agency receiving the report but withhold the reporter's name from the accused perpetrator.

To facilitate prompt investigation of life-threatening situations, most laws allow initial reports to be made verbally. MANDATED REPORTERS are usually required to file a full written report within a certain period of time. Many jurisdictions have established toll-free 24-hour HOTLINES to facilitate reporting. In addition, to these local services there are two hotlines that serve the entire United States.

Reporting laws usually require or specifically permit certain professionals to report cases of suspected maltreatment to the agency charged with investigation. In many jurisdictions, anyone who has reason to suspect that a child is being abused or neglected is legally obligated to report. About 50% of all reports of child abuse and neglect are made by friends, relatives or neighbors. Mandated reporters are usually granted immunity from civil

---

BASIC ELEMENTS OF REPORTING LAWS

- Who is required to report
- What should be reported
- Where or to whom it should be reported
- How much evidence is necessary to trigger a report
- Penalties for failure to report
- Immunity from prosecution for "good faith" reports
- Suspension of privileged communication laws

---

or criminal prosecution for reports made in good faith. Penalties, ranging from a small fine to imprisonment, are often imposed on mandated reporters who fail to report suspected abuse or neglect.

While reporting laws are usually clear about who is required to report suspected maltreatment, they are often vague about exactly what kinds of injuries/behavior should be reported. Many local statutes define abuse and neglect in broad terms or not at all. Conditions specifically mentioned range from serious physical injuries to vaguely defined MENTAL INJURIES and NEGLECT.

In Canada, Britain and the United States, lack of specificity in the types of injuries that should be reported has sometimes led to charges of frivolous reporting. Some critics believe that failure to define clearly abuse and neglect overburdens child protection agencies and causes some families to be subjected to needless invasions of privacy. Proponents of present laws argue that a broad definition of abuse and neglect is necessary to cover all situations that might seriously harm a child. This view holds that it is better to tolerate some overreporting than to run the risk of failing to identify children in need of help.

res gestae   See EXCITED UTTERANCE.

resilience of abused children   Experts say that some children are more resilient in the face of abuse than others, including children who have been severely abused. Factors affecting resilience appear to include

- The temperament of child (easygoing children are more resilient)

- The ability to avoid abusive parents and "make themselves invisible"
- Whether children have another adult or adults who they can rely upon
- An ability to separate the abuse from themselves and not blame themselves for the abuse

Interestingly, the factors that enable a child to adapt to an abusive environment can also make it difficult in some cases for the child to adapt to an adoptive family or to a nonabusive environment. Tactics that worked well in the abusive home, such as avoidance of a parent, lying when necessary to avoid abuse, emotional detachment and other reactions, may be seen as maladaptive in the adoptive home. Experts say that new adoptive parents should realize that the child needs to learn that the survival strategies that worked well for him or her in the past are not necessary and are a hindrance in a healthy family.

res ipsa loquitur   This legal doctrine is borrowed from the evidentiary law of negligence. It is invoked in child abuse or neglect cases and permits use of circumstantial evidence. This admissible evidence only infers that abuse or neglect has occurred, but as the term implies, "the thing speaks for itself." Evidence of this sort presented to the court includes, for example, medical reports or X-rays detailing the condition of a suspected victim of abuse or neglect.

See also EVIDENTIARY STANDARDS.

retardation   See MENTAL RETARDATION.

retinal hemorrhage   A blow to the body causes blood to rush out of the impacted area into surrounding vessels. This rapid increase in pressure causes capillaries to rupture. A blow to the head or chest causes small clots to form inside of or in front of the retina. Evidence of these hemorrhages remains present for up to two weeks.

Since retinal hemorrhages are often caused by head trauma, the child should also be examined for the presence of SUBDURAL HEMATOMA.

reversible growth failure   See DWARFISM.

reversible hyposomatotropic dwarfism   See DWARFISM.

rickets   Lack of sufficient quantities of vitamin D causes rickets, a condition that disturbs the normal development of bones. Rickets may occur as a result of nutritional neglect.

See also NEGLECT.

role reversal   Parents who abuse or neglect their children often have unrealistically high expectations for their behavior. Sometimes these parents engage in a reversal of roles in which the child becomes the comforter and caretaker of the parent while the parent largely ignores his or her parental responsibilities. Evidence of role reversal may be seen in young children who demonstrate a kind of PSEUDOMATURITY, shouldering responsibilities normally assumed by much older children or adults. Parents, on the other hand, may be unable to give emotional support and direction.

Role reversal may also be seen in cases of INCEST. The child assumes the role of sexual partner to the parent and, frequently, takes on other responsibilities normally performed by the spouse. Being forced prematurely to act as an adult, the child is denied the opportunity to follow the normal pattern of maturation. The child's own developmental needs are suppressed, leading to what is often referred to as the loss of childhood.

Some mental health experts speculate that parents may be repeating their own childhood in which they assumed a parental role. An alternate explanation is that parents who, as children, were not required to accept responsibility and were protected from the consequences of their actions are, as adults, unable to function maturely. It is likely that both types of childhood experience can contribute to role reversal; however, different treatment approaches might be taken depending upon the parent's specific developmental deficit.

See also PARENTIFIED CHILD.

runaways Studies of children and adolescents who run away from home show that many are running away from abuse. One study of runaway youths found that 73% of females and 38% of males reported having been abused. A 1998 study of 26 teenage runaways living in a New England shelter revealed that most reported that they left their homes only as a last resort and after having been physically, sexually or emotionally abused.

Ironically, some teenagers may actually increase their chances of abuse by leaving home. Runaways are often easy prey for adults seeking to lure them into prostitution. Unable to secure a job that pays enough to support them, both males and females are enticed by the promise of large sums of money in exchange for engaging in illicit activities. In addition to sexual exploitation, youths living on the streets are often robbed or assaulted. Most runaways do not live far from home, and several studies have revealed that the wide majority reside less than 100 miles from their families.

See also ADOLESCENT ABUSE; SEXUAL ABUSE; THROWAWAY CHILDREN.

McCormack, Arlene, Mark-David Janus, and Ann Wolbert Burgess. "Runaway Youths and Sexual Victimization: Gender Differences in an Adolescent Runaway Population." *Child Abuse and Neglect* 10 (1986): 387–395.

Schaffner, Laurie. "Searching for Connection: A New Look at Teenaged Runaways." *Adolescence* 33 (Fall 1998): 619–627.

sadism   Sadism is a relatively rare form of sexual perversion in which sexual gratification is derived by hurting or humiliating another person. Though assaults involving sadism comprise a very small proportion of all child SEXUAL ABUSE, highly publicized accounts of MYSOPEDIC OFFENDERS have led to a public misconception concerning their prevalence.

The overwhelming majority of sadistic sexual offenses are committed by men. When sadistic assaults occur they are likely to result in physical injury or, in extreme cases, death. Sexual pleasure is derived from the victim's visible suffering. The sadist usually exerts much greater force than would be necessary to overpower the child. Though usually described as a sexual offense, sadism actually combines physical, psychological and sexual abuse.

Some psychodynamically oriented therapists have explained sadism as a PROJECTION of the attacker's own self-hatred. By punishing the child the perpetrator symbolically punishes himself.

scalds   The most frequent type of abusive BURNS of children is a wet burn, or scald. Over one-fourth of all reported scalds can be likened to abuse. Most nonaccidental scalds are caused by overheated tap water. At 130 degrees Fahrenheit, a full thickness scald can occur on an adult in 30 seconds; at 150 degrees in two seconds. A child's thin skin burns even more quickly.

Abusive scalds often have different patterns than accidental scalds. Forcing a child to sit in a bathtub of hot water may result in a "donut burn," where the center of the buttocks is protected by the relative coolness of the tub while the surrounding area is burned. Glove or stocking burns are most likely to result from the hand or foot being forcibly held in hot water. When scalds are caused by splash-ing, careful observation of burn marks can reveal the direction from which the hot liquid came. This evidence should be compared to the caretaker's account for inconsistencies.

A study of scald victims revealed that 71% of the cases in which the child was brought to treatment by someone other than the primary caretaker were the result of abuse. Of children whose treatment was delayed two hours or more, 70% were found to be victims of abusive burns.

See also BURNS.

scapegoating   In abusive families, often one child in a family is singled out as the recipient of the most abuse. Reasons for this type of selection are complex and varied. Usually scapegoating begins at a very early age, sometimes at birth. Infants who are irritable, colicky and who do not respond well to parental nurturing may become targets for abuse. Premature infants are more likely to become scapegoats than those carried to full term.

Scapegoating is frequently described as an interactive process in which the child's physical, social or psychological characteristics combine with those of the parent to increase the likelihood of abuse. Children perceived as difficult, unresponsive or hyperactive are at risk. Other traits can include psychological impairment, learning disabilities, physical defects or chronic illness.

Caretakers of scapegoated children range from normally capable persons under stress to those with severe PSYCHOPATHOLOGY. Parents may perceive a particular child as reflecting their own defects or inadequacies. In such situations the parent's self-hatred is misdirected toward the child. The child has become a symbol of all the parent dislikes in him or herself.

Maltreatment by caretakers is quickly internalized by children. Scapegoated children come to have low self-esteem and see themselves as bad and deserving of punishment. As they grow older many of these children actually seek punishment by acting out at home or in school. They may also invite abuse from peers by taunting and provoking them. Because the children see themselves as deserving of abuse they offer only token self-defense when they are subsequently attacked.

As they grow older, victims of severe scapegoating continue to have difficulty in establishing close relationships with peers, teachers and others. Prolonged treatment is often required to help these children develop a capacity for displaying warmth toward themselves and others.

scurvy   Scurvy, a result of vitamin C deficiency, increases susceptibility to bruising and is often mistaken for BATTERED CHILD SYNDROME. Conversely, many cases of child battering were misdiagnosed as scurvy during the late 19th and early 20th centuries by physicians who failed to consider the possibility of abuse or who wished to protect the parents.

sealing of records   Many jurisdictions require a court order to examine criminal records of youthful offenders. Such records are considered "sealed."

Sealing of records is a controversial issue. Many youth advocates believe that by restricting access to court records adolescents will be protected from negative labeling and discrimination in school or in later employment. Others believe sealing makes it difficult to identify serious offenders who pose a threat to society. When the youthful offender has a history of abusing other children, sealing of criminal records may prevent parents, school officials and law enforcement officers from taking steps to protect younger children adequately.

Under certain circumstances records of adult offenders may be sealed or expunged. While sealing of adult records is less common, many of the same arguments, for and against, apply.

secondary prevention   See PREVENTION.

secrecy   SEXUAL ABUSE that continues for an extended period of time usually involves an element of secrecy. The abuser may bribe or coerce the victim not to tell about their encounters. Children themselves may maintain secrecy about abuse due to embarrassment, fear of being punished, fear of parental rejection or abandonment or, in the case of very young children, simply because they do not have sufficient verbal capacity to explain the problem. Some therapists speculate that enforced silence may be related to later development of nonverbal means of coping with stress, such as SUBSTANCE ABUSE, withdrawal or depression.

In cases of INCEST, secrecy may extend to other members of the family. Often the mother is accused of being a PASSIVE ABUSER, silently condoning sexual activity between the father and a child. Reasons for this phenomenon are complex and not fully understood. The mother may tacitly encourage the child to act as a substitute in order to avoid sexual relations with the father. In other cases, she may fear abandonment or reprisal.

Failure to report known abuse not only makes one a silent partner to maltreatment but also increases the harm to the child. Studies suggest that psychological damage from abuse is related to the length of time the child was abused.

seductive behavior   Seductive or inappropriate sexual behavior toward an adult may be a sign that a child has been sexually abused (see SEXUAL ABUSE). Sexually victimized children often learn that in order to gain the attention or affection of an adult they must appeal to them sexually. Such behavior, once learned, may be directed toward adults other than the abuser, increasing the risk of further abuse.

Seductive behavior may range from overly affectionate kissing, stroking, massaging etc. to overt sexual advances such as fondling the genitals or making sexual comments. Children who act seductively toward adults are often blamed for initiating sexual activity with them. Claims of seduction by a child have frequently been introduced in court as a defense against charges of child molestation. Others cite this apparent sexual aggressiveness as evidence that children enjoy sex with adults. Such claims notwithstanding, sexual relations between an adult and a child are considered to be an abusive act on the part of the adult and are outlawed in the United States and most countries around the world.

Experts in the treatment of child sexual abuse stress that seductive behavior on the part of children is learned from adults. The child who feels unloved may find that this is the only way to get the affection he or she craves. Starved for affection, the child may interpret sexual exploitation by an adult as genuine affection. As the child grows older, sexual submissiveness often gives way to intense anger toward the adult and/or self-loathing often manifesting itself in depression and SELF-DESTRUCTIVE BEHAVIOR.

self-destructive behavior In the general population, self-destructive acts by children are rare. Among neglected, and especially abused, children the incidence of such behavior is much higher. Studies have shown that up to 40% of abused children exhibited self-destructive tendencies compared with 2% of children with no history of abuse or neglect.

Abused children are more likely to engage in a range of harmful activities, including provocative acts designed to elicit punishment, accident proneness and suicide attempts. Self-destructive acts usually follow parental beatings or separation from the parent—real or threatened.

Neglected children display two to three times the amount of self-harming behavior as their peers who have not experienced abuse or neglect. Physically and sexually abused victims are even more likely than neglected children to exhibit this behavior—eight to 10 times more. Though neglected children share many of the same negative environmental conditions suffered by abused children, they are less likely to be subjected to physical violence and SCAPEGOATING.

Children who are punished frequently and brutally will assume they are bad and deserving of punishment. They often cannot connect the punishment with any specific behavior and consequently develop a general sense of self-hatred, unworthiness

and low SELF-ESTEEM. These feelings form the basis of later aggressive and self-destructive behavior.

See also ADULTS ABUSED AS CHILDREN.

self-esteem Feelings of low self-worth are often cited as both the cause and result of child abuse. Several psychiatric studies of abusive parents have found them to have unusually negative images of themselves. Many clinicians and researchers believe parents' low self-esteem can be attributed to abusive or neglectful treatment they received as children. These parents may project their feelings onto children by constantly punishing or degrading them (see PROJECTION). In turn, their children may grow up to be abusive parents.

Building self-esteem is often one of the most important goals in the treatment of abusers. In some cases, treatment may involve a process known as REPARENTING, in which parents receive instruction and nurturance from a trained older adult. In a sense, the parents take on another parent who can give the positive feedback and modeling they did not receive as children.

Abused children often develop a distorted view of themselves, seeing virtually everything they do as bad. Parental abuse and neglect is interpreted by the child as confirmation of perceived badness. Many children become so invested in this negative self-image that they stubbornly resist the efforts of therapists, foster parents and others to change this false view. For this reason, long-term psychotherapeutic treatment of abused children is sometimes necessary to eliminate this distorted sense of self.

self-help groups The number of people involved in self-help groups has grown dramatically since the 1950s. Alcoholics Anonymous, perhaps the most famous self-help organization, has thousands of groups around the world. Many mutual aid groups have patterned themselves after AA's 12-step program. Others are less structured, simply providing a forum for people with similar concerns to share experiences and emotional support.

The characteristic that distinguishes self-help from other educational groups is the degree of responsibility exercised by members. Self-help groups are totally controlled by their members.

Parents Anonymous is the largest organization of groups for parents who abuse their children. Several groups for victims of sexual abuse have formed since the late 1970s.

Self-help has proven effective in helping parents who want to control abusive impulses. Members often make themselves available to one another in times of crisis, serving as a safety valve for explosive emotions. A desire to change is essential for members of self-help groups. Though child abuse agencies often refer parents to such groups, membership is voluntary.

Groups also serve an important educational function. Parents learn coping skills from others with similar experiences. Victims of sexual abuse often learn they are not alone in their feelings of low self-esteem, guilt or similar reactions.

Though self-help groups can be very effective they are not for everyone. Abusers who are not motivated to change may need more structured assistance. In some cases, specialized treatment is necessary in addition to participation in a self-help group.

self-incrimination   See MIRANDA WARNINGS.

sentencing   The final phase of a criminal trial is pronouncement of the judge's order of punishment for a convicted defendant. Persons convicted of criminal charges related to child abuse or neglect may be imprisoned, fined or placed on probation. Actual sentences vary widely and depend on several factors, including local statutes, whether the crime is classed as a FELONY or MISDEMEANOR and the severity of the act. Sentencing occurs only in criminal trials and does not directly involve victims of maltreatment. The corresponding phase of civil court proceedings is the DISPOSITION.

sequelae   Children suffer many consequences of abuse and neglect. Aftereffects of maltreatment are sometimes referred to collectively as *sequelae*. The most obvious effects of abuse are physical trauma such as cuts, bruises or broken bones. Less apparent results of abuse include psychological harm, internal physical injuries such as brain damage, or impaired growth. Victims of sexual abuse may experience extreme feelings of low self-worth, sexual dysfunction in adulthood, an inability to trust others and similar sequelae of exploitation.

Aftereffects of abuse may appear as a delayed reaction many years after the traumatic incident. While some pedophiles (see PEDOPHILIA) argue that sex with children is not harmful, reports of adults who were sexually victimized as children indicate that the experience can have severe and long-lasting consequences.

Protection of children from further abuse, while essential, does not address the consequences of previous abuse. Treatment of psychological damage is often a time-consuming and expensive process. If left untreated, victims of abuse may continue to suffer from the aftereffects of abuse and may grow up to become abusers themselves.

See also NEGLECT; PSYCHOLOGICAL/EMOTIONAL MALTREATMENT; PHYSICAL ABUSE; SEXUAL ABUSE.

service plan   After completion of an ASSESSMENT, the child protection worker develops a plan for addressing specific problems and creating a safe environment for the abused child. The service plan (sometimes called a case plan) is often developed with the assistance of a MULTIDISCIPLINARY TEAM. If feasible, the abused child and his or her family is also involved in the planning process.

The first step in developing a service plan is setting realistic goals for the child and family. Treatment or service goals correspond directly to specific problems identified in the assessment. Goals may be described as proposed solutions to these problems. Some service plans make a distinction between short- and long-term goals.

Next in the planning process is the creation of measurable, time-limited objectives. Objectives are the standards by which progress toward identified goals can be monitored. Another way of viewing objectives is as a set of specific actions that must be taken to achieve a particular goal.

The final phase of service planning involves identifying and selecting the kinds of help the child and family will need in order to achieve the service goals. A wide range of services may be required to achieve the desired goals. Some examples of assistance that can be included in the service plan are: CATEGORICAL AID; HOMEMAKER SERVICES or PARENT AIDES; individual, family or marital counseling; temporary FOSTER CARE; and legal aid.

Service plans that set reasonable goals and have the family's support are the most likely to succeed. Families who are actively involved in the planning process usually have more confidence in the plan and tend to cooperate more fully in its implementation.

sex offenders, convicted Individuals who have been convicted in a court of the crime of sexually abusing children and adolescents. Sexual abuse can be defined as having engaged in unsolicited acts such as sexual fondling, sexual talk and sexual intercourse. (Each state has its own laws on how sexual abuse of a minor is defined. See APPENDIX VI for more information on state laws.) Once convicted of a sex crime, these individuals are required in all states to register with the state registry as a sex offender.

Some convicted sex offenders are adolescents, and they may be considered juveniles under the law, obtaining a lesser sentence than an adult would receive for the same crime. In such cases, they may *not* be required to register with the state as sex offender, even when the offense was severe, as with rape. This issue has caused considerable distress among the families of children who were abused and traumatized by adolescent sex offenders.

In 2005, according to the National Center for Missing & Exploited Children, there were 563,806 registered sex offenders in the United States. Some experts believe that sex offender registration should provide additional information on the nature and extent of the past crime(s) of the perpetrator, to avoid panic among the population that all sex offenders are aggressive and even homicidal. Others disagree that details of the types of crime are needed.

Some individuals and organizations believe that a federal database of all registered sex offenders in the United States, available through the Internet, would provide significantly more protection to families and children than only a state-by-state system database. The reason for this is that sex offenders may simply move to another state, where there is no record of their crimes and where they may continue to prey on children in the new location.

Even if the sex offender remains in the state where he committed the crime(s), it is believed (and is logical to assume) that the most dangerous sexual predators are the *least* compliant with state laws, and in many states, the burden for registration or of the notification of a move to another location (and other requirements) lies with the perpetrator. Dangerous and repeated child predators are unlikely to comply with such requirements.

Perpetrators are more likely than others to have been sexually victimized as children themselves; however, sexual victimization in children does not mean that the victimized child will grow up to become a sex offender. Individuals who are taking drugs, particularly cocaine or methamphetamine, have an increased risk for sexually abusing children. It should be noted that most sex offenders are known to children, such as family friends or neighbors. Few sexual assaults are committed by strangers to the child.

Most research on sex offenders has used information on males who were incarcerated for sex offenses. Based on such research, some "fixated" offenders are aroused exclusively by children, whom they seek out as sexual partners, while others ("regressed offenders") have sexual relations with both adults and children. It is believed that among the group who is also sexually aroused by adults, it is only when they feel threatened by an adult or do not have access to an adult sexual partner that these type of sex offenders may turn to children for their sexual gratification. However, a common motive of *all* sex offenders is a need for intimacy, power or control.

Said Cynthia Crosson-Tower in her book, *Understanding Child Abuse and Neglect*, the fixated offender "has failed to develop normally; he sees himself as a child and finds no gratification in the accomplishment of adult tasks. As children, these perpetrators' needs were unmet, and having lost faith in adults they now look to children to meet their dependency and nurturing needs. They find themselves at ease with children and become 'sexually addicted' to them."

In contrast, said Crosson-Tower, the regressed pedophile "is often married, and, in fact, may prefer an adult partner if she validates his need to feel adequate. When relationships with peers are too conflictual, he chooses children. Frequently the onset of his molestation behavior can be traced to a crisis in his life. His relationship with a child becomes an impulsive act that underlies his desperate need to cope." According to Crosson-Tower, the regressed offender may abuse children less often than the fixated offender. She noted "If their [the regressed offenders' lives] are relatively conflict free, the abusers may act only infrequently."

Though research on recidivism (repeat crimes) is fragmentary and inconclusive, many experts view the child sexual offender as particularly resistant to any treatment, and some believe that they are altogether untreatable. Others disagree, and they actively seek treatment for sex offenders.

Some male sex offenders agree to chemical CAS-TRATION, in which they are given medications to suppress their testosterone levels. In some cases, this treatment may be court-ordered. Surgical castration is considered too harsh a punishment to impose; however, some sex offenders have willingly undergone surgical castration to decrease or eliminate their sexual urges toward children.

Sex offenders who have assaulted a large number of children are generally thought to be less likely to benefit from treatment than offenders who have a less extensive history of the sexual abuse of children.

Male Sex Offenders

Most convicted sex offenders are males. Some sex offenders abuse children in their own or extended family, while others abuse children and adolescents from outside their family. Some sex offenders abuse children as young as infants and toddlers, such as very young children in their own family or extended family. (See INCEST.) Others assault non-related children whom they may be babysitting or with whom they have another association, such as being a coach, teacher, member of the clergy or another individual.

Female Sex Offenders

Some women are arrested and incarcerated for sex offenses against children, such as female teachers who sexually abused students. In some cases, females who sexually offend children, particularly adolescent males, receive a significantly more lenient sentence than male sex offenders receive for the same crime. This disparity is explained at least in part by the societal perception that sexual abuse against young teenage girls by adult males is much worse than sexual abuse of young teenage boys by adult females. Yet studies have shown that young teenage boys who have engaged in sexual acts with adult women suffer a significant risk of depression and other problems in adulthood.

Very few women have been required to undergo civil commitment, in which they are confined to a hospital, jail or other institution because they are a major risk for sexually abusing children if they are released into the community.

Types of female sex offenders According to a chapter in *Child Sexual Abuse* (Thomson Gale, 2005), there are three primary types of female sex offenders. First, is the "teacher-lover," who enjoys sex with underage boys, some as young as 12 or younger. She perceives herself as a "Mrs. Robinson" type of character and often imagines herself in love with the boy. As a result, this type of sex offender does not see her behavior as harmful. Many women who fit this category also have a SUB-STANCE ABUSE problem.

The second type primarily sexually abuses her own children, particularly daughters. However, some sex-offending women abuse other children, often children that they are babysitting. These women may be pedophiles, or they may be sadists. In one case, a female sex offender abused small children who were not yet verbal, slapping them until their nose bled or their teeth cut their mouth. These actions gave the offender sexual pleasure. This behavior was stopped when the woman abused a four-year-old child who reported the abuse to others.

The third type of female sex offender is the "male-coerced" or "male-accompanied" offender. This type sexually abuses children in the company of men.

Some female offenders provide alcohol or drugs to their victims before molesting them. It is also true that many male sex offenders use drugs or alcohol to help them seduce their child victims.

Registration of Sex Offenders

Whether sex offenders are males or females, nearly all must register as sex offenders. Each state has its own laws on how to handle sex offenders. In general, sex offenders may not work with children in any capacity, and thus they may not get jobs driving a school bus, working in the school cafeteria, teaching children under age 18, and so forth. If the sex offender relocates, he or she must inform law enforcement authorities in the new location of his or her sex-offender status and also provide new contact information. Sex offenders are generally banned from living near any areas where children congregate, such as schools, parks, playgrounds and other locations.

See ABUSERS; ADULTS ABUSED AS CHILDREN; CENTRAL REGISTRY; CIVIL COMMITMENT LAWS; CLERGY, ABUSE BY; MEGAN'S LAW; PEDOPHILIA; SEXUAL ABUSE.

Crosson-Tower, Cynthia. *Understanding Child Abuse and Neglect.* Boston: Allyn and Bacon, 2005.
Dolan, Maura. "Child Sexual Abuse by Females Is a Growing Problem." In *Child Sexual Abuse.* Detroit, Mich.: Greenhaven Press, 2005, pp. 96–103.

sexual abuse   A form of maltreatment that refers to the involvement of a child in sexual activity with an adult that provides a psychological, sexual and/or financial benefit to the perpetrator. Sexual abuse may also be committed by a person *under* the age of 18 when that person is either significantly older than the victim or when the perpetrator is in a position of power or control over another child. About 1.2% of children in the United States were sexually abused in 2003, according to *Child Maltreatment 2003*, an annual federal report. In some cases, sexual abuse is perpetrated by a highly trusted individual, such as a member of the clergy.

Sexual abuse is predominantly a male crime. Ninety percent of all child sexual molestation is committed by men, and 95% of female victims are victimized by men. Men are responsible for approximately 80% of all sexual abuse of boys. Both boys and girls who are sexually abused experience a significantly greater risk for substance abuse, depression and suicide in adulthood.

Sexual abuse includes molestation, STATUTORY RAPE, CHILD PROSTITUTION, CHILD PORNOGRAPHY, sexual exposure, INCEST and other sexually exploitative activities. Sexual abuse does not necessarily include intercourse but usually does include some sexual touching. (One exception is sexual talk over the Internet or on the cell phone or home phone, for the purpose of sexually arousing the perpetrator. Often this behavior ultimately leads to direct sexual contact.)

The greater percentages of sexual abuse are not perpetrated by parents. Of parental abusers committing all types of abusive acts against children, less than 3% commit sexual abuse. Among others who commit any form of child abuse, the highest percentage of sex abusers are friends and neighbors; of friends and neighbors who maltreat children in some way, nearly 76% are sex abusers. Among abusive relatives who are not parents, nearly 30% commit sexual abuse. (See Table I.)

Incidence of Sexual Abuse

According to the Administration on Children, Youth and Families in *Child Maltreatment 2003*, a total of 906,000 children were abused in 2003, and of this number, about 10% of the children were sexually abused. Most children (60%) were neglected, while about 20% were physically abused and 5% were emotionally maltreated. About 17% of the children had a finding of "other," such as ABANDONMENT, congenital drug addiction or other state categories of maltreatment. (Note that some children were maltreated in several different categories.)

Specific examples of forms of sexual abuse are included in the chart.

Disclosure of Abuse by Children

Many parents refuse to believe that a family member or another person they know could actually commit an act of sexual abuse. In a study of 384 adults (reported in a 1999 issue of *Child Welfare*) who had been physically, sexually or emotionally abused by family members as children, in most cases the disclosure of the abuse to a family member did

TABLE I
PHYSICAL ABUSE, NEGLECT AND SEXUAL ABUSE OF CHILD VICTIMS OF MALTREATMENT, 2003,
BY PERCENTAGE AMONG DIFFERENT CATEGORIES OF CHILD ABUSERS

	Parent	Other relative	Foster parent	Residential facility staff	Child day-care provider	Unmarried partner of parent	Friend or neighbor
Physical abuse only	11.0	10.4	16.9	19.0	12.9	16.6	3.4
Neglect only	62.0	37.5	50.0	46.3	48.4	37.0	9.7
Sexual abuse only	2.7	29.9	6.3	11.5	23.0	11.5	75.9
Psychological maltreatment only, other only or unknown only	9.1	5.8	7.3	8.4	2.5	14.4	2.7
Multiple maltreatments	15.2	16.4	19.6	14.7	13.1	19.6	8.3
Total percent	100.0	100.0	100.0	100.0	100.0	100.0	100.0

Source: Adapted from Administration on Children, Youth and Families, *Child Maltreatment 2003.* Children's Bureau, U.S. Department of Health and Human Services, Washington, D.C., 2005, page 68.

not end the abuse. Of 249 cases of disclosure, 60% of the respondents said that the abuse continued. Even worse, 20% said that the abuse accelerated after the disclosure. Fifteen percent said that the abuse temporarily abated, and only 5% said that the abuse stopped altogether after they revealed the abuse to a family member.

Individuals who disclosed abuse said family members either ignored the information or responded ineffectually. Others said that they were blamed or not believed and that the parent sided with the abuser. In one case, an adult disclosed severe physical abuse to a school nurse, who refused to provide any help. One individual told the family doctor, who reported the information to the parents rather than to child welfare authorities or the police.

It is hoped that today's MANDATED REPORTER laws help to prevent school nurses and physicians from shirking their responsibility to report suspected abuse to PROTECTIVE SERVICE staff. However, in one study in *Ambulatory Pediatrics* in 2005, of pediatricians who reported child abuse, many were reluctant to talk to protective service staff, particularly if they had ever been sued before for reporting child abuse.

Of the adults in the study who said that they had reported their disclosure of the abuse in childhood to adults, they reported that the adults most likely to believe them were as follows: friends or neighbors (91%), a nonparent relative (89%), mothers (61%) and professionals or officials (50%).

Child and Adolescent Reactions to Sexual Abuse

Children differ in their reactions to sexual abuse. Clinical and empirical studies indicate that sexually victimized children are more likely to be fearful, anxious, depressed, angry and hostile than non-abused

---

TYPE OF CHILD SEXUAL ABUSE

- Anal intercourse
- Anilingus—oral contact with the anus
- Cunnilingus—oral contact with the female genitals
- Encouraging a child to engage in sexual activity with other children for the benefit of an adult
- Child's caretaker is involved in prostitution
- Exhibitionism—deliberate display of the genitals to a child, usually for the sexual gratification of the perpetrator
- Fellatio—oral contact with the male genitals
- Forcing or encouraging a child to touch an adult's genitals
- Genital intercourse—without force
- Genital touching—including clothed and unclothed touching, fondling of the male or female genitals
- Intentional sexual touching of the breasts, buttocks or thigh, clothed or unclothed
- Rape—forceful genital intercourse
- Sexual intercourse between adults in the presence of a child
- Sexual kissing
- Taking sexually explicit photographs of a child

children. Of these children, 20% to 40% show signs of significant emotional disturbance following the abuse. Child victims sometimes exhibit inappropriate sexual behavior as a result of the abuse.

Excessive sexual curiosity, open masturbation and exposure of the genitals are frequently observed in young victims of sexual abuse. Older children and adolescents may become promiscuous or display inappropriately seductive behavior toward adults, and they are at greater risk of delinquency. Young girls and older boys seem to be the most seriously affected by this type of abuse.

Children often feel extremely guilty about their involvement in sexual abuse. Even in cases where there has been a brutal assault, a child may feel that she or he was in some way responsible for or deserving of the abuse. The abuser may have told the child that the sexual relationship was the child's fault or may have told the child that the behavior was normal, contrary to what the child suspects or later learns. The child may then perceive himself or herself as a bad person with a secret.

Guilty feelings are almost universal among incest victims should their parents get a divorce, and they often feel personally responsible for the breakup of their parents' marriage. It is important for family members and therapists to tell abused children that the marital breakdown was *not* the child's fault in any way and that the abuser was entirely at fault.

Conversely, some incest victims perceive themselves as holding the family together by preventing a divorce. In such cases, for example, the abused daughter may become, in effect, a surrogate wife filling a role that the mother is unable or unwilling to play (see ROLE REVERSAL). Guilt can also appear as a by-product of the confusing and often contradictory feelings of children who were abused by incestuous contact with a family member.

Though sexual contact is frequently painful and frightening for a child, there is sometimes an element of pleasure in such contact. A child may enjoy the exclusive and deceptively warm attention of an adult, especially when he or she feels unloved or unworthy of love. Having taken any enjoyment in sexual acts can be a source of intense guilt for the child, which is experienced long after the abuse has stopped.

Demographics of Sexually Abused Children

White children (about 9%) are most at risk for sexual abuse, followed by Hispanic children (7%). Most research indicates that girls are at a much greater risk for sexual abuse than boys; however, a retrospective study published in the *American Journal of Preventive Medicine* in 2005 challenged that premise, in a large study in which childhood sexual abuse was reported by 25% of females and 16% of males.

Risk Factors

Studies have identified several factors that may place some children at greater risk than others.

Dysfunctional families Marital conflict, separation and divorce were found to be more prevalent in the families of sexually abused girls. Specifically, these girls were more likely to have lived *without* their natural father and more likely to have lived *with* a stepfather. Mothers of victimized girls were more likely to have been employed outside the home or to be ill or disabled.

In contrast, studies have shown that victimized boys were more likely than their female counterparts to come from an impoverished environment, to be physically abused as well as sexually abused and to suffer their abuse at the hands of someone outside the family. Some experts believe sexual abuse of boys is less likely to be reported than abuse involving girls.

Social Isolation

Another factor associated with sexually abused children is social isolation. These children often have fewer friends than their peers and may be isolated in other ways as well. It is not clear, however, whether this phenomenon is a contributing factor or a result of abuse.

Emotional issues

Clinical evidence indicates that abuse victims are often depressed and withdrawn. Sexually victimized children also tend to report, more often than their peers, a poor relationship with their parents. Mothers are most frequently reported as the parent with whom the relationship is most strained. The absence of the mother greatly increases the risk to girls. Those living without their mothers are three times more likely to suffer sexual abuse than those whose mothers are present.

Sexually Abused Runaways

In an effort to avoid further sexual and/or physical abuse, many abused adolescents run away from home. Ironically, these teens may actually increase their likelihood of being sexually abused. A study of runaways in a Canadian shelter found that 71% of female and 38% of male runaways had been sexually victimized. The authors speculated that much of the abuse occurred *after* the child left home. Adolescents or children living on the streets are particularly vulnerable to sexual assault and may, in desperation, turn to CHILD PROSTITUTION as a means of financial support and survival.

Impact of Childhood Sexual Abuse

Ohene et al. studied sexual abuse and the impact of the child's age at the time of the abuse, reporting on their findings in a 2005 issue of *Sexually Transmitted Diseases*. Based on 2,175 adolescent subjects, 311 teenagers reported a history of current or past sexual abuse. About half of the adolescents were sexually abused at or younger than the age of 10. The researcher found that abuse at or before the age of 10 was also associated with a greater number of lifetime and recent sexual partners. Also, the odds of contracting a sexually transmitted disease in adolescence were 2.5 times greater when sexual abuse occurred before age 10.

In another study of childhood sexual abuse, published in the *American Journal of Public Health* in 2005, the researchers studied the age at first injection among injection drug users, and they found that childhood sexual abuse was associated with an earlier initiation of injection drug use. The majority (63%) of the subjects were male. In this study, 5.4% had been forced to have sex before age 13, and 7.2% were compelled to have sex between the ages of 13 and 17.

Said the researchers, "Although further investigation is needed to fully elucidate the association between sexual abuse and the initiation of substance use, we can conclude that childhood sexual abuse is strongly associated with early initiating of injection drug use and vulnerability to HIV infection among these young injection drug users. Furthermore, we observed, as have other researchers, that sexual abuse is associated with higher rates of trading sex for money or drugs. Whether or not the relation between sexual abuse and the initiation of injection drug use is causal, childhood sexual abuse can be considered a valuable marker of risk for behaviors that comprise the health of young adults."

Perpetrators of Sexual Abuse

About 70% of sexual abusers are known to children before the abuse takes place. (See ABUSERS.) A child's relationship to the offender is an important predictor of the duration of abuse. When the offender is previously unknown to the child, the abuse is likely to be limited to one incident per child, such as with an exhibitionistic episode. This type of offender is likely to have a large number of victims. In contrast, incestuous abuse often involves repeated molestations of the same child over a period of three to four years.

Most sexual abuse of children is perpetrated by heterosexual men who are considered "normal" by others. Of these offenders, 80% engaged in their first act of sexual abuse before the age of 30. Though alcohol or drug intoxication is often blamed for the abuse, less than one-third of these offenders are drug- or alcohol-dependent.

Adolescent Sexual Abusers

Many incarcerated adult SEX OFFENDERS began their sexually abusive behavior as adolescents. Some professionals who work with sex offenders believe that the seriousness of sexual assaults committed by adolescents has been minimized. Some argue that the failure of court- and youth-serving institutions to intervene effectively in such behavior has prevented young offenders from receiving treatment at a critical period. Repeat adult offenders have proven to be especially resistant to treatment. Treatment providers believe that these adult offenders may have been more amenable to intervention at an earlier age.

Another problem associated with the failure to recognize the seriousness of sexual abuse perpetrated by adolescents is that offenses often go undocumented. In the absence of a record of past assaults, each offense may be treated as an isolated incident. Young offenders can sometimes engage in a number of assaults before being charged with a criminal offense.

Though relatively little research has been done on the problem of adolescent sex offenders, most treatment providers agree that it is important for them to be held accountable for their behavior. Further, most providers believe that the treatment should be specific to the problem and should combine individual treatment with peer group and family counseling. Court involvement can be helpful in making sure offenders follow through with treatment recommendations.

A large number of adolescent sexual offenders are themselves victims of sexual abuse. This fact suggests that, as with PHYSICAL ABUSE, there may be a cyclical pattern to sexual abuse. Most psychotherapists believe early intervention with victims as well as offenders is an effective way to break the cycle of abuse.

Child Pornography and the Sexual Abuse of Children

Researchers have found a link between the use of child pornography and sexual abuse of children, although not all adults who use child pornography are also sex offenders.

A perpetrator of sexual abuse may have information on a computer which is received or sent through the Internet and which links him or her to the sexual abuse of children. Said Kimberly J. Mitchell, Janis Wolak and David Finkelhor in their chapter on Internet sex crimes against minors in *Child Victimization*, "The possession of child pornography was an element in at least two-thirds of Internet sex crimes against minors. The child pornography was of a serious nature. Most offenders possessed images of children between the ages of 6 and 12, and these images depicted the sexual penetration of minors."

The Parental Role in Non-Parental Sexual Abuse

According to Cynthia Crosson-Tower in her book, *Understanding Child Abuse and Neglect*, parents may fail to perceive possible harm from a perpetrator of sexual abuse for the following key reasons:

- They may have an emotional bond with the perpetrator (a trusted family friend or babysitter).

- The sexual abuse may not be in parent's frame of reference (they cannot imagine anyone sexually abusing a child).
- They may be unaware of the dangers of possible abuse of individuals met through the Internet.
- They may need the services of the potential abuser (day care, school or babysitting).
- They may trust the potential abuser (a coach, youth-group leader or member of the clergy).
- They may fail to provide adequate supervision for the child.
- They may feel unable to supervise the child (as with latchkey children left home alone after school).
- They may be absorbed in their own problems.
- The child may initiate separation from the parent, as with children who wander off or run away.

Common Myths and Confusions about Sexual Abuse

Many popular myths exist concerning the child molester and the victimized child. The common image of a sexual offender is that of a stranger, a "dirty old man" in a trench coat. However, statistics show that most offenders are under 30 years of age and are also known (and may be related) to the victim. Some people also assume that they will somehow *know* if a person is capable of sexually abusing a child. However, child sex offenders may be very adept at concealing their behavior and may evince no apparent guilt. (They may also feel no guilt about their behavior.)

Another area of confusion centers on the nature of child sexual abuse. While most people acknowledge that sexual relations between an adult and a child are harmful, there is disagreement over the age at which a person is able to give informed consent to sexual relations. However, the legal age of consent—when a person may legally consent to sex and below which consensual sex is considered STATUTORY RAPE—varies from state to state.

Another myth is that although it is traumatic for a female child to have consensual sex with an adult male, underage sex is a positive experience for young boys. According to a 1996 report in the

Journal of the American Academy of Child and Adolescent Psychiatry, male child victims who have experienced sex with an adult can be severely traumatized and depressed and even suicidal.

History

In many different cultures, the sexual victimization of children has actually been institutionalized and permitted by law, although worldwide pressure against such abuse is increasingly apparent and effective. Even more frequently, sexual abuse has flourished despite laws and mores that nominally prohibit such behavior. The sale and prostitution of children is still commonly practiced in many parts of the world.

In ancient Greek and Roman society, CASTRATION was practiced as a way of making boys more sexually attractive to adult males. Young girls and boys were present in approximately equal numbers in brothels of the period.

Child marriage has been widely practiced throughout history and still frequently occurs in some countries. Until the third century A.D. Talmudic law permitted the betrothal of girls beginning at the age of three years and one day. Subject to the father's permission, sexual intercourse was the method of sealing marital intentions with such a young girl.

For most of recorded history children—girls in particular—have been afforded the legal status of parental property. The rape of a young girl was often treated as a property offense against the father. Because the rapist had reduced the child's ability to bring a large dowry, he was required to reimburse the father for the lost income. In some cases, the man was forced to marry his victim. In modern days, in some countries, girls who have been raped are murdered because the family perceives that the girl has brought shame to the family, and this is the only way they perceive that family honor can be restored.

Victimization of children continued in medieval Europe. In 15th-century France, the legal age of consent (the age at which the child was deemed competent to marry or engage in sexual relations) was six.

Widespread abuse also was alleged to have occurred at the hands of clergy in convents and during confessional. Many young girls were cruelly executed for alleged fornication with the devil. His-

torians speculate that these girls may actually have been sexually assaulted by the same men who put them to death.

The lust for sexual relations with children appears to have been a major preoccupation with Victorian men. Prostitution flourished in 19th-century London, and the practice of deflowering young virgins was described as obsessional. London brothels were remarkable for their large numbers of young girls. An estimated 58% of the illegal prostitutes in Vienna during this period were minors. Child pornography also became a popular item in the Victorian era, a phenomenon that shows no signs of diminution even today.

During the 19th century in the United States, Chinese girls were bought and sold at prices ranging from $1,500 to $3,500. Prior to the abolition of slavery, black children were treated as sexual property and frequently brutalized by their white owners.

Many American, British, French and German children were victims of SEXUAL TRAFFICKING during the late 19th century. These children, most of them around the ages of 12 and 13, were often exported to Hong Kong, Thailand, India and various South American countries. Unfortunately, sexual trafficking still occurs worldwide, although there are active efforts to combat it by human rights groups and many governments.

Undeterred by public outcry against it, the demand for child pornography still provides a stimulus for exploitation. A significant proportion of prostitution around the world involves minors. And child marriage continues to be commonplace in India and some other countries.

Despite laws prohibiting the sexual misuse of children, sexually abusive practices continue to flourish in modern society in many different forms. A significant proportion of prostitution around the world involves minors, and child marriage continues to be commonplace in India, Africa and some other countries. In addition, practices such as CLITORDECTOMY are considered important or mandatory in some cultures, whereas in Western nations, they are regarded as sexually abusive.

Medical Indications of Sexual Abuse

According to the 1999 article "Guidelines for the Evaluation of Sexual Abuse of Children," in *Pedi-*

atrics, if a child has any of the following sexually transmitted diseases (STDs), it is diagnostic for sexual abuse: SYPHILIS, GONORRHEA, HUMAN IMMUNO-DEFICIENCY VIRUS (HIV) or chlamydia. (Some STDs may be transmitted during childbirth from mother to child.) A diagnosis of *Trichomonas* is highly suspicious of sexual abuse, and if the child has anogenital warts or herpes, it is suspicious for sexual abuse.

Laboratory studies should be performed as soon after a sexual attack as possible, preferably within 72 hours. According to the *Pediatrics* article, for girls, "the genital examination should include inspection of the medial aspects of the thighs, labia majora and minora, clitoris, urethra, periurethal tissue, hymen, hymenal opening, fossa navicularis, and posterior fourchette." For boys, "the thighs, penis, and scrotum should be examined for bruises, scars, chafing, bite marks, and discharge." In addition, the anus of both boys and girls should be examined in various positions to check for bruising, tearing and dilation. Pain or bleeding in the genital or anal area can indicate abuse.

Sexually molested children may exhibit somatic symptoms that appear to be unrelated to physical aspects of the abuse. As a result, secondary complaints may include

- Sleep disturbance
- Abdominal pain
- Enuresis (bed-wetting)
- Vomiting
- Loss of appetite

Experts also believe that behavioral indicators in children may indicate sexual abuse; for example, as in the case of a child with precocious sexual knowledge beyond his or her developmental stage. Although it is true that children watch television and movies that may provide them with images of explicit behavior, few children initiate sexual behavior with adults or animals, despite what they may have seen on TV, and thus, when it occurs, such behavior is cause for concern.

Possible behavioral signs of sexual abuse of a child include the following:

- Inappropriate knowledge about sex for the child's age

- The display of inappropriate sexual behavior in play with toys or others

Some signs of sexual abuse in an adolescent are promiscuous behavior, abuse of drugs or alcohol, prostitution, depression and SUICIDE threats.

According to Sirotnak, Moore and Smith in their chapter on childhood sexual abuse in *Understanding the Medical Diagnosis of Child Maltreatment: A Guide for Nonmedical Professionals,* behavioral indicators of having experienced sexual abuse vary depending on the age of the child. For example, a three-year-old girl may show some signs of trauma, have nightmares, wet the bed (when bed-wetting is not normal for the child) and may not wish to be in a room with or especially alone with a particular relative.

A five-year-old boy may fondle peers and attempt to undress them and may also use sexually explicit language in preschool or kindergarten. He may draw sexually explicit pictures and withdraw from normal play activities.

The authors said that a medical history must always be taken and that it is best to seek a medical examination for possible sexual abuse when the abuse may have occurred within the past 72 hours or if the child has pain and/or bleeding from the urethra, vagina or rectum. Painful urination or pain when the child walks or sits should also be checked out immediately.

They noted that the siblings of suspected sexual abuse should also be examined for possible sexual abuse. However, they noted that not all children who are suspected of being sexually abused were actually abused. Said the authors, "A common report might be the preverbal or very young child who returns from a parent weekend visit and a guardian thinks the genital area is red or irritated—both nonspecific findings. This might be caused from poor hygiene, infections or nonspecific vaginitis, non-abusive trauma, or nothing alarming at all."

Factors Affecting the Degree of Trauma in the Sexually Abused Child

The degree of trauma to the child who has been sexually abused is affected by various factors, according to Crosson-Tower. (See Table II.) For example, when the child is abused by an acquain-

TABLE II
FACTORS INFLUENCING DEGREE OF TRAUMA (WITH SEXUAL ABUSE)

| Factor | Incestual | Extrafamilial | | |
		Acquaintance	Stranger	Online victimization
Continues for a long period of time	Probable	Possible, but often not as long as in familial	Usually not	Possible
Close emotional bond	Almost always	Possible, but not always	Usually not	Often develops through online contacts
Involves penetration	More likely, due to progression and duration	Possible, but may not	Possible, but may not. If penetration, usually forcible rape	If offender and child meet, possible
Is accompanied by aggression	Majority of cases are not	Possible	Often	Usually not
Child's "participation" to some degree	Usually	Possible	Unlikely, but possible	Yes, the child is engaged and learns to trust through online contacts.
Child is cognizant of taboo against or violation	Possible in older children	Possible	Probable (due to admonishments about strangers)	Often not, due to being in security of home

Source: Crosson-Tower, Cynthia. *Understanding Child Abuse and Neglect.* 6th ed. Boston: Allyn and Bacon. Copyright © 2005 by Pearson Education. Reprinted by permission of the publisher.

tance or stranger, the abuse usually does not occur over a long period of time, as it usually does in an incestuous relationship. In addition, the child may have a close emotional bond in an incestuous relationship, which is unlikely when the abuser is an acquaintance or a stranger.

Treatment

In addition to ensuring that the sexual abuse ends, treatment may also include psychotherapy for the abused child and sometimes for other family members as well. Studies indicate that cognitive-behavioral therapy, centering on the issue of sexual abuse, appears to be more successful than "nondirective" therapy, in which the client talks about whatever comes to mind. Another important factor is parental support during treatment. A study of 43 children who were sexually abused revealed that the children who fared best were those whose parents were supportive of therapy for the 12-month period following the beginning of therapy.

Prevention

Systematic efforts to prevent the sexual abuse of children are relatively new. Current prevention programs are directed primarily toward school-age children. These programs employ a variety of approaches, including structured school curricula, children's books, films, puppet shows, theater performances and talks by well-known sports or media celebrities.

Most programs attempt to familiarize children with the concept of sexual abuse by defining "bad" behaviors or situations. Children are taught to recognize inappropriate touching, and they are alerted to simple actions that they can take to prevent such abuse. Frequently, they are encouraged to tell another trusted adult about the abuse. They may also be taught various methods of resistance, including verbal refusal (saying no), running away and even martial arts techniques.

Other prevention efforts focus on parents and professionals. Parents are taught how to educate their children about sexual abuse. Instruction often includes suggestions for the detection of abuse and what to do if sexual abuse is discovered. Professional training of teachers, physicians, police and mental health workers has followed similar lines, often emphasizing detection.

See also ADULTS ABUSED AS CHILDREN; CHILD ABUSE; CIVIL COMMITMENT LAWS; CLERGY, ABUSE BY; DEPRESSION; FAMILY VIOLENCE; GENITAL HERPES; INTERNET AND CHILD SEX ABUSE; PEDIATRICIANS; PEDOPHILIA; PRISONS, CHILD VICTIMIZERS IN; RAPE; SEX OFFENDERS, CONVICTED; SEXUAL TRAFFICKING; SEXUALLY TRANSMITTED DISEASE; SYPHILIS; TRUSTED PROFESSIONALS, CHILD ABUSE BY.

Administration on Children, Youth and Families. *Child Maltreatment 2003.* Children's Bureau, U.S. Department of Health and Human Services, Washington, D.C., 2005.

Briere, John et al., eds. *The APSAC Handbook on Child Maltreatment.* Thousand Oaks, Calif.: Sage Publications, 1996.

Committee on Child Abuse and Neglect, American Academy of Pediatrics. "Guidelines for the Evaluation of Sexual Abuse of Children: Subject Review." *Pediatrics* 103, no. 1 (January 1999): 186–191.

Cohen, Judith, A., and Anthony P. Mannarino. "Interventions for Sexually Abused Children: Initial Treatment Outcome Findings." *Child Maltreatment* 3, no. 1 (February 1998): 17–26.

Crosson-Tower, Cynthia. *Understanding Child Abuse and Neglect.* Boston: Allyn & Bacon, 2005.

Dube, Shanta R., et al. "Long-Term Consequences of Childhood Sexual Abuse by Gender of Victim." *American Journal of Preventive Medicine* 28, no. 5 (2005): 430–438.

Giardino, Angelo P., M.D., and Martin A. Finkel, D.O. "Evaluating Child Sexual Abuse." *Pediatric Annals* 34, no. 5 (May 2005): 382–394.

Gunn, Veronica L., M.D., Gerald B. Hickson, M.D., and William O. Cooper, M.D. "Factors Affecting Pediatricians' Reporting of Suspected Child Maltreatment." *Ambulatory Pediatrics* 5, no. 2 (March–April 2005): 96–101.

Lewis, Angela, ed. *Child Sexual Abuse.* New York: Thomson Gale, 2005.

Mitchell, Kimberly J., Janis Wolak, and David Finkelhor. "Internet Sex Crimes against Minors." In *Child Victimization.* Kingston, N.J.: Civic Research Institute, 2005, pp. 2-1–2-17.

Ohene, Sally-Ann, M.D., et al. "Sexual Abuse History, Risk Behavior, and Sexually Transmitted Diseases: The Impact of Age at Abuse." *Sexually Transmitted Diseases* 32, no. 6 (June 2005): 358–363.

Ompad, Danielle C., et al. "Childhood Sexual Abuse and Age at Initiation of Injection Drug Use." *American Journal of Public Health* 95, no. 4 (2005): 703–709.

Palmer, Sally E., et al. "Responding to Children's Disclosure of Familial Abuse: What Survivors Tell Us." *Child Welfare* 78, no. 2 (March 1, 1999): 259–282.

Peluso, Emanuel, and Nicholas Putnam. "Case Study: Sexual Abuse of Boys by Females." *Journal of the American Academy of Child and Adolescent Psychiatry* 35, no. 1 (January 1996): 51–54.

Sirotnak, Andrew P., Joyce K. Moore, and Jean C. Smith. "Child Sexual Abuse." In *Understanding the Medical Diagnosis of Child Maltreatment: A Guide for Nonmedical Professionals.* 3rd ed. New York: Oxford University Press, 2006, pp. 105–147.

sexual dysfunction Victims of child SEXUAL ABUSE often experience sexual difficulties in later life. Adult survivors of sexual abuse may report difficulty becoming aroused, pain during intercourse, inability to achieve orgasm or extreme physical revulsion during sex. Because some of their first sexual experiences involved force, coercion or exploitation many survivors come to associate these dynamics with all sexual encounters. Some adults experience flashbacks during which the sexual abuse is vividly recalled.

Subsequent reactions to sexual abuse range from total avoidance of all intimate relationships to frenetic, promiscuous sexual activity. In an effort to avoid painful memories or future exploitation some victims of sexual molestation close themselves off from any relationship that may lead to intimacy. Others, seeking to prove that they are in control of their sexuality or perhaps reacting to feelings of worthlessness and guilt, develop a pattern of compulsive sexual behavior. Some experts believe female survivors may see their sexuality as a way of gaining power over men and thereby regaining control of themselves. Though they are often extremely active sexually, survivors who exhibit this reaction usually achieve little pleasure from sex and have difficulty experiencing true intimacy with their sexual partner.

Males who are sexually victimized by a man often display hypermasculine behavior in an effort to prove to themselves and others that they are heterosexual. Abuse by an adult of the same sex is often accompanied by intense self-doubt concerning the victim's sexual orientation. Victims commonly feel responsible in some way for the abuse. When the assailant is of the same sex the child often believes that since the adult was attracted to him, he must be homosexual. If the child has internalized negative attitudes toward homosexuality the fear of homosexuality may intensify guilt feelings leading to even greater distress over sexuality.

Survivors of child sexual abuse often lack knowledge of how intimate relations develop. Children who are forced into sexual behavior prematurely may learn how to relate only sexually. These children may have difficulty relating to peers on a level appropriate to their age. Incest survivors often complain of being robbed of their childhood because they were prevented from developing the kind of family and peer relationships considered an important part of healthy development. The inability to develop intimacy often leads to later marital and/or sexual dysfunction.

Expert help and a supportive environment is usually necessary to help the survivor overcome problems related to sexual abuse. A number of self-help and formal therapy groups are available for the adult survivor. As awareness of the lasting effects of such victimization grows, more adults are seeking help in overcoming problems related to child sexual abuse.

sexual exploitation   Child sexual exploitation involves the use of children as prostitutes, models for pornographic purposes or objects of sexual molestation. Exploitation is usually, but not exclusively, undertaken for the economic gain of an adult. No reliable estimates of the incidence of sexual exploitation are available. Recent estimates of sexual abuse often fail to include victims of pornography or prostitution. Law enforcement officials believe the sexual exploitation of children to be one of the most underreported crimes.

See CHILD PORNOGRAPHY; CHILD PROSTITUTION; SEXUAL ABUSE.

sexually transmitted disease (STD)   Presence of a sexually transmitted disease in a child under the age of puberty is a strong indicator of SEXUAL ABUSE. It is extremely rare for such diseases to be contracted in any way other than by sexual contact. (Although newborn infants may contract some venereal diseases from their mothers during the birth process.) A thorough physical examination for possible sexual abuse should include taking cultures from the genitals, mouth and anus. A blood test is necessary to detect syphilis.

See also GONORRHEA; HERPES GENITAL; SYPHILIS; WARTS, VENEREAL.

sexual trafficking   A form of modern slavery that involves the buying and selling of children and adults (primarily females) for the purpose of their forcible use for sexual purposes. This is a practice that has occurred since ancient times. In the late 19th and early 20th centuries, CHILD PROSTITUTION and the enslavement of children and adults was a source of great public concern in Europe and in North America, where it was estimated that 60,000 children per year were kidnapped or lured into prostitution.

Human trafficking continues in the 21st century, although it is illegal in the United States and most other countries. An estimated half of all trafficked people are children. According to the Federal Bureau of Investigation (FBI) in the United States, human trafficking worldwide generates an estimated $9.5 billion in annual revenues. Human trafficking is also linked to drug trafficking, money laundering and document forgery.

The *Trafficking in Persons Report,* released in June 2005 by the State Department in the United States, estimated that there are 600,000–800,000 people trafficked between countries worldwide each year. These statistics do not, however, include individuals who are trafficked within their own countries. When individuals trafficked both inside and outside of their countries are considered, it is estimated that 2–4 million people are trafficked each year.

According to a 2005 Congressional Research Service report, it is believed that more than 14,500 children are trafficked into the United States each year. In Canada, according to a 2005 issue of the

Canadian Medical Association Journal, it is estimated by the Royal Canadian Mounted Police that 800 people are trafficked into Canada each year, although this estimate may be low.

Worldwide, the greatest numbers of trafficked children are believed to come from Albania. According to the Anti-Trafficking Directorate at the Ministry of Public Order in Albania, an estimated 4,000 children were trafficked from 1992 to 2000 from Albania. Other experts regard this estimate as very low. These children were primarily trafficked to ITALY and GREECE for the purposes of sexual exploitation, as well as to use the children for begging and slave labor.

Trafficked Children

Although most trafficked children and adolescents are females who are sexually exploited, boys are sometimes exploited for sexual purposes as well as for their labor. Male children are purchased or kidnapped from India, Pakistan and Bangladesh so that they can work as camel jockeys. Boys are also sometimes compelled into prostitution, especially into child sex tourism.

Traffickers obtain children and adolescents through promises of jobs, trickery or outright kidnapping. Once the children are in another country or in another part of their own country where they are isolated, they are usually threatened with beatings and even death unless they comply with the wishes of the trafficker. The trafficker may also tell children that if they do not cooperate, their families will be harmed or killed. Trafficked children and adolescents may be drugged into compliance.

They may be told that their parents sold them to the traffickers, whom they must now obey. (Sometimes this is a true statement.) Sometimes parents willingly give their children to traffickers, based on lavish promises of employment for the child, who will then be able to send money back to the impoverished families. These promises are not fulfilled.

Significant numbers of runaway children and adolescents in all countries are known to be lured or coerced into prostitution. They are often vulnerable because they need food and shelter, and the trafficker convinces gullible children that he or she will become a close and helpful friend to them. They may then slowly groom the child into prostitution or may quickly compel the child into prostitution.

United Nations Definition of Trafficking

As defined by the United Nations Protocol to Prevent Trafficking in Persons, especially Women and Children, trafficking is defined as

> The recruitment, transportation, transfer, harboring or receipt of persons, by means of threat or use of force or other forms of coercion, of abduction, of fraud, of deception, of the abuse of power or of a position of vulnerability or of the giving or receiving of payments or benefits to achieve the consent of a person having control over another person, for the purpose of exploitation. Exploitation shall include, at a minimum, the exploitation of the prostitution of others or other forms of sexual exploitation, forced labor or services, slavery or practices similar to slavery, servitude or the removal of organs.

The Trafficking Victims Protection Act of 2000 in the United States defined trafficking and also suggested actions to combat this practice. This law defined the "severe form of trafficking in persons" as

> (a) sex trafficking in which a commercial sex act is induced by force, fraud, or coercion, or in which the person induced to perform such an act has not attained 18 years of age; or
> (b) the recruitment, harboring, transportation, provision, or obtaining of a person for labor or services, through the use of force, fraud, or coercion for the purpose of subjection to involuntary servitude, peonage, debt bondage, or slavery.

According to the U.S. Department of State, the Trafficking Victims Protection Reauthorization Act of 2003 added the requirement that foreign governments would provide statistical data on the number of trafficking-related investigations, prosecutions, convictions and sentences. Based on the data provided for 2004, there were 6,885 prosecutions worldwide in 2004 and 3,025 convictions worldwide.

European Report on Trafficked Children

Some reports have described how and why children are trafficked in Europe. The ECPAT Law Enforcement Group provided data on the sexual trafficking of children in the 2004 report *Joint East West Research on Trafficking in Children for Sexual Purposes in Europe: The Sending Countries.* For example, in Russia, modeling agencies recruit young women who seek modeling jobs, but often these girls or women are trafficked in order to sexually exploit them. In the Ukraine, girls are sold for the equivalent of between $2,000 to $10,000 each. Most are sold to clients in the Arab Emirates, Canada, Cyprus, Germany, Italy, Japan, Turkey and the United States.

According to the report, children may also face re-trafficking, such as when they are returned to their families after being sexually exploited but are unable to integrate with these families. They are then re-trafficked by those who again exploit them.

In Albania, there are many blood feuds between families, and children may be compelled to leave school and go into hiding, away from revenge killers, who may seek to traffick them.

The prices that are paid for trafficked children vary, but in general, in western European countries, there is a demand for young boys, and in Moldova, there is a demand for virgin girls. In general, traffickers receive a higher price for adolescent girls than for adult women. However, even infants may be trafficked, usually to buyers who want to use them at a later age as brides for their male children. This practice is common among countries in which there is a gender imbalance, such as India and China.

Children from all countries who are sexually trafficked are also used to create child pornography, which is often bought and sold on the INTERNET. Sometimes pedophiles have their sexual acts with minors filmed, and then they sell (or give away) the photographs or videotapes on the Internet.

Health Risks of Trafficked Children

Children and adolescents who are trafficked face many health risks. They are usually raped repeatedly and are at high risk for contracting a sexually transmitted disease. They also face beatings that may cause serious physical injuries, such as broken bones, cuts and burns. Adolescents may be compelled to have unwanted abortions, under unsafe conditions.

Victims often experience trauma, anxiety and depression, and they may be suicidal. Mental abuse is common, and some victims suffer mental breakdowns. Many victims are denied any medical care, and if they become too ill to work, they may be killed.

Individual Signs of Trafficking

Included in the *Trafficking in Persons Report,* some signs of potential victims of trafficking are as follows:

- Evidence of being controlled and/or evidence of an inability to move or leave a job
- Bruises or other signs of physical abuse
- Fear or depression in the victim
- The victim does not speak on his or her own behalf and/or does not speak the local language
- The victim has no passport or any other forms of identification or documentation

Questions to Ask Persons Who Are Suspected Victims of Human Trafficking

According to the *Trafficking in Persons Report,* some questions that may help determine whether or not someone is a victim of human trafficking are as follows:

- What type of work do you do?
- Are you being paid?
- Can you leave your job if you want?
- Can you come and go as you please?
- Have you or your family been threatened?
- What are your work and living conditions like?
- Where do you sleep and eat?
- Do you have to ask permission to eat/sleep/go to the bathroom?
- Are there locks on your doors/windows so you cannot get out?
- Has identification or documentation been taken from you?

Child Sex Tourism

Individuals who travel to other countries and have sex with minors are participants in what is known as child sex tourism. Sometimes the primary or sole purpose of the trip is to engage in sex with children. Some experts estimate that a million children may be sexually exploited by child sex tourism in their own or other countries. The perpetrator travels to another country and engages in sex acts with children. Tourists usually assume that the sex will be anonymous and plentiful, with few (if any) restrictions.

Tourists may rationalize their abusive acts by telling themselves that the children in the other country enjoy sex and/or need the money that they earn from engaging in child prostitution. However, in most cases, the children receive little or no money, and they are compelled to prostitute themselves. (The idea that children in other countries are more sexually interested than children in the tourists' own countries is ignorant.)

Tourists may be unaware that they are at a high risk for contracting sexually transmitted diseases from the children, who may have been abused by many others. At least 32 countries ban child sex tourism, and individuals who sexually exploit children in other countries may be prosecuted for this crime in their own countries.

Victims May Be Maltreated or Stigmatized by Authorities

In many countries, children who have been trafficked and identified by the police are subject to arrest and prosecution. Sometimes the police themselves are involved with child trafficking, receiving payoffs.

In some countries, such as Albania, trafficked children are called prostitutes rather than victims, while their traffickers are referred to as protectors, tutors or exploiters. Often the children are deported, with little or no money and in the company of other children. They may be returned to their parents or relatives, although the likelihood of this occurrence is remote in many countries.

In some countries, the names of child prostitutes are listed in the newspaper. Because of the GUILT AND SHAME for their past acts of prostitution and/or participation in child pornography or use of drugs, children may believe that no one in their families wants them—and they may be correct in this perception.

According to the 2004 ECPAT report, most countries fail to realize that minor victims should be entitled to special protection from traffickers. The report said that "when faced with a minor who is being sexually exploited, the police and the public tend to see only a prostituted person, and not a child. There is a general perception, clearly emerging from the Eastern European reports, that young boys and girls who are prostituted are engaging in anti-social behaviour; the young people are not seen as victims of exploitation in need of protection. In several reports it is said that the reaction to such children is to treat them in the same way as adult prostitutes, and to simply arrest and deport them."

In some countries, trafficked children younger than a certain age (such as age 13) are placed in orphanages when they are identified, while older trafficked children are deported back to their country of origin, often in groups of other deported adolescents and adults.

See also AUSTRALIA; CANADA; CHILD ABUSE; CHILD MOLESTER; CHILD PORNOGRAPHY; CHINA, PEOPLE'S REPUBLIC OF; CONVENTION ON THE RIGHTS OF THE CHILD; CRIMINAL PROSECUTION; DENMARK; FRANCE; GERMANY; HAGUE CONVENTION ON THE CIVIL ASPECTS OF INTERNATIONAL CHILD ABDUCTION; HOMELESSNESS; INDIA; JAPAN; KIDNAPPING; PEDOPHILIA; PHYSICAL ABUSE; PSYCHOLOGICAL/EMOTIONAL MALTREATMENT; SEXUAL ABUSE; SEXUALLY TRANSMITTED DISEASE; STATUTORY RAPE; SWEDEN; TURKEY.

El-Rashidi, Yasmine. "Ride 'Em, Robot: Qatar Offers Solutions to a Jockey Shortage." *Wall Street Journal* CCXLVI, 68 (October 3, 2005): A2, A12.

Miko, Francis T. "Trafficking in Persons. The U.S. and International Response." Washington, D.C.: Congressional Research Service, updated June 24, 2005.

O'Briain, Muireann, Anke van den Borne, and Theo Noten, eds. *Joint East West Research on Trafficking in Children for Sexual Purposes in Europe: The Sending Countries.* Amsterdam, Netherlands: ECPAT Europe Law Enforcement Group, 2004.

Office of the Under Secretary for Global Affairs. *Trafficking in Persons Report.* Washington, DC: U.S. Department of State, June 2005. Available online. http://www.usembassy.it/pdf/other/RL30545.pdf. Downloaded October 27, 2005.

Omelaniuk, Irena. "Trafficking in Human Beings." New York: Population Division, Department of Economic and Social Affairs, United Nations Secretariat, July 8, 2005. Available online. http://www.un.org/esa/population/publications/ittmigdev/2005/P15_Iomelaniuk.pdf. Downloaded on October 27, 2005.

Stewart, Donna E., and Gajic-Veljanoski. "Trafficking in Women: The Canadian Perspective." *Canadian Medical Association Journal* 173, no. 1 (July 5, 2005): 25–26.

shaken infant syndrome A form of child abuse that is caused by the violent shaking of an infant and which can result in severe disabilities for the child or even death. The force of this shaking is so intense that the baby's brain bounces against the skull, causing a severe head injury. This form of PHYSICAL ABUSE, also known as shaken baby syndrome, was formerly called whiplash shaken infant syndrome. It is estimated that as many as 1,600 children experience shaken infant syndrome each year in the United States, and about 30% of these children die.

Parents and caretakers sometimes express their extreme frustration toward a crying, and/or irritable infant, whom they may assume is uncooperative or acting purposely to annoy them, by shaking the baby to try to make the baby stop crying or whining. However, the child usually reacts by crying louder in fear or pain, and the shaking may escalate to a dangerous level very rapidly.

Infants in their first six months of life are the most likely victims of shaken infant syndrome. During infancy, the head is the heaviest in proportion to the baby's total body weight and more so than at any other time in life. This fact, coupled with the relatively weak supporting neck muscles of the baby, makes this age group very sensitive to the sudden backward-forward motions associated with whiplash.

Shaking of a baby and the resultant SEQUELAE (aftereffect) were first differentiated from the BATTERED CHILD SYNDROME by radiologist John Caffey in the early 1970s. Dr. Caffey cited cases in which infants and children who showed no external signs of battering or abuse had suffered serious head and spinal cord injuries, and, in several instances,

death. Coffey said these injuries were caused by shaking. Some physicians today, however, argue that the diagnosis may be made too rapidly and, if incorrect, may affect the medical care that an ill child receives. Some doctors are dubious about this diagnosis altogether.

Coffey's closer examination showed that many of these infants suffered SUBDURAL HEMATOMA, retinal hemorrhaging and damage to the periosteum of the long bones. Further study revealed links between the shaking and permanent brain damage, mental retardation, blindness, visual loss, motor deficits, seizures and hypopituitarism. The injury that is most frequently associated with the shaking of infants is subdural hematoma.

If the child dies, the cause of death is most frequently uncontrollable intracranial hypertension. An autopsy reveals skull fractures in approximately 25% of infants with shaken infant syndrome, often in the posterior parietal bone or the occipital bone or in both areas.

Symptoms and Diagnostic Path

In the short term, the immediate effects of shaking an infant may include the following symptoms:

- Vomiting
- Concussion
- Bluish or pale skin
- Respiratory distress
- Seizures
- Unconsciousness
- Death
- Retinal hemorrhage
- Lethargy
- Irritability

If the child does not die after being shaken violently, the following long-term consequences may occur:

- Blindness or visual deficits
- Learning disabilities
- Mental retardation
- Cerebral palsy

- Motor delays
- Hypopituitarism (insufficient production of pituitary hormone that may result in inadequate production of other important hormones)
- Paralysis
- Learning disabilities

The physician may also find bruising and burn marks, and there may be other forms of abuse present. If a spinal tap is performed, it often reveals bloody fluid rather than the normally clear spinal fluid.

A thorough medical/social history and a complete physical examination by a physician who is familiar with the syndrome and with the subtle signs of head injury will increase the likelihood of an accurate diagnosis. Careful fundiscopic examination is an important tool for detecting retinal hemorrhages. In recent years, the use of computed tomography (CT) has greatly increased the ability to detect the presence of subdural hematoma.

In addition, magnetic resonance imaging (MRI) may also be useful in differentiating a shaken baby form of abuse from a spontaneous subarachnoid hemorrhage.

Ann-Christine Duhaime, M.D., et al., in a 1998 article in the *New England Journal of Medicine*, said,

> The majority of abused infants in fact have clinical, radiologic, or autopsy evidence of blunt impact to the head. Thus, the term "shaking-impact syndrome" may reflect more accurately than "shaken-baby syndrome" the usual mechanism responsible for these injuries. Whether shaking alone can cause the constellation of findings associated with the syndrome is still debated, but most investigators agree that trivial forces, such as those involving routine play, infant swings, or falls from a low height are insufficient to cause the syndrome. Instead, these injuries appear to result from major rotational forces, which clearly exceed those encountered in normal child-care activities.

These authors also stated that "The most consistent finding in cases of the shaking-impact syndrome is the presence of subdural and subarachnoid blood. Hemorrhage therefore is both a marker for the threshold of force required to cause the injury and a likely pathophysiologic contributor to the resultant brain damage."

Problems Sometimes Occur with Diagnosis

The diagnosis should be made carefully because sometimes it is immediately assumed, based on little evidence, that the child is a victim of shaken baby syndrome when other medical problems in fact may be causing the infant's distress or death. For example, in one case described in the *Journal of American Physicians and Surgeons* in 2005, in 1997, a father of a 10-week-old infant took his sick baby to the emergency room, where the child subsequently died.

The child had been born prematurely, to a mother with gestational diabetes, a urinary tract infection and group B streptococcus. The baby suffered from hyperbilirubinemia (too much bilirubin, a substance derived from hemoglobin), a potentially toxic condition. After the baby was discharged, he was frequently congested. He was still ill when he later received four vaccines, which is generally inadvisable for an ill baby.

According to the autopsy, the cause of death was "subdural hemorrhage, due to Shaken Baby Syndrome," and it was also ruled a homicide. Since the child was alone with his father, it was assumed that he was the perpetrator.

The baby's father insisted that he was innocent, refusing to accept a plea offer and ultimately being sentenced to life imprisonment. Subsequent to the trial, medical experts from Australia, the United Kingdom and the United States reviewed the infant's medical records, and they all agreed that the baby had died of medical causes. These experts also said there were problems with the autopsy.

In 2003, the baby's mother filed a complaint with the Florida Department of Heath, listing 25 problems and charges against the pathologist who did the autopsy. The father also filed a complaint. A probable cause panel met, and they upheld 12 of the complaints filed by the mother, put the pathologist on probation and banned him from performing autopsies.

At an evidentiary hearing in 2004, the judge reversed the guilty verdict because of errors and omissions in the records; for example, such as failing to record information on the birth records or hospitalizations of the baby, as well as the vaccinations while the baby was sick. At that time, the vaccine that the baby was given was associated with 72 reports to the Vaccine Adverse Event Reporting System (VAERS), for an association with five deaths, 36 emergency room visits and seven hospital admissions.

It was also noted that the autopsy report stated that the child was a three-month-old black male infant; however, the baby was a 10-week-old white male.

Said Dr. Yazbak, "Testimony by pathologists about autopsy results can help condemn innocent persons to life imprisonment or even death. The autopsy table is accepted as the altar of truth by physicians and courts alike. Yet, as this case shows, medical examiners are fallible, and autopsy reports must always be analyzed critically."

This case was also discussed at length in an article by Jane M. Orient, M.D., in the *Journal of American Physicians and Surgeons* in 2005. She said,

If child abuse is suspected, a careful differential diagnosis must be done, after a nonthreatening medical interview—as opposed to a police interrogation—of the parents and caregivers. The physician should consider the possibility of a vaccine reaction. Fundus photography and levels of plasma ascorbic acid and whole-blood histamine are indicated (on admission, before vitamin repletion) as part of the medical workup and the forensic investigation. At autopsy, evidence of blunt head trauma should be sought with special care, and the neck and cervical [upper spinal] cord should be carefully examined.

Treatment Options and Outlook

The prognosis for an infant who has been severely shaken is poor. Most infants who live are severely disabled and will require care for the rest of their lives because of induced mental retardation and/or cerebral palsy. The only treatment is emergency care immediately after the shaking incident, to stop the internal bleeding and relieve the increased intracranial pressure on the baby's brain.

Risk Factors and Preventive Measures

Parents with anger management problems, immaturity or other issues that may lead them to shake their baby need help before the incident occurs, although it may be very difficult to determine the intensity of their anger and frustration. They may need help in understanding that it is normal for babies to cry and in interpreting what the child's different cries may mean. Families that think there may be a pending abuse problem should not wait for an incident to happen, but should help the at-risk caretaker and/or report any child abuse indicators to state protective service officials.

The "Nanny Baby Murder" Case

The most famous case of shaken baby syndrome involved Louise Woodward, a British nanny who was accused and convicted of second-degree murder in 1997 in the death of American baby Matthew Eappen. Woodward's primary defense was the contention that the child had a previous brain injury, and for some reason, that injury began to "rebleed," leading to the child's death.

The judge subsequently overturned the verdict and found Woodward guilty of involuntary manslaughter, sentencing her only to the time she had already served. This decision created great controversy, and 50 physicians expert in the diagnosis and treatment of child abuse challenged the judge's action and published their findings on the Internet, stating that the medical evidence "overwhelmingly supported a violent shaking/impact episode on the day in question, when Matthew was in the sole custody of Ms. Woodward." The doctors stated the "rebleed theory" was a "courtroom diagnosis" rather than a medical diagnosis.

See also INFANTICIDE; SUDDEN INFANT DEATH SYNDROME.

Duhaime, Ann-Christine, et al. "Nonaccidental Head Injury in Infants—The 'Shaken-Baby Syndrome.'" *New England Journal of Medicine* 338, no. 25 (June 18, 1998): 1,822–1,829.

Orient, Jane M., M.D. "Reflections on 'Shaken Baby Syndrome': A Case Report." *Journal of American Physicians and Surgeons* 10, no. 2 (Summer 2005): 45–50.

Yazbak, F. Edward, M.D. "Post-Mortem on a 'Shaken Baby Syndrome' Autopsy." *Journal of American Physicians and Surgeons* 10, no. 2 (Summer 2005): 51–52.

Sheppard-Towner Infancy and Maternity Act This legislation, passed in 1921, established the first United States program to provide major funding to alleviate a wide range of problems suffered by infants and young children as a result of nutritional deficiency, generally poor health and lack of adequate care, The act was sponsored by the Children's Bureau, an agency established in 1912 during an era of social reform.

sibling abuse Violence between siblings is widespread in Western culture. Interestingly, such assaults constitute a relatively small proportion of all child abuse cases reported to investigative authorities. This fact in part reflects a belief that sibling violence is a normal part of family life that should be handled without outside interference. Underreporting may also be due to a tendency to cite parents for failing to protect the victimized sibling rather than labeling the child as the abuser. Parents may also fear that reporting would lead to the removal of the abused (or abusive) child from the family home. Denial is an important factor in the parents' failure to protect a child adequately from sibling attacks. Parents are often embarrassed or afraid to report abusive behavior in their children. Parents may also fear that reporting would lead to the removal of both the abused and the abusive children from the family home. They may also fear being blamed for perpetrating or allowing the abuse themselves. Once convinced that a child is at risk of serious harm, however, most parents are able to intervene effectively.

Brother-on-brother violence is more commonly observed than brother-sister violence. Sister-brother violence is not common. Least common is sister-sister violence. Brother-brother violence is often unreported and seen as "roughhousing" and typical male behavior.

Although sibling abuse has been estimated to be the most frequent manifestation of family violence, it is the least likely to result in death. Family factors that may result in abuse of a sibling are

- Lack of supervision
- Children who are treated as favorites versus children treated negatively
- Parents who ignore indications or obvious proof of minor forms of abuse by a sibling, thus tac-

itly signaling the abuse may continue and even escalate
- Severe family stress
- Alleged abuse may not be substantiated
- Medical or emotional illness in the family

Sometimes abuse is alleged but is not occurring, so investigation is important. Authors John Caffaro and Allison Conn-Caffaro cited in their book the case of a seven-year-old boy accused of constantly biting his 11-year-old brother to the point of drawing blood. The younger child actively denied the biting. After probing further, the therapists learned that the older child was actively jealous of the younger child, who was clearly enjoying a preferential status in the family. Bite impressions were taken the next time the wounds appeared and it was discovered that the older child was biting himself and blaming his brother in order to gain parental attention.

Risk Factors

Caffaro and Conn-Caffaro cited the following as risk factors for sibling offenders:

- Offender's thinking errors that distort or minimize abusive behavior
- History of victimization by parent, older sibling or persons outside the immediate family
- Inadequate impulse control, empathic deficits and emotional immaturity
- Willingness to use coercion or force to control victim (sadistic, cruel behavior)
- Drug or alcohol use
- Dissociative reactions to trauma

They also identified the following factors common to sibling victims:

- Large developmental, physical or intellectual differences between siblings
- Victim's dependence on an older, more powerful sibling
- Lack of other, supportive relationships
- Prior history of victimization
- Lack of sex education

Sexual Abuse Committed by a Sibling

Sexual contact between siblings, though legally defined as INCEST, often does not result in a report of child abuse. Exploratory sexual contact between young children is usually seen as a normal part of their sexual development. Sexual abuse by adolescents may be passed off by parents or therapists as experimentation. Many professionals who work with adolescents are reluctant to label them as SEX OFFENDERS.

However, when one or both siblings are adolescents or when the sexual contact results in trauma, infection or pregnancy, then the situation is usually viewed with greater alarm.

The amount of sibling-to-sibling sexual abuse is thought to be greatly underreported. Parents may view it as harmless sexual play or may be embarrassed to talk about it with others outside the family. In some cases, sexual abuse by a sibling can have more harmful effects on the victim than an incident involving an extrafamilial offender, especially if allowed to continue over an extended period of time.

Sexual abuse by a sibling perpetrator often involves a high degree of coercion. As with other forms of incest, this type of exploitation may make it difficult for the victim to form trusting relationships and may result in marital difficulty and a sexual dysfunction later in life.

Caffaro, John V., and Conn-Caffaro, Allison. *Sibling Abuse Trauma: Assessment and Intervention Strategies for Children, Families, and Adults.* New York: The Haworth Maltreatment and Trauma Press, 1998.

SIDS See SUDDEN INFANT DEATH SYNDROME.

situational abuse and neglect Situational abuse and neglect refers to circumstances over which the parents or caretakers have little control. POVERTY and discrimination are such conditions and often are associated with abuse or neglect. Though programs such as Temporary Assistance for Needy Families and HEAD START have helped reduce the effects of such circumstances, many children throughout the world still suffer from the effects of discrimination and poverty.

skeletal survey When child battering is suspected, a skeletal survey is often conducted to search for signs of previous battering. Physicians look for signs of multiple FRACTURES of the types most likely to result from abusive treatment. Careful examination of these X-rays can reveal OSSIFICATION resulting from previous fractures.

sleep deprivation Children who are severely abused, physically or psychologically, often do not get adequate sleep and the sleep that they do experience is troubled. Sleep deprivation often impairs intellectual functioning and makes children irritable and distractable. Negative behaviors resulting from a lack of sleep may make children more susceptible to abuse by a parent or caretaker.

In severe cases of sleep deprivation, secretion of the growth hormone somatotropin is inhibited, causing psychosocial DWARFISM. Cases of abuse-related dwarfism are rare. Once normal sleep patterns are reestablished, children usually experience a period of rapid growth, which in most cases reverses growth inhibition. In a study published in a 1997 issue of the *Journal of the American Academy of Child and Adolescent Psychiatry*, researchers compared 19 prepubertal children who had experienced substantiated abuse with 15 non-abused control children and 10 children diagnosed with depression. They found that physically abused children had the most difficulty falling to sleep and experienced more troubled sleep. For example, the abused children were "twice as active at night as controls." Sexually abused children also experienced more sleep problems than the control group or the depressed group. About half of the abused children experienced impaired sleep and five of the abused children (about 26%) had sleep problems severe enough to be considered a clinical sleep disturbance.

The researchers also noted that sleep problems in children could indicate abuse and said,

> Thus, if a child presents with impaired sleep, abuse (particularly physical abuse) should be considered as part of the differential formulation. Likewise, when evaluating a child who has been abused, sleep should be carefully assessed for clinically significant impairments. It is conceivable that early intervention tar-

geted at abused children with sleep disruption may help diminish long-term intractable insomnia.

slick but sick syndrome   The term *slick but sick* was coined by psychologist Logan Wright and describes the capacity of some abusive parents to hide underlying PSYCHOPATHOLOGY. By comparing convicted child batterers with a carefully matched control group of nonabusing parents, Wright was able to distinguish personality differences between the two groups. On certain psychological tests, batterers gave responses very similar to nonbatterers when the socially desirable answer to a question was logical or apparent. However, answers to the Minnesota Multiphasic Personality Inventory (MMPI), a less-apparent, empirically devised measure of psychopathology, showed that battering parents were actually much more disturbed than they appeared initially. The ability of abusive parents to present themselves as more healthy than they may actually be has been used to explain the often confusing evidence obtained in clinical studies of child abusers. Other researchers have emphasized the importance of societal pressures and stresses over the individual psychopathology of the abuser. The latter hypothesize that almost any parent or caregiver under certain stressful conditions will resort to child abuse. Proponents of the belief that child abusers are emotionally disturbed point to phenomena like the slick but sick syndrome to explain abusive behavior by adults who appear healthy. Others believe that some parents are abusive due to their own deficits and some are untreatable.

social abuse   Children often suffer as victims of poverty and discrimination. Most child advocates believe societies, and the governments that represent them, have a responsibility to provide for the safety and well-being of children and families. These responsibilities may include protecting children from all forms of physical, sexual and psychological maltreatment (including racial discrimination), making sure children are well nourished, have adequate housing and receive necessary medical care. Failure by society to provide for children's basic needs is sometimes referred to as social abuse. Though social abuse is not addressed by child abuse

laws, many experts believe it is an indirect cause of much child abuse and neglect.

social isolation   Abusive or neglectful parents tend to be isolated from helping networks. Social isolation may be externally imposed in the case of a parent who is ostracized by neighbors and relatives or internally imposed by the parent's choice. Frequent changes of residence may contribute to social isolation. Abused children may also engage in social WITHDRAWAL, turning inward and isolating themselves from peers, family members and others.

Neglectful parents are significantly less likely to belong to an organization such as a church or parent-teacher association. They also have fewer close friends and tend to socialize less often.

One explanation for social isolation is that neglectful parents may be suffering from depression, which renders them incapable of normal social functioning. Another is that parents use detachment from others as a defense. While fearing rejection, they avoid forming close relationships. This may also explain their difficulty in forming a strong attachment to their own children.

A number of methods are used to reduce social isolation and encourage the formation of a network of supporting friends. Individual, group and family therapy may help reduce psychological blocks to developing reciprocal relationships. Groups such as Parents Anonymous serve as helping networks and encourage members to be available to one another whenever help is needed.

social learning model of child abuse   Some theorists explain child abuse as a result of a learned pattern of relating to others. As children, parents may learn violent ways of expressing anger or frustration. Later these maladaptive coping mechanisms may be reflected in a range of aggressive behavior, including child abuse. Social learning theorists often look to parental models as the source of much, but not all, social learning. In contrast to a psychoanalytic approach, which postulates that early experiences leave largely unchangeable emotional imprints, social learning theory holds open the possibility of learning new ways of parenting.

Social Security Act This federal legislation was initially passed in 1935 and has been amended several times to provide for establishment of various social programs, many of which directly relate to child and family welfare.

Title IV of the act supports state welfare services, i.e., day care, foster care and varied preventive and protective programs. Provisions of Title IV also ensure that child support is paid by absent parents and provide for establishment of paternity. Originally, Title IV also encompassed funding for states' Aid to Families with Dependent Children programs, now the Temporary Aid to Needy Families (TANF) program.

Title V designates monies in support of Maternal and Child Health and other health care services for children from low-income families. Title XIX funds MEDICAID, a medical assistance program for low-income people. Title XX establishes state grants for service programs such as prevention of child abuse and neglect; preserving, rehabilitating and reuniting families; and referring individuals to institutions where appropriate.

sodomy Though the term can refer to any form of sexual intercourse considered to be unnatural according to societal standards, sodomy is most commonly used to refer to anal intercourse between two males. In the context of child SEXUAL ABUSE, sodomy is used to describe anal intercourse between an adult male and a child of either sex.

In addition to the emotional trauma caused by sexual abuse, sodomy can also result in physical harm to children. Sodomy is especially painful for young children who are likely to suffer anal tears or enlargement. Diseases such as gonorrhea and syphilis can also be conveyed through anal intercourse. Presence of a SEXUALLY TRANSMITTED DISEASE in a child is strong, but all too frequently overlooked, evidence of sexual abuse.

Children who have been subjected to sodomy may be reluctant to reveal their victimization but may complain of anal discomfort and may soil undergarments or exhibit other somatic and behavioral signs of trauma.

See also ENCOPRESIS.

soiling See ENCOPRESIS.

Sovereign Immunity, Doctrine of See DOCTRINE OF SOVEREIGN IMMUNITY.

spanking See AVERSIVE CONDITIONING.

special child See TARGET CHILD.

splitting Splitting refers to an intrapsychic process often employed by children who have been abused, Unable to understand how a parent can be both good and bad, children split positive and negative attributes and see others and themselves as either good or bad. This process may lead to the creation of scapegoats or a PARENTIFIED CHILD.

In the case of a child who sees the parent as only good and therefore incapable of doing wrong, the child interprets the parent's abusive behavior as a reflection of his or her own badness. The child may then become a willing scapegoat, actually seeking out punishment.

The parentified child, identifying with the good parent, seeks to fill the role of the neglectful or abusive parent. Parentification is reflected in a kind of pseudomaturity that exceeds the child's years. Often taking on extra household responsibilities and working hard in school, this child cannot do enough to please. When abused or neglected by the parent, the child redoubles efforts to please.

spouse abuse Spouse abuse includes physical and mental injury of a wife or husband by their marital partner. Though spouse abuse refers to the victimization of either partner, the overwhelming majority of such abuse involves battering of wives by their husbands. The term is sometimes used to refer to abuse of an unmarried person by a live-in partner.

Wife battering appears to be closely associated with child abuse. One study of mothers and their children in battered women's shelters found that 70% of children had been abused or neglected. In most cases the husband was responsible for the child abuse. About one-fourth of the children were abused by both mother and father. A very small number were abused by the mother only.

See also FAMILY VIOLENCE; YO-YO SYNDROME.

staff flight Maintaining qualified, well-trained and experienced protective service workers is a constant struggle in agencies charged with investigating and treating child abuse. Turnover rate among staff in these agencies has been estimated at 85% per year. While efforts to improve working conditions, provide additional training and ensure higher salaries have helped, the stressful nature of protective service work continues to contribute to early staff burnout. Social workers and investigators often find themselves working alone in highly charged emotional situations. Abusive parents or caretakers, frightened and angry when confronted, often direct their anger toward the protective service employee. Working with children who have been abused can also prove to be frustrating and heart-wrenching work for the human service professional who is sometimes powerless to reverse the effects of abuse. Over a period of time, even the most highly motivated and best-trained protective services worker may become discouraged and alienated from his or her work.

standard of proof See EVIDENTIARY STANDARDS.

Stanley v. Illinois This case, decided by the United States Supreme Court in 1971, involved an unwed father who, upon the death of his children's mother, was not allowed custody of his three children. The state of Illinois invoked a law automatically making children of unmarried fathers wards of the state upon death of the mother. The father, Peter Stanley, petitioned the court for custody of his children, arguing that he had been denied equal protection under the law as granted in the Fourteenth Amendment to the U.S. Constitution.

The Supreme Court reversed the Illinois decision and granted custody to the father. *Stanley v. Illinois* is often cited as establishing the principle that prevents a state from separating children from their parents unless, by due process, the parent is proven to be unfit.

starvation One of the most extreme results of child neglect is death from starvation. Though rare in most Western countries, cases of starvation continue to surface every year. In some African countries where drought and war have severely restricted food supply, starving infants and children are a common sight. Starvation in third world countries is often described as a form of societal neglect. However, many experts are reluctant to characterize poverty-induced starvation as abuse or neglect.

In contrast to deaths from inadequate nutrition in developing countries, child starvation in developed countries is generally thought to be intentional. The most frequent victims are infants who appear to have been totally neglected. A high percentage tend to be born prematurely to mothers of low intelligence who already have large families. Though undernourished children usually respond quickly to proper care and nutrition in a hospital, they rarely receive such attention. Autopsies of starved infants usually show other evidence of gross neglect.

status offense The term *status offense* refers to an action that is considered to be a criminal or delinquent act when engaged in by a person under a certain age, usually 16 years. A status offense may involve repeatedly defying parents' wishes, running away from home or being truant from school. In the United States many states have eliminated legal sanctions for status offenses, opting instead for categories such as CHINS (Child In Need of Services) or FWSN (Families With Service Needs). These new categories allow for court intervention in difficult cases; however, the court's role is often to provide an ASSESSMENT, make recommendations and monitor compliance with those recommendations.

statutory rape Criminal (though often consensual) sexual intercourse between an adult and a minor child that is also a form of SEXUAL ABUSE. Many state laws do not use the term *statutory rape*, instead using such terms as *criminal sexual assault*, *sexual assault*, *felonious sexual assault* or *aggravated sexual assault*. In some states, statutory rape is considered a form of child abuse, while in others, it is not reportable as child abuse. Only five states, Georgia, Mississippi, Missouri, North Carolina and

Tennessee, specifically use the term *statutory rape* in their statutes, which often causes confusion when attempts to make state-by-state comparisons are made. In addition, Pennsylvania has a criminal offense of "statutory sexual assault," while Nevada criminalizes "statutory sexual seduction."

Note: It is best to contact an attorney who is expert in state law to obtain current information on the laws of a particular state. This entry is provided for information only and does not constitute legal advice.

Purpose of Statutory Rape Laws

Statutory rape laws were initially passed to protect the chastity of young females, and they have continued to evolve through the years. Such laws currently exist to protect minor children from coercive or exploitive sexual contact with adults. As many as half of the children who are born to minors are fathered by adult males, and often the sexual partners of these adolescent mothers are three to six or more years older than the teenage girls. Some experts believe that a stricter enforcement of statutory rape laws would translate into far fewer teenage pregnancies.

Prosecutions for Statutory Rape

In general, statutory rape cases are often prosecuted less vigorously than other cases of sexual abuse, although prosecutors may exercise their own discretion. Said Elstein and Smith in *Victim-Oriented Multidisciplinary Responses to Statutory Rape Training Guide,* "Law enforcement often assigns statutory rape cases a much lower priority than incest and forcible rape cases with young children. There is a belief among criminal justice officers that investigation and arrest are a waste of time because prosecutors will not prosecute except in the most egregious cases."

The authors also stated that if prosecution does occur, often the defendant will state that he or she did not know the victim was underage. The authors advised that questions asked in the investigation can derail this defense, such as asking whether the victim was picked up at school, asking whether the victim and the defendant discussed the school day, whether the defendant attended intramural sports events in which the victim participated and whether the defendant attended school dances or the victim's birthday party.

If the teenage victim has a child, there may be a clear link to the defendant, either through the naming of the father on the baby's birth certificate or during application for public assistance. Even if the teenager has a miscarriage or abortion, a DNA test may be conducted on the fetus before it is destroyed, in order to determine paternity.

In some cases, when a child is pregnant or infected with a sexually transmitted disease, this is grounds for suspecting abuse. For example, in Rhode Island, a physician or nurse practitioner must report to protective services if a child who is less than 12 years old is infected with a sexually transmitted disease. In Michigan, physicians must report all cases if a child younger than age 12 is pregnant or has a sexually transmitted disease. However, in California, pregnancy alone is not grounds for a suspicion of sexual abuse.

In some cases, prosecutors may decide against prosecution unless the minor is very young, despite state laws making sexual contact illegal between the minor and the adult. However, this view may increase the risk for unwanted pregnancies and health and emotional problems among adolescents. According to Elstein and Smith, "Teenagers are just as deserving of protection from illegal sexual relationships as children and adults, even if they present themselves as sullen, uncooperative, sexually provocative, and difficult. After all, statutory rape is against the law."

Confusion over Consent

In many cases, the minor has consented to the sexual contact and openly states this to be true; however, state law often prohibits sexual contact even with the minor's stated consent, sometimes depending on the age of the minor. In some cases, violation of the law is a felony, while in others, it is a misdemeanor. For example, if the age difference between the minor victim and the defendant is greater than three years in California, this is a felony offense. If it is less than a three-year age difference, it is a misdemeanor.

Reporting Requirements May Be Unclear

Despite the disparity in state laws, in his article for *American Family Physician,* Dr. Tunzi advised that if criminal violence has occurred to the minor, then it should be reported by physicians to law enforcement authorities. In addition, if domestic abuse has occurred between a minor and an adult, physicians should contact the state protective service office to report child abuse.

Differences between States Laws

According to a report prepared by the Lewin Group in 2004 for the Office of the Assistant Secretary for Planning and Evaluation in the Department of Health and Human Services on state laws on statutory rape, only 12 states have one age below which it is not legal for a person to consent to sex. In other states, the age of consent depends on other factors, such as the age of the defendant, the age of the victim and sometimes the age differences between the defendant and the victim.

In some states, sex between two minors is illegal, while in other states, statutory rape is defined as sex between a person younger than 18 years old and an adult who is four years or more older than the minor. In about a third of the states, the relationship between the adolescent and the perpetrator is considered in making the determination for or against statutory rape; for example, in some states statutory rape is only considered a reportable offense to PROTECTIVE SERVICE personnel if the perpetrator is someone who holds responsibility for the child and who had sex with the minor or who has knowingly allowed sex to occur between the minor and another adult.

The other two-thirds of the states outline the specific circumstances under which statutory rape must be reported, with wide variations between the states.

Four Key Factors Related to Laws on Statutory Rape

The report compiled for the Office of the Assistant Secretary for Planning and Evaluation included data on state laws on sex between minors and adults. (See table.) Four key factors were considered relevant to statutory rape law. One factor is the age of consent, or the age at which an individual can legally consent to sexual intercourse under any circumstances. In the majority of states, the age of consent is age 16.

The second factor, and one that is applicable in about half the states, is the minimum age of the victim, or the age below which an individual cannot consent to sexual intercourse under any circumstances. These ages range between 10 years and 16 years, depending on the state.

The third factor is the age differential between the victim and the defendant. The age differential between the victim and the defendant may be heavily or partly weighted in determining whether prosecution should occur. The age differentials may also vary with the victim's age; for example, in Washington, a person who is between the ages of 14 and 16 years may legally consent to sex if the defendant is less than four years older than the victim. However, the age differential drops to three years if the victim is younger than age 14. It decreases further to two years if the victim is younger than age 12.

The fourth factor related to state statutory rape laws is the minimum age of the *defendant* (the accused) in order to prosecute, or "the age below which an individual cannot be prosecuted for engaging in sexual activities with minors." Some states consider the age of the defendant in determining whether to prosecute. For example, in Nevada, the age of consent is 16 years, but voluntary sex with someone under age 16 is illegal only if the defendant is 18 years old or older.

"Cultural" and "Married" Arguments against Prosecution for Sex with Minors

According to Elstein and Smith in their training guide on statutory rape, defendants will sometimes try to thwart their prosecution by stating that sex between an adult and young teenager is normal in their own native culture. However, prosecutors need not accept this view. Said the authors,

A prosecutor in Imperial County, California, reported that the defense sometimes argues that a sexual relationship is not wrong if it is part of the girl's and man's culture of origin. The prosecutor counter argues that this is not true and uses testimony of university professors as expert witnesses to dispel cultural myths raised by the defense. A prosecutor in Santa Clara County, California, argues that to allow the excuse that society should ignore statutory rape cases because it is part of the couple's culture of origin is simply a way of turning our backs on victims.

STATE AGE REQUIREMENTS

State	Age of consent	Minimum age of victim	Age differential between the victim and defendant (if victim is above minimum age)	Minimum age of defendant in order to prosecute
Alabama	16	12	2	16
Alaska	16	n/a	3	n/a
Arizona	18	15	2 (defendant must be in high school) and < 19 years old	n/a
Arkansas	16	n/a	3 (if victim is < age 14)	20 (if victim is = 14)
California	18	18	n/a	n/a
Colorado	17	n/a	4 (if victim is less than 15), 10 (if victim is less than 17)	n/a
Connecticut	16	n/a [1]	2	n/a
Delaware	18[2]	16	n/a	n/a
District of Columbia	16	n/a	4	n/a
Florida	18	16	n/a	24 (if victim is = 16)
Georgia	16	16	n/a	n/a
Hawaii	16	14	5	n/a
Idaho	18[3]	18	n/a	n/a
Illinois	17	17	n/a	n/a
Indiana	16	14	n/a	18 (if victim is = 14)
Iowa	16	14	4	n/a
Kansas	16	16	n/a	n/a
Kentucky	16	16	n/a	n/a
Louisiana	17	13	3 (if victim is < 14), 2 (if victim is < 17)	n/a
Maine	16	14[4]	5	n/a
Maryland	16	n/a	4	n/a
Massachusetts	16	16	n/a	n/a
Michigan	16	16[5]	n/a	n/a
Minnesota	16	n/a	3 (if victim is < 13), 2 (if victim is < 16)	n/a
Mississippi	16	n/a	2 (if victim is < 14), 3 (if victim is < 16)	n/a
Missouri	17	14	n/a	21 (if victim is = 14)
Montana	16	16[6]	n/a	n/a
Nebraska	16	16[7]	n/a	19
Nevada	16	16	n/a	18
New Hampshire	16	16	n/a	n/a
New Jersey	16	13[8]	4	n/a
New Mexico	16	13	4	18 (if victim is = 13)
New York	17	17	n/a	n/a
North Carolina	16	n/a	4	12
North Dakota	18	15	n/a	18 (if victim is = 15)
Oklahoma	16	14	n/a	18 (if victim is > 14)
Ohio	16	13	n/a	18 (if victim is = 13)
Oregon	18	15	3	n/a
Pennsylvania	16	13	4	n/a
Rhode Island	16	14	n/a	18 (if victim is 14)

(continues)

(Table continued)

State	Age of consent	Minimum age of victim	Age differential between the victim and defendant (if victim is above minimum age)	Minimum age of defendant in order to prosecute
South Carolina	16	14	Illegal if victim is 14 to 16 and defendant is older than victim	n/a
South Dakota	16	10[9]	3	n/a
Tennessee	18	13	4	n/a
Texas	17	14	3	n/a
Utah	18	16	10	n/a
Vermont	16	16	n/a	16
Virginia	18	15	n/a	18 (if victim is = 15)
Washington	16	n/a	2 (if victim is < 12), 3 (if victim is < 14) 4 (if victim is < 16)	n/a
West Virginia	16	n/a	4 (if victim is 11)	16, 14 (if victim is < 11)
Wisconsin	18	18	n/a	n/a
Wyoming	16	n/a	4	n/a

Note: Some states have marital exemptions. This table assumes the two parties are not married to each other.

1 Engaging in *sexual intercourse* with someone who is less than 16 years of age is legal under certain circumstances. However, *sexual contact* with someone who is less than 15 years of age is illegal regardless of the age of the defendant.

2 Sexual acts with individual who is at least 16 years of age are only illegal if the defendant is 30 years of age or older.

3 Intercourse with a *female* who is less than 18 years of age is illegal regardless of the age of the defendant. However, *sexual acts not amounting to penetration* are legal under certain circumstances in cases where the victim is at least 16 years of age.

4 It is illegal to engage in a *sexual act* with someone who is less than 14 years of age regardless of the age of the defendant. However, *sexual contact* or *sexual touching* with someone who is less than 14 years of age is legal under some circumstances.

5 It is illegal to engage in a *sexual penetration* with someone who is less than 16 years of age. However, *sexual contact* with someone who is at least 13 years of age is legal under certain circumstances.

6 *Sexual intercourse* with someone who is less than 16 years of age is illegal regardless of the age of the defendant. However, *sexual contact* with someone who is at least 14 years of age is legal under certain circumstances.

7 Under the offense, "debauching a minor," it is illegal to debauch or deprave morals by lewdly inducing someone less than 17 years of age to carnally know any other person.

8 It is illegal to engage in a *sexual penetration* with someone who is less than 13 years of age regardless of the age of the defendant. However, *sexual contact* with someone who is less than 13 years of age is legal under certain circumstances.

9 Engaging in *sexual penetration* with someone who is at least 10 years of age and less than 16 years of age is legal under certain circumstances. However, *sexual contact* with someone who is less than 16 years of age is illegal regardless of the age of the defendant.

Source: Glosser, Asaph, Karen Gardiner, and Mike Fishman. *Statutory Rape: A Guide to State Laws and Reporting Requirements,* prepared for the Office of the Assistant Secretary for Planning and Evaluation, Department of Health and Human Services: Lewin Group, December 15, 2004. Available online. URL: http://www.kewin.com/Lewin_Publications/Human_Services/StateLawsReport.htm. Downloaded September 25, 2005.

This prosecutor reasoned that people who have come to the United States from other countries as residents are subsequently subject to the rules of the United States, and thus, they may not be exempt from some laws because these behaviors may be allowed in their country of origin.

In other cases, the teenager and adult marry in a state where such marriage is allowed before the prosecution for statutory rape is completed in their home state. In some states, marriage is a defense to statutory rape, such as in Alaska, the District of Columbia and West Virginia.

Sometimes when such a marriage occurs, said the authors, "This happens because some defendants think if they marry the teen, they will not be prosecuted. The Santa Clara County, California, district attorney decided that marriage would be viewed as a 'nonevent,' having no impact on the prosecution of the case." This is an area of controversy, with some believing that marriage indicates a true commitment of the older person, while others believe that even if marriage occurs, the past sexual abuse of a minor should not be considered acceptable.

Issues with the Victim

Some teenage victims do not think that sex was forced unless they have been beaten or physically assaulted in some manner. However, upon further investigation, it may be discovered that adolescents may have submitted to sex because they feared being beaten if they refused to submit to demands for sex or because they wished to avoid the adult's anger. These are forms of coercion.

In some states, a case is prosecuted but the victim need not testify, and sometimes they may not even be advised of the outcome of the case. Said Elstein and Smith, "While it is possible to obtain convictions with minimal contact with victims, it is not good practice. Victims have rights in most States to be kept informed by the prosecutor or the victim advocate about what is happening with the case."

In addition, the authors said that victims should be notified if the arrested defendant is released from jail. The adult may be so angry with the victim that he or she may seek the victim out in retaliation for the incarceration. If adolescent victims know that the defendant will be released, they can avoid the places that are known to be normally frequented by the defendant. Victims may also be able to arrange to avoid being left alone or even to stay elsewhere with family members or friends in order to avoid the defendant, at least until the trial has occurred or they feel safe.

Physicians' Position Paper on Abuse and Sexual Activity

In 2004, the American Academy of Family Physicians, the American Academy of Pediatrics, the American College of Obstetricians and Gynecologists and the Society for Adolescent Medicine released a position paper on sexual activity and child abuse in the *Journal of Adolescent Health.* According to this paper, most cases of sexual coercion and sexual abuse can be identified with a careful clinical assessment. Said the authors,

These cases include adolescents in a sexual relationship with a family member, a person of authority (e.g., teacher, leader of a youth organization, etc.), or a member of the clergy. Also included are adolescents who are incapacitated by mental illness, mental retardation, drugs or alcohol, and are unable to comprehend, make informed decisions about, or consent to, sexual activity. In addition, any intimate relationships that are violent should be considered abusive. Physicians and other health professionals must know their state laws and report such cases to the proper authority, in accordance with state law, after discussion with the adolescent and parent, as appropriate.

The authors pointed out that in addition to physical force, sometimes verbal coercion is used with adolescents, in addition to drugs and alcohol.

See also CHILD PROSTITUTION; INCEST; SEXUAL TRAFFICKING.

American Academy of Family Physicians, the American Academy of Pediatrics, the American College of Obstetricians and Gynecologists and the Society for Adolescent Medicine. "Protecting Adolescents: Ensuring Access to Care and Reporting Sexual Activity and Abuse." *Journal of Adolescent Health* 35 (2004): 420–423.

Elstein, Sharon G., and Barbara E. Smith. *Victim-Oriented Multidisciplinary Responses to Statutory Rape Training Guide.* Washington, D.C.: U.S. Department of Justice, 1998.

Glosser, Asaph, Karen Gardiner, and Mike Fishman. *Statutory Rape: A Guide to State Laws and Reporting Requirements,* prepared for the Office of the Assistant Secretary for Planning and Evaluation, Department of Health and Human Services: Lewin Group, December 15, 2004. Available online URL: http://www.kewin.com/Lewin_Publications/Human_Services/StateLawsReport.htm. Downloaded September 25, 2005.

Tunzi, Marc, M.D. "Curbside Consultation: Isn't This Statutory Rape?" *American Family Physician* 65, no. 9 (May 1, 2002). Available online at URL: http://www.aafp.org/afp/20020501/curbside.html. Downloaded September 10, 2005.

stifling   See OVERLAYING.

stimulation, tactile   See TACTILE STIMULATION.

stipulation At the beginning of a trial, lawyers for both parties may enter into an oral or written agreement concerning certain facts of the case that are uncontested, These facts may include names and addresses of persons involved, relationships among the parties, ages etc. The stipulation serves as a basis for introduction of EVIDENCE and limits debate to those areas about which there is clear disagreement.

stomach, turned See *OPU HULE.*

stress Stress of various kinds is frequently associated with child abuse and neglect. Factors such as marital difficulty, POVERTY, work-related problems and SOCIAL ISOLATION have all been found to be related to increased levels of child abuse. Despite the association between stress and abuse it may not be correct to say that stress causes abuse. Many parents under a great deal of stress do not abuse or neglect their children.

Murray Straus, a noted researcher of FAMILY VIOLENCE, emphasizes the importance of mediating factors in establishing the link between stress and child maltreatment. Parents who were abused by their parents, in particular by the father, or who witnessed violence between their parents were more likely to abuse their own children. Straus suggests that violent responses to stress are learned, not innate.

Parents under stress are usually not uncontrollably driven to abuse their children. Parents who are abusive are more likely to approve of physical violence as a means of settling disputes. Marital violence is a strong predictor of child abuse. Both of these findings support the idea that parents who approve of or who regularly use physical force as a way of coping also abuse their children more often. Stress may increase the likelihood that parents who approve of violence will abuse their children but does not, by itself, produce violence.

Though stress may not directly cause child abuse, increases in family and societal stress may result in higher levels of abuse. Periods of high unemployment are frequently accompanied by increased family violence. Extreme poverty appears to increase the likelihood of abuse. Interestingly, however, occupational status and level of education do not appear to be related to abuse.

Learning how to cope with stress effectively is an important part of the treatment for perpetrators of child abuse. In many cases, parents are taught specific alternatives to physical punishment as a method of discipline or releasing frustrations. Groups such as Parents Anonymous place a great deal of importance on establishing support networks for parents under stress. Parents who have a number of contacts outside the family are usually better able to cope with stress than those who are relatively isolated.

subdural hematoma Battering or shaking may result in intracranial hemorrhaging, causing blood to collect immediately beneath the skull. This collection of blood, known as subdural hematoma, is usually caused by the tearing of veins running from the cerebral cortex to the dural sinuses.

Subdural hematoma may occur on only one side of the brain (lateral) or on both sides of the brain (bilateral). Eighty percent of all subdural hematomas in children are bilateral.

Almost all subdural hematomas are caused by trauma induced by the head striking or being struck by a heavy object, or by the rapid jerking motion of the head when an infant is shaken.

Although the most frequent cause of death in battered infants, it may also be one of the most frequently overlooked injuries. The absence of external signs, even in the presence of massive internal bleeding, makes diagnosis difficult. Subdural hematoma can be detected through the presence of blood in the subdural and cerebrospinal fluid and through the use of cranial computed tomography (CT).

subgaleal hematoma A collection of blood immediately underneath the scalp, called subgaleal hematoma, can be the result of HAIR PULLING. Blood accumulation is caused by the rupture of blood vessels attacked to the outside of the cranium.

subpoena Witnesses and accused perpetrators of child abuse may be subpoenaed to testify in court. The most common type of subpoena is sometimes referred to by its Latin name, subpoena ad testificandum. This type of subpoena is a written document, issued by a court or authorized agency, that requires the recipient to appear in a specified court at a certain day and time. Subpoena is literally translated as "under penalty." Failure to comply with a subpoena can result in a fine or imprisonment.

A subpoena duces tecum, literally, under penalty take with you, requires the recipient to bring certain relevant documents to court. In child abuse or neglect cases this type of subpoena may be issued to a physician or mental health professional, requiring them to submit treatment records of the victim or alleged abuser. Normally such information is considered PRIVILEGED COMMUNICATIONS; however, in many jurisdictions child abuse reporting laws specifically abrogate such privileges when abuse or neglect is suspected.

substance abuse   The frequent abuse of alcohol and/or drugs. Substance abuse may develop into dependence (addiction.) Substance abusers have a greater risk of committing child abuse and neglect than non-abusers, and in an estimated one-third to two-thirds of abused children, substance abuse of their parents or other caretakers is a factor.

Some drugs, such as cocaine and methamphetamine, are more predictive of child abuse than others; for example, methamphetamine creates a hypersexuality in some users, who have a high risk of sexual abuse. Parents are rarely sexual abusers, and according to *Child Maltreatment 2003*, a report produced by the Department of Health and Human Services and published in 2005, parents sexually abused their children in only 3% of cases, while in nearly 76% of perpetrators of sexual abuse, the abusers were friends or neighbors. However, drugs can remove the normal inhibitions of parents. Although some drugs have a greater risk for the user committing child abuse, all illegal drugs and illicit use of prescription drugs in their parents or caregivers are dangerous for children. Alcohol abuse in parents or caregivers is also very dangerous for children.

Heavy drinking during pregnancy can produce a number of birth defects and abnormalities, including those associated with FETAL ALCOHOL SYNDROME.

Children Prostitution

Young runaways may be lured into drug usage by pimps. CHILD PROSTITUTION becomes a means of obtaining drugs that, in turn, offer escape from the experience of emotional pain and lowered self-esteem associated with this lifestyle. Conversely, sometimes adolescents who are already drug-addicted will become prostitutes in order to obtain money to pay for drugs.

Teenagers sometimes become prostitutes because of SEXUAL TRAFFICKING. In some cases, they are given and/or compelled to take drugs by sexual traffickers (or the individuals to whom they are sold), so that they will become easier to control. Child prostitutes may also be forced into CHILD PORNOGRAPHY.

Protective Service Workers

When protective service workers become involved in the life of a child because of abuse and/or neglect allegations, often they must talk to the child about parental substance use. According to Breshear et al. in their manual for child protective service workers, the following statements may be helpful to facilitate a discussion with children:

- Addiction is a disease. Your parent is not a bad person; he or she has a disease. Parents may do things that are mean or stupid when they drink too much or use drugs.

- You are not the reason your parent drinks or uses drugs; you did not cause this disease and you cannot stop it.

- There are a lot of kids like you. In fact, there are millions of kids whose parents are addicted to drugs or alcohol; some are in your school. You are not alone.

- You can talk about the problem. You do not have to feel scared or ashamed or embarrassed. Find someone you can trust. Most towns have groups of kids that meet and talk, such as Alateen. A counselor, teacher, foster parent or other adult you trust may be able to help find one of these groups. (The child welfare workers can provide support as well.)

Child Welfare Goals v. Clients' Substance Abuse Problems

One issue of concern is that the agencies which provide substance abuse treatment to addicted individuals often have goals that differ from those of child welfare agencies. For example, at the substance treatment center, the person who abuses substances is the "client," and that person's family is not of primary importance or may be of no importance at all to the work of the treatment center.

Yet, with the passage of the ADOPTION AND SAFE FAMILIES ACT, and the provisons that parental rights should be terminated if a child is in foster care for 15 of the last 22 months (or sometimes in a shorter period, such as one year, depending on state law), substance abusers may be very concerned about their children who are in foster care and whether they may lose their parental rights. Thus, the timeline of the substance treatment center, which may not stipulate a time limit for recovery (federal law does not require such a time limit) often is very different from the much shorter timeline of the child welfare agency.

In additon to differing goals of rehabilitative centers and child welfare staff, confidentiality constraints may prevent substance treatment centers from conferring with child welfare agencies, even if a child welfare worker initiated a parent's going into treatment.

Child welfare workers may also worry, with reason, about the substance abuser's ability to "stay clean." Some relapses may be acceptable to the substance treatment center, but relapses are often not acceptable to the child welfare organization, because the child protective service worker is worried about the child's safety if he or she returned to the substance-abusing parent.

See also ABUSERS; PARENTAL SUBSTANCE ABUSE.

Breshears, E. M., S. Yeah, and N. K. Young. *Understanding Substance Abuse and Facilitating Recovery: A Guide for Child Welfare Workers.* Rockville, Md.: U.S. Department of Health and Human Services, Substance Abuse and Mental Health Services Administration, 2004.

substantiation Refers to the confirmation of the abuse of a child. Substantiation usually refers to incidents of physical or sexual abuse. Some cases cannot be substantiated because there is insufficient evidence, thus the allegation is unproven and is called "unsubstantiated." In some states, some cases are alluded to as "indicated," which means that abuse is likely, although unproven.

Sometimes abuse is faked, as in the case when an older sibling bit his own hand repeatedly, blaming a younger brother, who denied the abuse. Only when bite-mark impressions were taken was it proven that the older brother was biting himself.

Substantiation can be more difficult to determine in the case of infants or very young children, where marks and bruising may not be present, but the child has nonetheless sustained injuries or even death as a result of shaking, suffocation or other means. Often medical personnel may be consulted to help determine whether abuse was present or not. Sometimes physicians disagree among themselves on whether a child was abused.

Statistical Data

According to the Administration on Children, Youth and Families in the U.S. Department of Health and Human Services in their *Child Maltreatment 2003* report (released in 2005), there were 419,962 cases of substantiated child abuse in the United States in 2003. The substantiated cases included 669,218 child victims. (Some investigations involved more than one child in the family). There were also 918,304 cases that were *not* substantiated. (See Table I, which includes data from 49 states on substantiated or unsubstantiated cases of child abuse.)

As can be seen from Table I, there are more than twice as many unsubstantiated than substantiated cases.

Professional and Nonprofessional Reporters of Abuse

Depending on who has reported the suspicions of child abuse or child maltreatment, there are marked differences between the numbers and percents of substantiated cases. Reports that are filed by professionals are much more likely to be substantiated than those that are filed by others, such as friends and neighbors. Some writers speculate that professionals may be more familiar with diagnostic procedures and legal definitions of abuse than nonprofessionals, and therefore they are much better able to judge when a report should be filed. It is also true that professionals are much less likely

TABLE I
STATE-BY-STATE INVESTIGATIONS OF SUBSTANTIATED
AND UNSUBSTANTIATED CHILD ABUSE,
UNITED STATES, 2003

State	Substantiated	Unsubstantiated
Alabama	6,147	10,552
Alaska	4,260	2,344
Arizona	3,319	24,782
Arkansas	5,646	13,298
California	No data	No data
Colorado	5,923	20,380
Connecticut	9,267	23,535
Delaware	1,022	4,023
District of Columbia	1,456	2,980
Florida	33,427	75,523
Georgia	26,152	45,349
Hawaii	2,035	1,859
Idaho	975	5,289
Illinois	16,340	42,736
Indiana	14,997	19,308
Iowa	8,861	15,311
Kansas	3,878	11,962
Kentucky	9,964	19,978
Louisiana	7,187	16,927
Maine	2,632	2,520
Maryland	No data	No data
Massachusetts	22,051	17,640
Michigan	16,921	57,754
Minnesota	6,164	6,518
Mississippi	4,126	11,872
Missouri	7,053	11,065
Montana	994	6,608
Nebraska	2,379	4,643
Nevada	2,688	10,514
New Hampshire	766	5,659
New Jersey	5,872	7,490
New Mexico	4,060	11,218
New York	45,897	103,950
North Carolina	17,417	42,080
North Dakota	766	No data
Ohio	18,619	35,706
Oklahoma	7,261	19,366
Oregon	6,510	8,516
Pennsylvania	4,571	19,030
Rhode Island	2,168	4,691
South Carolina	6,448	12,001
South Dakota	924	2,594
Tennessee	5,950	20,840
Texas	33,093	72,372
Utah	7,714	11,612

State	Substantiated	Unsubstantiated
Vermont	1,012	1,854
Virginia	4,513	3,467
Washington	4,037	12,028
West Virginia	5,836	12,004
Wisconsin	10,174	25,842
Wyoming	490	714
Total	419,962	918,034

Source: Adapted from Administration on Children, Youth and Families. *Child Maltreatment 2003*. Children's Bureau, U.S. Department of Health and Human Services, Washington, D.C., 2005, pages 1–16.

to file intentionally false reports. (Nonprofessionals may be more likely to file false reports because of a grudge between neighbors, family members and others.) Professionals may also be more cooperative with investigators and more likely to follow up on their reports.

Data included in *Child Maltreatment 2003* revealed that professionals had more than double the numbers of substantiated cases (68.6%) than nonprofessionals (31.4%). (See Table II.) In addition, professionals had about a third of the rate of intentionally false reports (26.6%) compared to nonprofessionals (73.4%). Of all the categories of professionals, legal, law enforcement and criminal justice personnel (which is one category) had the highest percent of substantiated cases, followed by educational personnel and social services personnel. Categories of professionals with the lowest rates of substantiation included foster-care providers, child day-care providers and mental health personnel.

Of nonprofessional reporters, the following categories had the lowest rates of substantiation: alleged perpetrators, alleged victims and friends or neighbors.

In considering cases of reports that were intentionally false, among professionals, the following categories had the highest rates of intentionally false reports: criminal justice personnel, educational personnel and social services personnel. Professional reporters with the lowest rates of intentionally false reporters were foster-care providers, mental health personnel and medical personnel.

Among nonprofessional reports that were intentionally false, those with the highest percent of

TABLE II
SUBSTANTIATED, UNSUBSTANTIATED AND INTENTIONALLY FALSE SOURCES OF CHILD MALTREATMENT REPORTS,
PROFESSIONALS V. NONPROFESSIONALS BASED ON DATA FROM 43 STATES

Report source	Substantiated		Unsubstantiated		Intentionally false	
Professionals	Number	Percent	Number	Percent	Number	Percent
Educational personnel	49,595	13.8	141,526	17.6	32	7.0
Legal, law enforcement, criminal justice personnel	95,985	26.7	86,888	10.8	35	7.6
Social services personnel	47,279	13.2	87,430	10.9	24	5.2
Medical personnel	38,956	10.9	60,607	7.5	19	4.1
Mental health personnel	9,440	2.6	25,920	3.2	11	2.4
Child day-care providers	2,895	0.8	9,512	1.2	No data	No data
Foster-care providers	2,207	0.6	6,918	0.9	1	0.2
Total professionals	**246,357**	**68.6**	**418,801**	**52.0**	**122**	**26.6**
Nonprofessionals						
Anonymous reporters	18,475	5.1	95,878	11.9	75	16.3
Other reporters	24,848	6.9	67,239	8.4	30	6.5
Other relatives	23,779	6.6	72,458	9.0	61	13.3
Parents	17,404	4.8	68,106	8.5	114	24.8
Friends or neighbors	12,015	3.3	54,134	6.7	44	9.6
Unknown reporters	13,794	3.8	21,311	2.6	7	1.5
Alleged victims	1,735	0.5	6,119	0.8	4	0.9
Alleged perpetrators	515	0.1	625	0.1	2	0.4
Total nonprofessionals	**112,565**	**31.4**	**385,870**	**48.0**	**337**	**73.4**
Total, professionals and nonprofessionals	**358,922**	**100.0**	**804,671**	**100.0**	**459**	**100.0**

Source: Adapted from Administration on Children, Youth and Families, *Child Maltreatment 2003*. Children's Bureau, U.S. Department of Health and Human Services, Washington, D.C., 2005, pages 18–19.

reports were parents, anonymous reporters and other relatives. Those nonprofessionals with the lowest rates of intentionally false reports were individuals who were classified as alleged perpetrators, alleged victims and unknown reporters.

Power of Protective Services Is Debated

Some groups have protested that PROTECTIVE SERVICE staff have far too much power and frequently remove a child from a home where abuse has not yet been substantiated and may not have occurred at all. Often the decision boils down to a combination of the skill, experience and intuition of the protective service personnel.

Unfortunately, when social services staff err on the side of assuming that abuse was either mild or nonexistent, in some cases the children have subsequently died from abuse, and a public outcry arises that the state should "do something" about this problem. Thus, it can be a difficult balancing act for social service staff, many of whom receive little training and experience very high turnover.

See also INVESTIGATION; SIBLING ABUSE; UNFOUNDED REPORTS.

Administration on Children, Youth and Families. *Child Maltreatment 2003*. Children's Bureau, U.S. Department of Health and Human Services, Washington, D.C., 2005.

substantive due process   See DUE PROCESS.

sudden infant death syndrome (SIDS)   The sudden death of an infant under one year of age that remains unexplained after a thorough investigation, including performance of a complete autopsy, examination of the death scene and a thorough review of the child's clinical history. SIDS is also known as crib death and cot death. An estimated 2,200 infants die of SIDS in the United States each year.

Until the 19th century, overlaying, or accidentally rolling over on a baby in bed, was considered the primary cause of sudden and non-abusive deaths of infants. (It is also currently known as an actual cause of SIDS, although "overlaying" is not the terminology that is used.) Overlaying was thought to be preventable, and it was punished by the early Roman Catholic and Anglican churches. In the 17th century, the *arcuccio* was invented to prevent overlaying. This arch made of wood and steel was placed over the baby to prevent suffocation. Failure to use this device was a punishable offense in some countries. References to the use of the *arcuccio* can be found as late as 1890.

Physicians, baffled by a lack of identifiable symptoms, have suspected many different causes for SIDS through history. The belief that death was related to an enlarged thymus gland subsequently led to the practice of preventive irradiation of the thymus gland during the 1930s and 1940s. This "safety" measure was later found to cause cancer. A large thymus gland is now considered a common characteristic of most infants.

Known Risk Factors for SIDS

Based on modern research, the following SIDS risk factors have been identified:

- A prone (on the stomach) position of the baby during naps or nighttime sleeping
- Maternal smoking during pregnancy (which triples the risk of SIDS in the baby after birth)
- Smoking of others in the home during infancy
- Sleeping on a soft surface
- Late or no prenatal care
- Young maternal age (under age 20)
- Male gender of the child
- Premature birth

In addition, higher rates of SIDS have been found among African Americans (two times the rate of the national average for SIDS) and American Indians/Alaska Natives (three times the national average). It is unknown if these higher rates are related to other SIDS factors, such as young maternal age, smoking, low birth weight and so forth. In addition, some research has found that black mothers, unmarried mothers and poor mothers are more likely to place their babies in the prone position, despite warnings to the contrary from physicians, family and friends.

According to the Policy Statement from the Task Force on Sudden Infant Death Syndrome, within the American Academy of Pediatrics (published in *Pediatrics* in November 2005), other risk factors for SIDS have also been identified. For example, according to this group, "bed sharing" may cause accidental suffocation or death, particularly in infants younger than 11 weeks old. The risk is increased with multiple bed sharers and is further increased if one of the bed sharers has consumed alcohol or is overtired. Sleeping with an infant on the couch is even more dangerous than sleeping with the infant in a bed. Instead, the experts recommend that the infant sleep in his or her own crib in the parents' room until the child is about six months old.

A new finding is that pacifiers for infants six months old or younger may provide a *protective* mechanism against SIDS, although the reason for this is unclear.

Another cause for SIDS is the use of pillows or soft mattresses, combined with the prone position.

In some cases, sudden infant deaths have been associated with fetal exposure to cocaine during pregnancy.

The Back to Sleep Campaign

The Back to Sleep Program Studies implicated several key factors in SIDS. One primary cause was attributed to a prone (facedown) sleeping position of the baby, and in 1994, pediatricians in the United States, the United Kingdom and other countries began massive programs to convince pregnant women and new mothers to place their babies in the supine (face-up) position. This program was named "Back to Sleep."

This action has resulted in a marked reduction in the number of SIDS cases, and according to physicians who reported on SIDS in a 1999 issue of *Current Opinion in Pediatrics,* "During the past decade the most exciting news about sudden infant death syndrome (SIDS) has been the dramatic effect of the supine sleep position in lowering the SIDS rate." However, some mothers continue to use the prone position for their infants.

Some pediatricians have stated that some mothers have interpreted the advice to mean that the baby should *never* be in the prone position; however, the preference for the back position is for when the child is sleeping, not when he or she is active. Also, if the child has gastroesophageal reflux or other airway disorders that may predispose them to choking when on their backs, a pediatric gastroenterologist may advise that the child sleep in the prone position.

Physicians also warn that if the child is being cared for by another caretaker or a day-care center, parents should inform them as well that the prone position is not acceptable while the baby is sleeping, and instead that the baby should be placed on his or her back. According to the Task Force on Sudden Infant Death Syndrome, about 20% of all SIDS deaths occur when the infant is in the care of someone other than the parents. This may be because the caretaker or child-care center places the child on the stomach rather than the back.

When Abuse Is the Cause

Some experts have contended that there is overdiagnosis of SIDS. In one study in the United Kingdom, Professor Roy Meadow of St. James's University Hospital in Leeds studied 71 children who had been diagnosed with death from natural causes or SIDS (42 from SIDS and 29 from natural causes) but were later found to have been murdered by their parents.

In more than 80% of these cases, the cause of death was smothering by the mother. In 27 of the cases, blood had been found in the mouth, nose or on the face of the child and 10 of the children had unusual bruises on the face or neck. Two of the children had fractured ribs and two had paper balls in their stomach. In addition, 29 of the children came from families in which other children had died.

Professor Meadow stated, "Many pediatric units are failing to heed warning signs and failing to protect some very vulnerable children. The sudden infant death syndrome has been used at times as a pathological diagnosis to evade awkward truths."

In some cases, physicians in the United Kingdom have used covert video monitoring of the parents in order to protect the child when there is suspicion of parental involvement in apparent life-threatening events, and they have found that some parents sought to suffocate their infants. In their article in *British Medical Journal* in 2004, Craft and Hall estimated that about 10% of all unexplained deaths may be caused by deliberate suffocation of infants. If the infant is bleeding from the mouth and nose, this may indicate deliberate suffocation.

Preventive Advice

According to the National Institute of Child Health & Human Development, the following ways are recommended to reduce the risk of SIDS among infants under the age of one year (and particularly between the ages of two and four months, when most SIDS deaths occur):

- Place the baby on the back to sleep, for naptime and at night.
- Place the baby on a firm sleep surface. Avoid pillows, quilts, sheepskins or other soft surfaces.
- Keep soft objects, toys and loose bedding out of the baby's crib or sleep area.
- Never allow smoking around the baby.
- Keep the baby close to where others sleep but not in the same bed, couch or chair. If the baby is breast-fed in bed, when breast-feeding is completed, place the infant on the back in a separate sleeping area, such as a crib, bassinet cosleeper (an infant bed that attaches to the adult bed).
- Give the baby a clean, dry pacifier when placing the child for sleep, but do not force it. If breast-feeding, do not use a pacifier until the baby is about a month old.
- Do not overheat the baby. Use light sleepwear and keep the room temperature at a level comfortable for an adult.

- Avoid products that claim to reduce the likelihood of SIDS. Few have been tested for effectiveness or safety. Ask your doctor if you are unsure if a product may be useful.

- Avoid home monitors to reduce the risk of SIDS because they are not useful for this purpose.

See also ABUSERS; CHILD ABUSE; FATALITIES; INFANTICIDE; MUNCHAUSEN SYNDROME BY PROXY; PHYSICAL ABUSE; SHAKEN INFANT SYNDROME.

Blackwell, C. C. et al. "Infection, Inflammation and Sleep: More Pieces to the Puzzle of Sudden Infant Death Syndrome (SIDS)." *APMLS: Acta Pathologica, Microbiolgica et Immunologica Scandinavica* 107, no. 5 (May 1999): 455–473.

Blatt, Steven D., et al. "Sudden Infant Death Syndrome. Child Sexual Abuse, and Child Development." *Current Opinion in Pediatrics* 11, no. 2 (April 1999): 175–186.

Carroll, John L. and Ellen S. Siska. "SIDS: Counseling Parents to Reduce the Risk." *American Family Physician* 57, no. 7 (April 1, 1998): 1,566.

Committee on Child Abuse and Neglect. "Distinguishing Sudden Infant Death Syndrome from Child Abuse Fatalities." *Pediatrics* 107, no. 2 (February 2001): 437–441.

Croft, A. W., and D. M. B. Hall. "Munchausen Syndrome by Proxy and Sudden Infant Death." *British Medical Journal* 32 (May 28, 2004): 1,309–1,312.

Dwyer, Terence, et al. "Tobacco Smoke Exposure at One Month of Age and Subsequent Risk of SIDS—A Prospective Study." *American Journal of Epidemiology* 149, no. 7 (April 1, 1999): 593–602.

Guntheroth, Warren G. *Crib Death: The Sudden Infant Death Syndrome.* Mount Kisco, N.Y.: Futura, 1982.

Malloy, Michael. "SIDS—A Syndrome in Search of a Cause." *New England Journal of Medicine* 251, no. 10 (September 2, 2004): 957–959.

Martin, Richard J., et al. "Screening for SIDS: A Neonatal Perspective." *Pediatrics* 103, no. 4 (April 1, 1999): 812.

National Institute of Child Health and Child Development. *Safe Sleep for Your Baby: Ten Ways to Reduce the Risk of Sudden Infant Death Syndrome (SIDS).* Available online. URL: http//www.nichd.nih.gov/SIDS/reduce_infant_risk.htm. Downloaded December 7, 2005.

Task Force on Sudden Infant Death Syndrome. "Diagnostic Coding Shifts, Controversies Regarding the Sleeping Environment, and New Variables to Consider in Reducing Risk." *Pediatrics* 116, no. 5 (November 2005): 1,245–1,255.

White, Caroline. "Some 'Cot Deaths' Are Child Abuse." *British Medical Journal* 318, no. 147 (January 16, 1999): 147.

suicide   Studies indicate that emotionally, physically or sexually abused children, particularly adolescents, are more prone to suicide attempts than are children who are not abused. If a child has made or threatens to make a suicide attempt, then the possibility of abuse should he considered. (See also ADOLESCENT ABUSE.) Studies also indicate that adults who were abused as children are more prone to suicide attempts.

In the case of an adolescent, often the abuser is someone known to the adolescent, such as a family member, stepfather or other individual. In some cases, the suicidal child may be reacting to emotional and sexual abuse that she or he (usually she) is suffering from at the hands of peers. For example, in a Canadian study reported in a 1997 issue of *Adolescence*, researchers studied 1,025 females from grades 7–12 in Alberta schools. They found that nearly a quarter (23%) of the girls had experienced at least one type of sexual assault (sexual touching, sexual threats, indecent exposure) and 4% had frequently experienced such harassment.

Of the 793 girls who had never experienced any sexual assaults, about 15% were emotionally disturbed and 1% were suicidal. If the assault happened once, as happened to 105 girls, the percentage of girls who were emotionally disturbed rose to 20%, and nearly 3% were suicidal. If the assaults happened a few times, as happened to 107 girls, the rate of emotional disturbances was about 21% but the suicide rate increased to nearly 5%. And when the assault was frequent (as happened to 20 girls), then 31% of the girls were emotionally disturbed and 10% were suicidal. Clearly, sexual harassment has a profound impact on adolescents.

See also ADULTS ABUSED AS CHILDREN.

Bagley, Christopher, et al. "Sexual Assault in School, Mental Health and Suicidal Behaviors in Adolescent

Women in Canada." *Adolescence* 32, no. 126 (Summer 1997): 361–366.

supervision The term *supervision* is used in three different ways when speaking of child abuse and neglect. First, supervision may refer to the responsibility for protecting and guiding a child, usually a parental responsibility. When a child protection agency invested with authority to intervene determines that a child's caretakers are not giving adequate supervision, it may assume responsibility for the child.

Supervision also refers to oversight of a case by the child protection worker. Under this meaning of the word the entire family is the subject of supervision. Such intervention is usually guided by a SERVICE PLAN that outlines specific tasks and objectives for the family. The primary function of the child protection worker is to ensure that the family is taking steps necessary for protection of the child.

Finally, the process by which cases are reviewed is also referred to as supervision. Case review usually involves a meeting between the child protection worker and his or her superior to discuss both the family's progress and the worker's management of the case. This type of supervision helps make sure proper procedures are followed and may delay or prevent BURNOUT. Ongoing support and instruction are particularly important for counteracting job-related stress and maintaining the morale of child protection workers.

supporting services Abusive and neglectful parents are often subject to social, emotional and economic stress. Prevention of further maltreatment of children may require addressing the underlying causes of family stress as well as direct treatment of the abuse.

Support services include a wide variety of human services that help families function more effectively. Impoverished families will benefit from economic assistance, possibly in the form of CATEGORICAL AID. Other services include vocational training, educational assistance, child care and recreation. In some cases, support services alone may be sufficient to reduce family stress to a manageable level.

suspended judgment See DISPOSITION.

swaddling The ancient custom of tightly wrapping infants in a long strip of cloth is still practiced in some cultures. Swaddling restricts the child's movements and is said by critics to be physically, socially and emotionally damaging. In Turkey, some mothers swaddle their infants and strap them to their backs while working or traveling. Though held to be abusive in most Western countries, swaddling is considered simply a convenient way of carrying an infant in other cultures.

Sweden According to the *Country Reports on Human Rights Practices,* released by the United States State Department in 2005, child abuse is a problem in Sweden. The National Council for Crime Prevention reported 8,198 cases of child abuse of children younger than age 15 in Sweden in 2004. In considering sexual abuse only, there were 467 reported cases of rape in 2004, up from 332 cases in 2003. In addition, there were 1,400 reported cases of sexual abuse in 2004, up from 1,043 cases in 2003.

Child abuse is illegal in Sweden as is slapping a child or spanking. (See CORPORAL PUNISHMENT.) In general, the sentence for slapping or spanking is a fine, counseling and monitoring by social workers. However, the authorities may remove a child from the home and place him or her into foster care if the circumstances warrant such action.

Incidents of child trafficking of children and adolescents sometimes occur, although it is not common in Sweden. Those who violate the law against sexual trafficking may be sentenced to two to 10 years in prison. The police reported eight cases of child trafficking in 2004, and most victims were ages 16 and 17. Most of the trafficked children came from Estonia.

Bureau of Democracy, Human Rights, and Labor. *Country Reports on Human Rights Practices, 2004: Sweden.* United

States State Department, released on February 28, 2005. Available online. URL: http://www.state.gov/g/drl/rls/hrrpt/2004/41710.htm. Downloaded September 1, 2005.

syphilis A genital ulcerative disease caused by the *Treponema pallidum* bacterium that may, if left untreated, eventually attack the heart, blood vessels, spinal cord, brain and bones as well as the genitals. It can be fatal if untreated. It should also be noted that infection with syphilis does not provide immunity to reinfection. If a person is treated and recovers from syphilis, the disease may be contracted yet again.

Syphilis facilitates the transmission of the HUMAN IMMUNODEFICIENCY VIRUS. Sexual intercourse is the primary method by which the syphilis bacterium is transmitted; however, infants may contract the disease from their pregnant mothers, before or during birth. Syphilis can be contracted through oral, anal or vaginal sex, through contact with open sores. If a woman contracts syphilis within four years of her pregnancy, the fetus will be infected in greater than 70% of the cases.

Children who present with syphilis usually have been victimized by SEXUAL ABUSE. Adolescents with syphilis may have been sexually abused or may be victims of STATUTORY RAPE.

In 2003, the number of syphilis cases in the United States increased to 7,177 cases (1,217 among women, 5,956 cases among men and four cases in which the gender of the infected person was not reported). The number of cases in 2002 was 6,862. In 2003, the rate of both primary and secondary syphilis among women was highest in women ages 20–24 years and men ages 35–39 years.

As a precaution, children adopted from countries outside the United States and Canada should be tested for syphilis. About 15% of children adopted from Russia and countries that comprise the former Soviet Union have been treated for congenital syphilis prior to adoptive placement. In general, children from China and Central American countries are at greatest risk, according to the third edition of *The Encyclopedia of Adoption.*

Children in foster care who have been or may have been sexually abused or had consensual sex

with others should also be tested. Syphilis is not common in infants and children, but among those who contract the infection, it can have devastating long-term consequences if it is unidentified and untreated.

Symptoms and Diagnostic Path

Painless chancres (pimples, blisters or open sores) appear about three weeks after infection. Fever, sore throat and joint pain are other symptoms that may occur. Early treatment with penicillin is usually effective; however, some penicillin-resistant strains have developed. Treatment can stop the disease but cannot reverse physiological damage done to the brain and spinal cord. Congenital syphilis passed to an infant from an infected mother can weaken the child's bones, causing lesions in the joints. These lesions are sometimes mistaken for assault-induced wounds. Blood tests and the presence of other symptoms can aid in an accurate diagnosis.

According to the Centers for Disease Control and Prevention (CDC), syphilis cannot be transmitted through contact with doorknobs touched by infected people or through hot tubs, bathtubs, shared eating utensils or clothing or toilet seats. Instead, syphilis is contracted through direct contact with a syphilis sore and may be transmitted through oral, anal or vaginal sex. Pregnant women can transmit syphilis to their fetuses.

Stages of Syphilis

There are three stages of syphilis: primary, secondary and late (tertiary) stage. Each stage has different symptoms.

With the primary stage, the typical painless chancre sore (there is usually one sore, but some people have multiple chancres) appears in about two to six weeks and is usually located on the infected person's vagina, vulva or penis. The chancre may also appear on the tongue or lips. The chancre usually appears where the syphilis entered the body. The time from the initial infection with syphilis and the development of the chancre is about 21 days but ranges from 10 to 90 days from contact with an infected person.

In the second stage (secondary syphilis), the bacteria enter the bloodstream and spread throughout the body. With secondary syphilis, the patient experiences a rash that appears on one or more parts of the body. The rash of secondary syphilis may present as red, rough or reddish brown spots about the size of a penny, and they nearly always appear on the soles of the feet and palms of the hand. Rashes with a different appearance may present on other parts of the body. Other symptoms of secondary syphilis include sore throat, fever, swollen lymph glands, headache, weight loss, muscle aches and fatigue. There may also be patchy hair loss. Without treatment, the infection will progress to the tertiary stage. The secondary stage of syphilis may last from about one to two years.

In the third stage, some patients have latent syphilis, in which the disease is inactive. However, about a third of patients who have had untreated secondary syphilis will develop the complications of tertiary syphilis. In the latent or active third stage, syphilis is not contagious to others. It is within the third stage when the disease may damage the brain, nervous system, bones, heart, eyes, joints and other parts of the body. Mental illness, blindness and death may also occur in late-stage syphilis.

Syphilis is not contagious to others if the patient is in the third stage, although it is contagious during the primary and secondary stages.

Infants with Congenital Syphilis

Children born to mothers with syphilis may have symptoms at birth, but they often develop symptoms from two weeks to three months later. Their symptoms may include the following:

- Rashes
- Fever
- Weakened crying
- Yellowish skin (jaundice)
- Anemia (low red blood cell count)
- Skin ulcers
- Swollen liver and spleen

Individuals who provide care to infected infants should take special care, because the sores that develop are contagious. In some rare cases, the syphilis infection is not detected in infants, and when children become older children or adolescents, they may develop the symptoms of late-stage syphilis, such as damage to their brains, bones, teeth, eyes and ears.

Tests for Syphilis

The Venereal Disease Research Laboratory (VDRL) microscopic slide test or the rapid plasma reagin (RPR) are the primary tests to detect the presence of syphilis. A positive finding on either test is then confirmed with highly specific tests, such as fluorescent treponemal antibody absorption and micro-agglutination-*T. pallidum.*

Treatment Options and Outlook

If the disease is detected in the early stages, syphilis is treated with antibiotics, usually given as intramuscular injections. Syphilis can damage the eyes and ears, and children who contracted syphilis at or after birth (congenital syphilis) should receive eye examinations performed by an ophthalmologist, as well as hearing tests performed by a specialist. Dental treatment is indicated because even treated syphilis can lead to dental malformations.

If the person has had syphilis for more than a year before it is treated, it is more difficult to treat, and additional doses of antibiotics will be required. Treatment will not repair the damage that was already caused to the body by syphilis.

Risk Factors and Preventive Measures

The best way to avoid contracting syphilis is to refrain from sexual contact with infected people. Children born to infected mothers should be treated as soon as possible. They may develop developmental delays and seizures and may die if treatment does not commence quickly. Children who have been sexually exposed to a person who has syphilis, children with any sore around the genital area, and children with any symptoms of the disease should be evaluated by a physician. In addition, children who are sexually active and report that they have any symptoms of any type of sexually transmitted disease or who know they have had sexual contact with a person infected with syphilis (or who may have been infected with syphilis) should be urged to obtain immediate medical treatment. If parents learn that a child is sexually active or plans to become so, the child should receive regular gynecological or male genital examinations. Physicians can check for sexually transmitted diseases during these examinations.

Miller, Laurie C., M.D., and Christine Adamec. *The Encyclopedia of Adoption.* 3rd ed. New York: Facts On File, 2006.

National Center for HIV, STD, and TB Prevention. *Sexually Transmitted Disease Surveillance 2003 Supplement.* Atlanta, Ga.: Centers for Disease Control and Prevention, December 2004. Available online URL: http://www.cdc.gov/std/Syphilis2003syphsurvsupp2003.pdf. Downloaded October 16, 2005.

tactile stimulation Touching and holding infants appears to be important for their healthy sensory and emotional development. Early studies of HOSPITALISM led researchers to conclude that, in addition to adequate food and shelter, close physical and emotional contact with a nurturing adult is essential for normal development. Infants who did not receive such contact appeared dull and listless. Several eventually died despite availability of sufficient food, shelter and medical care.

Some experts speculate that FAILURE-TO-THRIVE SYNDROME is due not only to inadequate nutrition but to a lack of tactile stimulation as well. Parents who fail to develop an attachment to their infant may be cold and physically rejecting. Deprived infants can often be recognized by their eagerness to be held by strangers at a time when others their age demonstrate a normal fear of strangers.

Parents who were neglected as children often have a difficult time learning how to hold and touch their babies. Often they must be taught how to touch, rock and soothe their infants. Those who were physically or sexually abused must often overcome negative associations with physical contact. Some early intervention programs focus on teaching high-risk parents how to touch, hold and care for their infants in a positive and mutually enjoyable way.

See also EMOTIONAL NEGLECT.

target child Typically, in an abusive family, one child is singled out as the target of abuse. Reasons for selection of a particular child are not fully understood. In some cases, the child may be considered difficult or frustrating, for example, an infant who cries frequently; in other cases the child may have a physical deformity or simply be considered unattractive by the parent. Through a process known as SCAPEGOATING, the child becomes identified to the parent(s) as a "problem child." Because the target child may, indeed, be difficult to care for, he or she may be accused of causing the abuse. Attempts to rationalize abuse of a target child often result in BLAMING THE VICTIM. Focusing on the abused child's negative behavior may divert attention from the parent's inappropriate or brutal handling of the situation.

Treatment of the abuser seeks to change negative attitudes toward the target child. Often, peer support groups such as Parents Anonymous and parent training are helpful in presenting different ways in which parents can respond to frustrating situations.

team, community See COMMUNITY TEAM.

teenage pregnancy In a study reported in a 1998 issue of *Pediatrics* on 1,026 African-American women, most of whom were age 17 and 18, the researchers found a significant link between sexual abuse and early first intercourse and early pregnancy. Researchers found the sexually abused females had intercourse seven months earlier than non-abused women and their first pregnancy occurred 10 months earlier than those of the women who were not sexually abused. The women who had not been sexually abused had a first intercourse at the age of 15.5 years and their first pregnancy occurred at age 17.3 years.

The researchers defined childhood sexual abuse as nonconsensual sexual contact before age 13, including any of the following: intercourse, the child being touched on genitals or breasts or the child being forced to touch the genitals of the perpetrator. They found that more than 12% of the women had experienced an incidence of sexual abuse before age 13.

The researchers also looked at the incidence of physical and emotional abuse and age at first intercourse and pregnancy but did not find a significant relationship.

See also SEXUAL ABUSE.

Kevin Fiscella, et al. "Does Child Abuse Predict Adolescent Pregnancy?" *Pediatrics* 101 (April 1998): 620–624.

termination of parental rights   The severing by a court of all legal ties between a parent and a child. The parent may willingly sever the parental rights, as when a child is voluntarily placed for adoption by parents who know or believe that they cannot care for their children. The termination of parental rights may also be involuntary, as when the court determines that it is in the best interest of an abused or neglected child for the termination of parental rights to be made, whether the parents wish it so or not.

Once parental rights have been terminated by the court, the child may be adopted by another family. In some circumstances, the child will remain with or be transferred to the care of other relatives or a legal guardian. In many cases, foster children whose parental rights were terminated will then be adopted by their foster parents. They will not leave the household to which they have become accustomed, despite their change in legal status from foster child to adopted child. (However, this change is reportedly very significant in the minds of most former foster children and their new adoptive parents.)

The criteria for an involuntary termination of parental rights vary according to the state. (See APPENDIX V for a state-by-state listing of the grounds for terminating parental rights involuntarily.)

In general, parental rights may be terminated in the United States for the following reasons:

- Abandonment
- Severe alcohol or drug abuse by the parent(s)
- Serious mental illness or developmental delay of the custodial parent

- Repeated abuse or neglect of the child
- When other children in the family have been tortured or killed
- When the child has been in foster care for 15 of the past 22 months.

Some states terminate parental rights because of the parents' alcohol or drug abuse or because the children have been exposed to alcohol, drugs and/or have been encouraged or compelled to engage in sexual acts with adults.

States may terminate parental rights early, if there are special circumstances, such as the abandonment of an infant.

Child advocates differ in their ideas about the process of the termination of parental rights. Some believe that children should remain with the biological parents in all but clearly life-threatening or permanently and severely damaging situations. Supporters of this view emphasize the need for more and better interventions to help maintain the child at home.

Another point of view focuses on the potential danger to the child of remaining in an abusive situation, as well as the damaging effects of frequent or prolonged foster-care placement. This group believes that the decision of whether to terminate parental rights should be made relatively quickly to avoid long periods of uncertainty and to free the child for adoption at an earlier age if the parent (or other caretaker) is unable to resolve the problem that led to the abuse and/or neglect of the child.

Some experts believe that some abusive and/or neglectful parents are "untreatable." These parents do not acknowledge that their abuse or neglect was wrong, and they clearly have no intention of changing their behavior, despite what actions are taken and what help is offered by well-meaning and hardworking social workers. In such cases, the termination of parental rights is usually the best solution for the child.

See also ABUSERS; ADULTS ABUSED AS CHILDREN; FOSTER CARE; NEGLECT; PHYSICAL ABUSE; SEXUAL ABUSE.

tertiary prevention   See PREVENTION.

testimony Most EVIDENCE produced in trials related to child abuse and neglect takes the form of testimony. This type of evidence includes any written or spoken statement made under oath to establish a fact. Testimony is usually given in court in the presence of both the plaintiff and defendant. WITNESSES presenting testimony on behalf of one party are subject to questioning, or cross-examination, by the opposing party.

Usually, only testimony concerning facts directly observed or otherwise perceived by the witness are admissible in court. Hearsay testimony, involving observations made by persons other than the witness, is allowed only under certain circumstances. Some courts allow introduction of hearsay testimony in preliminary hearings. In such cases, an adult, usually the person who conducted the initial INVESTIGATION, is allowed to testify concerning the nature of alleged abuse. Judges usually allow this type of testimony in an effort to protect children from trauma associated with repeated court appearances.

Under the rules of *res gestae,* statements made during the excitement of an event may also be admitted as evidence. This rule is often referred to as the EXCITED UTTERANCE exception to the hearsay rule. Remarks made by a child to a teacher, parent, caseworker or similar party in a state of excitement following an abusive incident are allowed as testimony even though they are technically hearsay. Excited utterances are allowed under the theory that the urgency of the circumstances eliminates the element of self-interest, therefore increasing the likelihood that the statement is true. Timeliness is important in determining the admissibility of a res gestae statement. Statements made after a significant passage of time are not likely to be admitted as testimony. However, the precise amount of time allowed between the alleged abuse and the child's excited utterance is unclear. In at least one case, *State of Rhode Island v. Creighton,* The court accepted as evidence a statement made 14 hours after the event. The Rhode Island court reasoned that there was sufficient evidence in the record to establish that the victim was still under stress at the time of the statement.

Testifying in court can be a frightening experience for an adult. The experience may be terrifying

HINTS FOR TESTIFYING

- Dress appropriately.
- Prepare ahead of time.
- Do not memorize your testimony.
- Expect to feel anxious.
- Speak a little louder and slower than you feel is necessary.
- Be sincere and dignified.
- Speak clearly and distinctly.
- Use appropriate language.
- Answer the question that was asked.
- Let the attorney develop your testimony.
- If you do not know the answer to a question, say so. Do not guess.
- Do not make your testimony conform to other testimony you may have heard.
- When answering questions, look at the person asking the questions or at the judge or jury.
- Tell the truth.

How to survive cross-examination:
- Be careful about what you say and how you say it.
- Listen carefully to the question; do not answer it unless you understand it.
- If a question has two parts requiring different answers, answer it in two parts.
- Keep calm.
- Answer positively rather than doubtfully.
- If you are testifying as an expert, be prepared to reconcile or distinguish your opinion from opposing schools of thought.
- Do not close yourself off from supplying additional details.
- Do not allow yourself to be rushed.
- Do not get caught by a trick question.

Source: U.S. Department of Health and Human Services, Office of Human Development Services, Administration on Children, Youth and Families, Children's Bureau, National Center on Child Abuse and Neglect, *Child Protection: The Role of the Courts* (Washington, D.C.: Government Printing Office: 1980; [OHDS] 80-30256), 1980; page 59.

for a child. Victims of SEXUAL ABUSE are frequently asked to describe embarrassing and traumatic experiences in a large, formal courtroom in the presence of the alleged assailant. Some experts characterize the formal process of testifying in court as equally traumatic as the abuse itself.

Recently, steps have been taken to make the process of testifying less traumatic to the child.

Some courts attempt to reduce the number of court appearances required of a child. Provisions for separate waiting rooms prevent children from having to share a room with defense witnesses. Increasingly, courts allow children to testify IN CAMERA, on videotape or through closed-circuit television. These methods of testifying may eliminate some of the trauma of a court appearance. Measures that interfere with the defendant's right to cross-examine a witness are not permitted.

In sexual abuse trials, NATURAL DOLLS may be used as aids to testimony. Children are often embarrassed to talk about genitalia and may use idiosyncratic terminology. Use of anatomically correct dolls can both reduce embarrassment and allow for clearer testimony. However, the use of such dolls is controversial because some experts consider it leading.

Others who may testify in child abuse hearings include anyone who may have observed the abuse, police or child protection workers who conducted the initial investigation, character witnesses and relevant experts.

testimony, videotaped   See VIDEOTAPED TESTIMONY.

therapeutic day-care centers   Specialized day-care centers that provide both supervision and treatment of abused children are a valuable resource for child protection. Structured treatment usually focuses on behavioral and educational problems of children who have been abused. Therapeutic day care may be used by children in FOSTER CARE or while children remain at home. Usually, families of children in therapeutic day care are simultaneously receiving treatment at the center or from an outside provider.

throwaway children   A significant proportion of children labeled as runaways are actually throwaways. The term *throwaway* refers to a child who is forced or encouraged to leave home by parents or caretakers. This form of extreme NEGLECT affects adolescents as well as younger children. An estimated 10% to 20% of children housed in runaway shelters are throwaways. Though the throwaway is often labeled a problem child, the parent's inability or unwillingness to care for him or her is a significant factor in the child's behavioral difficulty.

Tinker v. Des Moines Independent School District   In 1965, a group of school children was prohibited by the Des Moines, Iowa, School District from wearing black armbands to protest hostilities in Vietnam. Students who wore the armbands were suspended from school. The children, through their parents, filed a petition in U.S. District Court to prohibit the school system from disciplining them for expression of their political beliefs. After a hearing, the court found in favor of the school district, citing their right to take reasonable actions to prevent a disturbance. This decision was appealed to the U.S. Supreme Court, which in 1969 reversed the lower court's decision, holding that children as well as adults have a right to freedom of speech under the First Amendment to the Constitution of the United States.

The Supreme Court's ruling in *Tinker v. Des Moines* established an important legal precedent for children's rights. By ruling that children are entitled to specific rights, the court recognized them as independent individuals with their own interests. Though subsequent decisions have modified the scope of children's rights, the principles confirmed in this case have afforded children much greater legal protection than they had previously enjoyed.

tithingman   In 17th-century Massachusetts, most communities, divided into church parishes, relied on a tithingman to determine whether families met responsibilities toward their members and toward society in general. A tithingman (whose presence was based on English tradition) could arrest individuals for legal infractions and could intervene in family disputes. A tithingman was responsible for judging whether parents were fulfilling their duties toward their children. The concept was devised as a way of ensuring social order rather than as a means of protecting children. Parents who did not act responsibly were seen as threats to community welfare.

toe tourniquet syndrome Emotionally disturbed parents have been known to strangle their children's appendages, such as toes or fingers, by tying hair or thread around the base. Restricted blood flow can cause severe pain and may result in loss of the appendage.

This relatively rare practice is apparently related to a superstitious belief of unknown origin. Most frequent victims of this form of abuse are infants from six weeks to 10 months of age. When toe tourniquet syndrome is suspected, evidence may be found in the form of loose threads or hairs in bed-clothing or garments. Thorough examination by a physician may also help determine the cause of injury.

trafficking, sexual See SEXUAL TRAFFICKING.

trauma The term *trauma* is most often used to describe an injury, wound or shock, of any kind, to the body. PHYSICAL ABUSE often leaves visible signs of trauma on a child's body.

Trauma can also refer to a painful or damaging emotional experience. This kind of trauma is present in virtually all types of child abuse. Emotional trauma is usually concomitant with physical trauma but may endure long after all signs of physical injury have disappeared. Victims of child abuse often report nightmares, flashbacks or panic attacks long after the danger of abuse is gone.

Support and therapy groups are available in many areas to help both child and adult survivors of abuse overcome the effects of emotional trauma associated with abuse.

trauma X This is another name for child abuse, most frequently used in medical facilities. Some hospitals use the term *trauma X* to refer to a child abuse and neglect program. For instance, the Trauma X Team at Boston Children's Hospital was an early example of a MULTIDISCIPLINARY TEAM.

treatment for maltreated children Specialized treatment provided to abused and neglected children in order to begin to restore their physical and emotional well-being. Abused children should receive medical services and individual counseling to cope with the abuse. The child's safety and well-being should be the ultimate goal of all treatment for abuse or neglect.

In the United States, many state and local government agencies sponsor specialized treatment services for the victims of abuse. Child abuse treatment units are often attached to hospitals, community mental-health centers or child welfare agencies.

Treating Child Victims

The diagnosis and planning for the treatment of abuse and neglect usually should be carried out by a MULTIDISCIPLINARY TEAM that includes professionals with specialized training in pediatrics, psychiatry, psychology, social work and child protection. In some cases, a child protection worker is responsible for providing all or most treatment directly. More often, treatment may take many different forms and is provided by professionals with an array of different skills.

If the child has been placed in foster care, a series of specific treatment goals are included in a SERVICE PLAN. Progress toward goals is monitored by the caseworker, and the caretaker's progress toward achieving these goals forms the basis for decisions to return the child to the parent or caretaker or take other actions, up to and including the involuntary TERMINATION OF PARENTAL RIGHTS.

Victims of SEXUAL ABUSE may also require special treatment. Sexually abused children must be helped to overcome the tendency to blame themselves for their abuse and to learn new ways of relating to adults. Sexual abuse victims have been forced to assume inappropriate adult roles, such as surrogate spouse, lover or prostitute. Treatment may focus on helping children learn to be children again. Overcoming feelings of low self-esteem and fear of emotional attachment are also important tasks.

Treating Perpetrators of Abuse

When parents or other family members are responsible for maltreatment, family therapy as well as individual therapy is often recommended to try to prevent further danger to the child. Perpetrators of abuse outside the family usually receive individual psychiatric treatment.

Specific methods employed to assist the families of children who have been abused or neglected include individual counseling, group counseling, marital or family counseling, educational treatment (such as parent education), a friendly visitor (usually a peer who can provide emotional support), psychotherapy, therapeutic day care or day treatment, HOMEMAKER SERVICES and SELF-HELP GROUPS.

Treatment of certain types of abusers may need to be highly specialized. For example, many SEX OFFENDERS have proven to be resistant to traditinal methods of psychiatric treatment, although some may respond to a combination of behavioral and group therapy. In some cases, medications are used to suppress the testosterone of male sex offenders, which is sometimes called chemical CASTRATION.

Adults Abused as Children

Adults who were physically and/or sexually abused as children, as well as those who were neglected in childhood, often carry emotional scars into adulthood. Therapy may provide significant relief.

Until recently, sexual abuse was shrouded in secrecy. Many adults who were molested as children received no treatment. Adults sexually abused as children often suffer sexual dysfunction, DEPRESSION, debilitating anxiety and difficulty forming emotional attachments.

See also ABUSERS; ADULTS ABUSED AS CHILDREN; CHILD ABUSE; INCEST; NEGLECT; PHYSICAL ABUSE; PSYCHOLOGICAL/EMOTIONAL MALTREATMENT; SEXUAL ABUSE.

trusted professionals, child abuse by   Physical, sexual or psychological abuse perpetrated by a professional, such as a coach, teacher, physician, counselor or member of the clergy. (See CLERGY, SEXUAL ABUSE BY.) In most cases, the abuse is most likely to be sexual in nature. These individuals are often in a position with ready access to children, and where children (and parents) are likely to trust them.

See also ABUSERS; PEDOPHILIA; SEX OFFENDERS, CONVICTED; SEXUAL ABUSE.

trust funds   See CHILDREN'S TRUST FUNDS.

turned stomach   See *OPU HULE.*

Turkey   According to the *Country Reports on Human Rights Practices,* released by the United States State Department in 2005 on behavior that occurred in 2004, there are some problems in Turkey with child abuse, as well as with honor killings and trafficking in adolescents and children for the purpose of prostitution or forced labor.

Honor Killings

Adolescents and young women are sometimes victims of honor killings, which are murders of a female by the members of her immediate family because she is regarded as unchaste. The girl or woman may have become pregnant out of wedlock from consensual sex, or she may have been sexually assaulted. In either case, she is believed to have defiled the family honor. It is estimated that there are dozens of honor killings each year, and these killings are the most common among conservative Kurdish families.

The Turkish parliament enacted a law under which honor killings are regarded as aggravated homicides, for which the sentence is life imprisonment; however, it is unclear whether judges are imposing this sentence. Also, since there is a sentence reduction for juveniles, some families assign the honor killing to a young male relative.

In one case of an honor killing in Istanbul, Nuran Halitogullar was killed by her brother and her father. She had been kidnapped and raped earlier that year, and a family council decided that she must be killed to restore the family's honor. The father was charged, and the case is ongoing as of this writing. In another case, Emine Kizilkurt, 14, who had been raped by her neighbor, was killed by her brother. He was sentenced to life imprisonment. In addition, the court sentenced eight other family members to jail terms because of their collusion in the honor killing.

Suicides

Some human rights organizations have reported a high rate of SUICIDE among Turkish girls, primarily because of forced marriages and economic problems.

Sexual Trafficking and Forced Labor

Turkish law bans trafficking in humans, as well as forced labor, however such practices do occur, according to the State Department. In 2003, the police raided Adana, a city in the south of Turkey, and freed more than 20 victims from forced labor camps, including orphaned minors or elderly people with mental and physical disabilities. Child protective service staff returned the children to their families.

Some people, especially adolescents and young women, emigrate to Turkey from other countries, believing that they will work as dancers, domestic servants, waitresses or in other jobs. Many use fraudulent documents to enter the country. Traffickers then steal the documents and rape the victims, threaten their families, and force them into prostitution. In one case, a 17-year-old Romanian woman described that when she was in the ninth grade, she was offered a job in Istanbul as a babysitter or housekeeper. Upon her arrival, she was taken to a hotel with other Romanian girls, her documents were destroyed, and she was told she would be killed if she talked to the police. The girl was compelled to have intercourse with 200 people over eight months before her situation was discovered and the abuse ended.

In general, adolescents and young women from Moldova, Ukraine, Romania and Russia had the greatest risk of being trafficked in 2003.

There is also a problem about whether law enforcement authorities take trafficking cases seriously. According to the State Department, it has been reported that the Turkish government continued to process trafficking cases as they would cases of voluntary prostitution and illegal immigration, and often did not pursue the traffickers. One measure taken by the government was to print warnings in visa applications in Russian to direct victimized immigrants to an emergency law-enforcement hotline. It is unknown if this warning has been effective, but since many trafficked children and women have illegal documents and also are in great fear of their captors, the warning may have dubious value.

Bureau of Democracy, Human Rights, and Labor. *Country Reports on Human Rights Practices, 2004: Turkey.* United States State Department, released on February 28, 2005. Available online. URL: http://www.state.gov/g/drl/rls/hrrpt/2004/41713.htm. Downloaded September 1, 2005.

underground networks   In the United States, several informal networks of safe homes shelter parents and children fleeing court orders that give custody to an allegedly abusive ex-spouse. Typically, these networks serve children and their mothers who have been unsuccessful in convincing a court that the father sexually abused the child. Lacking proof of the father's unfitness, courts have awarded visitation rights or in some cases, sole custody of the child to the father. An unknown number of mothers have chosen to hide their child rather than subject the child to what they believe would be further abuse.

Underground networks appear to be loosely organized. Though little is known about them, an estimated five to 10 such organizations are now operating in the United States. Families who provide shelter for fugitive children and their parents often do so at great legal, personal and financial risk. Sometimes called "key masters," sheltering families must maintain strict secrecy to avoid arrest and to protect their guests.

Many experts in the field of child protection have criticized underground networks for encouraging illegal behavior and subjecting children to additional disruption. Groups representing divorced fathers maintain that many mothers simply do not want to share custody of the child and have leveled false accusations of sexual abuse in an effort to deny access to the father.

Supporters of underground networks argue that they are made necessary by a failure of the legal system. Sexual abuse of young children is often difficult to prove. In some cases judges may not fully understand the nature of child sexual abuse, in others prosecutors simply lack sufficient EVIDENCE. Convinced that the child was indeed molested by the father, some mothers decide to risk imprisonment to protect their child.

unfounded report   Child abuse reporting laws generally require designated persons to report *suspected* abuse or neglect to an investigatory agency. If, upon investigation of a report, the reported conditions are determined not to be neglectful or abusive as defined by law, a report may be designated "unfounded." Reports may also be judged unfounded when there is a lack of sufficient evidence to establish the occurrence or extent of a potentially harmful condition.

The terms *unfounded* and *unsubstantiated report* are frequently used interchangeably. Criteria for substantiation of a report vary according to how maltreatment is defined by local laws, EVIDENTIARY STANDARDS and the investigator's ASSESSMENT of the potential for harm.

In most cases, child protection authorities cannot intervene further on behalf of a child once a case is determined to be unfounded. In some jurisdictions, intervention may proceed with the parent's permission. Some experts believe that the system is flooded with unfounded reports which they believe take away workers and services from the individuals who need the most help. Child welfare expert Douglas Besharov (and others) said in a 1996 article for *Society,* "Laws against child abuse are an implicit recognition that family privacy must give way to the need to protect helpless children. But in seeking to protect children it is also too easy to ignore the legitimate rights of parents. Each year, about 700,000 families are put through investigations of unfounded reports. This is a massive and unjustified violation of parental rights."

Besharov and his colleagues say that the problem is not reports made from malice and says that at most, 4–10% of sexual abuse allegations were made with the knowledge that they were untrue.

Rather, it is well-intentioned, overly zealous people who turn in families for child abuse because of a possibility of abuse. As a result, caseworkers are so inundated with cases to investigate that they may not have an opportunity to check on children who are clearly being abused. Besharov et al. say, "These nationwide conditions help explain why from 25 to 50% of child abuse deaths involve children previously known to the authorities."

They also noted that there was a tendency for some experts to advise that when children were shy or withdrawn, then they might be abused and this possibility should be considered. Yet, the authors say, "only a minority of children who exhibit such behaviors have actually been maltreated."

The answer to decreasing the number of unsubstantiated cases is to educate the public as well as protective services workers on what constitutes abuse, including direct and circumstantial evidence. Reports of abuse should also be screened, particularly those made anonymously or by estranged or former spouses or by previous sources who reported abuse that was unfounded. The report may be accurate but should be evaluated first.

Besharov, Douglas, J., et al. "Child Abuse Reporting." *Society* 33 (May/June 1996).

Uniform Child Custody Jurisdiction Act (UCCJA)   Approved in 1968 by the National Conference of Commissioners on Uniform State Laws, the UCCJA was designed to protect children from child stealing by resolving issues of jurisdiction in child CUSTODY cases. The act attempted to ensure that the best interests of the child were met. In custody disputes involving the UCCJA, best interest was most often interpreted as the child's primary need for stability.

This act was replaced in 1997 by the Uniform Child Custody Jurisdiction and Enforcement Act.

United Nations Declaration of the Rights of the Child, 1959   On November 20, 1959, the United Nations General Assembly unanimously adopted this declaration, which asserts rights and freedoms for the world's children. It is probably the best known of all international statements concerning adult responsibilities and obligations toward children. The declaration was conceived as a way in which to make a positive statement concerning certain principles to which children are by right entitled. The preamble to the declaration establishes that due to physical and mental immaturity, children need special safeguards both before and after birth.

In 10 principles, the declaration states that all children have the following rights: to develop in a normal and healthy manner; to have a name and a nationality from birth; to enjoy adequate housing, nutrition, recreation and medical services, including special services for the handicapped; to enjoy, if possible, the care and nurturance of their parents; to have an education; to be protected against cruelty, neglect and abuse, racism, discrimination, exploitation and religious persecution. The declaration states further that children are to be raised "in a spirit of understanding, tolerance, friendship among all peoples, peace and universal brotherhood and in full consciousness" that their talents should he dedicated to serving fellow human beings.

The declaration is similar to the Universal Declaration of Human Rights, a previous world-body statement that did not specifically address the needs of children. In adopting the Declaration of the Rights of the Child, the United Nations General Assembly placed the groundwork for a more comprehensive document, the Draft Convention on the Rights of the Child, submitted to the world body in 1978. As of 2005, the United States has signed but not ratified the UN Declaration.

utterance, excited   See EXCITED UTTERANCE.

venereal disease See SEXUALLY TRANSMITTED DISEASE.

ventricular septal defect The partition that separates the left and right ventricles of the heart is occasionally damaged by battering. Though both the heart and lungs are normally protected by the rib cage, rapid compression caused by a blow to the thoracic region can cause serious injury. Damage to the septum of the heart inhibits proper functioning and can cause death.

verbal abuse PSYCHOLOGICAL/EMOTIONAL MALTREATMENT includes verbal abuse as well as other forms of restrictive and punitive behavior. Verbal abuse covers a range of spoken messages that can usually be grouped into the categories of rejecting, terrorizing or corrupting. This type of abuse often occurs in combination with other forms of maltreatment.

Studies show that consistent verbal abuse can have serious and lasting effects on children. Low self-esteem resulting from verbal harassment may promote a wide range of destructive and defeating behavior. Verbal and psychological abuse has also been associated with poor school performance and antisocial and self-destructive behavior.

While most child abuse laws do not specifically identify verbal abuse, many make provisions for psychological/emotional abuse or MENTAL INJURY. Substantiation of verbal abuse usually depends upon psychiatric and/or psychological evaluation of the child, coupled with documentation of the abuse itself.

verification Reports of suspected abuse and neglect must be investigated to determine whether there is sufficient cause to believe that a child has been abused or neglected. Verified reports of maltreatment are often referred to as FOUNDED REPORTS or substantiated abuse.

See also INVESTIGATION.

victim, blaming See BLAMING THE VICTIM.

victim, identification with See IDENTIFICATION WITH THE VICTIM.

Victims of Crime Act (P.L. 98-473) Beginning in 1985, the U.S. Congress created a victims' compensation and assistance fund. The fund, made up of fines levied against persons convicted of certain federal offenses, makes grants to victim assistance and compensation programs. These programs compensate victims of crime or their survivors for medical expenses, loss of income and funeral expenses. Victim assistance programs also offer services such as crisis intervention, HOTLINES, temporary shelter, counseling and other services. Funding priority is given to programs that serve victims of sexual assault, spouse abuse or child abuse.

videotaped testimony A number of states and local authorities now allow child victims of SEXUAL ABUSE to provide legal testimony via videotape. Sixteen states specifically regulate the circumstances under which such videotaping will be admissible in court. These states are as follows: Arizona, Colorado, Hawaii, Indiana, Iowa, Kansas, Louisiana, Michigan, Minnesota, Missouri, New York, North Dakota, Rhode Island, Texas, Utah and Wisconsin.

Advantages of Videotaping

If a child's testimony is videotaped early in the process he or she may be spared the trauma of giving repeated accounts of the abusive incident. Videotaping can also eliminate the stress and possible intimidation of testifying in the presence of the alleged abuser (often a family member or friend).

Disadvantages of Videotaping

Legal scholars disagree as to the fairness of allowing videotaped testimony. Many U.S. lawyers believe such testimony violates the accused's right to confront the witness, as set forth in the Sixth Amendment to the Constitution.

In an attempt to ensure procedural DUE PROCESS, some courts require that the defendant, the defendant's lawyer, the trial judge and prosecutor be present at the videotaping. Others allow taping without the defendant if the child appears in court for cross-examination.

Videotaped testimony is sometimes criticized as being subject to manipulation by both parties. Since taping is usually done with one camera, the jury does not have the opportunity to observe equally the actions of other people present at the time of the testimony (e.g., the defendant). Subtle clues such as body language and flushing of the skin may be difficult or impossible to observe on videotape.

In some cases, untrained family members or incompetent therapists have videotaped lengthy sessions with a child which clearly caused the child great distress. These videotapes may appear to a judge and jury that the family and/or therapists were leading or coaching the testimony and thus it becomes inadmissible in court.

Covert Videotaping

Sometimes videotaping is done without the knowledge of the person being videotaped because it is believed that an individual is a perpetrator of child abuse. This is true in the case of individuals suspected of MUNCHAUSEN SYNDROME BY PROXY as well as other abuse cases. Sometimes families secretly videotape their babysitter or nanny in their own home, to verify the child is receiving good care.

The legality of covert videotaping is beyond the scope of this essay and individuals or organizations considering covert videotaping of anyone in any location (including their own home or workplace) should obtain legal advice in advance.

violence, family   See FAMILY VIOLENCE.

voir dire   Literally, "to speak the truth." This legal procedure permits attorneys to question prospective jurors in child abuse and neglect cases for possible bias. It also establishes grounds on which expert witnesses can be questioned to determine their qualifications prior to TESTIMONY.

voluntary intervention   Some abusive parents seek help voluntarily. Increased accessibility of HOTLINES and SELF-HELP GROUPS has made it easier and less threatening for parents to request help. In most areas child protection agencies actively encourage self-referral. Since many abusive and/or neglectful parents are never reported, self-help programs may reach many families that would not otherwise have received help.

Parents who seek help voluntarily tend to be more highly motivated to change their behavior. When parents are reported by someone else, fear of prosecution or removal of their children often leads them to cover up problems rather than face them openly. Denying or minimizing abusive behavior often prevents perpetrators of abuse from benefiting from treatment.

Following an INVESTIGATION in which abuse or neglect is substantiated, parents may be given the opportunity to seek help voluntarily. In such cases, the child protection agency agrees not to seek court intervention if parents follow a mutually agreed upon plan of treatment.

wanton The term *wanton* is used in court proceedings to denote extremely reckless or malicious behavior. Perpetrators of abuse or neglect are often accused of willful and wanton acts against a child. Wanton acts are considered to be more serious than simple carelessness.

WAR See WORLD OF ABNORMAL REARING.

warrant A warrant is a document, issued by a judge, that authorizes arrest or detention of a person. Search of a particular place and seizure of specified items may also be authorized.

When particularly serious acts of maltreatment are committed or perpetrators fail to cooperate with child protection authorities a warrant may be sought from the court. In order to issue such a document the judge must be satisfied that there is reasonable cause to believe that a crime has been committed. United States law does not require that a hearing be held or that the subject of the warrant be notified prior to its issuance.

warts, venereal Condyloma acuminata, commonly known as venereal warts, is sometimes found in children who have been sexually abused. The warts are small, appear in clusters and may be found in any area involved in direct sexual contact. Appearance of condyloma acuminata in children is strong evidence of SEXUAL ABUSE. There is no reason to believe that this condition is acquired in any way other than by sexual contact.

Wetterling Act This act was named after Jacob Wetterling, a Minnesota child who was abducted in 1989 and has never been located. His parents subsequently learned that halfway houses in their city of St. Joseph housed just-released sex offenders. This fact was unknown to local police.

The Jacob Wetterling Crimes Against Children and Sexually Violent Offender Registration Act was included as part of the Federal Violent Crime Control and Law Enforcement Act of 1994. It requires the registration of convicted sex offenders in all states. All 50 states now have such registration systems. If an offender notifies the state that he plans to move to another state, the "old" state is required to notify the new state that the offender is coming.

The law also required states to create a database of child sex offenders. In 1996, U.S. Attorney General Janet Reno ordered a system to be developed to connect the 50 child sex offender registries.

According to Mike Welter, chief of the violent crimes section of the Illinois State Police, in an address at a national conference of sex offender registries in 1998, the law has already identified child sex offenders who were involved in Boy Scout troops. Said Welter, "The first two times we gave the list to the Greater Cook County Council, a scout leader was discovered on each list. They were removed from their posts, and an investigation is continuing as to whether any crimes were committed during their association with scout troops."

Welter said checks with other community youth groups have also identified sex offenders.

States differ on how long the offender must register. In some states, sexual predators must register for life. Other states require registration only for repeat offenders. Some states limit the registration period; for example, seven states limit registration to 10 years from the offender's parole date. A few states reduce the time to register if offenders can prove that they have been rehabilitated.

Federal law requires that all states must notify offenders of the registration requirement, verify the offender's address each year and notify law enforcement officials if an offender relocates.

See also MEGAN'S LAW; RAPE.

"National Conference on Sex Offender Registries: Proceedings of a BJS/SEARCH Conference." Bureau of Justice Statistics, April 1998, NCJ-168965.

willful   The term *willful* is often used in legal proceedings related to child abuse or neglect. It implies knowledge and understanding of an act as well as the intention that any consequences normally associated with that particular act should occur. In some cases, the acts must be proven to be willful before they are considered illegal or negligent.

Wilson, Mary Ellen   In 1873, a well-publicized case of child abuse involving an eight-year-old New York girl named Mary Ellen Wilson became a rallying issue of reformers. Because of the notoriety surrounding the Mary Ellen Wilson case, reformers established the New York Society for the Prevention of Cruelty to Children (NYSPCC) in 1874.

Mary Ellen was an illegitimate daughter of Thomas McCormack and had been boarded out until she was nearly two years old. She then was placed under the care of the Superintendent of the Out-Door Poor in New York. Her natural father and stepmother were given charge of Mary Ellen on the stipulation that they report annually to the city's Commissioners of Charities and Corrections. After her father's death, Mary Ellen's stepmother remarried, She was then abused and neglected by these stepparents, Francis and Mary Connolly.

Among the reports of her abuse were those that described her being kept chained to a bed and beaten with a rawhide cord by her stepmother. When neighbors heard her screams, they approached the police department but were unsuccessful in getting help for Mary Ellen. They then went to the local chapter of the American Society for the Prevention of Cruelty to Animals, and the group petitioned the court on her behalf. When the *New York Times* received information about the girl's mistreatment, it began newspaper coverage of the case.

Mary Ellen's stepmother, Mrs. Connolly, was convicted and sent to jail for one year as a result of her actions. Mary Ellen was sent to live at the Sheltering Arms children's home and was later indentured to a farmer.

The Guide to American Law Yearbook, 1987. St. Paul, Minn.: West Publishing Co., 1987.

Nelson, Barbara J. *Making an Issue of Child Abuse.* Chicago: University of Chicago Press, 1984.

Wisconsin v. Yoder   This 1972 ruling by the U.S. Supreme Court affirmed parents' rights to raise children according to their own religious beliefs. The case actually involved three respondents: Jonas Yoder, Adin Yutzy and Wallace Miller. All were followers of the Amish religious sect. At issue was the state's ability to prevent Amish families from removing children from public schools after completing the eighth grade. Though they received vocational training at home, the children were not enrolled in any public or private school. The respondents and other members of this sect believed formal high school education interfered with the religious development, and therefore the religious freedom, of their children. The Supreme Court agreed with them and overturned their convictions for violating Wisconsin's compulsory school attendance law.

Wisconsin v. Yoder is often seen as limiting the rather broad powers granted to the state in *Prince v. Massachusetts.*

See also PARENTS' RIGHTS; RELIGIOUS ASPECTS.

withdrawal   Children subjected to severe abuse may withdraw from social contact, appearing dull and listless. Typically, they avoid doing anything that might attract attention or arouse the anger of their parents. Withdrawn children often exhibit a robotlike compliance with parental demands, demonstrating their desire to do virtually anything to avoid further abuse.

Withdrawal and HYPERVIGILANCE are usually observed in children who have been victims of the most severe forms of physical abuse from an early age. These children may appear visibly anxious or afraid in the presence of their parents. In a hospital emergency room these symptoms are a signal to physicians and nurses to look for other signs of nonaccidental injury.

When removed from home, such children may continue to appear withdrawn. It may take several years in a safe and therapeutic setting before they are able to develop a close, trusting relationship with anyone.

witness Trials related to child abuse or neglect may include testimony from lay witnesses and EXPERT WITNESSES. The kind of testimony allowed by the court depends upon the type of witness.

Lay witnesses are required to have firsthand knowledge of facts to which they testify. Inferences or conclusions may not be drawn by such witnesses. Hearsay evidence, facts not directly observed or experienced by the witness, is usually not permitted. An exception to the rule against hearsay testimony is sometimes made in preliminary hearings to spare a child from trauma related to repeated court appearances. In such cases a third party may present testimony based upon the child's account of the alleged abuse.

When the reputation or character of the defendant or respondent is in question, a lay witness may be called to testify. In a dependency hearing such testimony may center on the parents' fitness to adequately care for the child. Character witnesses are usually asked to state their own qualifications to give testimony, their relationship with the party in question and their knowledge of that party's reputation in the community. Rumors and witnesses' personal opinions about the party are not admissible.

An expert witness is anyone who, in the judge's opinion, possesses special knowledge or skills beyond those of the judge or jury. Expert witnesses may be called by either party in a case or may be appointed by the court. Unlike lay witnesses, expert witnesses are allowed to make inferences and express opinions. Inferences or opinions must be within the witness's area of expertise. For example,

a psychologist may testify about the psychological effects of abuse but is not allowed to give an opinion concerning the extent of physical injuries.

The allegedly abused child may be called as a witness by either party. The judge is responsible for determining whether the child's testimony is admissible as evidence. A child's competence to testify is based on age, maturity and level of understanding. In some areas, the minimum age of witnesses is specified by law.

Child witnesses may be allowed to testify in judge's chambers, on videotape or on closed circuit television rather than in the courtroom. Alternative ways of testifying can help reduce trauma to the child caused by reliving abuse in a threatening setting before a large group of strangers as well as the alleged attacker. Attempts to reduce trauma to the child must be balanced with the defendant's right to cross-examine witnesses.

The petitioner (usually the state) is the first to call witnesses in a hearing. Questioning of witnesses takes the form of: (1) direct examination by the attorney calling the witness; (2) cross-examination by the opposing attorney; (3) rebuttal or redirect examination by the first attorney concerning issues raised in the cross-examination; and (4) recross-examination by the opposing attorney on issues raised in the rebuttal examination. After a party has called all its witnesses it rests its case. Under ordinary circumstances, once a party has rested its case it is not allowed to call additional witnesses.

See also ADJUDICATORY HEARING; COURT; CIVIL PROCEEDING; CRIMINAL PROSECUTION; EVIDENCE.

witness, expert See EXPERT WITNESS.

World of Abnormal Rearing (WAR) The concept of the world of abnormal rearing, known by the acronym WAR, was developed by pediatrician Ray E. Helfer. WAR describes a cyclical process in which children fail to learn basic interpersonal skills and later, as parents, are unable to teach such skills to their children. This dysfunctional pattern of development is not limited to children who are physically or sexually abused but includes those who suffer various kinds of emotional abuse and neglect.

Dr. Helfer stresses the importance of parents breaking the cycle by learning principles of interpersonal behavior not learned in childhood.

The basic skills necessary to healthy development are, according to Helfer: learning how to meet one's needs appropriately, the ability to delay gratification, learning that one is responsible for one's own actions but not those of others, the ability to make decisions and solve problems, learning how to trust others and developing the ability to separate feelings and actions.

Abused children often learn inappropriate or dysfunctional ways of meeting their needs. Children who are ignored or neglected may learn that abuse is the only form of attention available from parents. Because their needs are so frequently frustrated, some children do not learn to delay immediate gratification in hopes of obtaining a greater reward later. Such children enter adulthood lacking this important work and parenting skill.

Children must also learn to be responsible for their behavior. Most learn this principle from parental teaching and discipline. When discipline is sporadic or abusive, children become confused about the consequences of their actions. In many abusive families a ROLE REVERSAL takes place in which the child assumes the role of a parent's caretaker. The parent may be unable or unwilling to reciprocate. Forced to direct their attention to meeting a parent's needs, children are prevented from mastering tasks important to their own development.

Abuse further complicates the process of learning to differentiate between one's self and others. Because they are often punished or abandoned, the children may come to feel responsible for causing the maltreatment. If beaten or molested, the child assumes that he or she did something to deserve it. This inappropriate sense of guilt contributes to future self-destructive and abusive behavior.

Maltreated children usually have few choices. Feeling trapped, they develop a sense of helplessness that prevents them from learning constructive approaches to problem solving. As adults they may find themselves unable to make decisions and may feel they have little control over their lives.

The ability to trust is perhaps most difficult for maltreated children to develop. Exploited, battered or neglected, they learn to fear rather than trust. Inability to trust not only prevents children from developing loving relationships but makes it difficult for them to seek protection from abuse as well. Children may look with suspicion on a concerned adult's attempts to help. If carried into adulthood, the inability to trust may contribute to marital and child-rearing difficulties.

Finally, the ability to distinguish feelings from actions is an important developmental task. Children often lash out at others because they are angry. As they grow older they learn that being angry does not justify or compel such behavior. They learn other ways of expressing anger.

Abused children are frequent targets of adults who have not learned to separate feelings and actions (see TARGET CHILD). As adults these victims are likely to direct their own anger, frustration or sexual feelings at children without stopping to consider the wisdom of their actions.

Each of these abilities, if not mastered, can contribute to inadequate or abusive parenting. Parents cannot teach such developmental tasks if they have not learned them. Left unchecked, developmental deficits are passed from generation to generation, contributing to a cycle of abuse and neglect.

Helfer believes the WAR is best interrupted in childhood before severe damage is done. Various treatment and parent education programs have demonstrated that much can be done to break the cycle during adulthood as well.

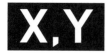

X-rays X-rays are nonluminous electromagnetic rays of very short wavelength. Discovered by the German physicist Wilhelm Roentgen, the X-ray achieved its name because of its then unknown properties. Because of its ability to penetrate opaque or solid substances, the X-ray is used in combination with photographic film for the study of internal body structures not normally visible. The study of the body through X-rays is known as radiology.

Brief exposure to X-rays produces a photograph of the bones often called an X-ray but more specifically known as a roentgenogram. The typical roentgenographic procedure transmits a small amount of radiation that has no harmful effects. Prolonged exposure to X-rays can, however, destroy body tissue.

Advances in pediatric radiology (see RADIOLOGY, PEDIATRIC) from the 1930s through the 1950s made it possible to determine both the type of force that caused a bone fracture and the approximate age of the injury. This information, along with other medical evidence, allowed physicians to check the validity of a caretaker's explanations of particular injuries. An especially important finding first reported by John Caffey was the combination of multiple FRACTURES of the long bones and SUBDURAL HEMATOMA. Caffey was one of the first to propose battering as the most likely cause for this combination of injuries. This observation was later expanded upon and publicized by C. Henry Kempe and others as the BATTERED CHILD SYNDROME.

Today a SKELETAL SURVEY is standard practice when child battering is suspected. Using barium sulfate (a tasteless compound that, when swallowed, appears as an opaque substance on a roentgenogram) physicians are also able to detect GASTROINTESTINAL INJURIES.

Other more recent medical advances such as computed tomography (CT scans) and magnetic resonance imaging (MRI) are also used in the identification of abuse-related trauma.

yo-yo syndrome Violent marital disputes can seriously affect the emotional, intellectual and physical well-being of children. A study of the effects of marital violence on children conducted by Britain's National Society for the Prevention of Cruelty to Children likened children to a yo-yo moving up and down in a pattern of restlessness and violence.

The name yo-yo syndrome has come to describe the situation of many children in violent households. Often shuttled back and forth between parents, these children suffer a range of problems directly related to their volatile environment. They are frequently blamed by parents for their marital problems and may be used as pawns in their parents' bitter disputes. If a child possesses traits similar to one parent he or she may become the victim of SCAPEGOATING by the other parent.

Though yo-yo children may also be physically abused or neglected, the psychological scars caused by the turbulence around them can be just as damaging. Yo-yo children usually feel responsible for family violence, engaging in self-destructive acts or attempting to serve as a buffer between parents.

Parents are often quite resistant to treatment, making it difficult to ensure a safe home environment for the child. It may be necessary to remove the child from home to prevent further trauma.

Moore, Jean G. "Yo-Yo Children—Victims of Matrimonial Violence." *Child Welfare* 54, no. 8 (1975): 557–566.

APPENDIXES

APPENDIX I
IMPORTANT ORGANIZATIONS

FEDERAL CLEARINGHOUSES WITH INFORMATION ON CHILDREN AND FAMILIES

Bureau of Justice Statistics
810 Seventh Street NW
Washington, DC 20531
(202) 307-0765
http://www.ojp.usdoj.gov/bis

Juvenile Justice Clearinghouse
P.O. Box 6000
Rockville, MD 20849-6000
(800) 851-3420
http://www.ojjdp.ncjrs.org

National Adoption Information Clearinghouse
330 C Street SW
Washington, DC 20447
(888) 251-0078
http://naic.acf.hhs.gov

National Clearinghouse for Alcohol and Drug Information
11426-28 Rockville Pike
Rockville, MD 20852
(800) 729-6686
http://www.health.org

National Clearinghouse on Child Abuse and Neglect Information
330 C Street SW
Washington, DC 20447
(800) FYI-3336
http://nccanch.acf.hhs.gov

National Clearinghouse on Families and Youth
P.O. Box 13505
Silver Spring, MD 20911-3505

(301) 608-8098
http://www.ncfy.com

National Criminal Justice Reference Services
P.O. Box 6000
Rockville, MD 20849-6000
(800) 851-3420
http://www.ncjrs.gov

ORGANIZATIONS WITH INFORMATION ON FOSTER CARE

American Foster Care Resources, Inc.
P.O. Box 271
King George, VA 22485
(540) 775-7410
http://www.afcr.com

American Humane Association
63 Inverness Drive East
Englewood, CO 80112
(303) 792-9900
http://www.americanhumane.org

Annie E. Casey Foundation
701 St. Paul Street
Baltimore, MD 21202
(410) 547-6600
http://www.aecf.org

Center for Child and Family Programs
Institute for the Study of Children, Families, and Communities
203 Boone Hall
Ypsilanti, MI 48197
(734) 487-0372
http://www.iscfc.emich.edu

Center for Child and Family Studies
College of Social Work
University of South Carolina
Columbia, SC 29208
(803) 777-9408
http://www.sc.edu/ccfs/

Center for Family Connections
350 Cambridge Street
Cambridge, MA 02141
(617) 547-0909
http://www.kinnect.org

Chapin Hall Center for Children
1313 East 60th Street
Chicago, IL 60637
(773) 753-5900
http://www.chapinhall.org

Children and Family Research Center
1203 West Oregon
Urbana, IL 61801
(217) 333-5837
http://cfrcwww.soial.uiuc.edu

Child Welfare League of America
Headquarters
440 First Street NW, Third Floor
Washington, DC 20001
(202) 638-2952
http://www.cwla.org

Foster Family-Based Treatment Association
294 Union Street
Hackensack, NJ 07601
(800) 414-FFTA
http://www.ffta.org

National Association of Foster Care Reviewers
P.O. Box 142501
Salt Lake City, UT 84114-2501
(801) 468-0121
http://www.nafcr.org

National Child Welfare Resource Center for Youth Development
College of Continuing Education
4502 East 41st Street
Building 4W
Tulsa, OK 74135
http://www.nrcys.ou.ed/nrcyd

National Foster Parent Association
7512 Stanich Avenue, #6
Gig Harbor, WA 98335
(800) 557-5238
http://www.nfpainc.org

ORGANIZATIONS WITH INFORMATION ON SUBSTANCE ABUSE

Al-Anon Family Group Headquarters
1600 Corporate Landing Parkway
Virginia Beach, VA 23454-5617
(888) 425-2666
http://www.al-anon.org

Alcoholic Anonymous World Services, Inc.
P.O. Box 459
Grand Central Station
New York, NY 10163
(212) 870-3400
http://www. alcoholics-anonymous. org

American Council on Alcoholism
1000 East Indian School Road
Phoenix, AZ 85014
(800) 527-5344
http://www.aca-usa.org

American Psychiatric Association
1000 Wilson Boulevard
Suite 1825
Arlington, VA 22209
(703) 907-7300
http://www.psych.org

American Psychological Association
750 First Street NE
Washington, DC 20002
(202) 336-5500
http://www.apa.org

Center for Substance Abuse Prevention
Substance Abuse and Mental Health Services Administration
5600 Fishers Lane
Rockville, MD 20857
(800) 729-6686
http://prevention.samhsa.gov

Center for Substance Abuse Treatment
Substance Abuse and Mental Health Services
     Administration
5600 Fishers Lane
Rockville, MD 20857
(800) 662-HELP
http://csat.samhsa.gov

Children of Alcoholics Foundation
164 West 74th Street
New York, NY 10023
(212) 595-5810, ext. 7760
http://www.coaf.org

**National Center on Substance Abuse and
     Child Welfare**
4940 Irvine Boulevard
Suite 202
Irvine, CA 92612
(714) 505-3525
http://www.ncsacw.samhsa.gov

**National Clearinghouse for Alcohol and
     Drug Information**
11426-28 Rockville Pike
Rockville, MD 20852
(800) 729-6686
http://www.health.org

**National Council on Alcoholism and Drug
     Dependence, Inc.**
22 Cortlandt Steet, Suite 801
New York, NY 10007-3128
(800) NCA-CALL or (212) 269-7797
http://www.ncadd.org

**National Institute on Alcohol Abuse and
     Alcoholism**
5635 Fishers Lane, MSC 9304
Bethesda, MD 20892
http://www.niaaa.nih.gov/

National Institute on Drug Abuse
National Institutes of Health
6001 Executive Boulevard
Room 5213
Bethesda, MD 20892-9561
(301) 443-1124
http://www.nida.nih.gov

**National Organization on Fetal Alcohol
     Syndrome**
900 17 Street NW, Suite 910
Washington, DC 20006
(202) 785-4585
http://www.nofas.org

**SAMHSA Fetal Alcohol Spectrum Disorders
     Centers for Excellence**
2101 Gaither Road, Suite 600
Rockville, MD 20850
(866) STOP-FAS
http://www.fascenter.samhsa.gov

**Substance Abuse and Mental Health Services
     Administration**
5600 Fishers Lane
Room 12-105, Parklawn Building
Rockville, MD 20857
(301) 443-8956
http://www.samhsa.gov/

ORGANIZATIONS INVOLVED WITH CHILDREN'S LEGAL CHILD WELFARE ISSUES

**American Bar Association Center on
     Children and the Law**
740 15th Street NW
Washington, DC 20005
(202) 662-1720
http://www.abanet.org/child

Legal Advocates for Permanent Parenting
3182 Campus Drive
Suite 175
San Mateo, CA 94403
(650) 712-1442
http://www.lapponline.org

National Association of Counsel for Children
1825 Marion Street, Suite 310
Denver, CO 80218
(303) 864-5320
http://www.nacchildlaw.org

National Center for Prosecution of Child Abuse
American Prosecutors Research Institute
99 Canal Center Plaza, Suite 510
Alexandria, VA 22314

(703) 549-9222
http://www.ndaa-apri.org/apri/programs/ncpca/
ncpca_home.html

National Center for State Courts
300 Newport Avenue
Williamsburg, VA 23185
(800) 616-6164
http://www.ncsconline.org

National Center for Youth Law
405 14th Street, 15th Floor
Oakland, CA 94612-2701
(510) 835-8098
http://www.youthlaw.org

National Conference of State Legislatures
7700 East First Place
Denver, CO 80230
(303) 364-7700
http://www.ncsl.org

**National Council of Juvenile and Family
    Court Judges**
P.O. Box 8970
Reno, NV 89507
(775) 784-6012
http://www.ncjfcj.org

**National Court-Appointed Special Advocate
    Association**
100 West Harrison Street, North Tower, Suite 500
Seattle, WA 98119
(206) 270-0072
http://www.nationalcasa.org

National Law Center for Children and Families
3819 Plaza Drive
Fairfax, VA 22030-4105
(703) 691-4626
http://www.nationallawcenter.org

National Legal Aid & Defender Association
1140 Connecticut Avenue NW, Suite 900
Washington, DC 20036
(202) 452-0620
http://www.nlada.org

**Resource Center on Domestic Violence, Child
    Protection and Custody**
P.O. Box 8970
Reno, NV 89507

(800) 527-3223
http://www.nal.usda.gov/pavnet/cf/cfrcdomv.htm

OTHER IMPORTANT ORGANIZATIONS

Alliance for Children and Families
11700 West Lake Park Drive
Milwaukee, WI 53224-3099
(414) 359-1040
http://www.alliancel.org

American Academy of Pediatrics
National Headquarters
141 Northwest Point Boulevard
Elk Grove Village, IL 60007
(847) 434-4000
http://www.aap.org

American Humane Association
63 Inverness Drive East
Englewood, CO 80112
(303) 792-9900
http://www.americanhumane.org

**American Professionals Society on the Abuse
    of Children**
P.O. Box 30669
CHO 3B-3406
Charleston, SC 29417
(877) 40A-PSAC
http://www.apsac.org

American Psychological Association
750 First Street NE
Washington, DC 20002
(202) 336-5500
http://www.apa.org

American Public Human Services Association
810 First Street NE, Suite 500
Washington, DC 20002
(202) 682-0100
http://www.aphsa.org/Home/News.asp

Association for Sexual Abuse Prevention
210 Pratt Avenue
Huntsville, AL 35801
(256) 533-5437
http://www.nationalcac.org/professionals/
    organizations/asap.html

Association for the Treatment of Sexual Abusers
4900 South West Griffith Drive, Suite 274
Beaverton, OR 97005
(503) 643-1023
http://www.atsa.com

Center on Child Abuse and Neglect
University of Oklahoma Health Sciences Center
P.O. Box 26901 CHO 3B 3406
Oklahoma City, OK 73190
(405) 271-8858
http://ccan.ouhsc.edu/

Centers for Disease Control and Prevention
1600 Clifton Road
Atlanta, GA 30333
(404) 639-3311
http://www.cdc.gov

Child Find of America, Inc.
P.O. Box 277
New Paltz, NY 12561
(914) 255-1848
http://www.childfindofamerica.org

Childhelp USA
15757 North 78 Street
Scottsdale, AZ 85260
(800) 4-A-CHILD or (480) 922-8212
http://www.childhelpusa.org

Child Molestation Research & Prevention Institute
1100 Piedmont Avenue, # 2
Atlanta, GA 30309
(404) 872-5152
http://www.childmolestationprevention.org

Children's Bureau
Administration of Children Youth and Families
1250 Maryland Avenue SW
Eighth Floor
Washington, DC 20024
http://www.acf.hhs.gov/programs/cb/

Children's Defense Fund
National Headquarters
25 E Street NW
Washington, DC 20001
(202) 628-8787
http://www.childrensdefense.org

Child Trends
4301 Connecticut Avenue NW
Suite 100
Washington, DC 20008
(202) 362-5580
http://www.childtrends.org

Child Welfare League of America
440 First Street NW, Third Floor
Washington, DC 20001
(202) 638-2952
http://www.cwla.org

Crimes Against Children Research Center
University of New Hampshire
126 Horton Social Science Center
Durham, NH 03824
(603) 862-1888
http://www.unh.edu/ccrc

Federation of Families for Children's Mental Health
9605 Medical Center Drive, Suite 280
Rockville, MD 20850
(240) 403-1901
http://www.ffcmh.org

International Society for Prevention of Child Abuse and Neglect
245 West Roosevelt Road
Building 6, Suite 39
West Chicago, IL 60185
(630) 876-6913
http://www.ispcan.org

Kempe National Children's Center
National Headquarters
1825 Marion Street
Denver, CO 80218
(303) 864-5300
http://www.kempecenter.org

Minnesota Center Against Violence and Abuse
School of Social Work, University of Minnesota
105 Peters Hall
1404 Gortner Avenue
St. Paul, MN 55108
(612) 624-0721
http://www.mincava.umn.edu

National Center for Assault Prevention
606 Delsea Drive
Sewell, NJ 08080
(908) 369-8972
http://www.ncap. org

National Center for Missing and Exploited Children
Charles B. Wang International Children's Building
699 Prince Street
Alexandria, VA 22314
(703) 274-3900
http://www.missingkids.com

National Center on Shaken Baby Syndrome
2955 Harrison Boulevard, # 102
Ogden, UT 84403
(801) 627-3399
http://www.dontshake.com

National Children's Advocacy Center
Administrative Offices
210 Pratt Avenue
Huntsville, AL 35801
(256) 533-5437
http://www.nationalcac.org

National Conference of State Legislatures
7700 East First Place
Denver, CO 80230
(303) 364-7700
http://www.ncsl.org

National Indian Child Welfare Association
5100 Southwest Macadam Avenue, Suite 300
Portland, OR 97239
(503) 222-4044
http://www.nicwa.org

Office for Victims of Crime
810 7th Street NW
Washington, DC 20531
(800) 851-3420
http://www.ojp.usdoj.gov/ovc

Parents Anonymous, Inc.
675 West Foothill Boulevard, Suite 220
Claremont, CA 91711
(909) 621-6184
http://www.parentsanonymous.org

Prevent Child Abuse America
500 North Michigan Avenue, Suite 200
Chicago, IL 60611
(312) 663-3520
http://www.preventchildabuse.org

Survivors of Incest Anonymous
World Service Office
P.O. Box 190
Benson, MD 21018
(410) 893-3322
http://www.siawso.org

Voices for America's Children
1000 Vermont Avenue NW, Seventh Floor
Washington, DC 20005
(202) 289-0777
http://www.voicesforamericaschildren.org

APPENDIX II
NATIONAL CHILD WELFARE RESOURCE CENTERS/ CHILDREN'S BUREAU RESOURCE CENTERS AND CLEARINGHOUSES

ARCH National Resource Network
The Chapel Hill Training-Outreach Project
800 Eastowne Drive, Suite 105
Chapel Hill, NC 27514
(919) 490-5577
http://www.archrespite.org

FRIENDS National Resource Center for Community-Based Resource Programs
800 Eastowne Drive, Suite 105
Chapel Hill, NC 27514
(919) 768-0162
http://www.friendsnrc.org

National Abandoned Infants Assistance Resource Center
University of California at Berkeley
1950 Addison Street, Suite 104 # 7402
Berkeley, CA 94720-7402
(510) 643-8390
http://aia.berkeley.edu

National Adoption Information Clearinghouse
Children's Bureau/ACYF
125 Maryland Avenue SW
Eighth Floor
Washington, DC 20024
(703) 352-3488
http://naic.acf.hhs.gov

National Child Welfare Center for Adoption
16250 Northland Drive, Suite 120
Southfield, MI 48075
(248)443-0306
http://www.nrcadoption.org

National Child Welfare Resource Center for Organizational Improvement
Edmond S. Muskie Institute
University of Southern Maine
400 Congress Street
P.O. Box 15010
Portland, ME 04112
(207) 780-5810
http://www.muskie.usm.maine.edu/helpkids

National Child Welfare Resource Center on Legal and Judicial Issues
ABA Center on Children and the Law
740 15th Street NW, Ninth Floor
Washington, DC 20005-1009
(202) 662-1720
http://www.abanet.org/child/rclji/home.html

National Clearinghouse on Child Abuse and Neglect Information
Children's Bureau/ACYF
1250 Maryland Avenue SE
Eighth Floor
Washington, DC 20024
(703) 385-7565
http://nccanch.acf.hhs.gov

National Data Archive on Child Abuse and Neglect
Beebe Hall-Family Life Development Center
Cornell University
Ithaca, NY 14853-4401
(607) 255-7799
http://www.ndacan.cornell.edu

**National Resource Center for Family
Centered Practice**
University of Iowa School of Social Work
100 Oakdale Campus W206 OH
Iowa City, IA 52242-5000
(319) 335-4965
http://www.uiowa.edu/~nrcfcp

**National Resource Center for Family-Centered
Practice and Permanency Planning**
Hunter College School of Social Work
129 East 79th Street
New York, NY 10021
(212) 452-7053
http://www.hunter.cuny.edu/socwork/nrcfcpp/

**National Resource Center for Youth
Services**
The University of Oklahoma
4502 East 41st Street, Building 4W
Tulsa, OK 74135
(918) 660-3700
http://www.nrcys.ou.edu

APPENDIX III
CHILD PROTECTIVE SERVICES OFFICES IN THE UNITED STATES

ALABAMA

Family Services
Alabama Department of Human Resources
50 North Ripley Street
Montgomery, AL 36130
(334) 242-9500
http://www.dhr.state.al.us

ALASKA

Office of Children's Services
Alaska Department of Health and Social Services
P.O. Box 110630
Juneau, AK 99811
(907) 465-3191
http://www.hss.state.ak.us

ARIZONA

Children, Youth and Families
Arizona Department of Economic Security
Site Code 750A, P.O. Box 6123
Phoenix, AZ 85005
(602) 542-3598
http://www.azdes.gov/asp

ARKANSAS

Division of Children and Family Services
Department of Health and Human Services
P.O. Box 1437, Slot S569
Little Rock, AR 72203-1437
(501) 682-8992
http://www.Arkansas.gov.dhs

CALIFORNIA

Children's Services Operations Bureau
Children and Family Services Division
Department of Social Services
Health and Human Services Agency
744 P Street, MS 3-90
Sacramento, CA 95814
(916) 651-8100
http://www.childsworld.ca.gov

COLORADO

Division of Child Welfare Services
Office of Children, Youth and Family Services
Department of Human Services
1575 Sherman Street
Denver, CO 80203
(303) 866-4365
http://www.cdhs.state.co.us

CONNECTICUT

Child Welfare Services
Department of Children and Families
505 Hudson Street
Hartford, CT 06106
(860) 550-6390
http://www.state.ct.us/dcf

DELAWARE

Office of Prevention and Early Intervention
Division of Family Services
Department of Services for Children, Youth, and
    Their Families
Delaware Youth and Family Center
1825 Faulkland Road
Wilmington, DE 19805
(303) 892-4513
http://www.state.de.us/kids

DISTRICT OF COLUMBIA

Licensing, Monitoring, Placement, and Support Services

Child and Family Service Agency
400 6th Steet SW
Fifth floor
Washington, DC 20024
(202) 442-6000
http://cfsa.dc.gov

FLORIDA

Florida Abuse Hotline

Department of Children and Families
1317 Winewood Boulevard
Tallahassee, FL 32399
(800) 962-2873
(850)487-6100
http://www.state.fl.us/cf_web

GEORGIA

Protective Services Unit

Social Services Section
Division of Family and Children Services
Department of Human Resources
2 Peachtree Street, Suite 29-213
Atlanta, GA 30303
(404) 657-3400
http://dhr.georgia.gov

HAWAII

Child Welfare Services Branch

Social Services Division
Department of Human Services
1390 Miller Street, Room 209
Honolulu, HI 96813
(808) 586-5667
http://www.state.hi.us/dhs

IDAHO

Division of Family and Community Services

Department of Health and Welfare
450 West State Street
Boise, ID 83720-0036
(208) 334-5500
http://www.healthandwelfare.idaho.gov

ILLINOIS

Department of Children and Family Services

100 West Randolph Street 6-200
Chicago, IL 60601
(312) 814-6800
http://www.state.il.us/dcfs

INDIANA

Division of Family and Children

Family and Social Services Administration
W364 Government Center South
402 West Washington Street
Indianapolis, IN 46204
(317) 232-4423
http://www.in.gov/fssa

IOWA

Division of Behavioral, Developmental, and Protective Services for Families, Adults, and Children

Department of Human Services
Hoover Building, Fifth Floor
1305 East Walnut Street
Des Moines, IA 50319
(800) 362-2178
(515) 281-5583
http://www.dhs.state.ia.us

KANSAS

Department of Social and Rehabilitation Services

Docking State Office Building, Room 551-S
915 SW Harrison Street
Topeka, KS 66612
(785) 368-4653
http://www.srskansas.org

KENTUCKY

Division of Protection and Permanency

Department for Community-Based Services
Cabinet for Health and Family Services
275 East Main Street
Frankfort, KY 40621
(502) 564-2136
http://chfs.ky.gov/dcbs/dpp/

LOUISIANA

Division of Child Welfare Program Development

Office of Community Services
Department of Social Services
33 Laurel Street

Baton Rouge, LA 70801
(225) 342-8631
http://www.dss.state.la.us

MAINE

Bureau of Child and Family Services
Department of Health and Human Services
221 State Street
Augusta, ME 04333
(207) 287-3707
http://www.maine.gov/dhs

MARYLAND

Social Services Administration
Department of Human Resources
Saratoga State Center
311 West Saratoga Street
Baltimore, MN 21201
(410) 767-7018
http://www.dhr.state.md.us

MASSACHUSETTS

Department of Social Services
Executive Office of Health and Human Services
24 Farnsworth Street
Boston, MA 02210
(617) 748-2239
http://www.mass.gov/dss

MICHIGAN

**Division of Child Protective Services and
      Foster Care**
Children's Services
Family Support Services
Family Independence Agency
P.O. Box 30037
Lansing, MI 48909
(517) 241-7521
http://www.michigan.gov/fia

MINNESOTA

Child Safety and Permanency Division
Department of Human Services
444 Lafayette Road
Saint Paul, MN 55155

(651) 296-2487
http://www.dhs.state.mn.us

MISSISSIPPI

Division of Family and Children's Services
Department of Human Services
750 North State Street
Jackson, MS 39202
(601) 359-4500
http://www.mdhs.state.ms.us

MISSOURI

Children's Services
Department of Social Services
221 West High Street
P.O. Box 1527
Jefferson City, MO 65102-1527
(573) 522-8024
http://www.dss.mo.gov

MONTANA

Child and Family Services Division
Department of Public Health and Human Services
P.O. Box 202951
Helena, MT 59620
(406) 444-9810
http://www.dphhs.state.mt.gov

NEBRASKA

Office of Protection and Safety
Department of Services
Health and Human Services System
P.O. Box 95044
Lincoln, NE 68508
(402) 471-8404
http://www.hhs.state.ne.us

NEVADA

Family Programs
Division of Child and Family Services
Department of Human Resources
505 East King Street, Room 600
Carson City, NV 89701-3708
(775) 684-4000
http://www.hr.state.nv.us

NEW HAMPSHIRE

Division of Children, Youth, and Families
Department of Health and Human Services
129 Pleasant Street

Concord, NH 03301
(603) 271-4837
http://www.dhhs.state.nh.us

NEW JERSEY

Division of Youth and Family Services
Department of Human Services
P.O. Box 717
Trenton, NJ 08625
(609) 292-6920
http://www.state.nj.us/humanservices

NEW MEXICO

Protective Services Division
Children, Youth, and Families Department
P.O. Drawer 5160
Santa Fe, NM 87502
(505) 827-8400
http://www.cyfd.org

NEW YORK

Office of Central Services
Division of Development and Prevention Services
Office of Children and Family Services
52 Washington Street, Room 324N
Rensselaer, NY 12144-2796
(518) 473-7793
http://www.ocfs.state.ny.us

NORTH CAROLINA

Family Support and Child Welfare Services Section
Division of Social Services
Department of Health and Human Services
325 North Salisbury Street
2406 Mail Service Center
Raleigh, NC 27699
(919) 733-9467
http://www.dhhs.state.nc.us

NORTH DAKOTA

Child Abuse and Neglect Program
Children and Family Services Division
Department of Human Services
State Capitol, Judicial Wing
Bismarck, ND 58505
(701) 328-4806
http://www.state.nd.us/humanservices

OHIO

Protective Services Section
Bureau of Family Services
Office for Children and Families
Department of Job and Family Services
30 East Broad Street, 32nd Floor
Columbus, OH 43215-3414
(614) 466-6282
http://jfs.ohio.gov

OKLAHOMA

Child Protective Services
Children and Family Services Division
Department of Human Services
P.O. Box 25352
Oklahoma City, OK 73125
(405) 521-2283
http://www.okdhs.org

OREGON

Child Protective Services
Children, Adults, and Families
Department of Human Services
500 Summer Street HE, E-68
Salem, OR 97301
(503) 945-7001
http://www.oregon.gov/DHS

PENNSYLVANIA

Department of Public Welfare
P.O. Box 2675
Harrisburg, PA 17105
(717) 787-4756
http://www.dpw.state.pa.us

RHODE ISLAND

Division of Child Protective Services
Department of Children, Youth, and Families
101 Friendship Street
Providence, RI 02903-3716
(401) 528-3502
http://www.dcyf.ri.gov

SOUTH CAROLINA

Child Protective and Preventive Services
Office of Policy and Operations
Department of Social Services
P.O. Box 1520

Columbia, SC 29202
(803) 898-7318
http://www.state.sc.us/dss

SOUTH DAKOTA

Child Protection Services
Division of Program Management
Department of Social Services
700 Governors Drive
Pierre, SD 57501
(605) 773-3227
http://www.state.sd/us/social/CPS

TENNESSEE

Department of Children's Services
Cordell Hull Building, Seventh Floor
436 Sixth Avenue North
Nashville, TN 37243-1290
http://www.state.tn.us/youth

TEXAS

**Department of Family and Protective
   Services**
Mail Code E-557
P.O. Box 149030
Austin, TX 78714
(512) 438-3312
http://www.dfps.state.tx.us

UTAH

Division of Child and Family Services
Department of Human Services
120 North 200 West, Room 319
Salt Lake City, UT 84103
(801) 538-4100
http://www.dhs.utah.gov

VERMONT

Department for Children and Families
Agency of Human Services
103 South Main Street
Waterbury, VT 05671
(802) 879-5901
http://www.ahs.state.vt.us

VIRGINIA

Division of Family Services
Department of Social Services
7 North Eighth Street
Richmond, VA 23219
(804) 726-7530
http://www.dss.virginia.gov

WASHINGTON

Placement and Permanency Services
Division of Program and Policy Development
Children's Administration
Department of Social and Health Services
P.O. Box 45710
Olympia, WA 98504
(360) 902-7953
http://www1.dshs.wa.gov

WEST VIRGINIA

Division of Children and Adult Services
Office of Children and Family Policy
Bureau for Children and Families
Department of Health and Human Resources
350 Capitol Street, Room 691
Charleston, WV 25301
(304) 558-7980
http://www.wvdhhr.org

WISCONSIN

Bureau of Programs and Policies
Division of Children and Family Services
Department of Health and Family Services
1 West Wilson Street
Madison, WI 53702
(608) 266-6799
http://dhfs.wisconsin.gov

WYOMING

Protective Services Division
Department of Family Services
Hathaway Building, Third Floor
2300 Capitol Avenue
Cheyenne, WY 82002
(307) 777-6137
http://dfsweb.state.wy.us

APPENDIX IV
CHILD ABUSE REPORTING NUMBERS AND WEB SITES

ALABAMA

(334) 242-9500
http://www.dhr.state.al.us/page.asp?pageid=304

ALASKA

(800) 478-4444
http://www.hss.state.ak.us/ocs/

ARIZONA

(888) 767-2445
http://www.de.state.az.us/dcyf/cps

ARKANSAS

(800) 482-4964
http://www.state.ar.us/dhs/chilnfam/child_
    protective_services.htm

CALIFORNIA

(916) 445-2771
http://www.dss.cahwnet.gov/cdsseb/FindServic_
    716.htm

COLORADO

Contact local agency or ChildHelp USA at: (800)
    422-4453 or TDD (800) 222-4453
http://www.cdhs.state.co.us/cyf/child_welfare/
    cw_home.htm

CONNECTICUT

(800) 842-2288
TDD: (800) 624-5518
http://www.state.ct.us/dcf/HOTLINE.htm

DELAWARE

(800) 292-9582
(302) 577-6550
http://www.state.de.us/kids

DISTRICT OF COLUMBIA

(877) 671-7233
(202) 671-7233

FLORIDA

(800) 962-2873
http://www5.myf1orida.com/cf_web/myflorida2/
    healthhuman/childabuse

GEORGIA

Contact local agency or Childhelp USA at: (800)
    422-4453 or TDD (800) 222-4453
http://dfcs.dhr.georgia.gov/portal/site

HAWAII

Contact local agency or Childhelp USA at: (800)
    422-4453 or TDD (800) 222-4453
http://www.state.hi.us/dhs

IDAHO

(800) 926-2588

ILLINOIS

(800) 252-2873
(217) 785-4020
http://www.state.il.us/dcfs/foster/index.shtml.

INDIANA

(800) 800-5556
http://www.in/gov/dcs/protection/dfcchi.html

IOWA

(800) 362-2178
(515) 281-3240
http://www.dhs.state.ia.us/reportingchildabuse.asp

KANSAS

(800) 922-5330
(785) 296-0044

http://www.srskansas.org/services/child_protective_
services.htm

KENTUCKY

(800) 752-6200
(502) 595-4550
http://cfc.state.ky.us/help/child_abuse.asp

LOUISIANA

(225) 342-6832
http://dss.state.la.us/departments/ocs/child_welfare_
services.htm

MAINE

(800) 452-1999
(207) 287-2983
http://www.maine.gov/dhhs/bcfs/abuse.htm

MARYLAND

(800) 332-6347
http://www.dhr.state.md.us/cps

MASSACHUSETTS

(800) 792-5200
(617) 232-4882

MICHIGAN

(800) 942-4357
(517) 373-3572

MINNESOTA

(800) 422-4553
http://www.dhs.state.mn.us/CFS/Programs/
ChildProtection

MISSISSIPPI

(800) 222-8000
(601) 359-4991
http://www.mdhs.state.ms.us/fcs_prot.htm.

MISSOURI

(800) 392-3738
(573) 751-3448
http://www.dss.state.mo.us/dfs/csp.htm

MONTANA

(866) 820-5437
(406) 444-5900

NEBRASKA

(800) 652-1999
(402) 595-1324
http://www.hhs.state.ne.us/cha/chaindex.htm

NEVADA

(800) 992-5757
(775) 684-4400
http://www.dcfs.state.nv.us

NEW HAMPSHIRE

(800) 894-5533
(603) 271-6556
http://www.dhhs.state.nh.us/DHHS/BCP

NEW JERSEY

(877) 652-2873
(800) 835-5510
http://www.state.nj.us/humanservices/dyfs

NEW MEXICO

(800) 797-3260
(505) 841-6100
http://www.cyfd.org

NEW YORK

(800) 342-3720
(800) 369-2437
http://www.ocfs.state.ny.us/mainl/cps

NORTH CAROLINA

Contact local agency or Childhelp USA at: (800)
422-4453 or TDD (800) 222-4453
http://www.dhhs.state.nc.us/dss/srv/cserv_protect.
htm

NORTH DAKOTA

(701) 328-2316
http://www.state.nd.us/humanservices/services/
childfamily/cps

OHIO

Contact local agency or Childhelp USA at: (800)
422-4453 or TDD (800) 222-4453
http://jfs.ohio.gov/ocf/

OKLAHOMA

(800) 522-3511
http://www.okdhs.org/dcfs/

OREGON

(800) 854-3508, ext. 2402
(503) 378-6704
(503) 378-5414
http://dhs.state.or.us/children/abuse/cps/cs_branches.
htm

PENNSYLVANIA

(800) 932-0313
(717) 783-8744
http://www.dpw.state.pa.us/Child/
ChildAbuseNeglect

RHODE ISLAND

(800) 742-4453
http://www.dcyf.ri.gov/chldwelfare.reporting.htm

SOUTH CAROLINA

(803) 898-7318
http://www.state.sc.us/dss

SOUTH DAKOTA

(605) 773-3227
http://www.state.sd.us/social/CPS

TENNESSEE

(877) 237-0004
http://www.state.tn.us/youth/cps/

TEXAS

(800) 252-5400
(512) 834-3784
http://www.tdprs.state.tx.us

UTAH

(800) 678-9399
http://www.hsdcfs.utah.gov

VERMONT

(800) 649-5285
http://www.dcf.state.vt.us/cdd/

VIRGINIA

(800) 552-7096
(804) 786-8536
http://www.dss.state.va.us/family/cps.html

WASHINGTON

(866) 363-4276
http://wwwl.dshs.wa.gov/ca/safety/prevAbuse.
asp?1

WEST VIRGINIA

(800) 352-6513
http://www.wvdhhr.org/report.asp

WISCONSIN

(608) 266-3036
http://www.dhfs.state.wi.us/Children/CPS

WYOMING

Contact local agency or Childhelp USA at: (800)
422-4453 or TDD (800) 222-4453
http://dfsweb.state.wy.us

APPENDIX V

STATE-BY-STATE GROUNDS FOR INVOLUNTARY TERMINATION OF PARENTAL RIGHTS, 2005

This appendix discusses grounds under state laws to involuntarily terminate parental rights, usually because of abuse, neglect, abandonment and other grounds that cause harm to children, such as the abuse and neglect of other children or the long-term alcohol or drug-induced incapacity of the parent(s). Other grounds for termination may be a long-term felony conviction, the mental illness of a parent, the failure to provide financial support to a child and so on.

The Adoption and Safe Families Act (ASFA) requires state agencies to terminate parental rights when children have been in foster care for 15 of the most recent 22 months as well as in other cases, such as when a child is an abandoned infant or the parent has murdered another child or the child's other parent or has solicited such a murder or when the parent has committed a felony assault that has caused serious physical harm to the child or to another child of the parent.

Exceptions to ASFA may be made, such as when the child is in the care of another relative, when it is believed that terminating parental rights is not in the child's best interests and when the parent has not been provided with services required by the case plan toward reunification of the parent with the child.

Note that this appendix is provided for information only and should not be used for legal purpose. Attorneys in the state should be consulted on current law.

ALABAMA

- The parent has abandoned the child.
- The parent is unable to discharge his or her parental duties due to
  - Emotional illness, mental illness or mental deficiency

- Use of alcohol or controlled substances
- A conviction and incarceration for a felony
- The parent has tortured, abused or severely maltreated the child.
- The parent's conduct or neglect has resulted in serious physical injury to the child.
- The parent has subjected the child to an aggravated circumstance, including, but not limited to, abandonment, torture, chronic abuse, substance abuse or sexual abuse.
- Reasonable efforts to rehabilitate the parent have failed.
- The parent has been convicted of
  - Murder or voluntary manslaughter of another child of the parent
  - Aiding, abetting, attempting or soliciting to commit murder or voluntary manslaughter of another child of the parent
  - A felony assault that results in serious bodily injury to the child or another child of the parent
- The parent has failed to support the child when financially able to do so.
- The parent has failed to maintain regular visitation, contact or communication with the child.
- Parental rights to another child have been involuntarily terminated.

ALASKA

- The parent has abandoned the child.
- The parent is unable to discharge his or her parental duties due to
  - Emotional illness, mental illness or mental deficiency

- Use of alcohol or controlled substances
- A conviction and incarceration for a felony
- The parent has subjected the child to circumstances that pose a substantial risk of harm, including, but not limited to, abandonment, torture, chronic mental injury, chronic physical harm or sexual abuse.
- The parent's conduct or neglect has resulted in serious physical or mental injury to the child.
- When the child has been in foster care for 15 of the most recent 22 months, and reasonable efforts to rehabilitate the parent have failed.
- The parent has been convicted of
  - Homicide of a parent of the child or a child
  - Aiding, abetting, attempting or soliciting to commit a homicide of a parent of the child or a child
  - A felony assault that resulted in serious bodily injury to a child
- The child has been sexually abused as a result of the parent's conduct or failure to protect the child.
- The parent has willfully failed to provide the child with needed medical treatment.
- The child has committed an illegal act as a result of pressure, guidance or approval from the parent.
- Parental rights to another child of the parent have been involuntarily terminated, and conditions that led to the termination have not been corrected.

ARIZONA

- The parent has abandoned the child.
- The identity of the parent is unknown even after diligent efforts to identify and locate the parent.
- The parent is unable to discharge his or her parental duties due to
  - Emotional illness, mental illness, or mental deficiency
  - Chronic abuse of dangerous drugs, alcohol, or controlled substances
  - A conviction and incarceration for a felony
- The parent has neglected or willfully abused the child.

- The parent's conduct or neglect has resulted in serious physical or emotional injury to the child.
- The child has been in out-of-home placement for a total of nine months, and the parent has refused to participate in services that could remedy the circumstances that caused the placement.
- The child has been in out-of-home placement for a total of 15 months, and the parent has participated in services but has been unable to remedy the circumstances that caused the placement.
- The parent has been convicted of
  - Murder or manslaughter of another child of the parent
  - Sexual abuse, sexual assault of a child, sexual conduct with a minor or molestation of a child
  - Commercial sexual exploitation of a minor, sexual exploitation of a minor or luring a minor for sexual exploitation
  - Aiding, abetting, attempting or soliciting to commit murder or manslaughter or any of the crimes listed above
- A putative father has failed to establish paternity or respond to notice.
- Parental rights to another child of the parent have been involuntarily terminated within the preceding two years, and conditions that led to the termination have not been corrected.

ARKANSAS

- The parent has abandoned the child.
- The parent is unable to discharge his or her parental duties due to
  - Emotional illness, mental illness, or mental deficiency
  - A conviction and incarceration for a felony
- The parent has neglected or willfully abused the child.
- The parent's conduct or neglect has resulted in serious physical or emotional injury to the child.
- The child has been out of the parent's custody for 12 months, and reasonable efforts to rehabilitate the parent have failed.

- The parent has been convicted of
  - Murder or voluntary manslaughter of any child
  - Aiding, abetting, attempting or soliciting to commit murder or voluntary manslaughter of any child
  - A felony battery or assault that results in serious bodily injury to any child

- The parent has subjected the child to aggravated circumstances, which can mean
  - The child has been abandoned, chronically abused, subjected to extreme or repeated cruelty, or sexually abused.
  - A judge has determined that there is little likelihood that services to the family will result in successful reunification.
  - The child has been removed from the custody of the parent more than three times in the last 15 months.

- The parent has willfully failed to provide significant material support in accordance with the parent's means.
- The parent has failed to maintain meaningful contact with the child.
- Parental rights to another child of the parent have been terminated involuntarily.

CALIFORNIA

- The parent has abandoned the child.
- The parent is unable to discharge his or her parental duties due to
  - Mental disability
  - Extensive, abusive and chronic use of alcohol or drugs
  - Incarceration or institutionalization

- The parent has physically or sexually abused the child.
- The parent's conduct or neglect has resulted in serious physical injury to the child.
- The parent has refused reunification services.
- The parent has been convicted of a violent felony, indicating parental unfitness.

- The child has been left without any provision for his or her support.
- The parent has failed to visit or contact the child for six months.
- The whereabouts of the parent have been unknown for six months.
- Parental rights to another child of the parent have been involuntarily terminated.
- The parent has caused the death of another child through abuse or neglect.
- The parent has subjected the child to severe or repeated sexual or physical abuse.
- The child was conceived as a result of a sexual offense against a child.
- The parent willfully abandoned the child, and the abandonment itself constituted a serious danger to the child.

COLORADO

- The parent has abandoned the child.
- The parent has been found to be unfit due to
  - Emotional illness, mental illness, or mental deficiency
  - A single incident of serious bodily injury or disfigurement to the child
  - Use of alcohol or controlled substances
  - Long-term incarceration

- The parent has caused serious bodily injury or death to a sibling of the child due to abuse or neglect.
- The parent's conduct or neglect has resulted in grave risk of death or serious physical injury to the child.
- The parent has subjected the child to an aggravated circumstance, including, but not limited to abandonment, torture, chronic abuse, substance abuse or sexual abuse.
- Reasonable efforts to rehabilitate the parent have failed, or the parent has failed to reasonably comply with a treatment plan.
- The parent has been convicted of
  - Murder or voluntary manslaughter of another child of the parent

- Aiding, abetting, attempting or soliciting to commit murder or voluntary manslaughter of another child of the parent
- A felony assault that resulted in serious bodily injury to the child or another child of the parent
- The parent has neglected the child and is unable or unwilling to provide nurturing and safe parenting.
- The parent has failed to maintain regular visitation with the child.
- Parental rights to another child of the parent have been involuntarily terminated, unless the prior sibling termination resulted from a parent delivering the child to a firefighter or hospital, pursuant to the provisions of § 19-3-304.5.

CONNECTICUT

- The parent has abandoned the child.
- The parent has inflicted sexual abuse, sexual exploitation or severe physical abuse on the child or has engaged in a pattern of abuse of the child.
- The parent is unable or unwilling to benefit from reunification efforts.
- The parent was convicted of a sexual assault that resulted in the conception of a child. The court may terminate the rights of the parent to such child at any time after the conviction.
- A court has found that the parent has
  - Killed, through a deliberate, nonaccidental act, a sibling of the child
  - Requested, attempted, conspired or solicited to commit the killing of the child or a sibling of the child
  - Assaulted the child or sibling of the child, and such assault resulted in serious bodily injury to the child
- The parent has failed to maintain a reasonable degree of interest, concern or responsibility as to the welfare of the child.
- Parental rights to another child of the parent have been involuntarily terminated.

DELAWARE

- The parent has abandoned the child.
- The parent has abandoned a baby in accordance with Tit. 16 § 907A and failed to manifest an intent to exercise parental rights within 30 days.
- The parent is unable to discharge his or her parental duties due to
  - Mental incompetence
  - Extended or repeated incarceration
- The parent's conduct or neglect has resulted in serious physical injury to the child.
- The parent has subjected the child to torture, chronic abuse, sexual abuse or life-threatening abuse.
- Reasonable effort to rehabilitate the parent have failed.
- The parent has been convicted of
  - A felony-level offense against a person, and the victim was the child or any other child
  - Aiding, abetting, attempting or soliciting the commission of such offense
  - The offense of dealing in children (trafficking)
  - The felony-level offense of endangering children
- The parent has failed to support the child when financially able to do so.
- The parent has failed to maintain regular visitation, contact or communication with the child.
- Parental rights to another child of the parent have been involuntarily terminated.

DISTRICT OF COLUMBIA

- The parent has abandoned the child.
- Drug-related activity continues to exist in the child's home environment after intervention and services have been provided.
- The parent has been convicted of
  - Murder or voluntary manslaughter of a child's sibling or another child
  - Aiding, abetting, attempting or soliciting to commit such murder or voluntary manslaughter
  - A felony assault that has resulted in serious

bodily injury to the child, a child's sibling or another child

- The child has been subjected to intentional and severe mental abuse.
- Parental rights to another child of the parent have been involuntarily terminated.

FLORIDA

- The parent has abandoned the child.
- The parent is unable to discharge his or her parental duties due to extended incarceration or there has been a finding that the parent is a
  - Violent career criminal
  - Habitual violent felony offender
  - Sexual predator
- The parent has subjected the child to egregious conduct, including abuse, abandonment or neglect that is flagrant or outrageous by a normal standard of conduct.
- The parent has subjected the child to an aggravated child abuse, as defined in § 827.03, that includes sexual battery, sexual abuse or chronic abuse.
- Reasonable efforts to rehabilitate the parent have failed.
- The parent has been convicted of
  - Murder or voluntary manslaughter of another child of the parent
  - Aiding, abetting, attempting or soliciting to commit murder or voluntary manslaughter of another child of the parent
  - A felony assault that resulted in serious bodily injury to the child or another child of the parent
- Parental rights to another child of the parent have been involuntarily terminated.

GEORGIA

- The parent has abandoned the child.
- The parent is unable to discharge his or her parental duties due to
  - A medically verifiable deficiency of his or her

physical, mental or emotional health
  - Excessive or chronic use of alcohol or controlled substances
  - A conviction and incarceration for a felony
- The parent has physically, mentally or emotionally neglected the child, or there has been past neglect of the child or another child.
- The parent's conduct or neglect has resulted in serious physical injury to the child or in the injury or death of a sibling.
- The parent has subjected the child to egregious conduct, or there has been past egregious conduct toward the child or another child, of a physically, emotionally or sexually cruel or abusive nature.
- Reasonable efforts to rehabilitate the parent have failed.
- The parent has been convicted of
  - Murder or voluntary manslaughter of another child of the parent or the child's other parent
  - Aiding, abetting, attempting or soliciting to commit murder or voluntary manslaughter of another child of the parent or the child's other parent
  - A felony assault that resulted in serious bodily injury to the child or another child of the parent
- The parent has failed to comply with a court order to support the child for a period of 12 months or longer.
- The parent has failed to develop and maintain a parental bond with the child in a meaningful, supportive manner.
- The child has been in foster care for 15 of the past 22 months.
- Parental rights to another child of the parent have been involuntarily terminated.

HAWAII

- The parent has abandoned the child.
- The parent is unable to discharge his or her parental duties due to mental illness or mental deficiency.

- The parent has tortured the child.
- The parent has subjected the child to an aggravated circumstance.
- Reasonable efforts to rehabilitate the parent have failed.
- The parent has been convicted of
  - Murder or voluntary manslaughter of another child of the parent
  - Aiding, abetting, attempting or soliciting to commit murder or voluntary manslaughter of another child of the parent
  - A felony assault that resulted in serious bodily injury to the child or another child of the parent
- The parent has failed to provide care and support for the child for at least one year.
- The parent has failed to communicate with the child for at least one year.
- The parent has voluntarily surrendered care and custody of the child to another person for at least two years.
- The parent is not the child's natural or adoptive father.
- Parental rights to another child of the parent have been involuntarily terminated.

IDAHO

- The parent has abandoned the child.
- The parent is unable to discharge his or her parental duties, and such inability will continue for a prolonged, indeterminate period.
- The parent has been incarcerated with no possibility of parole.
- The parent has abused or neglected the child.
- The parent has caused the child to be conceived as a result of rape, incest, lewd conduct with a minor under 16 years of age or sexual abuse of a child under the age of 16 years.
- The parent has subjected the child to an aggravated circumstance, including, but not limited to, abandonment, torture, chronic abuse or sexual abuse.

- Reasonable efforts to rehabilitate the parent have failed.
- The parent has been convicted of
  - Murder or voluntary manslaughter of another child of the parent or the child's other parent
  - Aiding, abetting, attempting or soliciting to commit murder or voluntary manslaughter of another child of the parent or the child's other parent
  - A felony assault that resulted in serious bodily injury to the child or another child of the parent
- The presumptive parent is not the natural parent of the child.
- The parent has failed to maintain a relationship with the child for a period of one year.
- Parental rights to another child of the parent have been involuntarily terminated.

ILLINOIS

- The parent has abandoned the child.
- The parent is unable to discharge his or parental duties due to
  - Mental illness, mental deficiency, or developmental disability
  - A conviction and incarceration for a felony
- The parent has substantially and continuously or repeatedly neglected the child.
- The parent has been found, two or more times, to have physically abused any child or to have caused the death of any child by physical child abuse.
- The parent has subjected the child to an aggravated circumstance, including, but not limited to, abandonment, torture or chronic abuse.
- Reasonable efforts to rehabilitate the parent have failed.
- A child was born exposed to controlled substances, and a substance-exposed child was previously born to the same mother.
- The parent has been convicted of
  - Murder or voluntary manslaughter of any child

- Aiding, abetting, attempting or soliciting to commit murder or voluntary manslaughter of any child
- Aggravated battery or felony domestic battery that has resulted in serious bodily injury to any child
- Aggravated criminal sexual assault

- The parent has repeatedly and continuously failed to provide the child with adequate food, clothing and shelter, although financially able to do so.

- The parent has failed to maintain regular visitation, contact or communication with the child for a period of 12 months.

- A putative father has failed to establish paternity.

- A child has been in foster care for 15 of the most recent 22 months.

- Parental rights to another child of the parent have been involuntarily terminated.

INDIANA

- The parent has abandoned the child.

- The parent has been convicted of
  - Causing a suicide, involuntary manslaughter rape, criminal deviate conduct, child molesting, exploitation or incest, and the victim is a child of the parent or the parent of the child
  - Murder or voluntary manslaughter of another child of the parent or a parent of the child
  - Aiding, abetting, attempting or soliciting to commit any of the above offenses
  - Battery, aggravated battery, criminal recklessness or neglect of a dependent against the child or another child of the parent

- The child has been in foster care for 15 of the most recent 22 months.

- Parental rights to another child of the parent have been involuntarily terminated.

IOWA

- The parent has abandoned the child.

- The child is a newborn infant who was relinquished in accordance with Chapter 232B.

- The child has been in foster care for 15 of the most recent 22 months.

- The parent is unable to discharge his or her parental duties due to
  - Chronic mental illness
  - Severe, chronic substance abuse problems
  - A conviction and incarceration for a crime against a child, and it is unlikely that the parent will be released for a period of five years or longer
  - A conviction and incarceration for physically or sexually abusing or neglecting the child or any child in the household

- The parent's conduct or omissions has resulted in the physical or sexual abuse or neglect of the child.

- The parent has been convicted of
  - Child endangerment resulting in the death of the child's sibling
  - Three or more acts of child endangerment involving the child, a sibling or another child in the household
  - Child endangerment resulting in serious injury to the child, a sibling or another child in the household
  - Murder or voluntary manslaughter of another child of the parent
  - Aiding, abetting, attempting or soliciting to commit murder or voluntary manslaughter of another child of the parent
  - A felony assault that resulted in serious bodily injury to the child or another child of the parent

- The parent has subjected the child to aggravated circumstances.

- Reasonable efforts to rehabilitate the parent have failed.

- The parent has failed to maintain significant and meaningful contact with the child for a period of six consecutive months.

- Parental rights to another child of the parent have been involuntarily terminated, and there is evidence that the parent continues to lack the ability or willingness to respond to services.

KANSAS

- The parent is unfit by reason of conduct or condition.
- The parent has abandoned the child.
- The parent is unable to discharge his or her parental duties due to
  - Emotional illness, mental illness, mental deficiency or physical disability
  - Excessive use of alcohol, narcotics, or dangerous drugs
  - A conviction and incarceration for a felony
- There has been an unexplained injury or death of another child or stepchild of the parent.
- The parent has physically, mentally or emotionally neglected the child.
- The parent has subjected the child or another child to aggravated circumstances, including, but not limited to, abandonment, torture, chronic abuse, sexual abuse or chronic, life-threatening neglect.
- Reasonable efforts to rehabilitate the parent have failed.
- The parent has been convicted of
  - Murder or voluntary manslaughter of another child of the parent or the other parent of the child
  - Aiding, abetting, attempting or soliciting to commit murder or voluntary manslaughter of another child of the parent or the other parent of the child
  - A felony assault that resulted in serious bodily injury to the child or another child of the parent
- The parent has failed to pay a reasonable portion of the cost of substitute care for the child when financially able to do so.
- The parent has failed to assume care of the child in the home when able to do so.
- The parent has failed to maintain regular visitation, contact or communication with the child.
- Parental rights to another child of the parent have been involuntarily terminated.

KENTUCKY

- The parent has abandoned the child for a period of not less than 90 days.
- The parent is unable to discharge his or her parental duties due to
  - Mental illness or mental retardation
  - Alcohol or other drug abuse
- The parent has inflicted or allowed to be inflicted upon the child, by other than accidental means, serious physical injury.
- The parent has continuously or repeatedly inflicted or allowed to be inflicted upon any child physical abuse, sexual abuse, neglect or emotional injury, and such injury to the child named in the petition is likely to occur if parental rights are not terminated.
- The parent has subjected the child to aggravated circumstances, including one or more of the following:
  - The parent has not had or attempted contact with the child for a period of not less than 90 days.
  - The parent is incarcerated and will be unavailable to care for the child for at least one year.
  - The parent has sexually abused the child and refused available treatment.
  - The parent has engaged in abuse of the child that required removal from the home two or more times in the past two years.
  - The parent has caused serious physical injury.
- Reasonable efforts to rehabilitate the parent have failed.
- The parent has been convicted of
  - (In a criminal proceeding) having caused or contributed to the death of a child as a result of physical abuse, sexual abuse or neglect
  - Committing a felony assault that resulted in serious bodily injury to the child or another child of the parent
- The parent has failed to provide essential food, clothing, shelter, medical care or education to the child when financially able to do so.
- The child has been in foster care for 15 of the most recent 22 months.

- Parental rights to another child of the parent have been involuntarily terminated.

LOUISIANA

- The parent has abandoned the child.
- The parent has been incarcerated for an extended period of time and is unwilling or unable to provide care other than foster care for the child.
- The parent has subjected the child to abuse that is chronic, life-threatening or results in gravely disabling physical or psychological injury or disfigurement.
- The parent has subjected the child to sexual abuse.
- The parent has subjected the child or any other child in the household to egregious conduct or conditions, including but not limited to, extreme abuse, cruel and inhuman treatment or grossly negligent behavior below a reasonable standard of human decency.
- Reasonable efforts to rehabilitate the parent have failed.
- The parent has been convicted of
  - Murder or voluntary manslaughter of another child of the parent
  - Murder or unjustified intentional killing of the child's other parent
  - A felony that has resulted in serious bodily injury to the child or another child of the parent
  - Rape, sodomy, aggravated incest, torture or starvation
  - Aiding, abetting, attempting or soliciting to commit any of the above crimes
- The parent has failed to provide significant contributions to the care and support of the child for any period of six consecutive months.
- The parent has failed to maintain regular visitation, contact or communication with the child for any period of six consecutive months.
- The parent has committed a felony rape that resulted in the conception of a child.

- The parent has relinquished a newborn infant in accordance with the law.
- Parental rights to another child of the parent have been involuntarily terminated.

MAINE

- The parent has abandoned the child.
- The parent is unable to discharge his or her parental duties due to a chronic substance abuse problem.
- The parent has subjected the child to aggravated circumstances, including but not limited to, rape, gross sexual conduct or assault, sexual abuse, incest, aggravated assault, kidnapping, promotion of prostitution, abandonment, torture, chronic abuse or any other treatment that is heinous or abhorrent to society.
- Reasonable efforts to rehabilitate the parent have failed.
- The parent has been convicted of any of the following crimes, and the victim was any child in the parent's household:
  - Murder, felony murder or manslaughter
  - Aiding, conspiring or soliciting to commit murder or manslaughter
  - A felony assault that resulted in serious bodily injury
- The parent has failed to take responsibility for the child within a reasonable period of time.
- Parental rights to another child of the parent have been involuntarily terminated.

MARYLAND

- The parent has abandoned the child.
- The parent has a disability that renders the parent consistently unable to care for the child for long periods of time.
- The parent has subjected the child to torture, chronic abuse, sexual abuse or chronic and life-threatening neglect.
- The child was born exposed to cocaine, heroin or a derivative thereof.

- The parent has committed acts of abuse or neglect toward any child in the family.
- Reasonable efforts to rehabilitate the parent have failed.
- The parent has been convicted of
  - A crime of violence, as defined in § 14-101 of the Criminal Law article, against the child, another child of the family or any person who resides in the household
  - Aiding, abetting, conspiring or soliciting to a crime described above
- The child has been in foster care for 15 of the most recent 22 months.

MASSACHUSETTS

- The parent has abandoned the child.
- The parent is unable to discharge his or her parental duties due to
  - Mental illness or deficiency
  - Alcohol or drug addiction
  - Incarceration for extended period of time
- The parent has subjected the child to aggravated circumstances, including but not limited to, sexual abuse or exploitation or severe or repetitive conduct of a physically or emotionally abusive nature.
- Reasonable efforts to rehabilitate the parent have failed.
- The parent has been convicted of
  - Murder or voluntary manslaughter of another child of the parent
  - Aiding, abetting, attempting or soliciting to commit murder or voluntary manslaughter of another child of the parent
  - A felony assault that results in serious bodily injury to the child or another child of the parent
- The parent has failed to support the child when financially able to do so.
- The parent has failed to maintain regular visitation, contact or communication with the child.
- The child has been in foster care for 15 of the immediately preceding 22 months.

MICHIGAN

- The parent has abandoned the child.
- The parent is incarcerated for a period exceeding two years and has not provided for the child's care.
- The parent's conduct or neglect has resulted in physical injury or sexual abuse to the child or a sibling of the child.
- The parent has abused the child or a sibling of the child, and the abuse included one or more of the following
  - Criminal sexual conduct involving penetration, attempted penetration or assault with intent to penetrate
  - Battering, torture or other severe physical abuse
  - Loss or serious impairment of an organ or limb
  - Life-threatening injury
  - Murder or voluntary manslaughter
  - Aiding, abetting, attempting, conspiring or soliciting to commit murder or voluntary manslaughter
- Reasonable efforts to rehabilitate the parent have failed.
- The parent has failed to support the child when financially able to do so.
- The parent has failed to maintain regular visitation, contact or communication with the child.
- Parental rights to another child of the parent have been involuntarily terminated, and attempts to rehabilitate the parents have been unsuccessful.

MINNESOTA

- The parent has abandoned the child.
- The parent has been diagnosed as chemically dependent and has failed to successfully complete a treatment plan.
- The parent has substantially, continuously and repeatedly neglected the child.
- The parent has subjected the child to egregious harm of a nature, duration or chronicity that indicates a lack of regard for the child's well-being.

- Reasonable efforts to rehabilitate the parent have failed.
- The parent has been convicted of
  - Murder or voluntary manslaughter of another child of the parent
  - Aiding, abetting, attempting or soliciting to commit murder or voluntary manslaughter of another child of the parent
  - An assault with a deadly weapon with the infliction of substantial bodily injury to the child or another child of the parent
  - Assault with a past pattern of child abuse
  - Assault with a victim under the age of four years
- The parent has failed to provide necessary support to the child when ordered to do so and financially able to do so.
- The parent has failed to maintain contact with the child for six months and has not demonstrated an interest in the child.
- A putative father has failed to register with the fathers' adoption registry.
- The child has been in foster placement for a cumulative period of 12 months within the preceding 22 months, and the parent has failed to correct the conditions that led to the placement.
- Parental rights to another child of the parent have been involuntarily terminated.

MISSISSIPPI

- The parent has abandoned the child.
- The parent is unable to discharge his or her parental duties due to
  - Severe mental deficiencies, mental illness or physical incapacitation
  - Alcohol or drug addiction
- The parent has been responsible for a series of abusive incidents concerning one or more children.
- There is an extreme and deep-seated antipathy by the child toward the parent that was caused at least in part by the parent's serious neglect, abuse or prolonged and unreasonable absence.

- The parent has subjected the child to an aggravated circumstance, including, but not limited to, abandonment, torture, chronic abuse, substance abuse or sexual abuse.
- Reasonable efforts to rehabilitate the parent have failed.
- The parent has been convicted of
  - Murder or voluntary manslaughter of another child of the parent
  - Aiding, abetting, attempting or soliciting to commit murder or voluntary manslaughter of another child of the parent
  - A felony assault that results in serious bodily injury to the child or another child of the parent
- The parent has been convicted of any of the following offenses against any child
  - Rape, sexual battery, exploitation or touching of a child for lustful purposes
  - Felonious abuse or battery of a child
  - Carnal knowledge of a stepchild, an adopted child or the child of cohabiting partner
- The parent has failed to exercise reasonable available visitation with the child.
- The parent has made no contact with a child under the age of three years for six months or a child three years of age or older for a period of one year.
- Parental rights to another child of the parent have been involuntarily terminated.

MISSOURI

- The child is an abandoned infant.
- The parent is unable to discharge his or her parental duties due to
  - A mental condition
  - Chemical dependency
  - A conviction of a felony that would deprive the child of a stable home for a period of years
- The parent's conduct or neglect has subjected the child to a substantial risk of physical or mental harm.
- The parent has subjected any child in the family to a severe act or recurrent acts of physical,

emotional or sexual abuse, including an act of incest.

- The child was conceived and born as a result of an act of forcible rape.
- Reasonable efforts to rehabilitate the parent have failed.
- The parent has been convicted of
  - Murder or voluntary manslaughter of another child of the parent
  - Aiding, abetting, attempting or soliciting to commit murder or voluntary manslaughter of another child of the parent
  - A felony assault that resulted in serious bodily injury to the child or to another child of the parent
- The parent has failed to contribute to the cost of care and maintenance of this child when financially able to do so.
- The parent has failed to maintain regular visitation or other contact with the child.
- The child has been in foster care for 15 of the most recent 22 months.
- Parental rights to another child of the parent have been involuntarily terminated within or immediately preceding three years.

MONTANA

- The parent has abandoned the child.
- The parent is unable to discharge his or her parental duties due to
  - Emotional illness, mental illness, or mental deficiency
  - A history of violent behavior by the parent
  - Use of intoxicating liquor or a narcotic or dangerous drug
  - A judicially ordered long-term confinement of the parent, including incarceration of more than one year
- The parent's conduct or neglect has resulted in the death or serious physical injury of a child.
- The parent has subjected the child to aggravated circumstances, including but not limited to, aban-

donment, torture, chronic abuse, sexual abuse or chronic severe neglect.

- Reasonable efforts to rehabilitate the parent have failed.
- The parent has been convicted of
  - Deliberate homicide of a child
  - Aiding, abetting, attempting or soliciting to commit deliberate homicide of a child
  - Aggravated assault against a child
  - Neglect of a child that resulted in serious bodily injury
- The parent is convicted of a felony in which sexual intercourse occurred; as a result, the child was born.
- A putative father has failed to contribute to the support of the child for an aggregate period of one year, to establish substantial relations with the child or to register with the putative father registry.
- Parental rights to another child of the parent have been involuntarily terminated, and the circumstances related to the termination are relevant to the parent's ability to adequately care for the child at issue.

NEBRASKA

- The parent has abandoned the child for six months or more.
- The parent is unable to discharge his or her parental duties due to mental illness or mental deficiency, and such condition will likely continue for a prolonged, indeterminate period.
- The parent has substantially and continuously or repeatedly neglected the child.
- The parent is unfit by reason of debauchery, habitual use of intoxicated liquor or narcotic drugs or repeated lewd and lascivious behavior.
- The parent has inflicted, by other than accidental means, serious physical injury upon the child.
- The parent has subjected the child to aggravated circumstance, including, but not limited to, abandonment, torture, chronic abuse or sexual abuse.

- Reasonable efforts to rehabilitate the parent have failed.
- The parent has been convicted of
  - Murder or voluntary manslaughter of another child of the parent
  - Aiding, abetting, attempting or soliciting to commit murder or voluntary manslaughter of another child of the parent
  - A felony assault that results in serious bodily injury to the child or another minor child of the parent
- The parent has failed to provide necessary care and subsistence for the child when financially able to do so.
- The child has been in out-of-home placement for 15 of the most recent 22 months.
- Parental rights to another child of the parent have been involuntarily terminated.

NEVADA

- The parent has abandoned the child for 60 days or more.
- The parent is unable to discharge his or her parental duties due to
  - Emotional illness, mental illness, or mental deficiency
  - Excessive use of intoxicating liquors, controlled substances or dangerous drugs
  - A conviction for a felony, if the facts of the crime are of such a nature to indicate the unfitness of the parent
- The parent has subjected the child to conduct of a physically or sexually cruel or abusive nature.
- The parent's conduct or neglect has resulted in substantial bodily injury to the child.
- Reasonable efforts to rehabilitate the parent have failed.
- The parent has committed, aided, abetted, attempted or solicited to commit murder or voluntary manslaughter.
- The parent has failed, although physically and financially able, to provide the child with adequate food, clothing, shelter, education or other necessary care.
- The parent has, for the previous six months, had the ability to contact the child and made no more than token efforts to do so.
- A putative father has failed to establish paternity.
- The child is less than one year of age and was delivered to a provider of emergency services pursuant to law.
- Parental rights to another child of the parent have been involuntarily terminated.

If the child has been placed outside his or her home, and has remained in that placement for 14 of any 20 consecutive months, the best interest of the child must be presumed to be served by termination of parental rights.

NEW HAMPSHIRE

- The parent has abandoned the child.
- The parent is unable to discharge his or her parental duties due to
  - Mental illness or mental deficiency
  - Incarceration for a felony offense
- The parent knowingly caused, or permitted another to cause, severe sexual, physical, mental or emotional abuse of the child.
- Reasonable efforts to rehabilitate the parent have failed.
- The parent has been convicted of
  - Murder or manslaughter of another child of the parent or the child's other parent
  - Attempting, soliciting or conspiring to commit murder or manslaughter of another child of the parent or the child's other parent
  - A felony assault that resulted in serious bodily injury to the child, another child of the parent or the child's other parent
- The parent has substantially and continuously neglected to provide the child with necessary subsistence, education and other necessary care when financially able to do so.

- The parent has failed to maintain regular communication with the child.
- The child has been in out-of-home placement for 12 of the most recent 22 months.

NEW JERSEY

- The parent has abandoned the child.
- The parent has subjected the child to aggravated circumstances of abuse, neglect, cruelty or abandonment.
- Reasonable efforts to rehabilitate the parent have failed.
- The parent has been convicted of
  - Murder, aggravated manslaughter or manslaughter of another child of the parent
  - Aiding, abetting, attempting or soliciting to commit the above murder, aggravated manslaughter or manslaughter of the child or another child of the parent
  - Committing or attempting to commit an assault or similarly serious criminal act that resulted, or could have resulted, in the death or significant bodily injury to the child or another child of the parent
- Parental rights to another child of the parent have been involuntarily terminated.

NEW MEXICO

- The parent has abandoned the child.
- The parent has subjected the child to aggravated circumstances, including those circumstances in which the parent has
  - Attempted, conspired to cause or caused great bodily harm to the child or great bodily harm or death to the child's sibling
  - Attempted, conspired to cause or caused great bodily harm or death to another parent, guardian, or custodian of the child
  - Attempted, conspired to subject or subjected the child to torture, chronic abuse or sexual abuse
- The child has been abused or neglected, and the conditions and causes of the abuse or neglect are unlikely to change in the near future.

- Reasonable efforts to rehabilitate the parent have failed or would be futile.
- Parental rights to another child of the parent have been involuntarily terminated.

NEW YORK

- The parent has abandoned the child for a period of six months.
- The parent is unable to discharge his or her parental duties due to
  - Mental illness or mental retardation
  - Hospitalization or institutionalization for use of drugs or alcohol
- The parent has severely or repeatedly abused the child.
- The parent has substantially and repeatedly or continuously failed to maintain contact with or plan for the future of the child for a period of more than one year.
- An incarcerated parent has failed to cooperate with efforts to assist the parent to plan for the future of the child or to plan and arrange visits with the child.
- The parent has subjected the child to aggravated circumstances, where the child has been either severely or repeatedly abused.
- Reasonable efforts to rehabilitate the parent have failed.
- The parent has been convicted of
  - Murder or manslaughter, or the attempt to commit such crime, and the victim or intended victim was the child, another child of the parent or a child who was the parent's legal responsibility
  - Criminal solicitation, conspiracy or facilitation of murder or manslaughter, and the victim or intended victim was the child, another child of the parent or a child who was the parent's legal responsibility
  - Assault or aggravated assault upon a person less than 11 years old, or an attempt to commit any such crime, and the victim or intended victim was the child, another child of the parent or a child who was the parent's legal responsibility

- Parental rights to another child of the parent have been involuntarily terminated.

NORTH CAROLINA

- The parent has willfully abandoned the child for six months.
- The parent is unable to discharge his or her parental duties due to
  - Mental illness or mental retardation
  - Substance abuse
- The parent has abused or neglected the child.
- The parent has subjected the child to aggravated circumstances, including, but not limited to: abandonment, torture, chronic abuse or sexual abuse.
- Reasonable efforts to rehabilitate the parent have failed.
- The parent has been convicted of
  - Murder or voluntary manslaughter of another child of the parent or another child residing in the home
  - Aiding, abetting, attempting or soliciting to commit murder or voluntary manslaughter of the child, another child of the parent, or another child residing in the home
  - A felony assault that results in serious bodily injury to the child, another child of the parent or another child in the home
- The child is in foster care, and the parent, for a period of six months, has failed to pay a reasonable portion of the cost of the care when financially able to do so.
- The noncustodial parent has failed, for a period of one year, to pay for the care, support and education of the child as required by the custody agreement.
- A putative father has failed to establish paternity or provide substantial financial support for the child.
- Parental rights to another child of the parent have been involuntarily terminated, and the parent lacks the ability or willingness to establish a safe home.

NORTH DAKOTA

- The parent has abandoned the child.
- The parent has subjected the child to aggravated circumstances, which mean circumstances in which a parent
  - Abandons, tortures, chronically abuses or sexually abuses a child
  - Fails to make substantial, meaningful efforts to secure treatment for addiction, mental illness, behavior disorder or any combination of those conditions
  - Engages in deviate sexual acts, sexual abuse or sexual imposition in which a child is the victim or intended victim
  - Has been incarcerated under a sentence for which the release date is after the child reaches his or her majority or, for a child under the age of nine years, after the child is twice his or her current age
- The causes and conditions of a child's deprivation are likely to continue and for that reason the child is suffering or will probably suffer serious physical, mental, moral or emotional harm.
- The parent has been convicted of
  - Murder, voluntary manslaughter, negligently causing the death of another or felony abuse or neglect of a child, and the victim is another child of the parent
  - Aiding, abetting, attempting, conspiring or soliciting to commit any of the above crimes in which the victim is a child of the parent
  - Aggravated assault that results in serious bodily injury to a child of the parent
- The child has been in foster care for at least 450 of the previous 660 nights.
- Parental rights to another child of the parent have been involuntarily terminated.

OHIO

- The parent has abandoned the child.
- The parent is unable to discharge his or her parental duties due to

- Chronic mental or emotional illness
- Mental retardation or physical disability
- Chemical dependency
- The parent is incarcerated for an offense committed against the child or a sibling of the child.
- The parent is incarcerated and thereby will not be available to care for the child for at least 18 months, or the parent is repeatedly incarcerated, and the repeated incarceration prevents the parent from providing care for the child.
- The parent has committed any abuse against the child or caused or allowed the child to suffer any neglect.
- Reasonable efforts to rehabilitate the parent have failed.
- The parent has been convicted of or pled guilty to
  - Murder, aggravated murder or voluntary manslaughter of another child of the parent or another child living in the household
  - Assault, aggravated assault or felonious assault of the child, a sibling or another child living in the household
  - Endangering children, rape, sexual battery, corruption of a minor, sexual imposition or gross sexual imposition, and the victim was the child, a sibling or another child in the household
  - A conspiracy or attempt to commit any of the offenses described above
- The parent has demonstrated a lack of commitment to the child by failing to regularly support, visit or communicate with the child when able to do so.
- The parent for any reason is unwilling to provide food, clothing, shelter and other basic necessities for the child or to prevent the child from suffering physical, emotional or sexual abuse or physical, emotional or mental neglect.
- The parent has placed the child at substantial risk of harm due to alcohol or drug abuse, and he or she has refused treatment.
- Parental rights to another child of the parent have been involuntarily terminated.

OKLAHOMA

- The parent has abandoned the child.
- The parent is unable to discharge his or her parental duties due to
  - Mental illness or mental deficiency
  - Extensive, abusive and chronic use of drugs or alcohol
  - Incarceration of a duration that would be detrimental to the parent-child relationship
- The parent has physically or sexually abused the child or a sibling of the child or has failed to protect the child from physical or sexual abuse.
- The child has been adjudicated a deprived child as a result of a single incident of severe sexual abuse, severe neglect or the infliction of serious bodily injury.
- The parent has inflicted chronic abuse, chronic neglect or torture on the child, a sibling or a child residing in the household.
- The child or a sibling has suffered severe harm or injury as a result of physical or sexual abuse.
- The child was conceived as a result of rape.
- Reasonable efforts to rehabilitate the parent have failed.
- The parent has been convicted of
  - Causing the death of a child as a result of physical abuse, sexual abuse or chronic abuse or neglect of such child
  - Murder or voluntary manslaughter of any child
  - Aiding, abetting, attempting or soliciting to commit murder or voluntary manslaughter of any child
  - A felony assault that resulted in serious bodily injury to the child or another child of the parent
- The parent has willfully failed, refused or neglected to contribute to the support of the child when financially able to do so.
- The parent has failed to maintain frequent and regular visitation, contact or communication with the child.
- The child has been in foster care for 15 of the most recent 22 months.

- Parental rights to another child of the parent have been involuntarily terminated, and the conditions that led to the termination have not been corrected.

OREGON

- The parent has abandoned the child.
- The parent is unable to discharge his or her parental duties due to
  - Emotional illness, mental illness or mental deficiency
  - Addictive or habitual use of intoxicating liquors or controlled substances
  - Criminal conduct that impairs the parent's ability to care for the child
- The parent has been found unfit by reason of a single or recurrent incident of extreme conduct toward any child. Such conduct can include
  - Rape, sodomy or sexual abuse of any child of the parent
  - Intentional starvation or torture of any child of the parent
  - Abuse or neglect that results in death or serious physical injury
  - Conduct by the parent to aid or abet another person who, by abuse or neglect, caused the death of any child
  - Conduct by the parent to attempt, solicit or conspire to cause the death of any child
  - Conduct by the parent that knowingly exposes any child of the parent to the storage or production of methamphetamines
- The parent has physically neglected the child.
- Reasonable efforts to rehabilitate the parent have failed.
- The parent has been convicted of
  - Murder or manslaughter of another child of the parent
  - Aiding, abetting, attempting or soliciting to commit murder or voluntary manslaughter of another child of the parent
  - A felony assault that result in serious bodily injury to the child or another child of the parent

- The parent has failed or neglected without reasonable or lawful cause to provide for the basic physical or psychological needs of the child for six months.
- The parent has failed to maintain regular visitation or other contact with the child.
- Parental rights to another child of the parent have been involuntarily terminated, and the conditions that led to the previous action have not been corrected.

PENNSYLVANIA

- The parent has abandoned the child.
- The parent has refused or failed to discharge parental duties.
- The repeated and continued incapacity, abuse, neglect or refusal of the parent has caused the child to be without essential parental care, control or subsistence.
- The parent is the presumptive but not the natural father of the child.
- The parent is the father of a child conceived as a result of rape or incest.
- The parent has subjected the child or another child of the parent to aggravated circumstances, including, but not limited to: physical abuse resulting in serious bodily injury, sexual abuse or aggravated physical neglect.
- Reasonable efforts to rehabilitate the parent have failed.
- The parent has been convicted of any of the following offenses where the victim was a child:
  - Criminal homicide
  - Felony aggravated assault, rape, statutory sexual assault, involuntary deviate sexual intercourse, sexual assault or aggravated indecent assault
  - Misdemeanor indecent assault
  - Attempt, solicitation or conspiracy to commit any of the offenses listed above
- In the case of a newborn child, the parent has failed for a period of four months to maintain substantial and continuing contact and to provide substantial financial support for the child.

- The child has been removed from the home for 12 months or more, and the conditions that led to the removal continue to exist.
- Parental rights to another child of the parent have been involuntarily terminated.

RHODE ISLAND

- The parent has abandoned the child.
- The parent is unable to discharge his or her parental duties due to
  - Institutionalization, including imprisonment, of such duration that the parent cannot care for the child for an extended period of time
  - A chronic substance abuse problem
- The parent has subjected the child to conduct of a cruel or abusive nature.
- The parent has subjected the child to aggravated circumstances, including, but not limited to: abandonment, torture, chronic abuse or sexual abuse.
- The child has been in the custody of the department for at least 12 months, and reasonable efforts to rehabilitate the parent have failed.
- The parent has been convicted of
  - Murder or voluntary manslaughter of another child of the parent
  - Aiding, abetting, attempting or soliciting to commit murder or voluntary manslaughter of another child of the parent
  - A felony assault that results in serious bodily injury to the child or another child of the parent
- The parent has willfully neglected to provide proper care and maintenance for the child when financially able to do so.
- The parent has failed to communicate with the child.
- Parental rights to another child of the parent have been involuntarily terminated, and the parent continues to lack the ability to respond to services.

SOUTH CAROLINA

- The parent has abandoned the child.
- The parent is unable to discharge his or her parental duties due to

- Mental illness, mental deficiency, or extreme physical incapacity
- Drug or alcohol addiction
- The parent has tortured, abused or severely maltreated the child.
- The parent's physical abuse of the child has resulted in death or serious physical injury to the child requiring admission to a hospital.
- The parent has subjected the child to aggravated circumstances, including, but to limited to: abandonment, torture, severe or repeated abuse or neglect or sexual abuse.
- Reasonable efforts to rehabilitate the parent have failed.
- The parent has been convicted of
  - Murder or voluntary manslaughter of another child of the parent
  - Aiding, abetting, attempting or soliciting to commit murder or voluntary manslaughter of another child of the parent
  - A felony assault that results in serious bodily injury to the child or another child of the parent
- The parent has been convicted of the murder of the child's other parent.
- The parent has willfully failed to support the child for a period of six months, when financially able to do so.
- The parent has willfully failed to visit the child for a period of six months.
- The presumptive legal father is not the biological father of the child.
- The child has been in foster care for 15 of the most recent 22 months.
- Parental rights to another child of the parent have been involuntarily terminated.

SOUTH DAKOTA

- The parent has abandoned the child for at least six months.
- The parent is incarcerated and unavailable to care for the child for a significant period of time.
- The parent has a documented history of abuse or neglect associated with chronic alcohol or drug abuse.

- The parent has subjected the child or another child to abandonment; torture; sexual abuse; chronic physical, mental or emotional injury; or chronic neglect, if the neglect was a serious threat to the safety of the child or another child.
- The parent has committed any of the following crimes:
  - Murder, felony murder or manslaughter
  - Rape, incest, sexual exploitation of children or abuse of or cruelty to minors
  - Aggravated assault against the child or another child of the parent
- The parent has exposed the child to or demonstrated an inability to protect the child from substantial harm or risk for substantial harm, and the child or another child
  - Has been removed from the parents' custody on at least one previous occasion
  - Has been removed from the parent's custody on two separate occasions, and the Department of Social Services offered or provided services on each of those occasions
- Parental rights to another child of the parent have been involuntarily terminated.

TENNESSEE

- The parent has abandoned the child.
- The parent has been found to be mentally incompetent to adequately provide care for the child.
- The parent has committed severe child abuse against the child or any sibling or half-sibling.
- The parent has been incarcerated for a sentence of more than two years for conduct against the child.
- The parent has been incarcerated for a criminal act for a sentence of 10 or more years, and the child is under the age of eight years at the time the sentence is entered.
- The parent has been convicted of or found civilly liable for the intentional and wrongful death of the child's other parent or legal guardian.
- The parent has subjected the child to aggravated circumstances.

- Reasonable efforts to rehabilitate the parent have failed.
- The parent has committed
  - Murder or voluntary manslaughter of a sibling or half-sibling of the child
  - Aiding, abetting, attempting or soliciting to commit murder or voluntary manslaughter of the child or any sibling or half-sibling
  - A felony assault that results in serious bodily injury to the child or any sibling or half-sibling
- The child has been in foster care for 15 of the most recent 22 months.
- The parent has failed to support the child in accordance with the child support guidelines.
- The parent has failed to seek reasonable visitation with the child, or when visitation has been granted, he or she has failed to visit.
- A person has failed to establish paternity within 30 days after notice of alleged paternity.
- Parental rights to another child of the parent have been involuntarily terminated.

TEXAS

- The parent has abandoned the child.
- The parent is unable to discharge his or her parental duties due to
  - Mental illness, emotional illness or mental deficiency
  - Use of a controlled substance
  - Incarceration for not less than two years
- The parent knowingly placed or allowed the child to remain in conditions or surroundings or with persons who engaged in conduct that endangered the physical or emotional well-being of the child.
- Reasonable efforts to rehabilitate the parent have failed.
- The parent has been convicted of being criminally responsible for the death or serious injury of a child or any of the following crimes against a child:
  - Murder or capital murder

- Indecency with a child, assault, sexual assault, aggravated assault or aggravated sexual assault
- Injury to a child, elderly individual or disabled individual
- Abandoning or endangering a child
- Prohibited sexual conduct, sexual performance by a child or possession or promotion of child pornography
- The parent is the father of a child conceived as a result of a sexual offense.
- The parent has failed to support the child in accordance with the parent's ability for one year.
- The father abandoned the mother of the child during her pregnancy and failed to provide adequate support or medical care for the mother and has failed to support the child since birth.
- An alleged father has filed to register with the paternity registry or to respond to notice.
- The parent has been the major cause of
  - The child's failure to be enrolled in school as required by law
  - The child's absence from home without the consent of the parent or guardian for a substantial length of time or without the intent to return
- The parent has been the cause of the child being born addicted to alcohol or a controlled substance.
- The parent voluntarily delivered the child to a designated emergency infant care provider.
- The parent has failed to maintain regular visitation, contact or communication with the child.
- Parental rights to another child of the parent have been involuntarily terminated.

UTAH

- The parent has abandoned the child.
- The parent is unable to discharge his or her parental duties due to
  - Emotional illness, mental illness or mental deficiency
  - Habitual or excessive use of intoxicating liquors, controlled substances or dangerous drugs

- A conviction and incarceration for a felony, and the sentence will deprive the child of a normal home for more than one year
- A history of violent behavior
- The parent has subjected the child to conduct of a physically, emotionally or sexually cruel or abusive nature.
- The parent's substantiated abuse or neglect has resulted in sexual abuse, injury or death of a sibling of the child.
- The parent has subjected the child to a single incident of life-threatening or gravely disabling injury or disfigurement.
- Reasonable efforts to rehabilitate the parent have failed.
- The parent has committed or aided, abetted, attempted, conspired or solicited to commit murder or voluntary manslaughter of a child or child abuse homicide.
- The parent has repeatedly or continuously failed to provide the child with adequate food, clothing, shelter, education or other care necessary for his or her physical, mental and emotional health and development.
- The parent has failed to communicate with the child.
- The parent has met the terms and conditions of a safe relinquishment of a newborn child.
- Parental rights to another child of the parent have been involuntarily terminated.

VERMONT

- In the case of a child under the age of six months, the parent did not exercise parental responsibility once he or she knew or should have known of the child's birth or expected birth. In making a determination under this subdivision, the court shall consider all relevant factors, which may include the respondent's failure to
  - Pay reasonable parental, natal and postnatal expenses in accordance with his or her financial means
  - Make reasonable and consistent payments, in accordance with his or her financial means, for the support of the child

- Regularly communicate or visit with the minor
- Manifest an ability and willingness to assume legal and physical custody of the minor
- In the case of a child over the age of six months at the time the petition is filed, the respondent did not exercise parental responsibility for a period of at least six months immediately preceding the filing of the petition. In making a determination under this subdivision, the court shall consider all relevant factors, which may include the respondent's failure to
  - Make reasonable and consistent payments, in accordance with his or her financial means, for the support of the child, although legally obligated to do so
  - Regularly communicate or visit with the minor
  - During any time the minor was not in the physical custody of the other parent, to manifest an ability and willingness to assume legal and physical custody of the minor
- The respondent has been convicted of a crime of violence or has been found by a court of competent jurisdiction to have committed an act of violence that violated a restraining or protective order, and the facts of the crime or violation indicate that the respondent is unfit to maintain a relationship of parent and child with the minor.
- An alleged father has failed to establish paternity.

VIRGINIA

- The parent has abandoned the child.
- The parent is unable to discharge his or her parental duties due to
  - Emotional illness, mental illness, or mental deficiency
  - Habitual abuse or addiction to intoxicating liquors, narcotics or other dangerous drugs
- The parent has subjected the child to aggravated circumstances, including, but not limited to: torture, chronic or severe physical abuse or chronic or severe sexual abuse. It includes the failure to protect the child from such conduct.

- Reasonable efforts to rehabilitate the parent have failed.
- The parent has been convicted of
  - Murder or voluntary manslaughter of a child of the parent, a child with whom the parent resided or the other parent of the child
  - Felony attempt, conspiracy or solicitation to commit any such offense
  - A felony assault that results in serious bodily injury, felony bodily wounding or felony sexual assault, and the victim was a child of the parent or a child residing with the parent
- The parent has failed to maintain continuing contact with the child for six months after the child has been placed in foster care.
- Parental rights to another child of the parent have been involuntarily terminated.

WASHINGTON

- The parent has abandoned the child.
- The parent is unable to discharge his or her parental duties due to
  - Psychological incapacity or mental deficiency
  - Use of intoxicating or controlled substances
- The parent has subjected the child to aggravated circumstances, that may include one or more of the following:
  - Conviction of the parent of rape, criminal mistreatment or assault of the child
  - Conviction of the parent of murder, manslaughter or homicide by abuse of the child's other parent, a sibling or another child
  - Conviction of the parent of attempting, soliciting or conspiring to commit any of the above crimes
  - Conviction of assault against a surviving child or another child of the parent
  - A finding that the parent is a sexually violent predator
  - Failure of the parent to complete available ordered treatment, and that failure has resulted in the termination of parental rights to another child

- Conviction of the parent of a sex offense or incest when a child is born of the offense
- The child has been found to be a dependent child, has been removed from the custody of the parent for at least six months, and there is little likelihood that conditions will be remedied so that the child can be returned to the parent in the near future.

WEST VIRGINIA

- The parent has abandoned the child.
- The parent is unable to discharge his or her parental duties due to
  - Emotional illness, mental illness or mental deficiency
  - Habitual abuse or addition to alcohol, controlled substances or drugs
- The parent has repeatedly or seriously injured the child physically or emotionally.
- The parent has sexually abused or exploited the child.
- The parent has subjected the child to an aggravated circumstance, including, but not limited to: abandonment, torture, chronic abuse or sexual abuse.
- Reasonable efforts to rehabilitate the parent have failed.
- The parent has
  - Committed murder or voluntary manslaughter of another child of the parent
  - Attempted or conspired to commit murder or voluntary manslaughter of another child of the parent
  - Committed a felonious assault that resulted in serious bodily injury to the child or another child of the parent
- Parental rights to another child of the parent have been involuntarily terminated.

WISCONSIN

- The parent has abandoned the child.
- The parent is unable to discharge his or her parental duties due to continuing parental dis-

ability due to mental illness or developmental disability.
- The parent has exhibited a pattern of physically or sexually abusive behavior that is a substantial threat to the health of child.
- The parent has caused death or injury to the child or children resulting in a felony conviction.
- The child was conceived as a result of sexual assault or incest.
- The parent has subjected the child to an aggravated circumstance, including, but not limited to: abandonment, torture, chronic abuse or sexual abuse.
- Reasonable efforts to rehabilitate the parent have failed.
- The parent has committed a serious felony against one of the parent's children, which may include
  - Intentional homicide, reckless homicide or felony murder
  - Aiding, abetting, attempting, conspiring or soliciting to commit intentional homicide, reckless homicide or felony murder
  - Battery, sexual assault, physical abuse, sexual exploitation or neglect of a child, incest with a child or soliciting a child for prostitution
  - Neglect of a child that results in the death of the child
- The parent has committed homicide or solicitation to commit homicide of the child's other parent.
- The parent has failed to assume parental responsibility for the child.
- The parent has failed to visit or communicate with the child for three months or longer.
- The parent relinquished the child when the child was 72 hours old or younger.
- Parental rights to another child of the parent have been involuntarily terminated.

WYOMING

- The parent has abandoned the child.
- The parent is incarcerated due to the conviction of a felony and a showing that the parent is unfit.

- The parent has subjected the child to aggravated circumstances, including, but not limited to: abandonment, torture, chronic abuse or sexual abuse.

- The parent has abused or neglected the child and reasonable efforts to rehabilitate the parent have failed.

- The child has been in foster care for 15 of the most recent 22 months, and there is a showing that the parent is unfit to have custody and control of the child.

- The child was relinquished to a safe haven provider, and neither parent has affirmatively sought the return of the child within three months.

- The parent has been convicted of
  - Murder or voluntary manslaughter of another child of the parent
  - Aiding, abetting, attempting, conspiring or soliciting to commit murder or voluntary manslaughter of another child of the parent
  - A felony assault that resulted in serious bodily injury to a child of the parent

- The child has been left in the care of another without provision for the child's support and without communication from the absent parent for at least one year.

- Parental rights to another child of the parent have been involuntarily terminated.

Source: Adapted from National Clearinghouse on Child Abuse and Neglect Information. "Grounds for Involuntary Termination of Parental Rights." Available Online. URL: http://nccanch.acf.hhs.gov/general/legal/statutes/groundterminall.pdf. Downloaded November 4, 2005.

APPENDIX VI
STATE DEFINITIONS OF ABUSE AND NEGLECT

There are federal laws on abuse and neglect, but each state also has its own laws to define what constitutes abuse and neglect. This appendix offers a summary of state laws on physical abuse, neglect, sexual abuse and emotional abuse.

ALABAMA

Physical Abuse

Abuse means harm or threatened harm to the health or welfare of a child through

- Nonaccidental physical injury
- Sexual abuse or attempted sexual abuse
- Sexual exploitation or attempted sexual exploitation

Neglect

Neglect means negligent treatment or maltreatment of a child, including the failure to provide adequate food, clothing, shelter, medical treatment or supervision.

Sexual Abuse

Sexual abuse includes

- The employment, use, persuasion, inducement, enticement or coercion of any child to engage in, or having a child assist any other person to engage in, any sexually explicit conduct
- Any simulation of the conduct for the purpose of producing any visual depiction of the conduct
- The rape, molestation, prostitution or other form of sexual exploitation of children
- Incest with children

Sexual exploitation includes

- Allowing, permitting or encouraging a child to engage in prostitution

- Allowing, permitting, encouraging or engaging in the obscene or pornographic photographing, filming or depicting of a child for commercial purposes

Emotional Abuse

Abuse includes nonaccidental mental injury.

ALASKA

Physical Abuse

Child abuse or neglect means the physical injury or neglect, mental injury, sexual abuse, sexual exploitation or maltreatment of a child under the age of 18 years by a person under circumstances that indicate that the child's health or welfare is harmed or threatened.

Neglect

Neglect means the failure by a person responsible for the child's welfare to provide necessary food, care, clothing, shelter or medical attention for a child.

Sexual Abuse

- Child abuse or neglect includes sexual abuse or sexual exploitation.
- Sexual exploitation includes the following conduct by a person responsible for the child's welfare:
  - Allowing, permitting or encouraging a child to engage in prostitution
  - Allowing, permitting or encouraging a child to engage in actual or simulated activities of a sexual nature that are prohibited by criminal statute

Emotional Abuse

Mental injury means a serious injury to the child as evidenced by an observable and substantial impairment in the child's ability to function in a developmentally appropriate manner, and the existence of that impairment is supported by the opinion of a qualified expert witness.

ARIZONA

Physical Abuse

Abuse means

- Inflicting or allowing the infliction of physical injury, impairment of bodily function or disfigurement
- Permitting a child to enter or remain in any structure in which chemicals or equipment used for the manufacture of a dangerous drug is found

Neglect

Neglect or neglected means the inability or unwillingness of a parent, guardian or custodian of a child to provide that child with supervision, food, clothing, shelter or medical care if that inability or unwillingness causes substantial risk of harm to the child's health or welfare.

Sexual Abuse

Abuse includes

- Inflicting or allowing sexual abuse
- Sexual conduct with a minor
- Sexual assault
- Molestation of a child
- Commercial sexual exploitation of a minor
- Sexual exploitation of a minor
- Incest
- Child prostitution

Emotional Abuse

Abuse means the infliction of or allowing another person to cause serious emotional damage to the child, as evidenced by severe anxiety, depression, withdrawal or untoward aggressive behavior, and such emotional damage is diagnosed by a medical doctor or psychologist, and the damage has been caused by the acts or omissions of an individual having care, custody and control of a child.

ARKANSAS

Physical Abuse

Abuse means any of the following acts or omissions:

- Extreme or repeated cruelty to a juvenile
- Engaging in conduct that creates a realistic and serious threat of death, permanent or temporary disfigurement or impairment of any bodily organ
- Any injury that is any variance with the history given
- Any nonaccidental physical injury
- Any of the following intentional or knowing acts, with physical injury and without justifiable cause:
  - Throwing, kicking, burning, biting or cutting the child
  - Striking a child with a closed fist
  - Shaking a child
  - Striking a child on the face

Severe maltreatment means acts or omissions that may or do result in death, abuse involving the use of a deadly weapon, bone fracture, internal injuries, burns, immersions, suffocation, medical diagnosis of failure to thrive or causing a substantial and observable change in the behavior or demeanor of the child.

Neglect

Neglect means those acts or omissions that constitute

- Failure or refusal to prevent the abuse of the juvenile when such person knows or has reasonable cause to know the juvenile is or has been abused
- Failure or refusal to provide necessary food, clothing, shelter, education or medical treatment necessary for the juvenile's well-being
- Failure to take reasonable action to protect the juvenile from abandonment, abuse, sexual abuse, sexual exploitation, neglect or parental

unfitness where the existence of such condition was known or should have been known

- Failure or irremediable inability to provide for the essential and necessary physical, mental or emotional needs of the juvenile
- Failure to provide for the juvenile's care and maintenance, proper or necessary support or medical, surgical or other necessary care
- Failure, although able, to assume responsibility for the care and custody of the juvenile or to participate in a plan to assume such responsibility
- Failure to appropriately supervise the juvenile that results in the juvenile's being left alone at an inappropriate age or in inappropriate circumstances that put the juvenile in danger

Sexual Abuse

Sexual abuse means

- Sexual intercourse, deviate sexual activity or sexual contact by forcible compulsion
- Attempted sexual intercourse, deviate sexual activity or sexual contact
- Indecent exposure
- Forcing, permitting or encouraging the watching of pornography or live sexual activity

Sexual exploitation means allowing, permitting or encouraging participation or depiction of the juvenile in prostitution, obscene photographing or filming or obscenely depicting a juvenile for any use or purpose.

Emotional Abuse

Abuse means acts or omissions that result in injury to a juvenile's intellectual, emotional or psychological development, as evidence by observable and substantial impairment of the juvenile's ability to function within the juvenile's normal range of performance and behavior.

CALIFORNIA

Physical Abuse

Child abuse or neglect includes

- Physical injury inflicted by other than accidental means upon a child by another person

- Willful harming or injury of the child or the endangering of the person or health of the child
- Unlawful corporal punishment or injury

Willful harming or injuring of a child or the endangering of the person or health of a child means a situation in which any person willfully causes or permits any child to suffer, or inflicts thereon, unjustifiable physical pain or mental suffering, or having the care or custody of any child, willfully causes or permits the person or health of the child to be placed in a situation in which his or her person or health is endangered.

Neglect

Neglect means the negligent treatment or the maltreatment of a child by a person responsible for the child's welfare under circumstances indicating harm or threatened harm to the child's health or welfare. The term includes both acts and omissions on the part of the responsible person.

Severe neglect means the negligent failure of a person having the care or custody of a child to protect the child from severe malnutrition or medically diagnosed nonorganic failure to thrive. Severe neglect also means those situations of neglect where any person having the care or custody of a child willfully causes or permits the person or health of the child to be placed in a situation such that his or her person or health is endangered, including the intentional failure to provide adequate food, clothing, shelter or medical care.

General neglect means the negligent failure of a person having the care or custody of a child to provide adequate food, clothing, shelter, medical care or supervision where no physical injury to the child has occurred.

Sexual Abuse

- Sexual abuse means sexual assault or sexual exploitation as defined below.
- Sexual assault includes rape, statutory rape, rape in concert, incest, sodomy, lewd or lascivious acts upon a child, oral copulation, sexual penetration or child molestation.
- Sexual exploitation refers to any of the following:

- Depicting a minor engaged in obscene acts; preparing, selling, or distributing obscene matter that depicts minors; employing a minor to perform obscene acts

- Knowingly permitting or encouraging a child to engage in, or assisting others to engage in, prostitution or a live performance involving obscene sexual conduct, or to either pose or model alone or with others for purposes of preparing a film, photograph, negative, slide, drawing, painting or other pictorial depiction, involving obscene sexual conduct

- Depicting a child in, or knowingly developing, duplicating, printing or exchanging any film, photograph, videotape, negative or slide in which a child is engaged in an act of obscene sexual conduct

Emotional Abuse

Serious emotional damage is evidenced by states of being or behavior including, but not limited to, severe anxiety, depression, withdrawal or untoward aggressive behavior toward self or others.

COLORADO

Physical Abuse

Abuse or child abuse or neglect means an act or omission in one of the following categories that threatens the health or welfare of a child:

- Any case in which a child exhibits evidence of skin bruising, bleeding, malnutrition, failure to thrive, burns, fracture of any bone, subdural hematoma, soft tissue swelling or death and either

  - Such condition or death is not justifiably explained

  - The history given concerning such condition is at variance with the degree or type of such condition or death

  - The circumstances indicate that such condition may not be the product of an accidental occurrence

- Any case in which, in the presence of a child, on the premises where a child is found or where a child resides, a controlled substance is manufactured

Neglect

Child abuse or neglect includes a case in which a child is in need of services because the child's parent has failed to provide adequate food, clothing, shelter, medical care or supervision that a prudent parent would take.

A child is neglected or dependent if

- The child has been subjected to mistreatment or abuse, or the parent, guardian or legal custodian has allowed another to mistreat or abuse the child without taking lawful means to stop such mistreatment or abuse and prevent it from recurring.

- The child lacks proper parental care through the actions or omissions of the parent, guardian or legal custodian.

- The child's environment is injurious to his or her welfare.

- A parent, guardian or legal custodian fails or refuses to provide the child with proper or necessary subsistence, education, medical care or any other care necessary for his or her health, guidance or well-being.

- A parent, guardian or legal custodian has subjected another child or children to an identifiable pattern of habitual abuse.

- The parent, guardian or legal custodian has been the respondent in another proceeding in which a court has adjudicated another child to be neglected or dependent based upon allegations of sexual or physical abuse, or a court of competent jurisdiction has determined that such abuse or neglect has caused the death of another child.

- The pattern of habitual abuse and the type of abuse pose a current threat to the child.

Sexual Abuse

- Abuse or child abuse or neglect means any case in which a child is subjected to sexual assault or molestation, sexual exploitation or prostitution.

- Sexual conduct means any of the following:

  - Sexual intercourse, including genital-genital, oral-genital, anal-genital or oral-anal, whether between persons of the same or opposite sex or between humans and animals

- Penetration of the vagina or rectum by any object
- Masturbation
- Sexual sadomasochistic abuse

Emotional Abuse

- Abuse or child abuse or neglect means any case in which a child is subjected to emotional abuse.
- Emotional abuse means an identifiable and substantial impairment or a substantial risk of impairment of the child's intellectual or psychological functioning or development.

CONNECTICUT

Physical Abuse

Abused means that a child or youth

- Has been inflicted with physical injury or injuries by other than accidental means
- Has injuries that are at variance with the history given of them
- Is in a condition that is the result of maltreatment such as, but not limited to, cruel punishment

Neglect

- A neglected child or youth is one who
  - Is being denied proper care and attention, physically, educationally, emotionally or morally
  - Is being permitted to live under conditions, circumstances or associations injurious to the well-being of the child or youth
  - Has been abused
- Abuse includes
  - Deprivation of necessities
  - Malnutrition

Sexual Abuse

Abuse includes sexual molestation or exploitation.

Emotional Abuse

Abuse includes emotional maltreatment.

DELAWARE

Physical Abuse

Abuse shall mean any physical injury to a child by those responsible for the care, custody and control of the child through unjustified force, emotional abuse, torture, criminally negligent treatment, sexual abuse, exploitation, maltreatment or mistreatment.

Neglect

Neglect shall mean the failure to provide, by those responsible for the care, custody and control of the child, the proper or necessary education, nutrition, medical, surgical or any other care necessary for the child's well-being.

Sexual Abuse

Abuse includes sexual abuse and exploitation.

Emotional Abuse

Abuse includes emotional abuse.

DISTRICT OF COLUMBIA

Physical Abuse

Abused, when used in reference to a child, means

- Infliction of physical or mental injury upon the child
- Sexual abuse or exploitation of a child

The term *discipline* does not include

- Burning, biting or cutting a child
- Striking a child with a closed fist
- Inflicting injury to a child by shaking, kicking or throwing the child
- Nonaccidental injury to a child under the age of 18 months
- Interfering with a child's breathing
- Threatening a child with a dangerous weapon or using such a weapon on a child

Neglected child means a child

- Whose parent, guardian or custodian has failed to make reasonable efforts to prevent the infliction of abuse upon the child

- Who is without proper parental care or control, subsistence, education or other care or control necessary for his or her physical, mental or emotional health

- Whose parent, guardian or other custodian is unable to discharge his or her responsibilities to and for the child because of incarceration, hospitalization or other physical or mental incapacity

- Whose parent, guardian or custodian refuses or is unable to assume their responsibility for the child's care, control or subsistence, and the person or institution providing for the child states an intention to discontinue such care

- Who is in imminent danger of being abused and another child living in the same household has been abused

- Who has received negligent treatment or maltreatment

- Who has resided in a hospital located in the District of Columbia for at least 10 calendar days following the birth of the child, despite a medical determination the child is ready for discharge from the hospital, and the parent has not taken any action or made any effort to maintain a parental, guardianship or custodial relationship or contact with the child

- Who is born addicted or dependent on a controlled substance or has a significant presence of a controlled substance in his or her system at birth

- In whose body there is a controlled substance as a direct and foreseeable consequence of the acts or omissions of the child's parent

- Who is regularly exposed to illegal drug-related activity in the home

Negligent treatment or maltreatment means failure to provide adequate food, clothing, shelter or medical care that includes medical neglect, and the deprivation is not due to the lack of financial means of his or her parent, guardian or other custodian.

Sexual Abuse
Sexual abuse means

- Engaging in, or attempting to engage in, a sexual act or sexual contact with a child

- Causing or attempting to cause a child to engage in sexually explicit conduct

- Exposing the child to sexually explicit conduct

Sexual exploitation means a parent, guardian or other custodian allows a child to engage in prostitution, or engages a child or allows a child to engage in obscene or pornographic photography, filming or other forms of illustrating or promoting sexual conduct.

Emotional Abuse
Mental injury means harm to a child's psychological or intellectual functioning that may be exhibited by severe anxiety, depression, withdrawal, outwardly aggressive behavior or a combination of those behaviors, and that may be demonstrated by a change in behavior, emotional response or cognition.

FLORIDA

Physical Abuse
Abuse means any willful act or threatened act that results in any physical, mental or sexual injury or harm that causes or is likely to cause the child's physical, mental or emotional health to be significantly impaired.

Harm to a child's health or welfare can occur when any person inflicts, or allows to be inflicted upon the child, physical, mental or emotional injury and can include

- Purposely giving a child poison, alcohol, drugs or other substances that substantially affect the child's behavior, motor coordination or judgment or that results in sickness or internal injury

- Inappropriate or excessively harsh discipline

- Exposure to a controlled substance or alcohol

- Engaging in violent behavior that demonstrates a wanton disregard for the presence of a child and could reasonably result in serious injury to the child

Neglect
- Neglect occurs when
  - A child is deprived of, or is allowed to be deprived of, necessary food, clothing, shelter or medical treatment.

- A child is permitted to live in an environment when such deprivation or environment causes a child's physical, mental or emotional health to be significantly impaired or to be in danger of being significantly impaired.
- Neglect of a child includes acts or omissions.
- Harm to a child's health or welfare can occur by leaving a child without adult supervision or arrangement appropriate to the child's age or mental or physical condition.

Sexual Abuse

Sexual abuse of a child means one or more of the following acts:

- Any penetration, however slight, of the vagina or anal opening of one person by the penis of another person, whether or not there is an emission of semen
- Any sexual contact or intentional touching between the genitals or anal opening of one person and the mouth or tongue of another person
- The intentional masturbation of the perpetrator's genitals in the presence of a child
- The intentional exposure of the perpetrator's genitals in the presence of a child, or any other sexual act intentionally perpetrated in the presence of a child, if such exposure or sexual act is for the purpose of sexual arousal or gratification, aggression, degradation or other similar purpose
- The sexual exploitation of a child, which includes allowing, encouraging or forcing a child to solicit or engage in prostitution or engage in a sexual performance

Emotional Abuse

Mental injury means an injury to the intellectual or psychological capacity of a child as evidenced by a discernible and substantial impairment in the ability to function within the normal range of performance and behavior.

GEORGIA

Physical Abuse

Child abuse means physical injury or death inflicted upon a child by a parent or caretaker by other than accidental means.

Neglect

Child abuse means neglect or exploitation of a child by a parent or caretaker.

Sexual Abuse

Sexual abuse means a person employing, using, persuading, inducing, enticing or coercing any minor who is not that person's spouse to engage in any act that involves

- Sexual intercourse, including genital-genital, oral-genital or oral-anal, whether between persons of the same or opposite sex.
- Bestiality or masturbation
- Lewd exhibition of the genitals or pubic area of any person
- Flagellation or torture by or upon a person who is nude
- Condition of being fettered, bound or otherwise physically restrained on the part of a person who is nude
- Physical contact in an act of apparent sexual stimulation or gratification with any person's clothed or unclothed genitals, pubic area or buttocks or with a female's clothed or unclothed breasts
- Defecation or urination for the purpose of sexual stimulation
- Penetration of the vagina or rectum by any object except when done as part of a recognized medical procedure

Sexual exploitation means conduct by a child's parent or caretaker who allows, permits, encourages or requires that child to engage in prostitution or sexually explicit conduct for the purpose of producing any visual or print medium depicting that conduct.

Emotional Abuse

Not addressed in statutes reviewed.

HAWAII

Physical Abuse

Child abuse or neglect means the acts or omissions that have resulted in the physical health or welfare of the child, who is under the age of 18 years, to be harmed, or to be subject to any reasonably foreseeable, substantial risk of being harmed. The acts or omissions are indicated for the purposes of reports by circumstances that include but are not limited to

- When the child exhibits evidence of any of the following injuries, and such injury is not justifiably explained, or when the history given concerning such condition or death is at variance with the degree or type of such condition or death, or circumstances indicate that such condition or death may not be the product of an accidental occurrence:
  - Substantial or multiple skin bruising or any other internal bleeding
  - Any injury to skin causing substantial bleeding
  - Malnutrition or failure to thrive
  - Burns or poisoning
  - Fracture of any bone
  - Subdural hematoma or soft tissue swelling
  - Extreme pain or mental distress
  - Gross degradation
  - Death
- When the child is provided with dangerous, harmful, or detrimental drugs; provided that this paragraph shall not apply when such drugs are provided to the child pursuant to the direction or prescription of a practitioner

Neglect

Child neglect means when the child is not provided in a timely manner with adequate food, clothing, shelter, psychological care, physical care, medical care or supervision.

Sexual Abuse

Child abuse or neglect means when the child has been the victim of

- Sexual contact or conduct including, but not limited to, sexual assault
- Molestation or sexual fondling

- Incest
- Prostitution
- Obscene or pornographic photographing, filming or depiction or other similar forms of sexual exploitation

Emotional Abuse

Child abuse or neglect includes the acts or omissions that have resulted in injury to the psychological capacity of a child as is evidenced by an observable and substantial impairment in the child's ability to function.

IDAHO

Physical Abuse

Abused means any case in which a child has been the victim of conduct or omission resulting in skin bruising, bleeding, malnutrition, burns, fracture of any bone, subdural hematoma, soft tissue swelling, failure to thrive or death, and such condition or death is not justifiably explained, the history given concerning such condition or death is at variance with the degree or type of such condition or death or the circumstances indicate that such condition or death may not be the product of an accidental occurrence.

Neglect

Neglected means a child

- Who is without proper parental care and control, subsistence, education, medical or other care necessary for his well-being because of the conduct or omission of his parents, guardian or other custodian or their neglect or refusal to provide them
- Whose parents, guardian or other custodian are unable to discharge their responsibilities to and for the child and, as a result of such inability, the child lacks the parental care necessary for his health, safety, or well-being
- Who has been placed for care or adoption in violation of the law

Sexual Abuse

Abuse means any case in which a child has been the victim of sexual conduct, including rape, molestation, incest, prostitution, obscene or pornographic photographing, filming or depiction for commercial purposes, or other similar forms of sexual exploitation harming or threatening the child's health, welfare or mental injury to the child.

Emotional Abuse

Mental injury means a substantial impairment in the intellectual or psychological ability of a child to function within a normal range of performance and/or behavior, for short or long terms.

ILLINOIS

Physical Abuse

Abused child means a child whose parent, immediate family member, any person responsible for the child's welfare, any individual residing in the same home as the child or a paramour of the child's parent

- Inflicts, causes or allows to be inflicted, or creates a substantial risk of physical injury, by other than accidental means, that causes death, disfigurement, impairment of physical or emotional health or loss or impairment of any bodily function
- Commits or allows to be committed an act or acts of torture upon the child
- Inflicts excessive corporal punishment
- Commits or allows to be committed the offense of female genital mutilation
- Causes to be sold, transferred, distributed or given to the child under 18 years of age a controlled substance, except for controlled substances that are prescribed and dispensed to the child in accordance with the law

Neglect

Neglected child means any child who is

- Not receiving the proper or necessary nourishment or medically indicated treatment including food or care, not provided solely on the basis of the present or anticipated mental or physical impairment as determined by a physician, or otherwise is not receiving the proper or necessary support or medical or other remedial care as necessary for a child's well-being

- Not receiving other care necessary for his or her well-being, including adequate food, clothing and shelter
- A newborn infant whose blood, urine or meconium contains any amount of a controlled substance or a metabolite thereof

Sexual Abuse

Abused child means a child whose parent, immediate family member, any person responsible for the child's welfare, any individual residing in the same home as the child or a paramour of the child's parent commits or allows to be committed any sex offense against the child.

Emotional Abuse

Abused child includes impairment or substantial risk of impairment to the child's emotional health.

INDIANA

Physical Abuse

A child is a child in need of services, if, before the child become 18 years of age, the child's physical or mental health is seriously endangered due to injury by the act or omission of the child's parent, guardian or custodian.

Evidence that the illegal manufacture of a drug or controlled substance is occurring on property where a child resides creates a rebuttable presumption that the child's physical or mental health is seriously endangered.

Neglect

A child is a child in need of services if before the child becomes 18 years of age

- The child's physical or mental condition is seriously impaired or seriously endangered as a result of the inability, refusal or neglect of the child's parent, guardian or custodian to supply the child with necessary food, clothing, shelter, medical care, education or supervision.
- The child is born with fetal alcohol syndrome, or any amount, including a trace amount, of a controlled substance or a legend drug is in the child's body.

- The child has an injury, abnormal physical or psychological development or is at a substantial risk of a life-threatening condition that arises or is substantially aggravated because the child's mother used alcohol, a controlled substance or a legend drug during pregnancy.

A child in need of services includes a child with a disability who is deprived of nutrition that is necessary to sustain life or is deprived of medical or surgical intervention that is necessary to remedy or ameliorate a life-threatening medical condition, if the nutrition, medical or surgical intervention is generally provided to similarly situated children with or without disabilities.

Sexual Abuse
A child is a child in need of services if before the child becomes 18 years of age the child is the victim, lives in the same household as another child who was the victim or lives in the same household as the adult who was convicted of a sex offense as defined the criminal statutes pertaining to

- Rape
- Criminal deviate conduct
- Child molesting
- Child exploitation or possession of child pornography
- Child seduction
- Sexual misconduct with a minor
- Indecent exposure
- Prostitution
- Incest

A child is a child in need of services if before the child becomes 18 years of age the child's parent, guardian, or custodian allows the child

- To participate in an obscene performance
- To commit a sex offense prohibited by criminal statute

Emotional Abuse
A child is a child in need of services if the child's mental health is seriously endangered by the act or omission of the child's parent, guardian or custodian.

IOWA

Physical Abuse
Child abuse or abuse means any nonaccidental physical injury, or injury that is at variance with the history given of it, suffered by a child as the result of acts or omissions of a person responsible for the care of the child.

Neglect
Child abuse or abuse means

- The failure on the part of a person responsible for the care of a child to provide for the adequate food, shelter, clothing or other care necessary for the child's health and welfare when financially able to do so or when offered financial or other reasonable means to do so
- The presence of an illegal drug in a child's body as a direct and foreseeable consequence of the acts or omission of the person responsible for the care of the child
- The person responsible for the care of a child has, in the presence of the child, manufactured a dangerous substance or possesses a product containing ephedrine, its salts, optical isomers, salts of optical isomers, or pseudoephedrine, its salts, optical isomers, or salts of optical isomers, with the intent to use the product as a precursor or an intermediary to a dangerous substance.

Sexual Abuse
Child abuse or abuse means

- The commission of a sexual offense with or to a child
- Allowing, permitting or encouraging the child to engage in prostitution
- The commission of bestiality in the presence of a minor by a person who resides in a home with a child as a result of the acts or omissions of a person responsible for the care of the child

Emotional Abuse
Child abuse or abuse means any mental injury to a child's intellectual or psychological capacity as

evidenced by an observable and substantial impairment in the child's ability to function within the child's normal range of performance and behavior as the result of the acts or omissions of a person responsible for the care of the child, if the impairment is diagnosed and confirmed by a licensed physician or qualified mental health professional.

KANSAS

Physical Abuse

Physical, mental, or emotional abuse means the infliction of physical, mental or emotional injury, or the causing of a deterioration of a child, and may include, but shall not be limited to, maltreatment or exploiting a child to the extent that the child's health or emotional well-being is endangered.

Neglect means acts or omissions by a parent, guardian or person responsible for the care of a child resulting in harm to a child or presenting a likelihood of harm and the acts or omissions are not due solely to the lack of financial means of the child's parents or other custodian. Neglect may include but shall not be limited to

- Failure to provide the child with food, clothing or shelter necessary to sustain the life or health of the child
- Failure to provide adequate supervision of a child or to remove a child from a situation that requires judgment or actions beyond the child's level of maturity, physical condition or mental abilities and that results in bodily injury or a likelihood of harm to the child
- Failure to use resources available to treat a diagnosed medical condition if such treatment will make a child substantially more comfortable, reduce pain and suffering or correct or substantially diminish a crippling condition from worsening

Sexual Abuse

Sexual abuse means any act listed below, committed with a child, regardless of the age of the child:

- Unlawful sex act
- Rape

- Indecent liberties with a child or aggravated indecent liberties with a child
- Indecent solicitation of a child or aggravated indecent solicitation of a child
- Sexual exploitation of a child
- Aggravated incest

Emotional Abuse

Physical, mental, or emotional abuse means the infliction of physical, mental or emotional injury or the causing of a deterioration of a child and may include, but shall not be limited to, maltreatment or exploiting a child to the extent that the child's health or emotional well-being is endangered.

KENTUCKY

Physical Abuse

Abused or neglected child means a child whose health or welfare is harmed or threatened with harm when his parent, guardian or other person exercising custodial control or supervision of the child and

- Inflicts or allows to be inflicted upon the child physical or emotional injury by other than accidental means
- Creates or allows to be created a risk of physical or emotional injury to the child by other than accidental means

Physical injury means substantial physical pain or any impairment of physical condition.

Serious physical injury means physical injury that creates a substantial risk of death, causes serious and prolonged disfigurement, prolonged impairment of health or prolonged loss or impairment of the function of any bodily member or organ.

Neglect

Abused or neglected child means a child whose health or welfare is harmed or threatened with harm when his parent, guardian or other person exercising custodial control or supervision of the child

- Engages in a pattern of conduct that renders the parent incapable of caring for the immediate and ongoing needs of the child, including but not limited to, parental incapacity due to alcohol and other drug abuse

- Continuously or repeatedly fails or refuses to provide essential parental care and protection for the child, considering the age of the child

- Does not provide the child with adequate care, supervision, food, clothing, shelter, education or medical care necessary for the child's well-being

Sexual Abuse

Abused or neglected child means a child whose health or welfare is harmed or threatened with harm when a parent, guardian or other person exercising custodial control or supervision of the child

- Commits or allows to be committed an act of sexual abuse, sexual exploitation or prostitution upon the child

- Creates or allows to be created a risk that an act of sexual abuse, sexual exploitation or prostitution will be committed upon the child

Sexual abuse includes, but is not necessarily limited to, any contacts or interactions in which the parent or guardian uses or allows, permits or encourages the use of the child for the purposes of sexual stimulation of the perpetrator or another person.

Sexual exploitation includes, but is not limited to, allowing, permitting or encouraging the child to engage in prostitution or an act of obscene or pornographic photographing, filming or depicting of a child.

Emotional Abuse

Emotional injury means an injury to the mental or psychological capacity or emotional stability of a child as evidenced by a substantial and observable impairment in the child's ability to function within a normal range of performance and behavior with due regard to his or her age, development, culture and environment, as testified to by a qualified mental health professional.

LOUISIANA

Physical Abuse

Abuse means any one of the following acts that seriously endanger the physical, mental or emotional health of the child:

- The infliction, attempted infliction or, as a result of inadequate supervision, the allowance of the infliction or attempted infliction of physical or mental injury upon the child by a parent or any other person

- The exploitation or overwork of a child by a parent or any other person

Crimes against the child include homicide, battery, assault or cruelty to juveniles.

Neglect

Neglect means the refusal or unreasonable failure of a parent or caretaker to supply the child with necessary food, clothing, shelter, care, treatment or counseling for any injury, illness or condition of the child, as a result of which the child's physical, mental or emotional health is substantially threatened or impaired.

Sexual Abuse

Abuse includes any one of the following acts that seriously endanger the physical, mental or emotional health of the child:

- The involvement of the child in any sexual act with a parent or any other person

- The aiding or toleration by the parent or caretaker of the child's sexual involvement with any other person

- The aiding or toleration by the parent of the child's involvement in pornographic displays

- Any other involvement of a child in sexual activity constituting a crime under the laws of the state

Child pornography means visual depiction of a child engaged in actual or simulated sexual intercourse, deviate sexual intercourse, sexual bestiality, masturbation, sadomasochistic abuse or lewd exhibition of the genitals.

Crime against a child includes rape, sexual battery, incest, carnal knowledge of a juvenile, indecent behavior with a juvenile, pornography involving juveniles or molestation of a juvenile.

Emotional Abuse

Abuse includes any act that seriously endangers the mental or emotional health of the child or inflicts mental injury.

MAINE

Physical Abuse

- Abuse or neglect means a threat to a child's health or welfare by physical injury or impairment, by a person responsible for the child.
- Jeopardy to health or welfare or jeopardy means serious abuse or neglect, as evidenced by serious harm or threat of serious harm.
- Serious harm means serious injury.
- Serious injury means serious physical injury or impairment.

Neglect

- Abuse or neglect means a threat to a child's health or welfare by deprivation of essential needs or lack of protection by a person responsible for the child.
- Jeopardy to health or welfare or jeopardy means serious abuse or neglect, as evidenced by deprivation of adequate food, clothing, shelter, supervision or care, including health care, when that deprivation causes a threat of serious harm.

Sexual Abuse

- Abuse or neglect means a threat to a child's health or welfare by sexual abuse or exploitation by a person responsible for the child.
- Serious harm includes sexual abuse or exploitation.

Emotional Abuse

Abuse or neglect includes a threat to a child's health or welfare by mental or emotional injury or impairment by a person responsible for the child.

Serious harm includes serious mental or emotional injury or impairment that now, or in the future, is likely to be evidenced by serious mental, behavioral or personality disorder, including severe anxiety, depression, withdrawal, untoward aggressive behavior, seriously delayed development or similar serious dysfunctional behavior.

MARYLAND

Physical Abuse

Abuse means

- The physical or mental injury of a child by any parent or other person who has permanent or temporary care, custody or responsibility for supervision of a child, or by any household or family member, under circumstances that indicate that the child's health or welfare is harmed or at substantial risk of being harmed
- Sexual abuse of a child, whether physical injuries are sustained or not

Neglect

Neglect means leaving a child unattended or other failure to give proper care and attention to a child by any parent or other person who has permanent or temporary care or custody or responsibility for supervision of the child under circumstances that indicate

- That the child's health or welfare is harmed or placed at substantial risk of harm
- Mental injury to the child or a substantial risk of mental injury

Sexual Abuse

- Sexual abuse means any act that involves sexual molestation or exploitation of a child by a parent or other person who has permanent or temporary care, custody or responsibility for supervision of a child, or by any household or family member.
- Sexual abuse includes incest, rape, sexual offense in any degree, sodomy and unnatural or perverted sexual practices.

Emotional Abuse

Mental injury means the observable, identifiable and substantial impairment of a child's mental or psychological ability to function.

MASSACHUSETTS

Physical Abuse

- Injured, abused, or neglected child means a child under the age of 18 years who is suffering physical injury resulting from abuse inflicted upon him or her that causes harm or substantial risk of harm to the child's health or welfare.
- Abuse means the occurrence of one or more of the following acts between a parent and the other parent or between a parent and the child:
  - Attempting to cause or causing bodily injury

- Placing another in responsible fear of imminent bodily injury
- Serious incident of abuse means the occurrence of one or more of the following acts between a parent and the other parent or between a parent and the child:
  - Attempting to cause or causing serious bodily injury
  - Placing another in reasonable fear of imminent serious bodily injury
  - Causing another to engage involuntarily in sexual relations by force, threat or duress

Neglect

Injured, abused, or neglected child means a child under the age of 18 years who is suffering from neglect, including malnutrition, or who is determined to be physically dependent upon an addictive drug at birth.

Sexual Abuse

Injured, abused, or neglected child includes sexual abuse.

Emotional Abuse

Injured, abused, or neglected child means a child under the age of 18 years who is suffering emotional injury resulting from abuse inflicted upon him or her that causes harm or substantial risk of harm to the child's health or welfare.

MICHIGAN

Physical Abuse

- Child abuse means harm or threatened harm to a child's health or welfare that occurs through nonaccidental physical or mental injury, sexual abuse, sexual exploitation or maltreatment.
- Severe physical injury means brain damage, skull or bone fracture, subdural hemorrhage or hematoma, dislocation, sprains, internal injuries, poisoning, burns, scalds, severe cuts or any other physical injury that seriously impairs the health or physical well-being of a child.

Neglect

Child neglect means harm or threatened harm to a child's health or welfare by a parent, legal guard-

ian or any other person responsible for the child's health or welfare that occurs through either of the following:

- Negligent treatment, including the failure to provide adequate food, clothing, shelter or medical care
- Placing a child at an unreasonable risk to the child's health or welfare by failure to intervene to eliminate that risk when that person is able to do so and has, or should have, knowledge of the risk

Sexual Abuse

- Sexual abuse means engaging in sexual contact or sexual penetration with a child, as those terms are defined in the penal code.
- Sexual exploitation includes allowing, permitting or encouraging a child to engage in prostitution or allowing, permitting, encouraging or engaging in the photographing, filming or depicting of a child engaged in a sexual act.

Emotional Abuse

Child abuse includes mental injury.

MINNESOTA

Physical Abuse

Physical abuse means any physical injury, mental injury or threatened injury inflicted by a person responsible for the child's care on a child by other than accidental means, or any physical or mental injury that cannot reasonably be explained by the child's history of injuries or any aversive and deprivation procedures or regulated interventions that have not been authorized by law. Actions considered abuse include, but are not limited to, any of the following that are done in anger or without regard to the safety of the child:

- Throwing, kicking, burning, biting or cutting a child
- Striking a child with a closed fist
- Shaking a child under age three years
- Striking or other actions that result in any nonaccidental injury to a child under 18 months of age
- Unreasonable interference with a child's breathing

- Threatening a child with a weapon
- Striking a child under age one on the face or head
- Purposely giving a child poison, alcohol or dangerous, harmful or controlled substances that were not prescribed for the child by a practitioner, in order to control or punish the child; giving the child substances that substantially affect the child's behavior, motor coordination or judgment or that result in sickness or internal injury; or subjecting the child to medical procedures that would be unnecessary if the child was not exposed to the substances
- Unreasonable physical confinement or restraint not permitted by law including, but not limited to, tying, caging or chaining

Neglect

Neglect means

- Failure by a person responsible for a child's care to supply a child with necessary food, clothing, shelter, health, medical or other care required for the child's physical or mental health when reasonably able to do so
- Failure to protect a child from conditions or actions that seriously endanger the child's physical or mental health when reasonably able to do so
- Failure to provide for necessary supervision or child-care arrangements appropriate for a child after considering such factors as the child's age, mental ability, physical condition, length of absence or environment, when the child is unable to care for the child's own basic needs or safety, or the basic needs or safety of another child in their care
- Failure to ensure that a child is educated as required by state law, which does not include a parent's refusal to provide the parent's child with sympathomimetic medications
- Prenatal exposure to a controlled substance, used by the mother for a nonmedical purpose, as evidenced by withdrawal symptoms in the child at birth, the result of a toxicology test performed on the mother at delivery or the child at birth or medical effects or developmental delays during the child's first year of life that medically indicated prenatal exposure to a controlled substance

- Medical neglect that includes, but is not limited to, the withholding of medically indicated treatment from a disabled infant with a life-threatening condition.
- Chronic and severe use of alcohol or a controlled substance by a parent or person responsible for the care of the child that adversely affects the child's basic needs and safety

Sexual Abuse

Sexual abuse means the subjection of a child by a person responsible for the child's care, a person who has a significant relationship to the child or a person in a position of authority to any act that constitutes criminal sexual conduct. Sexual abuse includes any act that involves a minor that constitutes a violation of prostitution offenses. Sexual abuse also includes threatened sexual abuse.

Emotional Abuse

Emotional maltreatment means the consistent, deliberate infliction of mental harm on a child by a person responsible for the child's care that has an observable, sustained and adverse effect on the child's physical, mental or emotional development.

Mental injury means an injury to the psychological capacity or emotional stability of a child as evidenced by an observable or substantial impairment in the child's ability to function within a normal range of performance and behavior with due regard to the child's culture.

Neglect includes emotional harm from a pattern of behavior that contributes to impaired emotional functioning of the child that may be demonstrated by a substantial and observable effect in the child's behavior, emotional response or cognition that is not within the normal range for the child's age and stage of development, with due regard to the child's culture.

MISSISSIPPI

Physical Abuse

Abused child means a child whose parent, guardian, custodian or any person responsible for his or her care or support, whether legally obligated to do so or not, has caused or allowed to be caused upon the child nonaccidental physical injury or other maltreatment.

Neglect

Neglected child means a child

- Whose parent, guardian, custodian or any person responsible for his or her care or support neglects or refuses, when able to do so, to provide for him or her proper and necessary care or support; education as required by law; medical, surgical or other care necessary for his or her well-being

- Who is otherwise without proper care, custody, supervision or support

- Who, for any reason, lacks the special care made necessary for him or her by reason of his or her mental condition, whether said mental condition be mentally retarded or mentally ill

- Who, for any reason, lacks the care necessary for his or her health, morals or well-being

Sexual Abuse

- Abused child includes sexual abuse or sexual exploitation

- Sexual abuse means obscene or pornographic photographing, filming or depiction of children for commercial purposes, or the rape, molestation, incest, prostitution or other such forms of sexual exploitation of children under circumstances that indicate that the child's health or welfare is harmed or threatened.

Emotional Abuse

Abused child includes emotional abuse or mental injury.

MISSOURI

Physical Abuse

Abuse means any physical injury inflicted on a child by other than accidental means by those responsible for the child's care, custody and control.

Neglect

Neglect means failure to provide, by those responsible for the care, custody and control of the child, the proper or necessary support; education as required by law; nutrition; medical, surgical or any other care necessary for the child's well-being.

Sexual Abuse

Abuse includes sexual abuse.

Emotional Abuse

Abuse includes emotional abuse inflicted on a child by those responsible for the child's care, custody and control.

MONTANA

Physical Abuse

- Physical abuse means an intentional act or omission or gross negligence resulting in substantial skin bruising, internal bleeding, substantial injury to skin, subdural hematoma, burns, bone fractures, extreme pain, permanent or temporary disfigurement, impairment of any bodily organ or function or death.

- Child abuse or neglect means
  - Actual physical or psychological harm to a child
  - Substantial risk of physical or psychological harm to a child
  - Abandonment

- The term includes
  - Actual physical or psychological harm to a child or substantial risk of physical or psychological harm to a child by the acts or omissions of a person responsible for the child's welfare
  - Exposing a child to the criminal distribution of dangerous drugs, the criminal production or manufacture of dangerous drugs or the operation of an unlawful clandestine laboratory

- Physical or psychological harm to a child means the harm that occurs whenever the parent or other person responsible for the child's welfare inflicts or allows to be inflicted upon the child physical abuse, physical neglect or psychological abuse or neglect.

Neglect

Physical neglect means:

- Failure to provide basic necessities, including but not limited to, appropriate and adequate nutrition, protective shelter from the elements and appropriate clothing related to weather conditions

- Failure to provide cleanliness and general supervision
- Exposing or allowing the child to be exposed to an unreasonable physical or psychological risk to the child

Physical or psychological harm to a child means the harm that occurs whenever the parent or other person responsible for the child's welfare

- Causes malnutrition or a failure to thrive or otherwise fails to supply the child with adequate food or fails to supply clothing, shelter, education or adequate health care, though financially able to do so or offered financial or other reasonable means to do so
- Exposes or allows the child to be exposed to an unreasonable risk to the child's health or welfare by failing to intervene or eliminate the risk

Withholding of medically indicated treatment means the failure to respond to an infant's life-threatening conditions by providing treatment, including appropriate nutrition, hydration and medication, that in the treating physician's or physician's reasonable medical judgment will be most likely to be effective in ameliorating or correcting the conditions.

Sexual Abuse

- Sexual abuse means the commission of sexual assault, sexual intercourse without consent, indecent exposure, deviate sexual conduct, ritual abuse or incest.
- Sexual exploitation means allowing, permitting or encouraging a child to engage in a prostitution offense or allowing, permitting or encouraging sexual abuse of children.
- Physical or psychological harm to a child means the harm that occurs whenever the parent or other person responsible for the child's welfare commits or allows sexual abuse or exploitation of the child.

Emotional Abuse

- Psychological abuse or neglect means severe maltreatment through acts or omissions that are injurious to the child's emotional, intellectual or psychological capacity to function, including acts

of violence against another person residing in the child's home.

- Physical or psychological harm to a child means the harm that occurs whenever the parent or other person responsible for the child's welfare induces or attempts to induce a child to give untrue testimony that the child or another child was abused or neglected by a parent or other person responsible for the child's welfare.

NEBRASKA

Physical Abuse

Abuse or neglect means knowingly, intentionally or negligently causing or permitting a minor child to be placed in a situation that endangers his or her life or physical health, or to be cruelly confined or cruelly punished.

Neglect

Abuse or neglect means knowingly, intentionally or negligently causing or permitting a minor child to be deprived of necessary food, clothing, shelter or care; or left unattended in a motor vehicle if such minor child is six years of age or younger.

Sexual Abuse

Abuse or neglect means knowingly, intentionally or negligently causing or permitting a minor child to be

- Sexually abused
- Sexually exploited by allowing, encouraging or forcing such person to solicit for or engage in prostitution, debauchery, public indecency or obscene or pornographic photography, films or depictions

Emotional Abuse

Abuse or neglect means knowingly, intentionally or negligently causing or permitting a minor child to be placed in a situation that endangers his or her mental health.

NEVADA

Physical Abuse

- Abuse or neglect of a child, except as otherwise provided in this section, means physical or mental injury of a nonaccidental nature.

- Physical injury includes, without limitation,
  - A sprain or dislocation
  - Damage to cartilage
  - A fracture of a bone or the skull
  - An intracranial hemorrhage or injury to another internal organ
  - A burn or scalding
  - A cut, laceration, puncture or bite
  - Permanent or temporary disfigurement or loss or impairment of a part of organ of the body
- Excessive corporal punishment may result in physical or mental injury constituting abuse or neglect of a child.

Neglect

Negligent treatment or maltreatment of a child occurs if a child has been abandoned; is without proper care, control and supervision; lacks the subsistence, education, shelter, medical care or other care necessary for the well-being of the child because of the faults or habits of the person responsible for his welfare or his or her neglect or refusal to provide them when able to do so.

Sexual Abuse

Sexual abuse includes acts upon a child constituting

- Incest
- Lewdness with a child
- Sadomasochistic abuse
- Sexual assault
- Statutory sexual seduction
- Mutilation of the genitalia of a female child; aiding, abetting, encouraging or participating in the mutilation of the genitalia of a female child; or removal of a female child from this state for the purpose of mutilating the genitalia of the child

Sexual exploitation includes forcing, allowing or encouraging a child

- To solicit for or engage in prostitution
- To view a pornographic film or literature
- To engage in filming, photographing or recording on videotape, or posing, modeling or depicting a live performance before an audience that involves the exhibition of a child's genitals or any sexual conduct with a child

Emotional Abuse

Mental injury means an injury to the intellectual or psychological capacity or the emotional condition of a child as evidenced by an observable and substantial impairment of his ability to function within his or her normal range of performance or behavior.

NEW HAMPSHIRE

Physical Abuse

Abused child means any child who has been

- Sexually abused
- Intentionally physically injured
- Physically injured by other than accidental means

Neglect

Neglected child means a child

- Who is without proper parental care or control, subsistence, education as required by law or other care or control necessary for his or her physical, mental or emotional health, when it is established that his or her health has suffered or is very likely to suffer serious impairment, and the deprivation is not due primarily to the lack of financial means of the parents, guardian or custodian
- Whose parents, guardian or custodian are unable to discharge their responsibilities to and for the child because of incarceration, hospitalization or other physical or mental incapacity

Sexual Abuse

Sexual abuse means the following activities under circumstances that indicate that the child's health or welfare is harmed or threatened with harm:

- The employment, use, persuasion, inducement, enticement or coercion of any child to engage in, or having a child assist any other person to engage in, any sexually explicit conduct or any simulation of such conduct for the purpose of producing any visual depiction of such conduct

- The rape, molestation, prostitution or other form of sexual exploitation of children, or incest with children

Emotional Abuse

Abused child means any child who has been psychologically injured so that the child exhibits symptoms of emotional problems generally recognized to result from consistent mistreatment or neglect.

NEW JERSEY

Physical Abuse

Abused child means a child under the age of 18 years whose parent, guardian or other person having his or her custody and control

- Inflicts or allows to be inflicted upon such child physical injury other than accidental means that causes or creates a substantial risk of death, serious or protracted disfigurement, impairment of physical or emotional health or of the function of any bodily organ

- Creates or allows to be created a substantial or ongoing risk of physical injury to such child by other than accidental means that would be likely to cause death or serious or protracted disfigurement, or loss or impairment of the function of any bodily organ

- Unreasonably inflicts or allows to be inflicted harm, or substantial risk thereof, including the infliction of excessive corporal punishment or using excessive physical restraint under circumstances that do not indicate that the child's behavior is harmful to himself or herself, others or property

Neglect

Abused child means a child under the age of 18 years whose physical, mental or emotional condition has been impaired or is in imminent danger of becoming impaired as the result of the failure of his parent or guardian, or such other person having his or her custody and control, to exercise a minimum degree of care in supplying the child with adequate food, clothing, shelter, education or medical or surgical care though financially able to do so or though offered financial or other reasonable means to do so.

Sexual Abuse

Abused child means a child under the age of 18 years whose parent, guardian or other person having his or her custody and control commits or allows to be committed an act of sexual abuse against the child.

Emotional Abuse

Abused child means a child under the age of 18 years who is in an institution, excepting day schools, and who

- Has been so placed inappropriately for a continued period of time with the knowledge that the placement has resulted and may continue to result in harm to the child's mental or physical well-being

- Has been willfully isolated from ordinary social contact under circumstances that indicate emotional or social deprivation

NEW MEXICO

Physical Abuse

Abused child means a child

- Who has suffered or is at risk of suffering serious harm because of the action or inaction of the child's parent, guardian or custodian

- Who has suffered physical abuse inflicted or caused by the child's parent, guardian or custodian

- Whose parent, guardian or custodian has knowingly, intentionally or negligently placed the child in a situation that may endanger the child's life or health

- Whose parent, guardian or custodian has knowingly or intentionally tortured, cruelly confined or cruelly punished the child

Physical abuse includes, but is not limited to, any case in which the child exhibits evidence of skin bruising, bleeding, malnutrition, failure to thrive, burns, fracture of any bone, subdural hematoma, soft tissue swelling or death, and where

- There is not a justifiable explanation for the condition or death.

- The explanation given for the condition or death is at variance with the degree or nature of the condition or the nature of the death.

- Circumstances indicate that the condition or death may not be the product of an accidental occurrence.

Evidence that demonstrates that a child has been negligently allowed to enter or remain in a motor vehicle, building or any other premises that contains chemicals, materials or equipment used or intended for use in the manufacture of a controlled substance shall be deemed prima facie evidence of abuse of a child.

Neglect

Neglected child means a child

- Who has been abandoned by the child's parent, guardian or custodian

- Who is without proper parental care and control or subsistence, education, medical or other care or control necessary for the child's well-being because of the faults or habits of the child's guardian, or custodian, or the failure or refusal to provide them

- Who has been physically or sexually abused, when the child's parent, guardian or custodian knew or should have known of the abuse and failed to take reasonable steps to protect the child from further harm

- Whose parent, guardian or custodian is unable to discharge his or her responsibilities to and for the child because of incarceration, hospitalization or other physical or mental disorder or incapacity

- Who has been placed for care or adoption in violation of the law

Sexual Abuse

- Abused child means a child who has suffered sexual abuse or sexual exploitation inflicted by the child's parent, guardian, or custodian.

- Sexual abuse includes, but is not limited to, criminal sexual contact, incest or criminal sexual penetration, as those acts are defined by state law.

- Sexual exploitation includes, but is not limited to,

  - Allowing, permitting or encouraging a child to engage in prostitution

  - Allowing, permitting, encouraging or engaging a child in obscene or pornographic photographing

  - Filming or depicting a child for obscene or pornographic commercial purposes

Emotional Abuse

Abused child means a child who has suffered emotional or psychological abuse inflicted or caused by the child's parent, guardian or custodian.

NEW YORK

Abused child means a child less than 18 years of age whose parent or other person legally responsible for his or her care

- Inflicts or allows to be inflicted upon such child physical injury by other than accidental means that causes or creates a substantial risk of death, serious or protracted disfigurement, protracted impairment of physical or emotional health or protracted loss or impairment of the function of any bodily organ

- Creates or allows to be created a substantial risk of physical injury to such child by other than accidental means that would be likely to cause death, serious or protracted disfigurement, protracted impairment of physical or emotional health or protracted loss or impairment of the function of any bodily organ

Neglect

Neglected child means a child less than 18 years of age whose physical, mental or emotional condition has been impaired or is in imminent danger of becoming impaired as a result of the failure of his or her parent or other person legally responsible for his or her care to exercise a minimum degree of care

- In supplying the child with adequate food, clothing, shelter, education, or medical or surgical care, though financially able to do so or offered financial or other reasonable means to do so

- In providing the child with proper supervision or guardianship

- By unreasonably inflicting, or allowing to be inflicted, harm, or a substantial risk thereof, including the infliction of excessive corporal punishment

- By misusing drugs or alcoholic beverages to the extent that he or she loses self-control of his or her actions

- By any other acts of a similarly serious nature requiring the aid of the court

Sexual Abuse

Abused child means a child less than 18 years of age whose parent or other person legally responsible for his or her care commits, or allows to be committed, an act of sexual abuse against such child, as defined in title H, article 130 of the penal law.

Emotional Abuse

Impairment of emotional health and impairment of mental or emotional condition includes a state of substantially diminished psychological or intellectual functioning in relation to, but not limited to, such factors as failure to thrive, control of aggressive or self-destructive impulses, ability to think and reason, acting out or misbehavior, including incorrigibility, ungovernability or habitual truancy; provided, however, that such impairment must be clearly attributable to the unwillingness or inability of the respondent to exercise a minimum degree of care toward the child.

NORTH CAROLINA

Physical Abuse

Abused juvenile means any juvenile less than 18 years of age whose parent, guardian, custodian or caretaker

- Inflicts or allows to be inflicted upon the juvenile a serious physical injury by other than accidental means

- Creates or allows to be created a substantial risk of serious physical injury to the juvenile by other than accidental means

- Uses or allows to be used upon the juvenile cruel or grossly inappropriate procedures or cruel or grossly inappropriate devices to modify behavior

Neglect

Neglected juvenile means a juvenile

- Who does not receive proper care, supervision or discipline from his or her parent, guardian, custodian or caretaker

- Who is not provided necessary medical or remedial care

- Who lives in an environment injurious to his or her welfare

- Who has been placed for care or adoption in violation of law

In determining whether a juvenile is a neglected juvenile, it is relevant whether that juvenile lives in a home where another juvenile has been subjected to abuse or neglect by an adult who regularly lives in the home.

Sexual Abuse

Abused juvenile means any juvenile less than 18 years of age whose parent, guardian, custodian or caretaker commits, permits or encourages the commission of a violation of the following laws regarding sexual offenses by, with or upon the juvenile:

- First- and second-degree rape or sexual offense

- Sexual act by a custodian

- Crime against nature or incest

- Preparation of obscene photographs, slides or motion pictures of the juvenile

- Employing or permitting the juvenile to assist in a violation of the obscenity laws

- Dissemination of obscene material to the juvenile

- Displaying or disseminating material harmful to the juvenile

- First- and second-degree sexual exploitation of the juvenile

- Promoting the prostitution of the juvenile

- Taking indecent liberties with the juvenile, regardless of the age of the parties

Emotional Abuse

Abused juvenile means any juvenile less than 18 years of age whose parent, guardian, custodian or caretaker creates or allows to be created serious emotional damage to the juvenile. Serious emotional damage is evidenced by a juvenile's severe anxiety, depression, withdrawal or aggressive behavior toward himself/herself or others.

NORTH DAKOTA

Physical Abuse

Abused child means an individual under the age of 18 years who is suffering from serious physical harm or traumatic abuse caused by other than accidental means by a person responsible for the child's welfare.

Harm means negative changes in a child's health that occur when a person responsible for the child's welfare inflicts or allows to be inflicted upon the child physical or mental injury, including injuries sustained as a result of excessive corporal punishment.

Neglected child means a deprived child.

Deprived child means a child who

- Is without proper parental care or control, subsistence, education or other care or control necessary for the child's physical, mental, emotional health or morals, and the deprivation is not due primarily to the lack of financial means of the child's parent, guardian, or other custodian
- Has been placed for care or adoption in violation of law
- Is without proper parental care, control, education or other care and control necessary for the child's well-being because of the physical, mental, emotional or other illness or disability of the child's parent or parents, and that such lack of care is not due to a willful act of commission or act of omission by the child's parents, and care is requested by a parent
- Is in need of treatment and whose parents, guardian or other custodian have refused to participate in treatment as ordered by the juvenile court
- Was subjected to prenatal exposure to chronic and severe use of alcohol or any controlled substance in a manner not lawfully prescribed by a practitioner

- Is present in an environment subjecting the child to exposure to a controlled substance or drug paraphernalia

Sexual Abuse

- Abused child means an individual under the age of 18 years who is suffering from or was subjected to any sex offenses against a child.
- Harm means negative changes in a child's health that occur when a person responsible for the child's welfare commits, allows to be committed or conspires to commit against the child a sex offense.

Emotional Abuse

Harm means negative changes in a child's health that occur when a person responsible for the child's welfare inflicts or allows to be inflicted on the child a mental injury.

OHIO

Physical Abuse

Abused child includes any child who

- Is endangered as defined in the statute concerning endangering children, except that the court need not find that any person has been convicted under that section in order to find that the child is an abused child
- Exhibits evidence of any physical or mental injury or death, inflicted by other than accidental means, or an injury or death that is at variance with the history given of it
- Because of the acts of his or her parents, guardian or custodian, suffers physical or mental injury that harms or threatens to harm the child's health or welfare
- Is subjected to out-of-home care child abuse

Neglect

Neglected child includes any child

- Who lacks proper parental care because of the faults or habits of the child's parents, guardian or custodian
- Whose parents, guardian or custodian neglects the child or refuses to provide proper or necessary subsistence, education, medical or surgical care or

treatment or other care necessary for the child's health, morals or well-being

- Whose parents, legal guardian or custodian neglects the child or refuses to provide the special care made necessary by the child's mental condition

- Whose parents, legal guardian or custodian have placed or attempted to place the child in violation of state laws regarding the placement and adoption of children

- Who, because of the omission of the child's parents, guardian or custodian, suffers physical or mental injury that harms or threatened to harm the child's health or welfare

- Who is subjected to out-of-home care child neglect

Sexual Abuse

Abused child includes any child who is the victim of sexual activity, where such activity would constitute an offense, except that the court need not find that any person has been convicted of the offense in order to find that the child is an abused child.

Sexual conduct means vaginal intercourse between a male and female, anal intercourse, fellatio and cunnilingus between persons regardless of sex; and without privilege to do so, the inserting, however slight, of any part of the body of any instrument, apparatus or other object into the vaginal or anal cavity of another. Penetration, however slight, is sufficient to complete vaginal or anal intercourse.

Sexual contact means any touching of an erogenous zone of another, including without limitation, the thigh, genitals, buttocks, pubic region or, if the person is a female, a breast, for the purpose of sexually arousing or gratifying another person.

A person commits the crime of endangering children when the person does any of the following to a child: entice, coerce, permit, encourage, compel, hire, employ, use or allow the child to act, model or in any other way participate in or be photographed for the production, presentation, dissemination or advertisement of any material or performance that the offender knows or reasonably should know is obscene, sexually oriented or nudity-oriented matter.

Emotional Abuse

Mental injury means any behavioral, cognitive, emotional or mental disorder in a child caused by an act or omission that is described in state law and is committed by a parent or other person that is responsible for the child's care.

OKLAHOMA

Physical Abuse

- Abuse means harm or threatened harm to a child's health, safety or welfare by a person responsible for the child's health, safety or welfare, including sexual abuse and sexual exploitation.

- Harm or threatened harm to a child's health or safety includes, but is not limited to, nonaccidental physical injury.

Neglect

- Harm or threatened harm to a child's health or safety includes, but is not limited to,
  - Neglect
  - Failure or omission to provide protection from harm or threatened harm

- Neglect means failure or omission to provide
  - Adequate food, clothing, shelter, medical care and supervision
  - Special care made necessary by the physical or mental condition of the child

Sexual Abuse

- Harm or threatened harm to a child's health or safety includes, but is not limited to, sexual abuse or sexual exploitation.

- Sexual abuse includes, but is not limited to, rape, incest and lewd or indecent acts or proposals, as defined by law, by a person responsible for the child's health, safety or welfare.

- Sexual exploitation includes, but is not limited to,
  - Allowing, permitting or encouraging a child to engage in prostitution, as defined by law, by a person responsible for the child's health, safety or welfare
  - Allowing, permitting, encouraging or engaging in the lewd, obscene or pornographic photo-

graphing, filming or depicting of a child by a person responsible for the child's health, safety or welfare

Emotional Abuse

Harm or threatened harm to a child's health or safety includes, but is not limited to, mental injury.

OREGON

Physical Abuse

Abuse means

- Any assault of a child and any physical injury to a child that has been caused by other than accidental means, including injury that appears to be at variance with the explanation given of the injury
- Threatened harm to a child, which means subjecting a child to a substantial risk of harm to his or her health or welfare

Neglect

Abuse means negligent treatment or maltreatment of a child, including but not limited to, the failure to provide adequate food, clothing, shelter or medical care that is likely to endanger the health or welfare of the child.

Sexual Abuse

Abuse means

- Rape of a child, that includes but is not limited to, rape, sodomy, unlawful sexual penetration and incest
- Sexual abuse
- Sexual exploitation, including but not limited to,

  - Contributing to the sexual delinquency of a minor
  - Any other conduct that allows, employs, authorizes, permits, induces or encourages a child to engage in the performing for people to observe, or the photographing, filming, tape recording or other exhibition that, in whole or in part, depicts sexual conduct or contact, sexual abuse involving a child or rape of a child

- Allowing, permitting, encouraging or hiring a child to engage in prostitution

Emotional Abuse

Abuse means any mental injury to a child that shall include only observable and substantial impairment of the child's mental or psychological ability to function caused by cruelty to the child, with due regard to the culture of the child

PENNSYLVANIA

Physical Abuse

- Child abuse shall mean any of the following:

  - Any recent act or failure to act by a perpetrator that causes nonaccidental serious physical injury to a child under 18 years of age
  - Any recent act, failure to act or series of such acts or failures to act by a perpetrator that creates an imminent risk of serious physical injury to a child under 18 years of age

- Serious bodily injury means bodily injury that creates a substantial risk of death or causes serious permanent disfigurement or protracted loss or impairment of function of any bodily member or organ.
- Serious physical injury means an injury that causes a child severe pain or significantly impairs a child's physical functioning, either temporarily or permanently.

Neglect

Child abuse includes serious physical neglect by a perpetrator constituting prolonged or repeated lack of supervision or the failure to provide essentials of life, including adequate medical care, that endangers a child's life or development or impairs the child's functioning.

Sexual Abuse

Child abuse shall mean any of the following:

- An act or failure to act by a perpetrator that causes sexual abuse or sexual exploitation of a child under 18 years of age

- Any recent act, failure to act, or series of such acts or failures to act by a perpetrator that creates an imminent risk of sexual abuse or sexual exploitation of a child under 18 years of age

Sexual abuse or exploitation means the employment, use, persuasion, inducement, enticement or coercion of any child to engage in or assist any other person to engage in any sexually explicit conduct or any simulation of any sexually explicit conduct for the purpose of producing:

- Any visual depiction, including photographing, videotaping, computer depicting or filming, of any sexually explicit conduct

- The rape, sexual assault, involuntary deviate sexual intercourse, aggravated indecent assault, molestation, incest, indecent exposure, prostitution, statutory sexual assault or other form of sexual exploitation of children

Emotional Abuse

- Child abuse includes an act or failure to act by a perpetrator that causes nonaccidental serious mental injury to a child under 18 years of age.

- Serious mental injury means a psychological condition, as diagnosed by a physician or licensed psychologist, including the refusal of appropriate treatment, that

  - Renders a child chronically and severely anxious, agitated, depressed, socially withdrawn, psychotic or in reasonable fear that his or her life or safety is threatened

  - Seriously interferes with a child's ability to accomplish age-appropriate development and social tasks

RHODE ISLAND

Physical Abuse

Abused and/or neglected child means a child whose physical or mental health or welfare is harmed or threatened with harm when his or her parent or other person responsible for his or her welfare

- Inflicts or allows to be inflicted upon the child physical or mental injury, including excessive corporal punishment

- Creates or allows to be created a substantial risk of physical or mental injury to the child, including excessive corporal punishment

Neglect

Abused and/or neglected child means a child whose physical or mental health or welfare is harmed or threatened with harm when his or her parent or other person responsible for his or her welfare

- Fails to supply the child with adequate food, clothing, shelter or medical care, though financially able to do so or offered financial or other reasonable means to do so

- Fails to provide the child with a minimum degree of care or proper supervision or guardianship because of his or her unwillingness or inability to do so by situations or conditions such as, but not limited to, social problems, mental incompetency or the use of a drug, drugs or alcohol to the extent that the parent or other persons responsible for the child's welfare loses his or her ability or is unwilling to properly care for the child

Sexual Abuse

Abused and/or neglected child means a child whose physical or mental health or welfare is harmed or threatened with harm when his or her parent or other person responsible for his or her welfare

- Commits or allows to be committed against the child an act of sexual abuse

- Sexually exploits the child in that the person allows, permits or encourages the child to engage in prostitution

- Sexually exploits the child in that the person allows, permits, encourages or engages in the obscene or pornographic photographing, filming or depicting of the child in a setting that taken as a whole suggests to the average person that the child is about to engage in or has engaged in any sexual act, or that depicts any such child under 18 years of age performing sodomy, oral copulation, sexual intercourse, masturbation or bestiality

- Commits or allows to be committed any sexual offense against the child

- Commits or allows to be committed against any child an act involving sexual penetration or sexual contact, if the child is under 15 years of age; or if the child is 15 years or older, and (1) force or coercion is used by the perpetrator, or (2) the perpetrator knows or has reason to know that the victim is a severely impaired person or physically helpless

Emotional Abuse

Mental injury includes a state of substantially diminished psychological or intellectual functioning in relation to, but not limited to, such factors as failure to thrive, ability to think or reason, control of aggressive or self-destructive impulses, acting-out or misbehavior, including incorrigibility, ungovernability or habitual truancy. However, the injury must be clearly attributable to the unwillingness or inability of the parent or other person responsible for the child's welfare to exercise a minimum degree of care toward the child.

SOUTH CAROLINA

Physical Abuse

- Abused or neglected child means a child whose death results from, or whose physical or mental health or welfare is harmed or threatened with harm by, the acts or omissions of the child's parent, guardian or other person responsible for his or her welfare.

- Child abuse or neglect or harm occurs when the parent, guardian or other person responsible for the child's welfare inflicts or allows to be inflicted upon the child mental injury or engages in acts or omission that present a substantial risk of physical or mental injury to the child, including injuries sustained as a result of excessive corporal punishment.

- Physical injury means death or permanent or temporary disfigurement or impairment of any bodily organ or function.

Neglect

Child abuse or neglect or harm occurs when the parent, guardian or other person responsible for the child's welfare fails to supply the child with adequate food, clothing, shelter, education or supervision appropriate to the child's age and development or health care, though financially able to do so or offered financial or other reasonable means to do

so, and the failure to do so has caused physical or mental injury or presents a substantial risk of causing physical or mental injury.

Sexual Abuse

Child abuse or neglect or harm occurs when the parent, guardian or other person responsible for the child's welfare commits or allows to be committed against the child a sexual offense or engages in acts or omissions that present a substantial risk that a sexual offense would be committed against the child.

Emotional Abuse

Mental injury means an injury to the intellectual or psychological capacity of a child as evidenced by a discernible and substantial impairment of the child's ability to function when the existence of that impairment is supported by the opinion of a mental health professional or medical professional.

SOUTH DAKOTA

Physical Abuse

Abused or neglected child means a child

- Whose parent, guardian or custodian has subjected the child to mistreatment or abuse

- Who was subjected to prenatal exposure to abusive use of alcohol, any controlled drug or a substance not lawfully prescribed by a practitioner

Neglect

Abused or neglected child means a child

- Who lacks proper parental care through the actions or omissions of the child's parent, guardian or custodian

- Whose environment is injurious to his or her welfare

- Whose parent, guardian or custodian fails or refuses to provide proper or necessary subsistence, supervision, education, medical care or any other care necessary for the child's health, guidance or well-being

- Whose parent, guardian or custodian knowingly exposes the child to an environment that is being used for the manufacturing of methamphetamines

- Who is homeless, without proper care or not domiciled with the child's parent, guardian or custodian through no fault of the child's parent, guardian or custodian

Sexual Abuse

Abused or neglected child means a child who is subject to sexual abuse, sexual molestation or sexual exploitation by the child's parent, guardian, custodian or any other person responsible for the child's care.

Emotional Abuse

Abused or neglected child means a child who has sustained emotional harm or mental injury as indicated by an injury to the child's intellectual or psychological capacity, evidenced by an observable and substantial impairment in the child's ability to function within the child's normal range of performance and behavior, with due regard to the child's culture.

TENNESSEE

Physical Abuse

- Abuse exists when a person under the age of 18 years is suffering from, has sustained or may be in immediate danger of suffering from or sustaining a wound, injury, disability or physical or mental condition caused by brutality, neglect or other actions or inactions of a parent, relative, guardian or caretaker.
- Severe child abuse means
  - The knowing exposure of a child to or the knowing failure to protect a child from abuse or neglect that is likely to cause great bodily harm or death, and the knowing use of force on a child that is likely to cause great bodily harm
  - Specific brutality, abuse or neglect toward a child that in the opinion of qualified experts has caused or will reasonably be expected to produce severe psychosis, severe neurotic disorder, severe depression, severe development delay or retardation or severe impairment of the child's ability to function adequately in the child's environment, and the knowing failure to protect a child from such conduct.

- The knowing failure to protect the child from the commission of any such act toward the child
- Knowingly allowing a child to be present in a structure where the act of creating methamphetamine is occurring

Neglect

Neglected child means a child

- Who is under unlawful or improper care, supervision, custody or restraint by any person, corporation, agency, association, institution, society or other organization, or who is unlawfully kept out of school
- Whose parent, guardian or custodian neglects or refuses to provide necessary medical, surgical, institutional or hospital care for the child
- Who, because of lack of proper supervision, is found in any public place the existence of which is in violation of the law
- Who is in such condition of want or suffering or is under such improper guardianship or control as to injure or endanger the morals or health of the child or others

Sexual Abuse

Child sexual abuse means the commission of any act involving the unlawful sexual abuse, molestation, fondling or carnal knowledge of a child under 13 years of age that on or after November 1, 1989, constituted the criminal offense of

- Aggravated rape, sexual battery or sexual exploitation of a minor
- Criminal attempt for any of the offenses listed above
- Especially aggravated sexual exploitation of a minor
- Incest
- Rape, sexual battery or sexual exploitation of a minor

Child sexual abuse also means one or more of the following acts:

- Any penetration, however slight, of the vagina or anal opening of one person by the penis of another person, whether or not there is the emission of semen

- Any contact between the genitals or anal opening of one person and the mouth or tongue of another person

- Any intrusion by one person into the genitals or anal opening of another person, including the use of any object for this purpose

- The intentional touching of the genitals or intimate parts, including the breasts, genital areas, groin, inner thighs and buttocks, or the clothing covering them, of either the child or the perpetrator

- The intentional exposure of the perpetrator's genitals in the presence of a child, or any other sexual act intentionally perpetrated in the presence of a child, if such exposure or sexual act is for the purpose of sexual arousal or gratification, aggression, degradation or other similar purpose

- The sexual exploitation of a child, which includes allowing, encouraging or forcing a child to solicit for or engage in prostitution, or engage in sexual exploitation of a minor

Emotional Abuse

Mental injury means an injury to the intellectual or psychological capacity of a child as evidenced by a discernible and substantial impairment in the child's ability to function within the child's normal range of performance and behavior, with due regard to the child's culture.

TEXAS

Physical Abuse

Abuse includes the following acts or omissions by a person:

- Physical injury that results in substantial harm to the child, or the genuine threat of substantial harm from physical injury to the child, including an injury that is at variance with the history or explanation given and excluding an accident or reasonable discipline by a parent, guardian or conservator that does not expose the child to a substantial risk of harm

- Failure to make a reasonable effort to prevent an action by another person that results in physical injury or substantial harm to the child

- The current use by a person of a controlled substance, in a manner or to the extent that the use results in physical, mental or emotional injury to a child

- Causing, expressly permitting or encouraging a child to use a controlled substance

Neglect

Neglect includes the following acts or omissions by a person:

- Placing a child in or failing to remove a child from a situation that a reasonable person would realize requires judgment or actions beyond the child's level of maturity, physical condition or mental abilities and that results in bodily injury or a substantial risk of immediate harm to the child

- Failing to seek, obtain or follow through with medical care for a child, with the failure resulting in or presenting a substantial risk of death, disfigurement or bodily injury, or with the failure resulting in an observable and material impairment to the growth, development or functioning of the child

- The failure to provide a child with food, clothing or shelter necessary to sustain the life or health of the child, excluding failure caused primarily by financial inability unless relief services had been offered and refused

- Placing a child in or failing to remove the child from a situation in which the child would be exposed to a substantial risk of sexual conduct harmful to the child

- The failure by the person responsible for a child's care, custody or welfare to permit the child to return to the child's home without arranging for the necessary care for the child after the child has been absent from the home for any reason, including having been in residential placement or having run away

Sexual Abuse

Abuse includes the following acts or omissions by a person:

- Sexual conduct harmful to a child's mental, emotional or physical welfare, including conduct that constitutes the offense of indecency with a child, sexual assault or aggravated sexual assault

- Failure to make a reasonable effort to prevent sexual conduct harmful to a child
- Compelling or encouraging the child to engage in sexual conduct
- Causing, permitting, encouraging, engaging in or allowing the photographing, filming or depicting of the child if the person knew or should have known the resulting photograph, film or depiction of the child is obscene or pornographic
- Causing, permitting, encouraging, engaging in or allowing a sexual performance by a child

Emotional Abuse

Abuse includes the following acts or omissions by a person:

- Mental or emotional injury to a child that results in an observable and material impairment in the child's growth, development or psychological functioning
- Causing or permitting the child to be in a situation in which the child sustains a mental or emotional injury that results in an observable and material impairment in the child's growth, development or psychological functioning

UTAH

Physical Abuse

- Child abuse or neglect means causing harm or threatened harm to a child's health or welfare.
- Harm or threatened harm means damage or threatened damage to the physical or emotional health and welfare of a child through neglect or abuse and includes, but is not limited to, causing nonaccidental physical or mental injury.

Neglect

Harm or threatened harm means damage or threatened damage to the physical or emotional health and welfare of a child through neglect or abuse and includes, but is not limited to, repeated negligent treatment or maltreatment.

Sexual Abuse

- Harm or threatened harm means damage or threatened damage to the physical or emotional

health and welfare of a child through neglect or abuse and includes, but is not limited to, incest, sexual abuse, sexual exploitation or molestation.
- Sexual abuse means acts or attempted acts of sexual intercourse, sodomy or molestation directed toward a child.
- Sexual exploitation of minors means knowingly employing, using, persuading, inducing, enticing or coercing any minor to pose in the nude for the purpose of sexual arousal of any person or for profit, or to engage in any sexual or simulated sexual conduct for the purpose of photographing, filming, recording, or displaying in any way sexual or simulated sexual conduct, and includes displaying, distributing, possessing for the purpose of distribution or selling material depicting minors in the nude, or engaging in sexual or simulated sexual conduct.

Emotional Abuse

Harm or threatened harm means damage or threatened damage to the emotional health and welfare of a child through neglect or abuse.

VERMONT

Physical Abuse

- Abused or neglected child means a child whose physical health, psychological growth and development or welfare is harmed or is at substantial risk of harm by the acts of omissions of his or her parent or other person responsible for the child's welfare.
- Harm can occur by physical injury.
- Physical injury means death or permanent or temporary disfigurement or impairment of any bodily organ or function by other than accidental means.
- Sexual abuse includes the aiding, abetting, counseling, hiring or procuring of a child to perform or participate in any photograph, motion picture, exhibition, show, representation or other presentation that, in whole or in part, depicts sexual conduct, sexual excitement or sadomasochistic abuse involving a child.

Neglect

Harm can occur by failure to supply the child with adequate food, clothing, shelter or health care.

Sexual Abuse

- An abused or neglected child also means a child who is sexually abused or at substantial risk of sexual abuse by any person.

- Sexual abuse consists of any act or acts by any person involving sexual molestation or exploitation of a child, including but not limited to, incest, prostitution, rape, sodomy or any lewd and lascivious conduct involving a child.

- Sexual abuse also includes the aiding, abetting, counseling, hiring or procuring of a child to perform or participate in any photograph, motion picture, exhibition, show, representation or other presentation that, in whole or in part, depicts sexual conduct, sexual excitement or sadomasochistic abuse involving a child.

Emotional Abuse

- Harm can occur by emotional maltreatment.

- Emotional maltreatment means a pattern of malicious behavior that results in impaired psychological growth and development.

VIRGINIA

Physical Abuse

Abused or neglected child means any child less than 18 years of age whose parents or other person responsible for his or her care creates or inflicts, threatens to create or inflict or allows to be created or inflicted upon such child a physical injury by other than accidental means, or creates a substantial risk of death, disfigurement or impairment of bodily functions.

Neglect

Abused or neglected child means any child less than 18 years of age

- Whose parents or other person responsible for his or her care neglects or refuses to provide care necessary for his or her health

- Who is without parental care or guardianship caused by the unreasonable absence or the mental or physical incapacity of the child's parent, guardian, legal custodian or other person standing in loco parentis

Sexual Abuse

Abused or neglected child means any child less than 18 years of age whose parents or other person responsible for his or her care commits or allows to be committed any act of sexual exploitation or any sexual act upon a child in violation of the law.

Emotional Abuse

Abused or neglected child means any child less than 18 years of age whose parents or other person responsible for his or her care creates or inflicts, threatens to create or inflict or allows to be created or inflicted upon such child a mental injury, or creates a substantial risk of impairment of mental functions.

WASHINGTON

Physical Abuse

- Abuse or neglect means the injury or maltreatment of a child by any person under circumstances that indicate that the child's health, welfare and safety are harmed.

- Severe abuse means any of the following:

  - Any single act of abuse that causes physical trauma of sufficient severity that, if left untreated, could cause death

  - Any single act of sexual abuse that causes significant bleeding, deep bruising or significant external or internal swelling

  - More than one act of physical abuse, each of which causes bleeding, deep bruising, significant external or internal swelling, bone fracture or unconsciousness

Neglect

- Abuse or neglect means the negligent treatment of a child by any person under circumstances that indicate that the child's health, welfare and safety are harmed.

- Negligent treatment or maltreatment means an act or omission that evidences a serious disregard of consequences of such a magnitude as to constitute clear and present danger to the child's health, welfare and safety.

Sexual Abuse

- Abuse or neglect means the sexual abuse or sexual exploitation of a child by any person under circumstances that indicate that the child's health, welfare and safety are harmed.
- Sexual exploitation includes
  - Allowing, permitting or encouraging a child to engage in prostitution by any person
  - Allowing, permitting, encouraging or engaging in the obscene or pornographic photographing, filming or depicting of a child by any person

Emotional Abuse

Not addressed in the statutes reviewed

WEST VIRGINIA

Physical Abuse

Child abuse and neglect or child abuse or neglect means physical injury or sale or attempted sale of a child by a parent, guardian or custodian who is responsible for the child's welfare, under circumstance that harm or threaten the health and welfare of the child.

Imminent danger to the physical well-being of the child means an emergency situation in which the welfare or the life of a child is threatened. Such emergency situations exist when there is reasonable cause that the following conditions threaten the health or life of any child in the home:

- Nonaccidental trauma inflicted by a parent, guardian, custodian, sibling, babysitter or other caretaker
- A combination of physical and other signs indicating a pattern of abuse that may be medically diagnosed as battered child syndrome
- Sale or attempted sale of the child by the parent, guardian or custodian

Serious physical abuse means bodily injury that creates a substantial risk of death or causes serious or prolonged disfigurement, prolonged impairment of health or prolonged loss or impairment of the function of any bodily organ.

Neglect

Child abuse and neglect or child abuse or neglect means negligent treatment or maltreatment of a child by a parent, guardian or custodian who is responsible for the child's welfare, under circumstances that harm or threaten the health and welfare of the child.

Neglected child means a child

- Whose physical or mental health is harmed or threatened by a present refusal, failure or inability of the child's parent, guardian or custodian to supply the child with necessary food, clothing, shelter, supervision, medical care or education that is not due primarily to a lack of financial means
- Who is presently without necessary food, clothing, shelter, medical care, education or supervision because of the disappearance or absence of the child's parent or custodian

Sexual Abuse

Child abuse and neglect or child abuse or neglect means sexual acts of sexual exploitation of a child by a parent, guardian or custodian who is responsible for the child's welfare, under circumstances that harm or threaten the health and welfare of the child. Sexual abuse means the acts of sexual intercourse, sexual intrusion or sexual contact, when they occur under the following circumstances:

- As to a child who is less than 16 years of age, those acts that a parent, guardian or custodian shall engage in, attempt to engage in or knowingly procure another person to engage in with the child, notwithstanding that the child may have willingly participated in such conduct or the fact that the child may have suffered no apparent physical, mental or emotional injury as a result of such conduct
- As to a child who is 16 years or age or older, those acts that a parent, guardian or custodian shall engage in, attempt to engage in or knowingly procure another person to engage in with the child, notwithstanding the fact that the child may have consented to such conduct or the fact that the child may have suffered no apparent physical, mental or emotional injury as a result of such conduct

Sexual abuse also means any conduct whereby a parent, guardian or custodian displays his or her sex organs to a child or procures another person to display his or her sex organs to a child, for the purpose of gratifying the sexual desire of the person making such display, or of the child or for the purpose of affronting or alarming the child.

Sexual exploitation means an act whereby

- A parent, custodian or guardian, whether for financial gain or not, persuades, induces, entices or coerces a child to engage in sexual explicit conduct

- A parent, guardian or custodian persuades, induces, entices or coerces a child to display his or her sex organs for the sexual gratification of the parent, guardian, custodian or a third person, or to display his or her sex organs under circumstances in which the parent, guardian or custodian knows such display is likely to be observed by others who would be affronted or alarmed.

Emotional Abuse

Child abuse and neglect or child abuse or neglect includes mental or emotional injury of a child by a parent, guardian or custodian who is responsible for the child's welfare, under circumstances that harm or threaten the health and welfare of the child.

Imminent danger to the physical well-being of the child includes substantial emotional injury inflicted by a parent, guardian or custodian.

WISCONSIN

Physical Abuse

- Abuse means any of the following:
  - Physical injury inflicted on a child by other than accidental means
  - When used in referring to an unborn child, serious physical harm inflicted on the unborn child, and the risk of serious physical harm to the child when born, caused by the habitual lack of self-control of the expectant mother of the unborn child in the use of alcoholic beverages, controlled substances or controlled substance analogs, exhibited to a severe degree
- Physical injury includes, but is not limited to, lacerations, fractured bones, burns, internal injuries, severe or frequent bruising or great bodily harm

Neglect

Neglect means failure, refusal or inability on the part of a parent, guardian, legal custodian or other person exercising temporary or permanent control over a child, for reasons other than poverty, to provide necessary care, food, clothing, medical or dental care or shelter so as to seriously endanger the physical health of the child.

Sexual Abuse

Abuse means any of the following:

- Sexual intercourse or sexual contact
- A violation of the statute regarding the sexual exploitation of a child
- Permitting, allowing or encouraging a child to engage in prostitution
- A violation of the statute that prohibits causing a child to view or listen to sexual activity
- A violation of the statute that prohibits the exposure of the genitals to a child

Emotional Abuse

Abuse means emotional damage for which the child's parent, guardian or legal custodian has neglected, refused or been unable for reasons other than poverty to obtain the necessary treatment or to take steps to ameliorate the symptoms.

Emotional damage means harm to a child's psychological or intellectual functioning.

Emotional damage shall be evidenced by one or more of the following characteristics exhibited to a severe degree: anxiety, depression, withdrawal, outward aggressive behavior or a substantial and observable change in behavior, emotional response or cognition that is not within the normal range for the child's age and state of development.

WYOMING

Physical Abuse

Abuse with respect to a child means inflicting or causing physical injury, harm or imminent danger to the physical health or welfare of a child other than by accidental means including excessive or unreasonable corporal punishment.

Physical injury means any harm to a child, including but not limited to, disfigurement, impairment of any bodily organ, skin bruising if greater in magnitude than minor bruising associated with reasonable corporal punishment, bleeding, burns, fracture of any bone, subdural hematoma or substantial malnutrition.

Neglect

• Abuse with respect to a child means malnutrition or substantial risk of harm by reason of intentional or unintentional neglect.

• Neglect means a failure or refusal by those responsible for the child's welfare to provide adequate care, maintenance, supervision, education, medical, surgical or any other care necessary for the child's well-being.

Sexual Abuse

Abuse with respect to a child means the commission or allowing the commission of a sexual offense against a child, as defined by law.

Emotional Abuse

• Abuse with respect to a child means inflicting or causing mental injury, or harm to the mental health or welfare of the child.

• Mental injury means an injury to the psychological capacity or emotional stability of a child as evidenced by an observable or substantial impairment in his or her ability to function within a normal range of performance and behavior with due regard to his or her culture.

Source: Adapted from National Clearinghouse on Child Abuse and Neglect information, "Definitions of Child Abuse and Neglect: Summary of State Laws." Available online. URL: http://www.nccanch.acf.hhs.gov/general/legal/statutes/define.cfm. Downloaded December 10, 2005.

APPENDIX VII

ALCOHOL AND DRUG USE CONTINUUM AND IMPLICATIONS FOR RISKS FOR CHILD MALTREATMENT

Alcohol and Drug Use Continuum	Implications for Child Welfare/Examples of Risk to Children
Use of alcohol or drugs to socialize and feel effects; use may not appear abusive and may not lead to dependence; however, the circumstance under which a parent uses can put children at risk of harm.	• Use during pregnancy can harm the fetus • Use of prescription pain medication per the instructions from a prescribing physician can sometimes have unintended or unexpected effects—a parent caring for children may find that he or she is more drowsy than expected and cannot respond to the needs of children in his or her care
Abuse of alcohol or drugs includes at least one of these factors in the last 12 months: • Recurrent substance use resulting in failure to fulfill obligations at work, home or school • Recurrent substance use in situations that are physically hazardous • Recurrent substance-related legal problems • Continued substance use despite having persistent or recurrent social or interpersonal problems caused by or exacerbated by the substance	• Driving with children in the car while under the influence • Children may be left in unsafe care—with an inappropriate caretaker or unattended—while parent is partying • Parent may neglect or sporadically address the children's needs for regular meals, clothing and cleanliness • Even when the parent is in the home, the parents' use may leave children unsupervised • Behavior toward children may be inconsistent, such as a pattern of violence followed by remorse
Dependence, also known as addiction, is a pattern of use that results in three or more of the following symptoms in a 12-month period: • Tolerance—needing more of the drug or alcohol to get "high" • Withdrawal—physical symptoms when alcohol or other drugs are not used, such as tremors, nausea, sweating and shakiness • Substance is taken in larger amounts and over a longer period than intended • Persistent desire or unsuccessful efforts to cut down or control substance use • A great deal of time is spent in activities related to obtaining the substance, use of the substance or recovering from its effects • Important social, occupational or recreational activities are given up or reduced because of substance use • Substance use is continued despite knowledge of persistent or recurrent physical or psychological problems caused or exacerbated by the substance	• Despite a clear danger to children, the parent may engage in addiction-related behaviors, such as leaving children unattended while seeking drugs • Funds are used to buy alcohol or other drugs, while other necessities, such as buying food, are neglected • A parent may not be able to think logically or make rational decisions regarding children's needs or care • A parent may not be able to prioritize children's needs over his or her own need for the substance

Source: SAMHSA. *Understanding Substance Abuse and Facilitating Recovery: A Guide for Child Welfare Workers.* Available online. URL: http://www.ncsacw.samhsa.gov/files/508/understandingSAGUIDEDW.htm. Downloaded February 9, 2006.

BIBLIOGRAPHY

Adamec, Christine, and Laurie C. Miller, M.D. *The Encyclopedia of Adoption.* 3rd ed. New York: Facts On File, 2006.

Administration on Children, Youth and Families. *Child Maltreatment 2003.* Available online. URL: http://www.acf.hhs.gov/programs/cb/pubs/cm03/index.htm. Downloaded February 9, 2006.

Adoption and Foster Care Analysis and Reporting System (AFCARS). "The AFCARS Report: Preliminary FY 2003 Estimates as of April 2005." Available online. URL: http://www.acf.hhs.gov/programs/cb/publications/afcars/report10.pdf. Downloaded July 17, 2005.

American Academy of Family Physicians, the American Academy of Pediatrics, the American College of Obstetricians and Gynecologists and the Society for Adolescent Medicine. "Protecting Adolescents: Ensuring Access to Care and Reporting Sexual Activity and Abuse." *Journal of Adolescent Health* 35 (2004): 420–423.

Anda, Robert F., M.D., et al. "Adverse Childhood Experiences, Alcoholic Parents, and Later Risk of Alcoholism and Depression." *Psychiatric Services* 53, no. 8 (August 2002): 1,001–1,009.

Anderson, Mark, M.D., et al. "School-Associated Violent Deaths in the United States, 1994–1999." *Journal of the American Medical Association* 286, no. 21 (December 5, 2001): 2,695–2,702.

Ascione, Frank R., and Arkov, Phil. *Child Abuse, Domestic Violence and Animal Abuse: Linking the Circles of Compassion for Prevention and Intervention.* West Lafayette, Ind.: Purdue University Press, 1999.

Bagley, Christopher, et al. "Sexual Assault in School Mental Health and Suicidal Behaviors in Adolescent Women in Canada." *Adolescence* 32, no. 126 (Summer 1997): 361–366.

Baher, R. E., et al. *At Risk: An Account of the Work of the Battered Child Research Department.* London: Routledge and Kegan Paul, 1976.

Bakan, David. *Slaughter of the Innocents.* San Francisco, Calif.: Jossey-Bass, 1971.

Band, Isin, et al. "Self-Mutilating Behavior of Sexually Abused Female Adults in Turkey." *Journal of Interpersonal Violence* 13, no. 4 (August 1998): 427–438.

Bassuk, Ellen, and Lenore Rubin. "Homeless Children: A Neglected Population." *American Journal of Orthopsychiatry* 57, no. 2 (April 1987): 279–286.

Bellamy, Carol. *The State of the World's Children 2005: Childhood under Threat.* Available online. URL: http://www.unicef.org/sowc05/english/sowc05.pdf. Downloaded February 9, 2006.

Bensley, Lillian Southwick, et al. "Self-Reported Abuse History and Adolescent Problem Behaviors, Antisocial and Suicidal Behaviors." *Journal of Adolescent Health* 24, no. 3 (1999): 163–172.

Besharov, Douglas J. "An Overdose of Concern: Child Abuse and the Overreporting Problem." *Regulation* (November–December 1985): 25–28.

Beyer Kendall, Wanda D., and Monit, Cheung. "Sexually Violent Predators and Civil Commitment Laws." *Journal of Child Sexual Abuse* 13, no. 3 (2004): 41–57.

Blackwell, C. C., et al. "Infection, Inflammation and Sleep: More Pieces to the Puzzle of Sudden Infant Death Syndrome (SIDS)." *APMIS: Acta Pathologica, Microbiolgica et Inununologica Scandinavica* 107, no. 5 (May 1997): 455–473.

Blatt, M. D., et al. "Sudden Infant Death Syndrome, Child Sexual Abuse, and Child Development." *Current Opinion in Pediatrics* 11, no. 2 (April 1999): 175–186.

Briere, John, et al. *The APSAC Handbook on Child Maltreatment.* Thousand Oaks, Calif.: Sage Publications, 1996.

Bureau of Democracy, Human Rights, and Labor. *Country Reports on Human Rights Practices, 2004: Australia.* United States State Department. Available online. URL: http://www.state.gov/g/drl/rls/hrrpt/2004/41635.htm. Downloaded September 1, 2005.

———. *Country Reports on Human Rights Practices, 2004: China.* United States State Department. Available online. URL: http://www.state.gov/g/drl/rls/hrrpt/2004/41640.htm. Downloaded September 1, 2005.

———. *Country Reports on Human Rights Practices, 2004: Denmark.* United States State Department. Available online. URL: http://www.state.gov/g/drl/rls/hrrpt/2004/41678.htm. Downloaded September 1, 2005.

———. *Country Reports on Human Rights Practices, 2004: France.* United States State Department. Available online. URL: http://www.state.gov/g/drl/rls/hrrpt/2004/41681.htm. Downloaded September 1, 2005.

————. *Country Reports on Human Rights Practices, 2004: Germany.* United States State Department. Available online. URL: http://www.state.gov/g/drl/rls/hrrpt/2004/41683.htm. Downloaded September 1, 2005.

————. *Country Reports on Human Rights Practices, 2004: Greece.* United States State Department. Available online. URL: http://www.state.gov/g/drl/rls/hrrpt/2004/41684.htm. Downloaded September 1, 2005.

————. *Country Reports on Human Rights Practices, 2004: India.* United States State Department. Available online. URL: http://www.state.gov/g/drl/rls/hrrpt/2004/41740.htm. Downloaded September 1, 2005.

————. *Country Reports on Human Rights Practices, 2004: Italy.* United States State Department. Available online. URL: http://www.state.gov/g/drl/rls/hrrpt/2004/41688.htm. Downloaded October 19, 2005.

————. *Country Reports on Human Rights Practices, 2004: Japan.* United States State Department. Available online. URL: http://www.state.gov/g/drl/rls/hrrpt/2004/41644.htm. Downloaded September 1, 2005.

————. *Country Reports on Human Rights Practices, 2004: Sweden.* United States State Department. Available online. URL: http://www.state.gov/g/drl/rls/hrrpt/2004/41710.htm. Downloaded September 1, 2005.

————. *Country Reports on Human Rights Practices, 2004: Turkey.* United States State Department. Available online. URL: http://www.state.gov/g/drl/rls/hrrpt/2004/41713.htm. Downloaded September 1, 2005.

Bureau of Justice Statistics. National Conference on Sex Offender Registries: Proceedings of a BJS/Search Conference, April 1998. Available online. URL: http://www.ojp.usdoj.gov/bjs/pub/paf/ncsor.pdf. Downloaded February 9, 2006.

Burke, Anne, et al. "Child Pornography and the Internet: Policing and Treatment Issues." *Psychiatry, Psychology and Law* 9, no. 1 (2002): 79–84.

Caffaro, John V., and Allison Conn-Caffaro. *Sibling Abuse Trauma: Assessment and Intervention Strategies for Children, Families, and Adults.* Binghamton, N.Y.: Haworth Press, 1998.

Caffey, John. "Multiple Fractures in the Long Bones of Infants Suffering from Chronic Subdural Hematoma." *American Journal of Roentgenology, Radium Therapy, and Nuclear Medicine* 56 (1946): 163–173.

————. "On the Theory and Practice of Shaking Infants." *American Journal of Diseases of Children* 124, no. 2 (1972): 161–169.

————. "Some Traumatic Lesions in Growing Bones Other than Fractures and Dislocations: Clinical and Radiologic Features." *British Journal of Radiology* 30, no. 353 (1957): 225–238.

————. "The Whiplash Shaken Infant Syndrome: Manual Shaking by the Extremities with Whiplash-Induced Intracranial and Intraocular Bleedings, Linked with Residual Permanent Brain Damage and Mental Retardation." *Pediatrics* 54, no. 4 (1974): 396–403.

Carr, John. *Child Abuse, Child Pornography and the Internet.* London: NCH. Available online. URL: http://image.guardian.co.uk/sys-files/Society/documents/2004/01/12/pornographyreport.pdf. Downloaded September 23, 2005.

Carroll, John L., and Ellen S. Siska. "SIDS: Counseling Parents to Reduce the Risk." *American Family Physician* 57, no. 7 (April 1, 1998): 1,566.

Centers for Disease Control and Prevention (CDC). "Cases of HIV/AIDS, by Area of Residence, Diagnosed in 2004—33 Sites with Confidential Name-Based JIV Infection Reporting." *HIV/AIDS Surveillance Report* 16. Atlanta, Ga.: Department of Health and Human Services, Public Health Services, 2005. Available online. URL: http://www.cdc.gov/hiv/STATS/2004SurveillanceReport.pdf. Downloaded December 22, 2005.

Ceci, Stephen K., and Helen Hembrooke, eds. *Expert Witnesses in Child Abuse Cases: What Can and Should Be Said in Court.* Washington, D.C.: American Psychological Association, 1998.

Cohen, Judith A., and Anthony O. Mannarino. "Intervention for Sexually Abused Children: Initial Outcome Findings." *Child Maltreatment* 3, no. 1 (February 1998): 17–26.

Croft, A. W., and D. M. B. Hall. "Munchausen Syndrome by Proxy and Sudden Infant Death." *British Medical Journal* 32 (May 28, 2004): 1,309–1,312.

Crosson-Tower, Cynthia. *Understanding Child Abuse and Neglect.* Boston: Allyn & Bacon, 2004.

Daly, Martin, and Margo I. Wilson. "Some Differential Attributes of Lethal Assaults on Small Children by Stepfathers versus Genetic Fathers." *Ethnology and Sociobiology* 15 (1994): 207–216.

Drake, Brett, and Susan Zuravin. "Bias in Child Maltreatment. Revisiting the Myth of Classlessness." *American Journal of Orthopsychology* 68, no. 2 (April 1998): 295–304.

Dube, Shanta R., et al. "Childhood Abuse, Household Dysfunction, and the Risk of Attempted Suicide throughout the Life Span: Findings from the Adverse Childhood Experiences Study." *Journal of the American Medical Association* 286, no. 24 (December 26, 2001): 3,089–3,096.

————. Childhood Abuse, Neglect, and Household Dysfunction and the Risk of Illicit Drug Use: The Adverse Childhood Experiences Study." *Pediatrics* 111, no. 3 (March 2003): 564–572.

Duhaime, Ann-Christine, M.D., et al. "Nonaccidental Head Injury in Infants—The Shaken-Baby Syndrome." *New England Journal of Medicine* 338, no. 25 (1998): 1,822–1,829.

DiGiorgio-Miller, Janet. "Sibling Incest: Treatment of the Family and the Offender." *Child Welfare* 77, no. 3 (May 1998): 335–338.

Dwyer, Terence, et al. "Tobacco Smoke Exposure at One Month of Age and Subsequent Risk of SIDS Prospective Study." *American Journal of Epidemiology* 149 (April 1, 1999): 593–602.

Edens, J. F., et al. "Psychopathy and Institutional Misbehavior among Incarcerated Sex Offenders: A Comparison of the Psychopathy Checklist-Revised and the Personality Assessment Inventory." *International Journal of Forensic Mental Health* 1, no. 1 (2002): 49–58.

Edwards, Valerie J., et al. "Relationship between Multiple Forms of Childhood Maltreatment and Adult Mental Health in Community Respondents: Results from the Adverse Childhood Experiences Study." *American Journal of Psychiatry* 160, no. 8 (August 2003): 1,453–1,460.

El-Rashidi, Yasmine. "Ride 'Em, Robot: Qatar Offers Solutions to a Jockey Shortage." *Wall Street Journal* CCXLVI, 68 (October 3, 2005): A2, A12.

Elstein, Sharon G., and Barbara E. Smith. *Victim-Oriented Multidisciplinary Responses to Statutory Rape Training Guide.* Washington, D.C.: U.S. Department of Justice, 1998.

Esposito, Lesli. "Regulating the Internet: The New Battle against Child Pornography." *Case Western Reserve Journal of International Law* 30, no. 2 (April 1, 1998): 541–565.

Falk, Adam J. "Sex Offenders, Mental Illness and Criminal Responsibility: The Constitutional Boundaries of Civil Commitment." *American Journal of Law and Medicine* 25 (Spring 1999): 117–147.

Fagan, Peter J., et al. "Pedophilia." *Journal of the American Medical Association* 288, no. 19 (November 20, 2002): 2,458–2,465.

Feiner, Leslie. "The Whole Trust: Restoring Reality to Children's Narrative in Long-Term Incest Cases." *Journal of Criminal Law and Criminology* 87, no. 4 (Summer 1997): 1,385–1,429.

Finkelhor, David, and Richard Ormrod. "Child Pornography: Patterns from NIBRS." *Juvenile Justice Bulletin,* Office of Juvenile Justice and Delinquency Prevention, Office of Justice Programs, U.S. Department of Justice, December 2004, 1–8.

Finkelhor, David, and Richard Ormrod. "Prostitution of Juveniles: Patterns from NIBRS." Office of Juvenile Justice and Delinquency Prevention, Office of Justice Programs, U.S. Department of Justice. Available online. URL: http://www.ncjrs.org/pdffiles1/ojjdp/203946. pdf. Downloaded September 1, 2005.

Finkelhor, David, et al. "The Victimization of Children and Youth: A Comprehensive, National Survey." *Child Maltreatment* 10, no. 1 (February 2005): 5–25.

Fiscella, Kevin, et al. "Does Child Abuse Predict Adolescent Pregnancy?" *Pediatrics* 101 (April 1998): 620–624.

Frader, Joel F., et al. "Female Genital Mutilation." *Pediatrics* (July 1998): 153–156.

Frias-Armenia, Martha, and Laura Ann McCloskey. "Determinants of Harsh Parenting in Mexico." *Journal of Abnormal Child Psychology* 26, no. 2 (April 1998): 129–139.

Fuller, Tamara L., and Susan J. Wells. "Predicting Maltreatment Recurrence among CPS Cases with Alcohol and Other Drug Involvement." *Children and Youth Services Review* 25, no. 7 (2003): 553–569.

Garbarino, James. "Psychological Maltreatment Is Not an Ancillary Issue." *Brown University Child and Adolescent Behavior Letter* 14, no. 8 (August 1998).

Gelles, Richard J. "Child Abuse as Psychopathology: A Sociological Critique and Reformulation." *American Journal of Orthopsychiatry* 43 (July 1973): 611–621.

————. "Treatment-Resistant Families." In *Treatment of Child Abuse: Common Ground for Mental Health, Medical, and Legal Practitioners,* 304–312. Baltimore: Johns Hopkins University Press, 2000.

————. "Violence Towards Children in the United States." *American Journal of Orthopsychiatry* 48 (October 1978): 580–592.

Gelles, Richard J., and Ake W. Edfeldt. "Violence Towards Children in the United States and Sweden." *Child Abuse and Neglect* 10 (1986): 501–510.

Gelles, Richard J., and Murray Straus. "Determinants of Violence in the Family: Toward a Theoretical Integration." In Vol. 1 of *Contemporary Theories about the Family,* edited by W. Burr, et al. New York: Free Press, 1979.

————. *Intimate Violence.* New York: Simon and Schuster, 1988.

Gelles, Richard J., Murray Straus, and J. W. Harrop. "Has Family Violence Decreased? A Response to J. Timothy Stocks." *Journal of Marriage and the Family* 50, no. 1 (1988): 286–291.

Gershoff, Elizabeth Thompson. "Corporal Punishment by Parents and Associated Child Behaviors and Experiences: A Meta-Analytic and Theoretical Review." *Psychological Bulletin* 128, no. 4 (2002): 539–579.

Giardino, Angelo P., M.D., and Martin A. Finkel, D. O. "Evaluating Child Sexual Abuse." *Pediatric Annals* 34, no. 5 (May 2005): 382–394.

Gibbons, Claire B., et al. "Safety of Children Involved with Child Welfare Services." In *Child Victimization.* Kingston, N.J.: Civic Research Institute, 2005.

Glod, Carol A., et al. "Increased Nocturnal Activity and Impaired Sleep Maintenance in Abused Children." *Journal of the American Academy of Child and Adolescent Psychiatry* 36 (September 1997): 1,236–1,243.

Glosser, Asaph, Karen Gardiner, and Mike Fishman. *Statutory Rape: A Guide to State Laws and Reporting Requirements.* Available online. URL: http://www.kewin.com/Lewin_Publications/Human_Services/StateLawsReport.htm. Downloaded September 25, 2005.

Goldstein, Joseph, Anna Freud, and Albert J. Solnit. *Beyond the Best Interests of the Child.* New York: Free Press, 1979.

Greenfield, Lawrence. *Child Victimizers: Violent Offenders and Their Victims.* Available online. URL: http://www.ojp.usdoj.gov/bjs/pub/pdf/cvvoatv.pdf. Downloaded February 9, 2006.

Grinage, Bradley D., M.D. "Volitional Impairment and the Sexually Violent Predator." *Journal of Forensic Science* 48, no. 4 (July 2003): 1–8.

Gunn, Veronica L., M.D., Gerald B. Hickson, M.D., and William O. Cooper, M.D. "Factors Affecting Pediatricians' Reporting of Suspected Child Maltreatment." *Ambulatory Pediatrics* 5, no. 2 (March–April 2005): 96–101.

Gwinnell, Esther, M.D., and Christine Adamec. *The Encyclopedia of Addictions and Addictive Behaviors.* New York: Facts On File, 2005.

Haapasalo, Jaana, and Jenhi Aaltonen. "Child Abuse Potential: How Persistent?" *Journal of Interpersonal Violence* 14 (June 1999): 571–585.

Health Resources and Services Administration. "Bullying among Children and Youth with Disabilities and Special Needs." Available online. URL: http://stopbullyingnow.hrsa.gov/HHS-PSA/pdfs/SBN_Tip_24.pdf. Downloaded December 8, 2005.

———. "Children Who Bully." Available online. URL: http://stopbullyingnow.hrsa.gov/HHS_PSA/pdfs/SBN_Tip_1.pdf. Downloaded December 8, 2005.

———. "State Laws Related to Bullying among Children and Youth." Available online. URL: http://www.stopbullyingnow.hrsa.gov?HHS_PSA/pdfs/SBN_Tip_6.pdf. Downloaded December 9, 2005.

Henry, Darla L. "Resilience in Maltreated Children: Implications for Special Needs Adoption." *Child Welfare* 78, no. 5 (September 1999): 519–540.

Herman-Giddens, Marcia E. "Newborns Killed or Left to Die by a Parent." *Journal of the American Medical Association* 289, no. 11 (March 19, 2003): 1,425–1,429.

Hornor, Gail. "Domestic Violence and Children." *Journal of Pediatric Health Care* 19, no. 4 (2005): 206–212.

Howe, David. *Child Abuse and Neglect: Attachment, Development and Intervention.* New York: Palgrave Macmillan, 2005.

International Society for Prevention of Child Abuse and Neglect. *World Perspectives on Child Abuse.* 6th ed. Carol Stream, Ill.: International Society for Prevention of Child Abuse and Neglect, 2004.

Jackson, Rebecca L., Richard Rogers, and Daniel W. Shuman. "The Adequacy and Accuracy of Sexually Violent Predator Evaluations: Contextualized Risk Assessment in Clinical Practice." *International Journal of Forensic Mental Health* 3 (2004): 115–129.

"Japan's Study of Cot Death." *Pediatrics* 103, no. 6 (June 1999): A64.

Kairys, Steven W., Charles F. Johnson, and Committee on Child Abuse and Neglect. "The Psychological Maltreatment of Children—Technical Report." *Pediatrics,* 2002. Available online. URL: http://www.pediatrics.org/cgi/content/full/109/4/e8. Downloaded December 9, 2005.

Kelly, Michelle, L., and William Fals-Stewart. "Psychiatric Disorders of Children Living with Drug-Abusing, Alcohol-Abusing, and Non-Substance-Abusing Fathers." *Journal of the American Academy of Child & Adolescent Psychiatry* 43, no. 5 (May 2004): 621–628.

Kempe, C. Henry. "Pediatric Implications of the Battered Baby Syndrome." *Archives of Disease in Childhood* 46, no. 245 (1971): 28–37.

Kempe, C. Henry, and Ray F. Heifer, eds. *The Battered Child.* 3rd ed. Chicago: University of Chicago Press, 1980.

Kempe, C. Henry, et al. "The Battered-Child Syndrome." *Journal of the American Medical Association* 181 (1962): 17–24.

Kennedy Bailey, Rahn, M.D. "The Civil Commitment of Sexually Violent Predators: A Unique Texas Approach." *Journal of the American Academy of Psychiatry Law* 30 (2002): 525–532.

Kim, Christine H. "Putting Reason Back into the Reasonable Efforts Requirement in Child Abuse and Neglect Cases." *University of Illinois Law Review* 1999, no. 1 (1999): 287–325.

Knight, Laura D., M.D., and Kim A. Collins, M.D. "A 25-Year Retrospective Review of Deaths Due to Pediatric Neglect." *American Journal of Forensic Medicine and Pathology* 26, no. 3 (September 2005): 221–228.

Kropenske, Vickie, and Judy Howard. *Protecting Children in Substance-Abusing Families.* U.S. Department of Health and Human Services, Administration for Children and Families, National Center on Child Abuse and Neglect, 1994.

Krug, E. G., et al. eds. *World Report on Violence and Health.* Geneva, Switzerland: World Health Organization, 2002.

Kyle, Angelo D., and Bill Hansell. *The Meth Epidemic in America: Two Surveys of U.S. Counties: The Criminal Effect of Meth on Communities; The Impact of Meth on Children.* Available online. URL: http://www.naco.org/content/contentGroups/Publications/Press_Releases/Documents/Naco-MethSurvey.pdf. Downloaded February 9, 2006.

Lee, Li-Ching, Jonathan B. Kotch, and Christine E. Cox. "Child Maltreatment in Families Experiencing Domestic Violence." *Violence and Victims* 19, no. 5 (October 2004): 573–591.

Liang, Bryan A., and Wendy L. MacFarlane. "Murder by Omission: Child Abuse and the Passive Parent." *Harvard Journal in Legislation* 36, no. 2 (Summer 1999): 397–450.

Lieder, Holly S., et al. "Munchausen Syndrome by Proxy: A Case Report." *AACN Clinical Issues* 18, no. 2 (2005): 178–184.

Livingston-Smith, Susan, and Jeanne A. Howard. "The Impact of Previous Sexual Abuse on Children's Adjustment in Adoptive Placement." *Social Work* 39, no. 5 (September 1994): 491–501.

Loseke, Donileen R., Richard J. Gelles, and Mary M. Cavanaugh, eds. *Current Controversies on Family Violence,* 2nd ed. Thousand Oaks, Calif.: Sage Publications, 2005.

MacMillan, Harriet L., M.D., et al. "Prevalence of Child Physical and Sexual Abuse in the Community." *Journal of the American Medical Association* 278, no. 2 (July 9, 1997): 131–135.

Malloy, Michael. "SIDS—A Syndrome in Search of a Cause." *New England Journal of Medicine* 251, no. 10 (September 2, 2004): 957–959.

Martin, Richard J., et al. "Screening for SIDS: A Neonatal Perspective." *Pediatrics* 103, no. 4 (April 1, 1999): 812–813.

Miko, Francis T. *Trafficking in Persons: The U.S. and International Response.* Congressional Research Service. Available online. URL: http://www.usembassy.it/pdf/other/RL30545.pdf. Downloaded February 9, 2006.

Miller, Holly A., Amy E. Amenta, and Mary Alice Conroy. "Sexually Violent Predator Evaluations: Empirical Evidence, Strategies for Professionals, and Research Directions." *Law and Human Behavior* 29, no. 1 (February 2005): 29–54.

Mitchell, Kimberly J., Janis Wolak, and David Finkelhor. "Internet Sex Crimes against Minors." In *Child Victimization.* Kingston, N.J.: Civic Research Institute, 2005.

———. "Police Posing as Juveniles Online to Catch Sex Offenders: Is It Working?" *Sexual Abuse: A Journal of Research and Treatment* 17, no. 3 (July 2005): 241–267.

———. "The Exposure of Youth to Unwanted Sexual Material on the Internet: A National Survey of Risk, Impact, and Prevention." *Youth & Society* 34, no. 3 (March 2003): 330–358.

Moore, Joyce K., and Jean C. Smith. "Abuse by Burns." In *Understanding the Medical Diagnosis of Child Maltreatment: A Guide for Nonmedical Professionals,* 37–48. New York: Oxford University Press, 2006.

National Center for HIV, STD, and TB Prevention. *Sexually Transmitted Disease Surveillance 2003 Supplement.* Atlanta, Ga.: Centers for Disease Control and Prevention. Available online. URL: http://www.cdc.gov/std/Syphilis2003. Downloaded October 16, 2005.

National Center for Injury Prevention and Control. "Child Maltreatment Fact Sheet." Available online. URL: http://www.cdc.gov/ncipc/factsheets/cmfacts.htm. Downloaded November 4, 2005.

National Clearinghouse on Child Abuse and Neglect Information. "Recognizing Child Abuse and Neglect: Signs and Symptoms." Available online. URL: http://nccanch.acfs.gov/pubs/factsheets/sighs.pdf. Downloaded December 9, 2005.

National Institute of Child Health and Child Development. *Safe Sleep for Your Baby: Ten Ways to Reduce the Risk of Sudden Infant Death Syndrome (SIDS).* Available online. URL: http://www.nichd.nih.gov/SIDS/reduce_infant_risk.htm. Downloaded December 7, 2005.

O'Brian, Muireann, Anke van den Borne, and Theo Noten, eds. *Joint East-West Research on Trafficking in Children for Sexual Purposes in Europe: The Sending Countries.* Available online. URL: http://europa.eu.int/comm/justice_home/fsj/crime/forum/docs/ecpat_en.pdf. Downloaded February 9, 2006.

O'Connell Davidson, Julia. "Child Sex Tourism: An Anomalous Form of Movement?" *Journal of Contemporary European Studies* 12, no. 1 (April 2004): 31–46.

Office of Applied Studies. "Alcohol Dependence or Abuse among Parents with Children Living in the Home." Available online. URL: http://oas.samhsa.gov/2k4/ACOA/ACOA.htm. Downloaded February 9, 2006.

Office of Juvenile Justice and Delinquency Prevention. *Burn Injuries in Child Abuse.* Available online. URL: http://www.ncjrs.gov/pdffiles/91190-6.pdf. Downloaded February 9, 2006.

Office of the Under Secretary for Global Affairs. *Trafficking in Persons Report.* Available online. URL: http://www.usembassy.it/pdf/other/RL30545.pdf. Downloaded October 27, 2005.

Omelaniuk, Irena. "Trafficking in Human Beings." Available online. URL: http://www.un.org/esa/population/publications/ittmigdev/2005/P15_Iomelaniuk.pdf. Downloaded October 27, 2005.

Orient, Jane M., M.D. "Reflections on 'Shaken Baby Syndrome': A Case Report." *Journal of American Physicians and Surgeons* 10, no. 2 (Summer 2005): 45–50.

Ormrod, Richard K., and David Finkelhor. "Using New Crime Statistics to Understand Crimes Against Children—Child Pornography, Juvenile Prostitution, and Hate Crimes against Youth." In *Child Victimization.* Kingston, N.J.: Civic Research Institute, 2005.

Paintal, Sureshrani. "Banning Corporal Punishment of Children: A Position Paper." *Childhood Education* 76, no. 1 (October 1999): 36–39.

Palmer, Sally, et al. "Responding to Children's Disclosure of Familial Abuse: What Survivors Tell Us." *Child Welfare* 78, no. 2 (March 1, 1999): 259–282.

Pasqualone, Georgia A., and Susan Fitzgerald. "Munchausen by Proxy Syndrome." *Critical Care Nursing Quarterly* 22 (May 1999): 52–64.

Printz, Winterfeld, and J. P. Amy. "An Overview of the Major Provisions of the Adoption and Safe Families Act of 1997." *Protecting Children* 14, no. 3 (1998).

Randall, Peter. *Adult Bullying: Perpetrators and Victims.* London: Routledge, 1997.

Reece, Robert M., M.D., ed. *Treatment of Child Abuse: Common Ground for Mental Health, Medical, and Legal Practitioners.* Baltimore: Johns Hopkins University Press, 2000.

Rinehart, Deborah J., et al. "The Relationship between Mothers' Child Abuse Potential and Current Mental Health Symptoms." *Journal of Behavioral Health Services & Research* 32, no. 2 (2005): 155–166.

Sataline, Suzanne. "Catholic Parish Pays High Price for Independence." *Wall Street Journal* CCXLVI, 134 (December 20, 2005): A1, A9.

Schaffner, Laurie. "Searching for Correction: A New Look at Teenaged Runaways." *Adolescence* 33 (Fall 1998): 619–627.

Schene, Patricia A. "Past, Present, and Future Roles of Child Protective Services." *The Future of Children* 8, no. 1 (Spring 1998): 23–38.

Schusterman, G. R., J. D. Fluke, and Y. T. Yuan. *Male Perpetrators of Child Maltreatment: Findings from NCANDS.* Available online. URL: http://aspe.hhs.gov/hsp/05/child-maltreat/execsum.htm. Downloaded February 9, 2006.

Sirotnak, Andrew P., Joyce K. Moore, and Jean C. Smith. "Child Sexual Abuse." In *Understanding the Medical Diagnosis of Child Maltreatment: A Guide for Nonmedical Professionals.* 3rd ed. New York: Oxford University Press, 2006.

———. "Neglect." In *Understanding the Medical Diagnosis of Child Maltreatment: A Guide for Nonmedical Professionals.* New York: Oxford University Press, 2006.

Sokol, Robert J., M.D., Virginia Delaney-Black, M.D., and Beth Nordstrom. "Fetal Alcohol Spectrum Disorder." *Journal of the American Medical Association* 290, no. 22 (December 10, 2003): 2,996–2,999.

Spinelli, Margaret G., M.D. "Maternal Infanticide Associated with Mental Illness: Prevention and the Promise of Saved Lives." *American Journal of Psychiatry* 161, no. 9 (September 2004): 1,548–1,557.

Spitz, Rene A. "Hospitalism." *The Psychoanalytic Study of the Child* 1 (1945): 53.

———. "Hospitalism: A Follow-up Report." *The Psychoanalytic Study of the Child* 2 (1946): 113.

Stewart, Donna E., and Gajic-Veljanoski. "Trafficking in Women: The Canadian Perspective." *Canadian Medical Association Journal* 173, no. 1 (July 5, 2005): 25–26.

Straus, Murray A. "Children Should Never, Ever, Be Spanked No Matter What the Circumstances." In *Current Controversies about Family Violence.* 2nd ed. Thousand Oaks, Calif.: Sage Publications, 2004.

Straus, Murray A., and Richard J. Gelles. "Societal Change and Change in Family Violence from 1975 to 1985 as Revealed by Two National Surveys." *Journal of Marriage and the Family* 48, no. 3 (August 1986): 465–479.

———. *Physical Violence in American Families: Risk Factors and Adaptations to Violence in 8,145 Families.* New Brunswick, N.J.: Transaction Publishers, 1995.

Straus, Murray A., Richard J. Geiles, and Susan Steinmetz. *Behind Closed Doors: Violence in the American Family.* New York: Doubleday/Anchor, 1980.

Substance Abuse and Mental Health Services Administration. *Take Action against Bullying.* Available online. URL: http://www.mentalhealth.samhsa.gov/publications/allpubs/SVP-0056. Downloaded February 9, 2006.

Task Force on Sudden Infant Death Syndrome. "The Changing Concept of Sudden Infant Death Syndrome: Diagnostic Coding Shifts, Controversies Regarding the Sleeping Environment, and New Variables to Consider in Reducing Risk." *Pediatrics* 116, no. 5 (November 2005): 1,245–1,255.

Trocmé, Nico, et al. *Canadian Incidence Study of Reported Child Abuse and Neglect, 2003: Major Findings.* Available online. URL: http://www.phac-aspc.gc.ca/ncfv-cnivf/familyviolence/pdfs/childabuse_final_e.pdf. Downloaded December 15, 2005.

Tunzi, Marc, M.D. "Curbside Consultation: Isn't This Statutory Rape?" *American Family Physician* 65, no. 9 (May 1, 2002): Available online. URL: http://www.aafp.org/afp/20020501/curbside.html. Downloaded September 10, 2005.

Vig, Susan, Susan Chinitz, and Lisa Shulman, M.D. "Young Children in Foster Care: Multiple Vulnerabilities and Complex Service Needs." *Infants & Young Children* 19, no. 2 (2005): 147–160.

Walsh, Bill. *Investigating Child Fatalities,* Office of Juvenile Justice and Delinquency Prevention. Available online. URL: http://www.ncjrs.gov/pdf-filesl/ojjdp/209764.pdf. Downloaded February 9, 2006.

Watson, Malcolm W., et al. "Patterns of Risk Factors Leading to Victimization and Aggression in Children and Adolescents." In *Child Victimization.* Kingston, N.J.: Civic Research Institute, 2005.

Weinberger, Linda E., et al. "The Impact of Surgical Castration on Sexual Recidivism Risk among Sexually Violent Predatory Offenders." *Journal of the American Academy of Psychiatry Law* 33, no. 1 (2005): 16–36.

Westcott, Helen L., and David P. Jones. "Annotation: The Abuse of Disabled Children." *Journal of Child Psychology and Psychiatry and Allied Disciplines* 40 (May 1999).

White, Caroline. "Some 'Cot Deaths' Are Child Abuse." *British Medical Journal* 318 no. 7,177 (January 16, 1999): 147.

Willis, Brian M., and Barry S. Levy. "Child Prostitution: Global Health Burden, Research Needs, and Interventions." *Lancet* 359 (April 20, 2002): 1,417–1,422.

Wolak, Janis, David Finkelhor, and Kimberly H. Mitchell. *Child Pornography Possessors Arrested in Internet-Related Crimes: Findings from the National Juvenile Online Victimization Study.* Available online. URL: http://www.missingkids.com/en_US/publications/NC144.pdf. Downloaded September 25, 2005.

Wolak, Janis, David Finkelhor, and Kimberly Mitchell. "Internet-Initiated Sex Crimes against Minors: Implications for Prevention Based on Findings from a National Study." *Journal of Adolescent Health* 35 (2004): 424e11–424e20. Available online. URL: http://unh.edu/ccrc/pdf.cv71.pdf.

Wolfe, David A., et al. "Factors Associated with Abusive Relationships among Maltreated and Nonmaltreated Youth." *Development and Psychopathology* 10 (1998): 61–85.

Woiraich, Mark, et al. "Guidance for Effective Discipline." *Pediatrics* 101 (April 1998).

Yazbak, F. Edward, M.D. "Post-Mortem on a 'Shaken Baby Syndrome' Autopsy." *Journal of American Physicians and Surgeons* 10, no. 2 (Summer 2005): 51–52.

INDEX

Page numbers in **boldface** indicate major discussion of a topic.

A